A COMPREHENSIVE BOOK ON AUTISM SPECTRUM DISORDERS

Edited by **Mohammad-Reza Mohammadi**

A Comprehensive Book on Autism Spectrum Disorders
Edited by Mohammad-Reza Mohammadi

Published by InTech
Janeza Trdine 9, 51000 Rijeka, Croatia

Publishing Process Manager Marina Jozipovic

Technical Editor Teodora Smiljanic

Cover Designer InTech Design Team

Additional hard copies can be obtained from orders@intechopen.com

A Comprehensive Book on Autism Spectrum Disorders,
Edited by Mohammad-Reza Mohammadi
p. cm.
978-953-307-494-8

For EU product safety concerns:
IN TECH d.o.o., Prolaz Marije Krucifikse Kozulić 3, 51000 Rijeka, Croatia,
info@intechopen.com or visit our website at intechopen.com.

Meet the editor

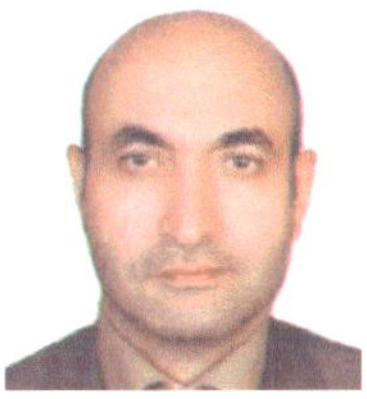

Professor Mohammad-Reza Mohammadi works as a child and adolescent psychiatrist at Tehran University of Medical Sciences (TUMS), and is the chair of Psychiatry and Psychology Research Centre of Iran. He has authored more than 160 articles, 23 books, and few book chapters. He obtained a diploma in Child and Adolescent Psychiatry as well as M.Phil. at the University of London, 1996 and 1997; in Cognitive Behavior Therapy at Middle Sex Hospital, University College of London (UCL) 1998. He is the founder and the Editor-in-chief of Iranian Journal of Psychiatry (IJP). He is also a member of Editorial Boards of many Iranian and International journals. He established University of Welfare and Rehabilitation Sciences in 1992, and has been the Head of National Research Centre for Medical Sciences of Iran (2001-2005). His research interests include epidemiological and clinical trial, cognitive behavior therapy and spiritual psychotherapy.

Contents

Preface

This book arose from experiences of learners, teachers, clinicians, children and adolescent psychiatrists and other professionals. It is an attempt to synthesize the humanistic and caring demands of our discipline with its pragmatic and scientific needs. This synthesis is written by clinicians, experts in child and adolescent psychiatry.

This book is an attempt to bring visibility to Autism Spectrum Disorders in child and adolescent psychological practices. The famous dictum of William Osler says: "Medicine is a science of uncertainty and an art of probability". This book could not have been written without the support and assistance of many people. Even for the most successful book editions there comes a time for the closure and a time for the new beginning. This book is the new beginning, offering readers new views and insights on Autism Spectrum Disorders.

The vision was to create a clinically focused book that would be useful to trainees and practitioners of different specialties. In that process, I have been able to apply what I have learned in thirty years of my career as a training director of Child and Adolescent Psychiatry as well as the Editor-in-chief of the psychiatric journal.

In addition, for nearly thirty years, numerous teachers and colleagues in the field; my students and followers (many of whom are now experts and academic leaders), children who have been our patients, together with their parents, have been unfailingly generous with sharing their experiences and insights. This introduction aims to communicate the clinical art and wisdom of child psychiatry, tied firmly to the science of our clinical disciplines in autism spectrum disorders. Each chapter highlights what we know about practices in assessment and treatment.

Finally, I am particularly grateful for all your questions, feedbacks, comments and suggestions.

Mohammad-Reza Mohammadi, M.D
Professor of Child and Adolescent Psychiatry, Tehran University of Medical Sciences
Director of Psychiatry and Psychology Research Center of Iran
Iran

Part 1

Language Assessment and Education

1

Language Assessment in Autism

Fernanda Dreux M.Fernandes, Cibelle A.H. Amato
and Daniela R.Molini-Avejonas
Universidade de São Paulo
Brazil

1. Introduction

Language development is strongly related to the linguistic and environmental contexts. There are individual differences in language development that relate to the onset period of certain abilities as well as to the rhythm of development and language characteristics. Those factors are associated to individual abilities and are deeply influenced by environmental aspects. The language acquisition process is dependent of a series of non-linguistic strategies and better language resources are usually available to further developed children. In this constant interaction the knowledge about language is constructed and used in different contexts. Those steps of language and communication development, however, do not occur always as expected. Some children transgress several of the steps and milestones of development. Language acquisition is considered a fundamental element of infantile development, potentiating also the social cognitive development (Amato & Fernandes, 2010).

Language is also considered an important diagnostic and prognostic factor in autism. Regardless of the theoretical perspective or etiology, the linguistic issues are important features of the descriptions of autism spectrum disorders, varying from lack of verbal communication to pedantic speech (Miilher & Fernandes, 2009). The identification of this group's language pattern would answer questions such as whether there are specific or underlying deficits and if they are common to all autistic children.

The exact nature of language impairments in the autism spectrum is still unclear, especially due to the variations of symptoms. Approximately half of the autistic children do not use language functionally and present persistent communicative delay. Other children present language development similar to normal children but with pragmatic inabilities such as difficulties varying communicative stiles according to the situations or the interlocutor, misunderstanding rhetoric expressions such as metaphors or irony (Roberts et al, 2004; Young et al, 2005; Bekaldi, 2006; Smith et al, 2007).

However, there is a general agreement that any therapeutic intervention proposal should be based on an individual language and communication profile, as detailed as possible (Bekaldi, 2006). Therefore, issues such as how and what to assess in an autistic child's communication are continually being addressed by several studies that provide some evidence about the available alternatives.

Jarrold et al. (1997) stated that evidence suggests that there are at least three differences between autistic and normal children's language: articulation abilities seem to be better developed then the other areas; verbal expression seem to be more advanced than verbal comprehension and lexical comprehension is superior than grammatical comprehension.

The identification of this group's language pattern would answer to questions such as if there are specific or underlying deficits and if they are common to all autistic children. Hetzroni & Tannous (2004) suggested that linguistic impairments are linked to one of the three language components (form, use and meaning) or to their association. Walenski et al (2006), however, stated that the linguistic profile of autistic subjects is defined by pragmatic and grammatical disorders and intact lexical abilities.

Several authors (Fernandes, 1994; Folstein & Rosen-Shedley, 2001; Volkmar & Pauls, 2003; Bekaldi, 2006; Smith et al, 2007) pointed out that the pragmatic inabilities are a central feature of autistic disorders and thus are the focus of many researches since the 1980 decade. However, since the beginning of the XXI century the interest about formal and semantic issues have been restored.

Generally, literature points out to grammatical, lexical and pragmatic deficits in autistic children. However, it is still not clear how these abilities relate and mutually interfere. Tager-Flusberg & Calkins (1990) reported that autistic children's grammatical abilities measured by the Index of Productive Syntax (IPSyn) and by the Mean Length of Utterance (MLU) are the same, either if spontaneous or imitative speech is analyzed. In the study by Rollins & Snow (1998) communicative intent with joint attention purposes was related to syntactic development. However, there was no correlation of the syntactic development with communicative intent with regulatory purpose. The authors concluded that apparently, autistic children's pragmatic abilities contribute to grammatical acquisition. Kjelgaard & Tager-Flusberg (2001) observed that autistic children presented lexical-syntactic and grammatical impairments in standardized tests. Condouris et al (2003) used standardized tests and spontaneous speech to assess autistic children's language performance and observed that the children presented impairments in formal aspects of language on both conditions. Among the grammatical measures used by the authors to spontaneous speech assessment, MLU was the one that presented the largest number of correlations with other measures and was considered a useful way to assess grammatical abilities. In the research by Paul et al (2004) autistic children presented the lowest performance in pragmatic and grammatical aspects including word combining, use of functional terms and grammatical markers, use of language to communicate personal experiences and share new information. Roberts et al (2004) reported that autistic children actually present grammatical deficits when compared to peers of the same chronological age. Eigsti et al (2007) observed syntactic delays in autistic children and stated that these children present an atypical developmental pattern, marked by inconsistent performance. Walensky et al (2006) pointed out that the main grammatical impairments refer to flexional morphology but that it is not clear if to morpho-phonology or to morpho-syntax. Evaluating the pattern of verbal abilities along seven years, Anderson et al (2007) found out that the linguistic development path followed a predictable pattern from two to nine years of age.

There are different methods of language assessment, each one with specific advantages and disadvantages. However, due to autistic children's characteristics such as lack of social engagement, the use of spontaneous speech samples may provide important information about their functional linguistic performance especially when environmental variables such

as familiarity and cognitive demand are controlled. Besides, this method also reflects language use's productivity (Tager-Flushberg, 2000; Condouris et al, 2004).
The aim of this chapter is not to present strict models of assessment protocols, but to present data and report results of different alternatives and suggestions for assessing language and communication in children of the autism spectrum. There are several options of tests and measures available to assess a few languages such as English, French and Spanish. But all the other languages need specific tools and parameters and demand adaptations by the speech and language pathologist. Some of the studies described discuss important issues involving language-specific adaptations and group-specific analysis criteria.

2. Core aspects of language assessment in ASD children

Determining which ones are the language aspects that should be systematically assessed in all ASD children is frequently a challenge to the speech and language pathologist (SLP). A comprehensive language assessment doesn't have to be necessarily exhaustive, but it must provide the necessary information to allow the determination of a complete profile of characteristics that will be the basis for diagnosis and intervention proposals.
Considering the areas of social, cognitive and linguistic development, necessarily impaired in autistic individuals, overall information about them is obviously necessary. But how the different linguistic systems are associated is an aspect that still demands further research.
Aiming to confirm the consistency of the assessment results, a study was conducted to verify and analyze the relation between grammatical, lexical and pragmatic development in autistic children in a period of 12 months of language therapy (Miilher & Fernandes, 2009). In this study, subjects were 10 individuals with diagnosis within the autism spectrum that were assessed and attended to language therapy on a specialized service. The average age on initial assessment was 7 years, 2 months. All were male and had received no prior language therapy. Video-taped samples of initial assessment, six and twelve months after language therapy onset were analyzed in regard to the Functional Communicative Profile (FCP) and communicative functions; Mean Length of Utterance (MLU) and Vocabulary. It totalized three samples per subject with a total number of 30 recordings with 30 minutes each. The Functional Communicative Profile (FCP) included the analysis of the number of communicative acts expressed and the communicative functions they expressed (among 20 possibilities). These communicative functions were divided in more interpersonal and less interpersonal according to Cardoso & Fernandes (2003). The FCP also considered the communicative means used to express each communicative act: verbal (emission with more than 75% of the correct form), vocal (emission with less than 75% of the correct form) and gestural (facial and body movements), adapted from Weterby & Prutting (1984). The communicative functions were also analyzed according to Halliday's (1978) proposal as: instrumental, regulatory, interactive, personal, heuristic and imaginative.
To the assessment of the Mean Length of Utterance (MLU) the same videotaped therapy sessions were used, providing the necessary 100 speech segments and singing and delayed echolalia were excluded from the analysis. The grammatical classes considered were: adverbs, adjectives, articles, conjunctions, prepositions, pronouns, nouns and verbs. Grammatical Morphemes (GM) were divided in two sub-groups: GM1 (nouns, verbs and articles) and GM2 (prepositions, conjunctions and pronouns). The total sum of GM1 and GM2 constituted the Total-MLU. The ratio of MLU-words and MLU-morphemes was also determined.

To the assessment of Vocabulary the same 100 speech segments described above were used. The terms of psychological state (physical, emotional, of desire and cognitive) and of designation (natural and cultural entity, body parts, action, artifacts, time and space location and people's names) were counted by occurrence. According to the studies by Lee & Rescorla (2002) and Perkins et al (2006), the number of different psychological state terms was also counted, besides its total occurrence.

The results have shown that, of the total assessed variables the ones with larger number of correlations were: MLU-words, verbs, GM1, MLU morphemes and proportion of interpersonal communicative acts.

MLU-words was the item with the largest number of correlations. MLU-words may be an indicator of the grammatical development as well as of the phrasal extension. However, they point out that, since it doesn't differentiate structure and morpho-syntactic complexity, MLU-words may be better used as a linguistic development indicator.

The grammatical variables associated with MLU-words were: type 1 Grammatical Morphemes (nouns, verbs and articles), MLU-morphemes and the word classes of adverbs, adjectives and verbs. Except for the grammatical variables the other variables seem to reflect rather the communicative use than the linguistic system. The MLU-words was larger in subjects with better pragmatic abilities and more social-emotional engagement during communicative exchange.

Generally MLU-words presented more associations with pragmatic variables than with lexical abilities. On the two first moments (1 and 2) when there was more use of the verbal communicative mean and of interpersonal communicative acts, the MLU-words was also larger. On the last two moments (2 and 3), larger numbers of communicative acts per minute and more use of communicative space are associated with larger the MLU-words. The association with the verbal communicative mean is not surprising once this is the main mean of utterance. However, the association to interactive factors is visible on the occupation of the communicative space and on the number of communicative acts per minute.

In what refers to the pragmatic variables, the second moment seems to have a transition role. On the first moment all the variables referred to each child's own performance, with internal parameters (number of communicative functions and number of interpersonal communicative acts). On the third moment the two variables referred to the child's performance in relation to an external parameter (acts per minute, where the parameter is the time and communicative space, where the parameter is the other). The second moment presented both types of parameters and seemed to function as a rehearsal to the third moment. That is, on the second moment the association between phrasal extension and performance factors with external and internal parameters coexists.

The strong statistical significance observed in the associations between lexical, grammatical and pragmatic aspects indicates the mutual influence of different aspects of language. Therefore, the language diagnosis must take all these aspects into account. The fact that the grammatical variables were the ones with the largest number of correlations may suggest that the formal aspects of language mediate the associations between meaning and function. However, any positive conclusion demands further investigation, with larger number of subjects and with users of different languages. Generally grammatical variables presented more associations with pragmatic variables then with lexical abilities. The positive correlations between grammatical variables and pragmatic abilities seem to reflect rather the communicative use of language than the linguistic system.

The spontaneous speech analysis showed the communicative functionality of the studied individuals and indicated that there was association of two types of variables of the same corpus. These results reinforce the use of samples of spontaneous communication as a useful alternative to the assessment of children of the autism spectrum, especially in situations where there are no language-specific tests available. The number of subjects imposes a limit to the generalization of the findings of this research and further research with larger more homogenous sample is desirable. But the analysis of the correlations between grammatical, lexical and functional aspects of language offers information to the determination of individual profiles of abilities and inabilities and therefore provides information to the clinical intervention in language therapy for children of the autism.

The consistency of results along the intervention period indicates that the results obtained reveal the profiles of abilities and the associations among them are not random observations, but close reports of each child's profile that were useful in the intervention process.

These results agree with other studies reported in the literature that demand careful consideration. The correlations with strong statistical significance show the association between lexical, grammatical and pragmatic aspects. As reported by Toppelberg & Shapiro (2000), the language components are linked and function harmonically, although independently.

The association between MLU-words and occupation of the communicative space shows the important role of the verbal communicative mean to the symmetry of the interactive setting, although they have been shown to be independent factors (Fernandes, 2000b).

The correlations regarding grammatical class also cannot be taken as a causal relation; a strong correlation suggests that the variables have important common ground (Bates & Goodman, 1999). Children do not learn the meaning of new words only by time-space contiguity clues; they focus on clues about the speaker's intentional references such as gaze direction (Bloom, 1997). Considering that verbs convey less evident meaning then most nouns, a larger use of verbs seem to indicate more attention to other people, what may suggest better social abilities not just in more attention to other people but also in more interactive interpersonal communication. While many nouns refer to concrete objects, verbs may refer to transient events or to complex changes with multiple organizational principles. The concepts conveyed through verbs can be more complex than those conveyed by nouns (Goldfield, 2000).

In most languages the nouns are apprehended by object concept mapping while the knowledge about verbs is language-specific. The role of self-other interaction is important in learning and using verbs and factors such as verbal meaning, social-pragmatic clues and input (frequency, positional salience and syntactic structural diversity on which they are used) have important influence on the order of verbal acquisition (Naigles & Hoff-Ginsberg. 1998).

Befi-Lopes et al (2007) in their study about the use of different kinds of verbs by Portuguese speaking Brazilian children stated that the evolution on the use of verbs agrees with the hypotheses that acquisition is based on the use and attention do contextual and semantic-syntactic clues.

Negative associations with the gestural mean may indicate one of two things: either the use of gestures is replaced by verbalization or the use of verbal utterances doesn't exclude the gestural delay that is observed even in children with better linguistic abilities. Perkins et al (2006) stated that even before the first year of life autistic children present delayed gestural communication that is a better diagnostic factor than word production or comprehension.

The third more frequent correlations observed in the study by Miilher & Fernandes (2009) involve MLU-morphemes, type 1 grammatical morphemes (GM-1) and the proportion of interpersonal communicative acts. MLU-morphemes presented correlations on the first and third moments with artifacts and with the total of designative terms. Artifacts are words that express entities that are dependent on the human action, as clock, house or others (Perkins et al 2006) and in several cases they are expressed by words that refer to objects. These words are included in the category of nouns whose maximum score is three points (morphemes that express gender, number and degree) and are the grammatical class with higher scoring possibilities on MLU according to Araujo & Befi-Lopes (2004) criteria. The study by Tager-Flusberg et al (1990) showed high correlation indexes with syntactic productivity and lexical diversity measures.

Nouns, verbs and articles are the basic phrasal components in Portuguese; this way the link between artifacts and designative terms and the use of the verbal communicative mean is not surprising. Besides this link with the language it is possible that the association with designative terms and artifacts is related to the fact that autistic children tend to speak about less complex, more concrete, events (Eigst et al, 2007) and therefore use more words that designate real objects as the artifacts. The correlation with interactivity indicates that the intention in socially participate in communicative situations is essential to the effective use of linguistic knowledge. The idea that the communicative effectiveness depends on the aspects of form and use (besides content) becomes clear through this association (Toppelberg & Shapiro, 2000; Hertzroni & Tannous, 2004).

The linguistic idiosyncrasies that are widely reported in literature (Eigst et al, 2007) may hide the fact that autistic children present communicative intent. Wetherby & Prutting (1984) reported that these individuals use interactive communicative acts, but that most of them have environmental consequences and the communicative acts with social consequences are less frequently used. The association of interpersonal communicative acts with other variables shows that there is a link between linguistic and social-pragmatic abilities as reported by several authors (Ninio & Snow, 1988; Bates & Goodman, 1999; Bishop, 2000). The correlation analysis do not determine the association path; that is, if the use of interactive communicative acts favors the use of certain lexical terms or larger MLU or if certain lexical terms and more complex utterances favor communicative interactivity. What can be stated is that there is an association and that it may be related to social-pragmatic structures that function as language facilitators (Bates & Goodman, 1999) or it may be a mechanism of reciprocal influence (Marcos, 2001; Garcia-Perez et al, 2008).

Therefore, the association between the various aspects of language (especially grammar, syntax and pragmatics) demands careful and sometimes individual analysis. The use of spontaneous interaction samples and language-specific criteria may provide significant data to the determination individualized of intervention proposals.

3. Specific assessment situations and groups

Language and communication are socially-related abilities and thus the child's communicative and linguistic performance is frequently socially influenced. Language assessment may have different purposes: it may be important to determine an ASD child's best possible performance or it may be useful to identify the specific difficulties that an ASD adolescent faces in a group situation. Therefore the communicative situations and interlocutors proposed to the language and communication assessment must be appropriate to its purpose. Different settings can be used, as peer-group or individual situations with the speech-language pathologist or with the mother or a sibling. Frequently the use of more than one situation provides the most significant results.

Three studies aimed to investigate different issues of language assessment: the identification of differences between verbal and non-verbal children; the analysis of different interlocutors and materials assessing language in ASD children and the language assessment of adolescents with ASD.

3.1 Communicative functionality of verbal and non-verbal autistic children

In this study (Amato & Fernandes, 2010) mothers were included in the data gathering process in order to identify the usual communicative context available to each child. The subjects were 20 autistic children with ages varying from 2:10 to 10:6, 17 of male gender and 3 females. They were all divided in two groups (verbal and non-verbal) filmed just once before the language assessment. The inclusion criteria in the verbal (V- 10 subjects) or in the non-verbal (NV- 10 subjects) groups was the medical report included in the referral documents. None of the subjects had prior speech and language assessment or intervention. All subjects were filmed for 30 minutes during a spontaneous play situation with their mothers that didn't receive any special instructions.

The results were considering regarding each child to allow better analysis of the results of a procedure that included mothers as the communicative interlocutor. The proportion of occupation of the communicative space didn't reveal significant differences between groups while the number of communicative acts produced per minute did. In both groups the gestural communicative mean was the most frequently used. This was the only communicative mean that didn't present significant differences between the groups. The results referring to the interpersonal communicative functions expressed, that is, the proportion of communication interactivity. Although there is a significant difference between the groups, the low proportion of interactive communicative acts in the communication of autistic children is an issue that must be carefully considered.

The analysis of the occupation of communicative space and of the number of communicative acts produced per minute by the subjects of this research shows variations in both aspects. The occupation of the communicative space indicates a certain balance in the mother-child communication. However, when the production of communicative acts is considered in relation to the sample's duration the data about both groups are different, suggesting that the reciprocity between mother and child forms the base from which communication develops. In the first aspect, communicative space occupation, the mother seems to be the agent of the balance.

The difficulties presented by autistic children with the interactive use of communication reinforces the notion that isolated and specific social and cognitive elements evolve together with the linguistic and non-linguistic communication development and there is a mutual interference in the process. The option of conducting the data gathering in communicative situations with the mothers provided a familiar interlocutor that probably allowed each child's best performance. The characterization of the functional communicative profile confirmed the areas of larger difficulties. The presence of large individual differences demands other studies comparing more homogeneous groups.

The interactive situation is a privileged one because each child has his/her own mother as a communicative partner. Knowing the child's communicative needs the mother works as a facilitator to the communication and places the child as the central focus of her attention (at least during the data gathering period). Prior studies (Chawarska et al, 2007; Clifforf & Dissanayake, 2008; Davis & Crter, 2008; Ruser et al, 2007; Scheeren & Stauder, 2008; Solomon et al, 2008) point out to the mother's important role as a communicative partner to the communication development process and eventually in the assessment processes. The mother represents a preferred partner to the child, determining an affective association that will generate symmetric communication patterns (Wachtel & Carter, 2008; Williams et al, 2005). Mothers use simple, repetitive speech, grammatically and semantically adjusted to the child's understanding and interest levels (Grindle et al, 2009). In this sense, the largest data dispersion referring to the non-verbal children with more than 3 years of age shows how difficult is this process undertaken by the mother, of building a symmetric communication and therefore of building her own role as a communicative partner.

Another research (Benson et al, 2008) studied the communication of autistic children in different contexts and observed variations in the use of the different communicative means according to the communicative partner. According to the authors when the interlocutor is less efficient (in the case of this study, a group situation without an adult's facilitation) the use of redundant communicative means is necessary, and so the gestural means may support what is conveyed by the verbal mean, for example. It follows the same principle identified in the present study.

The analysis of the use of the interpersonal communicative functions provides data about the child's interactive competence and the data presented show the autistic children's impairment in this domain. This observation confirms prior studies (Grindle et al, 2009) that concluded that autistic children are less responsive to interactive attempts and have less spontaneous communication. Other studies (Bara et al, 2001; Davis & Carter, 2008; Laugeson et al, 2009; Reed et al, 2007) report the severe impairment of autistic children in the interactive use of communication to specific functions.

3.2 Communicative profile with unknown interlocutors and materials

The knowledge about ASD children's performance with a trained speech and language therapist but unknown communication partner may provide information about the performance with new partners, adaptation to new situations and eventual generalization of learned abilities to unknown situations. This way of measuring, controlling and standardizing variables of spontaneous production from the therapeutic context to different situations is essential to provide objective data for language assessment and intervention with autistic children.

Therefore, the aim of this study was to determine the communicative performance of individuals of the autistic spectrum in non-familiar situations (with unknown material and communication partner) for a period of 15 minutes of interaction in free-play situations (Moreira & Fernandes, 2010). Subjects were 20 children and adolescents with ASD, with mean age of 9:7 years, were filmed during 15-minute free-play situations with an unknown speech therapist and unfamiliar toys and games and the results were compared to the ones obtained from sessions of free play with the therapists and familiar material.

The comparison of the variables analyzed has resulted in statistically significant differences between the Familiar (FS) and the Non-Familiar (NS) Situations regarding the number of communicative acts per minute and the number of responses, with higher results in the familiar situation.

There were no significant differences in what refer to the communicative means and to the interpersonal communicative functions. Just two non-interpersonal communicative

functions (Play and Non-Functional) were expressed with different frequencies during the different situations.
The comparison between the two different situations has shown few differences between the familiar and the non-familiar situations. The familiarity of the interlocutor and the material seems to interfere very little on the performance of ASD children. However, despite the small differences the familiar situation was the most effective since it has leaded to the occurrence of the largest number of communicative acts per minute and the greatest proportion of responses. Therefore if the aim of the assessment is to identify the best performance of the ASD child, the spontaneous, familiar situation with a known interlocutor seems to be the best alternative.

3.3 Assessment of adolescents in different situations

Another study was conducted, aiming to verify the communicative functional profile and the social-cognitive performance of adolescents with ASD in three different communicative situations: individual speech-language therapy, group activity with and without coordination during a 12 months period and to verify the associations between the results. Five low functioning adolescents with ASD, with ages varying from 12:4 years to 16:3 years, with no previous language therapy were selected. The communicative situations were determined and the communicative contexts varied according to the individual or group activities proposed by the adult or chosen by the subjects. During a twelve-month period two recording sets were performed, initial and final, for each subject. Each recording set was carried out in three different situations, lasting 30 minutes each. Situation I involved individual speech-language therapy; Situation II refers to a group with a coordinating adult (not the speech-language therapist) and in Situation III the group didn't have the adult's coordination.
In what refer to the communicative situations, it was possible to observe that the subjects presented similar communicative behaviors in the three of them. There was an increase in the number of communicative acts, differing only in relation to the average of occurrence, probably due to the dispute for the communicative space in group situations. Initially, the percentage of interpersonal communicative functions was lower in situation III, however in the end of the 12-month period this position was reversed with some participants presenting maximum scores. It is also possible to observe in situation III that the diversity of communicative functions used decreased while in the other situations (I and II) it didn't occur in the same way.
The results demonstrated that the performance throughout the different situations studied during the 12-month period presented variations in all analyzed items. When the functional communicative profile was investigated, the variable number of communicative acts may be once more confirmed as an interesting focus of assessment (Cardoso & Fernandes, 2003; Fernandes, 2003). The decrease of the variability of communicative functions verified in situation III may show the focus on communicative effectiveness, since in the other situations the same participants could experiment and exercise their communicative abilities, but in the situation with a symmetric interlocutor only more effective strategies were appropriate. It was also observed an association between the functional communicative profile and the social-cognitive performance, showing a strict correlation between language and cognitive development (Anderson et al, 2007; Cardoso & Fernandes, 2006; Fernandes & Ribeiro, 2000).

It could be observed that these adolescents seem to understand differences of each communicative situation and are able to adapt to them, changing the functional communicative profile according to the demands. In all situations there were changes in either the functional communicative profile and in the social-cognitive aspects, being possible to verify the association between the participants' performance in these two aspects. It is important to stress that the changes in the performance may be considered interconnected, however nonlinear.

Another aspect that should be considered is that the subjects of this study were low functioning adolescents without previous therapy, and the assessment criteria and instruments were appropriate to this specific group.

4. The use of objective measures to analyze spontaneous language samples

Due to autistic children's characteristics such as lack of social engagement, the use of spontaneous speech samples may provide important information about their functional linguistic performance especially when environmental variables such as familiarity and cognitive demand are controlled. Besides, this method also reflects language use productivity. The use of objective measures to analyze spontaneous communicative samples may lead to important and meaningful results. The Functional Communicative Profile (FCP) may be based on a 15 minute sample of filmed interaction and includes the analysis of the number of communicative acts expressed and the communicative functions they expressed. These communicative functions are divided in more interpersonal and less interpersonal. The FCP also considers the communicative means used to express each communicative act: verbal, vocal and gestural. Among the grammatical measures used to assess spontaneous speech, Mean Length of Utterance (MLU) presents a large number of correlations with other measures and is considered a useful way to assess grammatical abilities.

A more detailed description of these assessment suggestions is presented bellow.

4.1 Functional communicative profile

The communicative acts are the minimal units of analysis in the assessment of the Functional Communicative Profile (adapted from Wetherby & Prutting, 1984). A communicative acts starts when the interaction is initiated and ends when there is a shift on the attention focus or on the communicative turn.

The communicative means used to express each communicative act are divided in:

- Verbal (VE): emissions with more than 75% of the correct form,
- Vocal (V): emission with less than 75% of the correct form and
- Gestural (GE): facial and body movements.

The communicative functions considered (Fernandes, 2004) are 20 alternatives specifically described and that can be divided, according to Fernandes & Calinari (1999) as interactive (or interpersonal) and non-interactive (or less interpersonal):

- Interactive communicative functions: Object Request, Action Request, Social Routine Request, Consent Request, Information Request, Protest, Recognition of Other, Comment, Labeling, Expressive, Narrative, Joint Play, Protest Expression and Showing Of.
- Non-interactive communicative functions: Self Regulatory, Performative, Protest, Reactive, Non-Focused and Exploratory.

4.2 Linguistic complexity

A useful way to assess the linguistic complexity of non collaborative individuals is to analyze the Mean Length of Utterance (MLU) of samples of spontaneous communication. This is not a simple or effortless task but its applicability in several and different contexts, without any specific material, is undoubtedly a great advantage.

The analysis of MLU-w (mean length of utterance in words) identifies the medium number of words per utterance on a sample of 100 utterances. The analysis of MLU-m (mean length of utterance in morphemes) identifies the medium number of morphemes per utterance on a sample of 100 utterances. Obviously in situations where the subject produces very little oral language, the proportional number should be calculated.

Another important aspect to be considered is the need of specific parameters for each language and eventually for different groups, once grammatical differences interfere enormously on the number of morphemes of each utterance, regardless of its meaning (Befi-Lopes et al, 2007).

To the assessment of the Mean Length of Utterance (MLU) the same videotaped therapy sessions used to the analysis of the FCP can be used, providing the necessary 100 speech segments. Singing and delayed echolalia should be excluded from the analysis since they don´t represent the individuals grammatical performance.

The grammatical classes considered usually are: adverbs, adjectives, articles, conjunctions, prepositions, pronouns, nouns and verbs. And the Grammatical Morphemes (GM) can be divided in two sub-groups: GM1 (nouns, verbs and articles) and GM2 (prepositions, conjunctions and pronouns). The total sum of GM1 and GM2 constitutes the Total-MLU. The ratio of MLU-words and MLU-morphemes can also be determined.

4.3 Vocabulary

The analysis of formal aspects of autistic children's communication is still a challenge. Very few studies describe the lexical performance of ASD children and language- or group-specific parameters are also essential in this aspect of the overall language assessment. There are already general normality parameters in Portuguese (Andrade et al, 2000) and one study that analyzed ten ASD children aimed to describe their performance on a vocabulary task involving five semantic categories (clothing, animals, food, transport and household items) and has shown that the ASD children didn't relate to any parameter.

There is a clear need for more studies about the best way to access vocabulary in this population as well as about language- and group-specific parameters. Apparently the use of computer generated images facilitate the children's participation but the answers on a controlled situation do not always express the performance in real communicative situations.

5. Associations between language and communication and other aspects of development in ASD

Considering the associated areas of development, the complete language assessment of ASD children should include information about social and cognitive abilities as well. Therefore, aspects such as social-cognitive performance, social-communicative adaptation and meta-representation should be part of the procedure.

5.1 Social-cognitive performance

It is suggested that the social-cognitive aspects can be analyzed according to the criteria proposed by Molini & Fernandes (2003), adapted from Wetherby & Prutting (1984). The situation to determine the child's best performance in seven domains can vary according to the examiner's intentions and demands:

- Spontaneous situations: have the advantage of allowing repetitions as frequent as needed, but eventually to not include opportunities that demand the best performance.
- Use of pre-determined material: demands some time interval between assessments, but the selected material may facilitate the occurrence of behavior that otherwise wouldn't appear in spontaneous situations.
- Use of a pre-determined set of material and attitudes by the adult: demands a time interval of at least 1 year and sometimes the substitution of some of the material, but prompts behaviors in all the targeted areas.

The analysis identifies the children's best performance in the following areas:

Gestural Communicative Intent (GCI):

1. The child examines or manipulates objects and does not report to the adult.
2. The child expresses emotional reactions to objects/events, including clapping, smiling, making a face and hitting.
3. The child emits signs that are contiguous to the goal, to the child's own body or to the adult's body; the child reports to the adult.
4. The child repeats the same gesture until the purpose is achieved; the child reports to the adult.
5. The child modifies the gesture shape until the purpose is achieved, that is, the child repeats the gesture with an extra element; the child reports to the adult.
6. The child emits ritualized gestures that are not contiguous to the goal, to the child's body or to the adult's body, that is, the same gesture must be used in at least two occasions in the same communicative context to be qualified as a ritual; the child reports to the adult.

Vocal Communicative Intent (VCI):

1. The child vocalizes while he/she manipulates or examines an object or while ignores an object and does not report to the adult.
2. The child expresses emotional reactions to objects/events, including screams, laughs, crying.
3. The child emits vocal signs referring to an object or to the adult; the same sing must be used in at least two different communicative contexts.
4. The child repeats the same vocal sign until the purpose is achieved; the child reports to the adult.
5. The child modifies the vocal sign until the purpose is achieved, that is, the child repeats the gesture with an extra element; the child reports to the adult.
6. The child emits ritualized sounds, that is, the same sign must be used in at least two occasions in the same communicative context to be qualified as a ritual; the child reports to the adult.

Tool Use (TU):

1. The child uses a familiar instrument contiguous to the object as a way to obtain it.
2. The child uses a familiar instrument not contiguous to the object as a way to obtain it.

3. The child uses an unfamiliar instrument contiguous to the object as a way to obtain it.
4. The child uses an unfamiliar instrument not contiguous to the object as a way to obtain it.

Gesture Imitation (GI):

1. The child imitates familiar action schemes.
2. The child imitates complex gestures composed by familiar action schemes.
3. The child imitates unfamiliar visible gestures.
4. The child imitates unfamiliar invisible gestures and reproduces the adult's model in the first attempt when the model is no longer present.

Vocal Imitation (VI):

1. The child imitates familiar vocal sounds.
2. The child imitates familiar words.
3. The child imitates unfamiliar sound patterns.
4. The child imitates unfamiliar words and reproduces the adult's model in the first attempt when the model is no longer present.

Combinatory Play (CP):

1. The child uses simple motor schemes in objects.
2. The child manipulates physical features of the objects.
3. The child relates two objects.
4. The child relates three or more objects without sequential order.
5. The child combines at least three objects with sequential order.
6. The child combines more than three objects with sequential order.

Symbolic Play (SP):

1. The child uses simple motor schemes in objects.
2. The child manipulates physical features of the objects.
3. The child uses conventionally the realistic objects; he/she may or may not use invisible substances, applies the schemes only to him/herself.
4. The child uses miniatures conventionally; he/she may or may not use invisible substances, applies the schemes only to him/herself.
5. The child uses objects conventionally with invisible substances; applies the schemes to him/herself and to others.
6. The child uses one object by the other; applies the schemes to him/her and to others.

Wetherby & Prutting (1984) concluded that autistic children certainly present a delay in the acquisition of social-cognitive abilities and therefore present the behavioral, interactive and communication disorders that are typical of this syndrome.

Autistic children also present individual variations, that is, levels of social-cognitive performance vary within the pathology, but all of them present some kind of communicative intent, wheatear it is expressed by verbal, vocal or gestural means. Therefore it is essential to include these data in the discussions about the SLPs communicative attitudes during language therapy (Molini & Fernandes, 2003). The authors also report that there is a certain point of difficulty in the use of social cognitive abilities. The study has shown that autistic children seem to understand how the world functions but lack the ability to share their knowledge and use it spontaneously in every-day-life situations.

The social cognitive performance scores also clearly indicate associations with functional aspects of communication. Although there isn't a typical developmental pattern of autistic children the existing theories reaffirm the verbal and non-verbal language disorders and their associations with social and cognitive inabilities.

5.2 Social-communicative adaptation

The identification of each child's social-communicative adaptation may provide important information to support clinical decisions about intervention models and focus.
A useful proposal to determine the social-communicative adaptation of ASD children differentiates 4 levels with 4 stages each (Gutstein & Sheely, 2002):

- Level I: Beginner - stages: attuning, social reference, apprentice-guide and social adjustment.
- Level II: Apprentice - stages: variation, adaptation, synchronization and considering others.
- Level III: Challenger - stages: collaboration, co-creation, improvisation and shared perceptions.
- Level IV: Explorer - stages: perspectives, shared imagination, sharing ideas and friends.

According to this proposal the information can be obtained through interviews with parents or teachers or with the use of a questionnaire.

5.3 Meta-representation

The concept of meta-representation or "Theory of Mind" (ToM) describes the ability to assign thoughts and feelings to others with the objective of predicting and explaining behaviors (Frith, 1994).
There are no formal tests of meta-representation and probably the variety of the assessment procedures is the reason of the different results reported in the literature (Sparrevohn & Howie, 1995).
It is suggested that the failures in meta-representations are responsible for the inappropriate behavior of autistic children when interacting with others (Frith, 1994). The development of representational abilities would contribute to the improvement of experience exchanges and role variations (Beatson & Prelock, 2002).
It follows an example of the possible associations between functional communicative profile, social-cognitive performance, vocabulary and meta-representation in ASD children.
Subjects were 20 children between 6 and 13 years (mean age 8.9) and the procedures included the identification of the communicative profile and the best social-cognitive performance, through the analysis of 30 minutes of filmed interaction; the application of an expressive vocabulary test (specially constructed for Brazilian children) and four theory of mind tasks (as suggested by Sparrevohn and Howie, 1995), through the presentation of pictures on a computer screen.
Results involved the comparison of data of all subjects. It was possible to observe that, on most of the subjects, less than half of all communicative acts expressed had interpersonal functions. Children that expressed more interpersonal communicative acts also performed better at meta-representation tasks and social-cognitive abilities; they presented the greatest proportion of verbal use and less episodes of non-designation on the vocabulary test.
The sole comparison criteria in which it was possible to identify strong consistency on the correlation between data is the proportion of use of verbal mean of communication. It was

possible to identify a certain linearity that can be summarized by the notion that "the more verbal the autistic child is, the better his/her performance on the areas of social cognitive development, communicative functionality, lexical development and meta-representation". Individual data analysis, however, points to specific variations and correlations that cannot be overlooked.
Statistical analysis points to significant correlations (at 5%) that can be synthesized as follows:

- Greater proportion of use of verbal communicative means is positively correlated to greater proportion of interpersonal communicative functions expressed, better performance on verbal communicative intent and more usual verbal designations.
- Greater proportion of interpersonal communicative functions expressed is positively correlated to better performances on symbolic play and usual verbal designations.
- Better performance on verbal communicative intent is positively correlated to better performance on tool used and on combinatory play.
- Better performances on gestural imitation and on tool use are positively correlated to combinatory and symbolic play.

Autistic children's difficulties with the interactive use of communication, as mentioned by Stone & Caro-Martinez (1990) could also be observed in this study, since just 35% of the subjects expressed more than 50% of interpersonal communicative functions.
Despite the fact that data involving meta-representation didn't lead to statistical significance, they allow some interesting discussion. For example, although the complete false belief task was the most complex and the one that produced the greater number of wrong answers, it was also the one that generated the smaller number of non-answers. It may be due to the fact that it was the only task on which the material presented was concrete and not pictures, and it may be associated to the ideas of Bara et al (2001) that suggested that these children's difficulties are related to attention deficits that can be reduced by the use of concrete elements.
Data show that, of the 17 subjects that responded to any of the meta-representation tasks, none of them presented the right answer to all the questions. This data agree with the literature that suggests to a great difficulty of autistic children on theory of mind (for example, Frith, 1994; Leslie & Thaiss, 1992; Sparrevohn & Howie, 1995).
In respect to the correlation between the various results, the statistical analysis identified two strong correlations involving the increase on the proportion of use of verbal communication: the decrease on use of gestural communicative mean and the increase of usual verbal designations. This data correspond to the expected, as more verbal communication decreases the necessity of gestures, since for this subjects, the redundancy of communicative means doesn't increases the efficacy of communication. On the other side, various researches suggest that there is no correlation between communicative competency and the morphological abilities of these children (for example: Wetherby & Prutting, 1984; Bara et al, 2001).
The association between social-cognitive performance, functional communication profile and lexical abilities indicated that:

1. better results on vocal communicative intent were associated to greater proportion of verbal expression and less use of gestures, agreeing with the notion that communicative performance tends to be better when there is communicative intent (Carpenter & Tomasello, 2001);
2. better performance on combinatory play was related to less use of vocal communicative mean, a result that can be associated to the fact that both areas involve motor abilities, that can be altered in just some of these children (Mundy & Stella, 2001);

3. better results on symbolic play were related to greater use of interpersonal communicative functions, what seems to reinforce the use of these situations during language therapy with autistic children, as suggested by Gutstein & Sheely, 2002 and larger numbers of usual verbal designations, greater proportions of interpersonal communicative functions expressed and smaller proportions of the use of gestures were associated - this data can be due to the relation between lexical performance and language use, as proposed by Befi-Lopes, 2007.

The relatively small volume of statistically significant results should not lead to the depreciation of obtained data. Careful and detailed individual analysis is essential to the determination of consistent and efficient therapeutic procedures (Koegel, 2000; Wetherby & Prizant, 2001; Greenspan & Wieder, 2001).

Analysis of the aspects of vocabulary and meta-representation in children of the autistic spectrum may provide important information to the determination of therapeutic processes, when related to the functional communicative profile and social-cognitive performance. This data may help on the identification of each child's greater difficulties and better abilities.

6. Conclusion

The purpose of this chapter was to discuss the assessment of various aspects of language, once it is an essential diagnostic feature in ASD. The common impairment observed in individuals with ASD is in the functional use of communication, but MLU and vocabulary should also always be assessed. Specific groups (verbal and non-verbal individuals; children and adolescents) and situations (individual or group, familiar or non-familiar) should be specifically considered. Samples of spontaneous communication may provide data to objective measures of functional communicative profile, linguistic complexity and vocabulary that can be considered in the overall diagnosis as well as in intervention planning. The associations between the functional communicative profile and domains such as social-cognitive performance, meta-representation and social communicative adaptation have also been subject of several studies, as well as the best way to prompt the better performances during testing procedures. The results of these studies may support evidence-based proposals for language therapy with ASD children and the objective assessment of their outcomes.

The language assessment of ASD children may include the use of the protocols and criteria described or others suggested in the literature. Especially when dealing with a non-English speaking population the speech and language pathologist is frequently faced with challenges involving his/her practice consistency. Language assessment criteria, tools and procedures must be strictly adjusted to the language-specific characteristics and group differences and therefore demand careful consideration of weather it is appropriate to specific needs and demands.

7. References

Anderson, D.K., Lord, C., Risi, S., DiLavore, P.S., Shulman, C., Thurn, A., Welch, K. & Pickles, A. 2007. Patterns of growth in verbal abilities among children with autism spectrum disorder. *J Consult Clin Psychol*, Vol.75, No.4 (,2007), pp. 594-604. ISSN 0022-006X

Andrade, C.R.F.; Befi-Lopes, D.M., Fernandes, F.D.M. & Wertzner, H.F. 2000. *ABFW – Teste de linguagem infantil nas áreas de fonologia, vocabulário, fluência e pragmática*. Pró-Fono, ISBN 8585491.45-0, São Paulo, Brazil

Amato, C.A.H. & Fernandes, F.D.M. 2010. Interactive use of communication by verbal and non-verbal autistic children. *Pro Fono Rev Atual Cien.*,Vol.22, No.4, (December 2010), pp.373-378, ISSN 01045687

Araújo, K, & Befi-Lopes, D.M. 2004. Extensão média do enunciado em crianças entre 2 e 4 anos de idade: diferenças no uso de palavras e morfemas. *Rev Soc Bras Fonoaudiol.*, Vol.9, No.3, (September, 2004), pp.156-163, ISSN 1516-8034

Bara BG, Bucciarelli M & Colle L.2001. Communicative abilities in autism: evidence for attentional deficits. *Brain and Lang,* Vol. 77, No.2, (February, 2001), pp.216-240, ISSN 0093-934X

Bates, E. & Goodman, J.C. 1999. On the emergence of grammar from the lexicon. In: *The emergence of language.* MacWhinney, B. , editor, pp. 29-79, Laurence Eralbaum Associates, ISBN 0-8058-3010-3, Mahwah NJ USA

Beatson, J.E. & Prelock, P.A. 2002. The Vermont Rural Autism Project: Sharing experiences, shifting attitudes. *Foc Autism & Other Develop Disab,* Vol.17, No.1(March, 2002), pp. 48-54, ISSN 1088-3576

Befi-Lopes, D.M., Cáceres, A.M., & Araújo, K. 2007. Aquisição de verbos em pré-escolares falantes do português brasileiro. *Rev CEFAC,* Vol.9, No.4, (December, 2007), pp.444-452, ISSN 1516-1846

Belkadi, A. 2006. Language impairments in autism: evidence against mind-blindness. *SOAS Working Papers in Linguistic,* Vol.14, No.1 (February, 2006), pp.3-13, ISBN 0728602814

Benson, P., Karlof, K.L. & Siperstein, G.S. 2008. Maternal involvement in the education of young children with autism spectrum disorders. *Autism.* Vol. 12., No.1 (February 2008), pp. 47–63, ISSN 1362-3613

Bishop, D.V.M. 2000. How does the brain learn language? Insights from the study of children with and without language impairment. *Dev Med Child Neurol.,* Vol. 42, No. 1 (March 2000), pp.133-142, ISSN 0012-1622

Bloom, P. 1997. Intentionality and word learning. *Trends Cogn Sci.,* Vol.1, No.1 (March, 1997), pp. 9-12, ISSN 1364-6613

Cardoso, C., & Fernandes, F.D.M. 2003. Use of personal and non-personal communicative functions in ASD children. *Pro Fono Rev Atual Cien.,* Vol.15, No.3, (September, 2003), pp.279-86, ISSN 0104-5687

Cardoso, C. & Fernandes, F.D.M. 2006. Relations between social-cognitive performance and functional communicative profile in ASD adolescents. *Pró-Fono Rev Atual Cient,*V. 18, No.1, (March, 2006), pp. 89-98, ISSN 0104-5687

Carpenter, M. & Tomasello, M. 2001.Joint Attention, Cultural Learning and Language Acquisition. In: *Autism Spectrum Disorders – A Transactional Developmental Perspective,* A.M.Wetherby & B.M.Prizant, (Eds.), pp.62-72, Paul Brooks, ISBN 9781557664457, Baltimore, USA

Chawarska, K., Paul, R., Klin, A., Hannigen, S., Dichtel, L.E. & Volkmar, F. 2007. Parental Recognition of Developmental Problems in Toddlers with Autism Spectrum Disorders. *J Autism Dev Disord,* Vol.37, No.1, (March, 2007), pp.62–72, ISSN 0162-3257

Clifford, S.M. & Dissanayake, C. 2008. The Early Development of Joint Attention in Infants with Autistic Disorder Using Home Video Observations and Parental Interview. *J Autism Dev Disord,* Vol.38, No.4, (December, 2008), pp.791–805, ISSN 0162-3257

Condouris, K., Meyer. E., & Tager-Flusberg, H. 2003. The relationship between standardized measures of language and measures of spontaneous speech in children with autism. *Am J Speech Lang Pathol,* Vol.12, No.3, (June, 2003), pp. 349-58, ISSN 1058-0360

Davis N.O. & Carter AS. 2008. Parenting Stress in Mothers and Fathers of Toddlers with Autism Spectrum Disorders: Associations with Child Characteristics. *J Autism Dev Disord.,* Vol.38, No.7, (October, 2008), pp.1278–1291, ISSN 0612-3257

Eigsti, I.M., Bennetto, L., & Daldani, M.B. 2007. Beyond pragmatics: morphosyntactic development in autism. *J Autism Dev Disord*, Vol.37, No.6, (August 2007), pp.1007-1023, ISSN 0612-3257

Fernandes, F.D.M. 1994. A questão da linguagem em autismo infantil: uma revisão crítica da literatura. *Revista de Neuropsiquiatria da Infância e Adolescência*, Vol.2, No.3, (September, 1994), pp. 5-10, ISSN 1618-5342

Fernandes, F.D.M. & Galinari, H.S. 1999. Oficina de linguagem em hospital-dia infantil - primeiros relatos. *Pró-Fono Rev Atual Cient*, Vol.11, No.2, (August 1999), pp.85-91, ISSN 0104-5687

Fernandes, F.D.M. 2000. Aspectos funcionais da comunicação de crianças autistas. *Temas sobre Desenvolvimento*, Vol.9, No.51, (April, 2000), pp.25-35, ISSN 0103-7749

Fernandes, F.D.M. & Ribeiro, S,L. 2000. Investigação do desempenho sócio cognitivo durante a terapia fonoaudiológica de crianças autistas - o uso de procedimentos específicos. *J Bras Fonoaud*, Vol.1, No.4, (September, 2000), pp. 71 - 83, ISSN 1517-5308

Fernandes, F.D.M. 2003. Perfil comunicativo, desempenho sociocognitivo, vocabulário e meta-representação em crianças com transtorno do espectro autístico. *Pró-Fono Rev Atual Cient*, Vol. 15, No.3, (September, 2003), pp.267-278, ISSN 0104-5687

Folstein, S.E., & Rosen-Shedley, B. 2001. Genetics of autism: complex aetiology for a heterogeneous disorder. *Nature*, Vol. 414, No.2. (December, 2001), pp.943-55 ISSN 0028-0836

Frith U. 1994. Autism: beyond theory of mind. *Cognition*, Vol.1, No.3 (August 1994), pp.115-132, ISSN 0010-0277

García-Pérez,R., Hobson, R.P., & Lee, A. 2008. Narrative role-taking in autism. *J Autism Dev Disord.*, Vol.38, No.1, (February, 2008), pp.156-168, ISSN 0162-3257

Goldfield, B.A. 2000. Nouns before verbs in comprehension vs. production: the view from pragmatics. *J Child Lang*, Vol.27, No.3, (September, 2000), pp.501-20, ISSN 0305-0009

Greenspan, S.I. & Wieder, S. 2001.A developmental approach to difficulties in relating and communicating in autism spectrum disorders and related syndromes. In: *Autism Spectrum Disorders - A Transactional Developmental Perspective*, A.M.Wetherby & B.M.Prizant, (Eds), 279-306, Paul Brooks, ISBN 9781557664457, Baltimore, USA.

Grindle, C.F., Kovshoff, H., Hastings, R.P. & Remington, B. 2009. Parents' Experiences of Home-Based Applied Behavior Analysis Programs for Young Children with Autism. *J Autism Dev Disord*, Vol. 39, No.1, (February, 2009), p.42–56, ISSN 0162-3257

Gutstein, S. & Sheely, R. 2002. *Relationship Development Intervention for Children, Adolescents and Adults with Autism/ Asperger*. Future Horizons, ISBN-13 978 1 843107170, Arlington, Texas, USA

Halliday, M.A.K. 1978. *Language as Social Semiotic - the social interpretation of language and meaning*, University Park Press, ISBN 0839111835, Maryland, USA

Hetzroni,O.E., & Tannous,J. 2004. Effects of a computer-based intervention program on the communicative functions of children with autism. *J Autism Develop Dis.*,Vol.34, No.2 (April, 2004), pp.95-113, ISSN 0162-3257

Jarrold, C., Boucher, J., & Russell, J. 1997. Language profiles in children with autism: theoretical and methodological implications. *Autism*,Vol.3, No.1, (March, 1997), pp.57-76, ISSN1362-3613

Kjelgaard,M.M.,& Tager-Flusberg,H.2001.An investigation of language impairment in autism: implications for genetic subgroups. *Lang Cogn Process*, Vol.16, No.2-3, (July, 2001), pp. 287-308, ISSN 0169-0965

Koegel, L.K.2000. Interventions to facilitate communication in autism. *J Autism Develop Disord*, Vol.30, No.5, (August, 2000), pp.383-291, ISSN 0162-3257

Laugeson, E.A., Frankel, F., Mogil, C. & Dillon, A.R. 2009.Parent-Assisted Social Skills Training to Improve Friendships in Teens with Autism Spectrum Disorders. *J Autism Dev Disord*. Vol.39, No.3 (August, 2009), pp.596–606, ISSN 0162-3257

Lee, E.C., & Rescorla, L. 2002. The use of psychological state terms by late talkers at age 3. *Applied Psycholinguistic*, Vol.23, No.3, (October, 2002), pp.623-641, ISSN 0142-7164

Leslie, A.M. & Thais, P. 1992. Pretence and representation: the origins of theory of mind. *Psychol Review*, Vol.94, No.4, (December, 1992), pp. 412-426, ISSN 0033-295X

Marcos, H. 2001. Introduction: early pragmatic development. *First Lang*, Vol.21, No.2, (April, 2001), pp.209-218 ISSN 0149-7997

Miilher, L.P. & Fernandes, F.D.M. 2009. Habilidades pragmáticas, vocabulares e gramaticais em crianças com transtornos do espectro autístico. *Pró-Fono Rev Atual Cient*, Vol.21, No. 3, (September, 2009), pp. 309-314, ISSN 1516-8034

Molini, D.R, & Fernandes F;D.M. 2003. Communicative intent and tool use in children with psychiatric disorders, *Pro-Fono Rev Atual Cient*, Vol.15, No.2, (June, 2003), pp.149-158, ISSN 1516-8034

Moreira, C.R. & Fernandes, F.D.M. 2010. Assessing communication in the autistic spectrum: interference of familiarity in language performance. Rev Soc Bras Fonoaudiol, Vol.15, No. 3, (September, 2010), p. 430-435, ISSN - 1516-8034

Mundy, P. & Stella, J. 2001. Joint attention, social orienting, and nonverbal communication in autism. In: *Autism Spectrum Disorders – A Transactional Developmental Perspective*, A.Wetherby, B.Prizant, (Eds.), 55-77, Paul Brooks, ISBN 9781557664457, Baltimore, USA

Naigles, L.R., & Hoff-Ginsberg, E. 1998. Why are some verbs learned before other verbs? Effects of input frequency and structure on children's early verb use. *J Child Lang*, Vol.25, No. 1, (March, 1998), pp.95-120, ISSN 0305-0009

Ninio, A., & Snow, C.E. (1988). Language acquisition through language use: the functional sources of children's early utterances. In: *Categories and processes in language acquisition*, Y. Levy, I. Schlesinger, & Braine M.D.S. (Eds), pp.11-30, Erlbaum, ISBN 0805801510, Hillsdale, NJ, USA

Paul, R., Miles, S., Cicchetti, D., Sparrow, S., Klin, A., Volkmar, F., Colin, M., & Booker, S. 2004. Adaptative behavior in autism and pervasive developmental disorder-not otherwise specified: microanalysis of scores on the Vineland Adaptative Behavior Scale. *J Autism Develop Dis*, Vol.34, No.2, (April, 2004), pp.223-28, ISSN 0162-3257

Perkins, M.R., Dobbinson, S., Boucher, J., Bol, S., & Bloom, P.2006. Lexical knowledge and lexical use in autism. *J Autism Dev Disord*, Vol.36, No. 6, (August, 2006), pp.795-805, ISSN 0162-3257

Reed, P., Osborne, L;A & Corness, M. 2007. Brief Report: Relative Effectiveness of Different Home-based Behavioral Approaches to Early Teaching Intervention. *J Autism Dev Disord*. Vol.37, No.7, (November, 2007), pp.1815–1821, ISSN 0162-3257

Roberts,J.A., Rice,M.L., & Tager-Flusberg,H. 2004. Tense marking in children with autism. *Applied Psycholinguistics*, Vol. 25, No.3, (May, 2004), pp. 429-448, ISSN 0142-7164

Rollins, P. R., & Snow, C. E. 1998. Shared attention and grammatical development in typical and children with autism. *J Child Lang*, Vol.25, No.3, (September, 1998), pp.653-73, ISSN 0305-0009

Ruser, T.F; Arin, D., Dowd M., Putnam, S., Winklosky, B., Rosen-Sheidley, B., Piven, J., Tomblin, B., Tager-Flusberg, H. & Folstein, S. 2007. Communicative Competence in Parents of Children with Autism and Parents of Children with Specific Language Impairment. *J Autism Dev Disord*, Vol.37, No.6, (September, 2007), pp.1323–1336, ISSN 0162-3257

Scheeren, A.M. & Stauder, J.E.A. 2008. Broader Autism Phenotype in Parents of Autistic Children: Reality or Myth? *J Autism Dev Disord,* Vol. 38, No.1, (February, 2008), pp.276–287, ISSN 0162-3257

Smith, V., Mirenda, P., & Zaidman-Zait, A. 2007. Predictors of expressive vocabulary growth in children with autism. *J Speech Lang Hear Res,* Vol.50, No.1, (March, 2007), pp.149-160, ISSN 1092-4388

Solomon,M., Ono,M.,Timmer,S. & Goodlin-Jones,B. 2008. The Effectiveness of Parent–Child Interaction Therapy for Families of Children on the Autism Spectrum. *J Autism Dev Disord,* Vol.38, No.7, (October, 2008), pp.1767–1776, ISSN 0162-3257

Sparrevohn, R. & Howie, P.M. 1995. Theory of mind in children with autistic disorder: evidence of developmental progression and role of verbal ability. *J Child Psychol,* Vol.36, No.2, (February, 1995), pp.249-263, ISSN 0021-9630

Stone, W.L. & Caro-Martinez, L.M. 1990. Naturalistic observations of spontaneous communication in autistic children. *J Autism Develop Disord,* Vol.20, No.4, (August, 1990), pp.437-453, ISSN 0162-3257

Tager -Flusberg, H. 2000. The challenge of studying language development in children with autism. In: *Methods for studying language production,* N. Menn, N.B. Ratner (Eds.), pp.187- 213, Laurence Eralbaum Associates, ISBN 0-8058-3033-2, Mahwah, NJ, USA

Tager-Flusberg, H., & Calkins, S. 1999. Does imitation facilitate the acquisition of grammar? Evidence from a study of autistic, Down's syndrome and normal children. *J Child Lang,* Vol.17, No.3, (September, 1999),pp. 591-606, ISSN 0305-0009

Tager-Flusberg, H., Calkins, S., Nolin, T., Baumberger, T., Anderson, M. & Chadwick-Dias, A. 1990. A longitudinal study of language acquisition in autistic and Down syndrome children. *J Autism Dev Disord,* Vol.20, No.1, (January, 1990), pp.1-21, ISSN 0162-3257

Toppelberg, C.O., & Shapiro, T. 2000. Language disorders: a 10 year research update review. *J Am Acad Child Adolesc Psychiatry,* Vol.39, No.2, (March, 2000), pp.143-52, ISSN 0980-8567

Volkmar, F.R., & Pauls, D. 2003. Autism. *Lancet,* Vol.362, No.1133, (March, 2003), pp. 29-41, ISSN 0140-6736

Wachtel, K. & Carter, A.S. 2008. Reaction to diagnosis and parenting styles among mothers of young children with ASDs. *Autism,* Vol.12, No.5, (May, 2008), pp.575–594, ISSN 1362-3613

Walenski, M., Tager-Flusberg, H., & Ullman, M.T. 2006. Language in autism. In: *Understanding autism: from basic neuroscience to treatment,* S.O. Moldin & J. L. R. Rubenstein (eds), pp 87-103, Taylor & Francis Books, ISBN 10-0-8493-2732-6, London

Wetherby, A. & Prizant, B. 2001. Introduction to autism spectrum disorders. In: *Autism Spectrum Disorders – A Transactional Developmental Perspective,* A.Wetherby & B. Prizant, (Eds), pp.1-7, Paul Brooks ISBN 9781557664457, Baltimore, USA

Wetherby,A. & Prutting, C. 1984. Profiles of communicative and cognitive-social abilities in autistic children. *J.Speech Hear Res,* Vol.27, N.2, (April, 1981), pp.364-377, ISSN 1092-4388

Williams E., Kendell-Scott L. & Costall, A. 2005. Parents' experiences of introducing everyday object use to their children with autism. *Autism,* Vol.9, No.5, (August, 2005), pp.495–514, ISSN 0140-6736

Young, E.C., Diehl, J.J., Morris, D., Hyman, S.L., & Benneto, L. 2005. The use of two language tests to identify pragmatic language problems in children with autism spectrum disorders. *Lang Speech Hear Serv Sch.,* Vol. 36, No.1, (February, 2005), pp.62-72, ISSN 1092-4388

2

Language Therapy with Children with Autism Spectrum Disorders

Fernanda Dreux M.Fernandes, Daniela R.Molini-Avejonas and Cibelle A.H.Amato
Universidade de São Paulo
Brazil

1. Introduction

The role of language in Autism Spectrum Disorders (ASD) is a singular one because, contrary to other broad developmental disorders in which language impairments are a symptom or a consequence of other deficits, in the autism spectrum language disorders constitute one of the three diagnostic criteria. The diagnostic procedures always involve clinical observation and behavior identification. Although several hypothesis claim that this is a neurobiological disorder with a strong genetic component no biological marker for autism was identified (Gothem et al., 2007).

Pragmatic perspectives have been providing elements for the analysis of functional aspects of communication and it's relation with other aspects of development of children within the autistic spectrum for some decades (Bates, 1976 Bates, 1979; Eigsti et al., 2007; Halliday, 1978; Ingersol, 2006; Keen et al.,2007; Prizant, 1996; Rogers & Benetto, 2001; Rutter, 1983; Suttera et al., 2007; Tomasello et al., 1999; Wollner & Geller, 1982).

Several authors point out that some language and communication difficulties of children with autism will probably follow them throughout life, especially if they are not included in remediation programs (Grela & Mclaughlin, 2006; Koegel, 2000; Mandell & Salzer, 2007; Mesibov et al, 2007; Rogers et al., 2006; Ruhterford et al., 2007; Seroussi, 2002; Sigafoos et al. 1994; Whalen et al.,2006;).

The question about the possibility of identification of the best therapeutic approach for children with autism has also been frequently discussed on the literature (DiLalla & Rogers, 1994; Fernandes, 2000a; 2000b; Giddan et al, 1995; Kuschner 2007; Partington & Sundberg, 1998; Toth et al. 2006; Turner et al, 2006; Wetherby et al., 2001;).

The search for alternatives of more efficient language therapy approaches for autistic children has been the focus of several important researches. Several authors suggest that it seems premature to suppose that just one therapeutic approach is more effective than the others. They state that there is not one model effective for all children. It is suggested that the intervention should be individualized, in the sense of identifying the present level of development of each child and the profile of strong and weak points of each one (Gothem, 2007; Prizant & Rubin, 1999, Solomon et al, 2007; Mesibov & Shea, 2010; Vismara & Rogers, 2010).

The best therapeutic approach to children of the autism spectrum is still undetermined and probably depends on several factors such as individual profile, family characteristics, educational and intervention alternatives. The determination of the meaningful variables is essential to the better use of the available resources.

Most of the therapeutic intervention programs aim the development of functional speech and use a variety of techniques to achieve it: increasing motivation, use of directive reinforcements (positive or negative, depending on the proposal), variations of concrete stimulus, reinforcement of verbal communicative attempts, use of multiple examples and others. These intervention processes should address increasing spontaneity, varying communicative functions, using language socially and other aspects involved in communicative efficiency. The application of research results as the basis of therapeutic intervention proposals has resulted in studies about therapeutic processes and their outcomes, allowing improvement of evidence based practice.

This chapter will discuss the theoretical basis of language therapy within the pragmatics linguistic framework and describe different therapeutic models within the same approach as well as experiences of mother coaching and a follow-up study. Pragmatic theories are the mostly used framework to the analysis of autistic children's communication in the last decades. It is probably due to the fact that the studies evolved to the notion that the central language feature within the autism spectrum is related to the functional use of language, especially regarding its interface with social cognitive development. The pragmatics theories focus exactly on these areas of development (Bates, 1976; Hallyday, 1978) and therefore provide consistent support to the analysis as well as to the proposal of intervention programs.

The effectiveness of different therapeutic approaches suggests that any conclusion must take into account data about social and familiar contexts that play central roles in practical issues such as frequency of attendance, continuity of the intervention process and involvement with the therapeutic proposals.

It is premature and deceiving to suggest that one sole therapeutic approach is more effective than the others and that there is a method that is more effective with all children. It is suggested that the intervention program should be individualized, considering each child's actual development level and identifying personal profiles of abilities and inabilities.

The proposed therapeutic framework focus on the individual communicative profile that considers: the communication interactivity (including the number of communicative acts produced per minute and the proportion of more interpersonal communicative functions expressed); the communicative means (basically verbal, vocal and gestural communicative means, but it can be expanded to include written language or any form of sign language); initiative for interaction; discursive abilities (including conversational and joint attention strategies) and social cognitive performance. The individual profile is the base for individually designed language intervention processes they may include the formal aspects of language (such as speech articulation, vocabulary, grammatical complexity or reading comprehension skills).

With the support of research data, three alternative models will be discussed: individual therapy (based in building the communicative partnership through supportive interaction); language workshop (where two subjects allowed symmetric interaction and provided communicative challenges) and mother-child language therapy (designed to provide a more comprehensive intervention and improve communicative settings at home).

Anticipating some results, it can be stated that apparently peer communication situations provide a symmetry that is not obtained in situations with adults. This symmetry provides affective performance demands and communicative challenges in which subjects must use their communicative abilities. Therefore, it seems to be possible to use temporary controlled changes during the therapeutic process and maintaining the progress rhythm of in the long term.

On the other hand, language therapy process can also benefit from specific orientations to caretakers about language and communication processes focused on individual profiles of abilities and inabilities of each communicative dyad. The proposal of mother-child language therapy settings aims to create the possibility of a more comprehensive intervention process, especially improving the alternatives of more productive communicative settings at home. The inclusion of mothers in the therapeutic process during a set period of time, however, demands the determination of parameters indicating when to begin this type of intervention, its duration and the procedures for a long time support.

Clinical experience suggests that each individual goes through periods of development and balance, and some may even experience periods of regression - that are absolutely unique and can almost never be anticipated. Long term therapeutic processes, as is the case with autistic children, also demand consideration about the long term results obtained from short term interferences.

2. Different intervention models: Research data

The study was proposed to determine if there are more efficient intervention procedures to improve communication abilities of children with disorders of the autism spectrum and to identify possible differences in the functional communicative profile and in the social cognitive performance of 36 autistic children and adolescents receiving language therapy in three different models.

Based on the Pragmatic theories of Linguistics (Bates, 1976) and on previous research results (Cardoso & Fernandes, 2006; Fernandes, 2005), the therapeutic framework that was common to all the intervention procedures, regardless of its specific model, can be synthesized in some central points:

- Focus on the individual profile: the absence of chronological order of the developmental milestones is not altogether rare within the autism spectrum. Children that, for example, learn to read before being able to name the basic colors are fairly frequent among the ones with diagnosis within the autism spectrum. Therefore, the careful identification of individual's profile of abilities and inabilities is essential to determine a more efficient therapeutic design that will not overlook some impairment or place the focus on abilities already well developed.
- The communication interactivity must always receive careful attention. When a child doesn't speak, or does it with extreme difficulty, the attention is frequently drawn to improve the interaction. However, in the opposite situations, whether if the child has severe behavior problems or if he or she is extremely talkative (to the point of ignoring the listener), the therapeutic focus is easily directed towards other issues. Therefore, symmetric communicative situation, where all the participants share equally the communicative initiative and where most of the communication has interpersonal functions, is one of the most important aims of any intervention program.
- Verbal communication is the easiest, most common and most efficient form of human interaction and therefore it is, naturally, the foremost objective of language therapy. Several studies indicate that autistic children that can speak are frequently considered

more normal by their parents even when their performance in other areas is worse than that of non-speaking children. There are situations however, where the communication's content is more important than the form through which it is conveyed. For example, a child that verbally reproduces a sequence of train stations may communicate more personal contents through much less intelligible emissions or even gestures. The attention to all communicative means will contribute to more effective and personal exchanges.

- Natural and rich communication situations include opportunities and challenges to exercise communicative initiatives with real contextual results that will provide a natural feedback to each situation. The therapeutic setting, therefore, must be flexible and offer opportunities to problem solving while also being organized enough to avoid producing stress and anxiety. Another issue that must be considered is the flexibility of the therapist's role, avoiding situations when the adult always takes the communicative initiatives with questions, requests and comments.
- Naturalistic communicative situations and symbolic play games also favor the practice of discursive abilities such as turn taking, obtaining and maintaining attention, introducing a new topic, maintaining a topic, identifying and repairing communicative breakdowns, using linguistic markers of politeness and isotopy.

The three different models proposed to this study aim to address more directly some specific points:

- The individual therapy is mainly focused on building the communicative partnership, where a repertoire of shared information, interests and mutual knowledge favors the development of a supportive interaction. In these situations new acquired abilities can be safely exercised and used in various contexts.
- The main proposal of the mother-child language therapy situation is to provide a comprehensive intervention where successful experiences can be reenacted at home and the unsuccessful ones can be understood and avoided, improving the communicative settings offered to the child at home and in other environments.
- The language workshop proposes therapeutic sessions with two children and two adults (a therapist and an auxiliary). This situation allows more symmetric interactions with natural challenges, since the children may share interests as well as difficulties. This way the children may, for example, naturally dispute over a board game and must find ways to be understood by the other, despite his or her individual difficulty. In these situations usually the child uses more than one communicative mean to convey a single communicative function as a way to guarantee comprehension, and it may be an efficient way to exercise the use of a new alternative to communicate a certain meaning.

2.1 Study design and method

The participants were divided in three groups according to the received intervention model during a pre-determined time period of 20 weeks. The groups of language workshops, mother-child language therapy and individual therapy were determined according to clinical criteria. Subjects were 36 children and adolescents with mean age of 8 years and 3 months with psychiatric diagnosis included in the autism spectrum. All subjects had similar social-cognitive performance in the beginning of the study.

In group A subjects were included in language workshops. They were 10 participants with mean age of 9 years and 7 months (standard deviation 2.4). All of them were receiving language therapy for at least 6 months, and for a maximum of 1 year, prior to the study. They were paired according to developmental level and types of interests. They were included in language workshops for a six-month period, that is, 20 therapeutic sessions and after that they returned to individual sessions for another period of 20 sessions.

In group B the situation was of mother-child language therapy. There were 9 participants with mean age of 7 years and 11 months (standard deviation 4.6). All of them were receiving language therapy for at least 6 months, and for a maximum of 1 year, prior to the study. The subjects received language therapy with their mothers for a six-month period, that is, 20 therapeutic sessions. After that, they received individual sessions for another period of 20 sessions. In this group we had the lowest mean age - but this variable wasn't controlled, since prior studies discarded chronological age as a significant element to autistic children's performance.

Subjects in group C received only individual language therapy. This group had 17 participants with mean age of 9 years and 6 months (standard deviation 3.4). All of them were receiving language therapy for at least 6 months, and for a maximum of 1 year, prior to the study. They received individual language therapy sessions for a period of twelve months, that is, 40 sessions.

All the therapy processes had the same orientations: emphasize functional and inter-personal communication.

All participants were video recorded during play interaction situations with their therapists in three moments:

- Before starting the period of the modified language therapy situations.
- After the period of modified situations (20 sessions of double, with the mother or individual language therapy sessions).
- After the following period of 20 individual sessions.

The analysis of the Functional Communicative Profile (FCP) included the identification of the communicative means used (verbal, vocal, gestural); the communication interactivity (i.e. the proportion of interpersonal communicative functions); the proportion of initiative of communication; the number of communicative acts per minute and the occupation of the communicative space.

The Social Cognitive Performance (SCP) was determined in relation to the observed Vocal and Gestural Communicative Intent; Vocal and Gestural Imitation, Tool Use, Combinatory Play and Symbolic Play (adapted from Wetherby & Prutting, 1984).

The FCP progress indicators identified were:

- increase in the proportion of communication initiative,
- increase in the proportion of use of the verbal mean,
- decrease in the proportion of use of the gestural mean,
- increase in the communication interactivity,
- increase in the communication's symmetry.

The SCP progress indicators were identified by the improvement on the performance in each one of the 7 assessed domains. Each domain has different possible scores (adapted from Wetherby & Prutting, 1984):

- gestural communicative intent: from 1 to 6
- vocal communicative intent: from 1 to 6
- gestural imitation: from 1 to 4
- vocal imitation: from 1 to 4

- tool use: from 1 to 4
- combinatory play: from 1 to 6
- symbolic play: from 1 to 6

2.2 Results

A general overview of the results will be presented first, followed by the comparisons between the groups and between the different time periods. The, other results will be briefly presented.

Although the inclusion criteria for each group didn't consider the chronological age, there are no significant differences between the mean ages of the subjects of the different groups.

It could be observed that 2 of the subjects that attended only individual therapy (group C) didn't present any progress indicators in the Functional Communicative Profile (FCP), but this was the group where the largest number of progress indicators per subject was observed, although the difference between groups wasn't significant.

In what refer to the Social Cognitive Performance the smallest improvement was observed in the group that attended a period of language therapy with their mothers (group B). However, after the following period of individual language therapy these subjects' performance was similar to that of the subjects who attended language workshop and the children who attended only individual therapy presented the smaller overall progress index per subject.

The number of progress indicators for each subject of each group on the Functional Communicative Profile and on the Social - Cognitive Performance is presented in Table 1.

	N	1st to 2nd recording				2nd to 3rd recording				Mean of indexes per subject	
		Subjects with progress		Areas with progress		Subjects with progress		Areas with progress			
		FCP	SCP	FCP	SCP	FCP	SCP	FCP	SCP	FCP	SCP
Group A	10	10	6	23	14	9	8	13	22	3.6	3.6
Group B	9	8	3	15	6	9	9	16	31	3.4	3.1
Group C	17	15	12	34	21	15	12	31	28	3.8	2.8

Table 1. Total number of progress indexes on the Functional Communicative Profile (FCP) and on the social Cognitive Performance (SCP)

The analysis of the significance of the differences observed in the Functional Communicative Profile shows that the differences of the mean results are not significant for any of the variables referring to groups A and B. The differences between the means of all subjects on the first and second periods (i.e. after the second and the third recordings) weren't significant for either the number of subjects or the number of areas with progress. The only significant differences refer to group C, as can be verified in Table 2.

Considered variables	*(p) value*
1st and 2nd periods – number of subjects with progress	0.5
1st and 2nd periods – number of areas with progress	0.16
Areas with progress – groups A x B	0.36
Areas with progress – groups A x C	0.07
Areas with progress – groups B x C	0.03*
Subjects with progress – groups A x B	0.25
Subjects with progress– groups A x C	0.02*
Subjects with progress – groups B x C	0.02*

Significance level (p) ≤ 0.05

Table 2. Significance of the observed differences – Functional Communicative Profile

In what refer to the differences between the groups that were related to the Social Cognitive Performance, the data synthesized in Table 3 shows that the only significant differences observed were related to the groups A and C. It can be supposed the differences were consistent because they refer both to the number of subjects and to the number of areas with progress. This analysis also verified that the differences in the mean performances of all subjects in the first and second periods were not significant to neither of the considered pairs of variables.

Considered variables	*(p) value*
1st and 2nd periods – number of subjects with progress	0.07
1st and 2nd periods – number of areas with progress	0.13
Areas with progress – groups A x B	0.48
Areas with progress – groups A x C	0.02*
Areas with progress – groups B x C	0.31
Subjects with progress – groups A x B	0.35
Subjects with progress– groups A x C	0.06*
Subjects with progress – groups B x C	0.14

Significance level (p) ≤ 0.05

Table 3. Significance of the observed differences – Social Cognitive Performance

Other observed outcomes were:

- The situation that produced the best results in the number of communicative acts expressed per minute was the Language Workshop.
- Subjects of groups A and B presented similar performances in the use of communication means, demonstrated by an increase in the proportion of verbal mean use and a decrease in the use of gestures.
- The communication's interactivity increased in all groups after the first studied time interval (i.e., after the modified therapy situation). This increase was not observed after the second studied time interval.
- Most of the observable differences were not statistically significant. It is probably related to the great individual differences among children of the autism spectrum, what makes procedures that consider each subject as his own control the best alternative, but reduces the impact of group results.

- The group that presented more progress indicators was the language workshop - where the subjects received therapy in groups of two.
- The unexpected result was that there was no drop in the results obtained during the first six-month period on the following six-month period.
- Individual results indicate that a few subjects continued to show improvements afterwards.

2.3 Discussion

It is still premature and deceiving to suggest that one sole therapeutic approach is more effective than the others and that there is a method that is more effective with all children. The several variables that must be considered when verifying the results of therapeutic intervention with children of the autism spectrum demand a great amount of research and follow-up studies.

It was already mentioned that the intervention program were individualized, considering each child's actual development level and identifying personal profiles of abilities and inabilities. This information supported clinical decisions about the therapeutic intervention, strategies and approaches.

The subjects of this study were divided in groups according to subjective clinical criteria. The pairs were defined according to the children´s similarities (development and interests) and/or to their differences (calm/agitated, speaker/non-speaker) and responding to each one's objective demands referring to week-day and hour of appointment. The inclusion criterion of similar social cognitive performance was the only objective information used to determine the intervention groups. Probably an ideal research situation would consider exclusively objective criteria to determine the inclusion of each child in different intervention groups. But that is still not enough information about what are the most useful factors to predict intervention outcomes and therefore, no objective criteria that is ethically supported to determine inclusion criteria.

Data referring to the number of communicative acts per minute show that subjects that were attending language workshops presented greater development. Apparently peer communication situations provided a communication symmetry that is not obtained in situations with adults. This symmetry, by its turn, generates affective performance demands in which subjects must use their communicative abilities to obtain better results from each interaction and more effective communication exchanges.

The subjects of the three groups presented very similar averages regarding the number of communicative acts expressed per minute in the third recording. This data demands reasoning about individual development rhythm. If the progress and stabilization periods are carefully monitored, short term changes on the intervention process may be introduced aiming to generate new demands and therefore different opportunities for development.

The results presented by subjects of group A (i.e. those attending language workshops) indicate progresses in the period of therapy, reinforcing this model as a productive alternative of language therapy with autistic children. It could be observed that, during the period of language workshop, all subjects presented progress in the Functional Communicative Profile (FCP) while the same result in the Social Cognitive Performance (SCP) was observed just in 60% of the subjects. On the following period, the number of subjects with progress in SCP was very similar to those with progress in FCP and the number of areas with progress in the SCP was much larger than in the FCP. It seems to be a clear indication of the impact of symmetric interactive situations on the communicative and social-cognitive performance of children of the autism spectrum.

Subjects of group B (i.e. the ones whose mothers also participated in the therapy for six months) were the ones with higher indexes of progress on the Functional Communicative Profile (number of communicative acts expressed per minute and the proportion of verbal communicative mean use) and on the Social Cognitive Performance after the second six-month period. Two aspects must be considered: in this group was the one with the youngest children and it is expected that earlier intervention produces better results. On the other hand, it was hypothesized that the inclusion of the mothers in the intervention process would amplify the results of language therapy to other contexts and produce better long term results; and these results seem to confirm that hypothesis. It is possible to suggest the alternative hypothesis that, although the situations with the mothers are not the ones that offer the better opportunities to use communicative abilities, this situation apparently offers a safer environment for their practice.

On the other hand, however, just one third of the children receiving language therapy with their mothers presented progress in this first period of intervention and they were the ones with less areas of progress during this period. But interestingly, in the following period all this children presented progress in both areas, especially in the SCP. If we consider only the situations where the identification of some changes in behavior could be determined, subjects of group B were the ones who presented higher indexes of development in the areas of gesture and vocal communication intent and tool use in the second period.

One rationale that can be considered is that mothers tend to present a less challenging environment for their children but the intervention period allowed the better use of posterior situations. The use of communication opportunities that occur in daily situations evidently increases the impact of speech/language intervention in the development of each individual. Although more research results are necessary to determine exactly when and how to include mothers in language intervention programs it seems to be a useful alternative to be carefully considered, since in this study the therapy situation involving mothers was the one that produced the better results.

As mentioned before, in general, great individual differences among subjects with autistic spectrum disorders produce results where the group means values do not vary significantly. This does not disqualify the importance of the obtained results, since they confirm the need to identify individual ability and inability profiles in order to determine the most productive intervention procedures. The lack of significant differences between the results presented by subjects from the three groups keeps, on the other hand, individual therapy as a possible alternative for language therapy.

2.4 Conclusion

The main purpose of the present study was to verify the existence of observable differences in the functional communicative profile and in the social cognitive performance of autistic children and adolescents receiving language therapy in three different situations. The conclusions may be synthesized as follows:

- Variations were observed after a pre-determined experimental intervention period.
- Maintenance of the results were also observed after an equal period of regular speech-language therapy

- The obtained results indicate that temporary changes can be made in the therapeutic scheme for autistic children, as an alternative for obtaining better results.
- This type of intervention, however, requires specific control of the results after short periods of intervention.
- Results also reinforce the requirement for the adaptation of procedures to obtain individual profiles of abilities and inabilities as the basis to determine any intervention model.
- The inclusion of mothers in the therapeutic process during a set period of time is a proposal that requires other studies.
- These studies should aim at the search for parameters that indicate when to begin this type of intervention, its duration and the procedures for a long time support.
- Long term therapeutic processes, as is the case with autistic children, also demand consideration about the long term results obtained from short term interferences.
- The question about the possible identification of the best therapeutic approach to these children has yet to be further discussed.
- The effectiveness of different therapeutic approaches suggests that any comparison must take into account data about social and familiar contexts.

3. Results of systematized support-instructional groups with mothers

In order to study alternative ways to amplify the results of the language therapy intervention and considering that the language therapy process can benefit from specific orientations about language and communication processes focused on individual profiles of abilities and inabilities of each communicative dyad, another study was conducted focusing on specific orientations to mothers.

The actions directed towards families of autistic children, conducted by speech and language pathologists, require extreme caution so they keep the focus on the area that belongs to speech and language pathology and do not involve other areas that also deal with autistic manifestations.

In what refer specifically to studies about families with children with autistic spectrum disorders, a recent study reviewed the articles published over the past five years in the three most traditional journals specifically addressed to studies about infantile autism. The study revealed interesting data: less than 5% of the 1096 papers published refer to this theme, which certainly was not expected when we consider the impact of autistic children in family dynamics or the importance of family for diagnosis, intervention and education processes. On the other hand, more than half of these articles were published in the last 18 months.

The speech and language therapeutic process can be improved by specific orientations about the development of communication and language processes strongly focused on the individual profiles of abilities and inabilities of each mother-child dyad. But there are no reports of experiments conducted in this area. Thus, we proposed an initial study involving a systematic orientation to mothers of children of the autistic spectrum who attended weekly at the service and the verification of the results by the observation of the patients' development the quality of life reported by the mothers. It was hypothesized that systematic and specific orientations, held for short periods of time and with the possibility of return, may not only contribute to the communicative environment of the autistic child but also the understanding of the capabilities and difficulties of each child by their families.

Therefore, the purposes of this study were to investigate the interference of orientations offered to mothers in the process of communication and language development of autistic children and in their communicative and social-cognitive performance. Besides, it aimed to verify the interference of these orientations on the way these mothers observe their child, according to an adaptation of the Questionnaire of the World Health Organization Quality of Life (Barbosa & Fernandes, 2009).

3.1 Method

Subjects were 26 mother-child dyads who met the inclusion criteria and completed the entire study period. The inclusion criteria were:

- diagnosis included in the autistic spectrum,
- mother being the main responsible for bringing the child to speech and language therapy,
- child systematically attending weekly a specialized speech and language therapy service for at least six months with no interruptions larger than one week,
- age under 11 years (so that none of the subjects was characterized as a teenager at the end of study) and
- consent form signed by the responsible adult.

The mother groups were organized according to the children's therapy schedule. The average age of mothers at the onset of the study was 38:1y and the children's average age was 8:2y. In what refer to educational level, the majority of mothers (53%) had completed high school and six of them (23%) had higher education.

The children were filmed in regular speech and language therapy, playing with various types of toys with their therapist. These recordings were used to collect data on the Functional Communicative Profile and on the Social-Cognitive Performance of each child. Mothers were interviewed individually by specialized speech-language therapists that are familiar to them but not their son's or daughter's therapists. During the interview they were asked to sign the consent form and answer the protocols on quality of life.

To avoid the need for mothers to attend to the interviews at other times at the Speech and Language Pathology Service (and therefore avoiding the interference of economic and transport issues), the orientations were offered in 30 minute periods during their children's therapy. The completion of counseling sessions in pairs or triads provides more symmetrical communication situations since there is a common theme and a shared position. Thus, mothers were grouped according to the time of their children's therapy, regardless of their children's performance.

Each group was conducted by two speech and language therapists who were postgraduate in this specific area. There were five consecutive sessions of orientation, with each group of mothers. They were shown videos of their children interacting with the therapists, already known to them. The mothers who agreed or wished could also be videotaped with their children so that this material was discussed in this small group.

The goals of these orientation sessions were:

- Session 1. Presentation of the proposal, identification of "strengths" and "weaknesses" of each child; suggestion that each mother identify pleasant and unpleasant situations in every-day activities.
- Session 2. Identification of situations of productive and unproductive interaction between children and therapists; suggestion to compare them to everyday situations; resolution of doubts.

- Session 3. Identification of key elements in successful and productive situations and suggestions of possible expansion, multiplication or transfer; resolution of doubts.
- Session 4. Identification of key elements in the communication breakdowns and proposals for alternative procedures; resolution of doubts.
- Session 5. Individual reports on the impact of the orientations; solving questions.

After these initial five consecutive sessions, five other follow-up sessions were scheduled with a three-week interval. These sessions dealt about the same subjects of the initial sessions, according to the needs of each small group. After the last follow-up session, individual interviews were conducted with each mother, to resolve remaining questions. Two weeks after the last follow-up session the children were videotaped again with their therapists and various types of toys. These recordings were used to collect data on the functional communicative profile and social-cognitive performance of each child. The results of each session were recorded by the coaches of the groups after each session in the specific protocols and served as a basis for qualitative analysis of this process.

The individual differences between autistic children justify the use of a methodology in which the child is his or her own control. Thus, the statistical analysis makes point by point comparisons, referring to the two moments to data gathering regarding the children's performance with respect to (adapted from Wetherby & Prutting, 1984):

- number of communicative acts per minute,
- use of communicative space,
- communication interactivity,
- use of communicate means,
- gestural communicative intent,
- vocal communicative intent,
- gestural imitation,
- vocal imitation,
- tool use,
- combinatory play and
- symbolic play.

The analysis of data concerning the quality of life used the Tukey test to determine the statistical significance of differences between the responses for the different areas analyzed.

3.2 Results

The proposition of ten sessions with 26 mothers of autistic children, or 260 meetings, required extreme care while recording data. The recorded data of these sessions included the identification of the subject and the intervention, or the moment established by the group to the theme. There was great variation in the manner of each group's functioning, some participants seemed to exert a degree of leadership and proposed themes for discussion. On the other hand, other mothers seemed to comfortably accommodate in less active positions in the groups, although these were always small (two to four participants). The topics most frequently discussed were:

- difficulties with the child's behavior and the difficulties caused by them,
- questions about other professionals,
- reports of new achievements,
- school adjustment and doubts about it,
- reports on changes in medical management and their results,

- reports and questions on independence in relation to activities of daily living,
- observations about the process of speech therapy and
- questions involving aspects of sexuality.

About the intervention of the coordinator on each group and the dynamics established by the group, the reports revealed that the dynamics were the most common interaction on the same theme, often due to the fact that one of the group members have brought common themes. When participants brought individual questions, the coach sometimes answered directly, sometimes rephrased the question to include all (or most) of the group. In a few situations the participants said that the doubt brought by one of the members was common to the others, without the intervention of the therapist. Not all meetings ended with a conclusion and some participants showed frustration about it. Aiming to accept what appeared to be a need for closure, an interview was conducted individually extra, unplanned, to provide a moment of completion. Figure 1 summarizes the results of the number of areas with progress in the Functional Communicative Profile identified in each of the subjects in this study. It is possible to observe that among the five possible areas 65% of subjects (17) had between two and four areas with progress. Just one of the children didn't present any progress index. A separate analysis has shown that 96% of subjects presented progress in increasing the interpersonal communication.

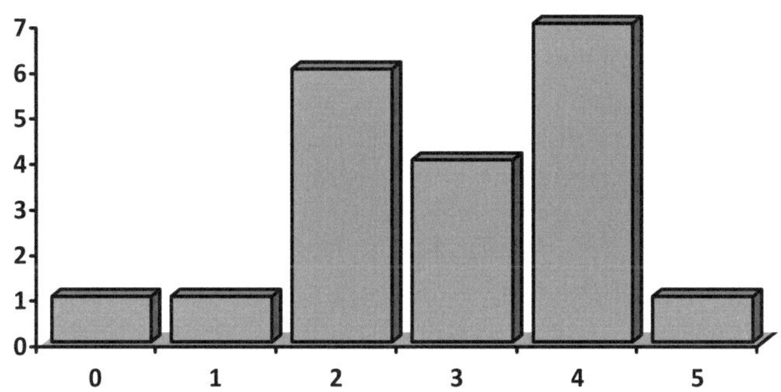

Fig. 1. Number of subjects and number of areas of progress in the Functional Communication Profile

Figure 2 presents data on the number of areas of progress when we analyzed Socio-Cognitive Performance. It is observed that among the seven areas surveyed, 61% of the participants showed progress in two to four areas. Also in this assessment one of the subjects showed no progress on any of the areas studied. However, the fact that this occurred on two different subjects, support the conclusion that 100% of them showed some progress in the areas studied. The statistical analysis of the answers to the Quality of Life Questionnaire showed statistically significant differences between subjects (mothers). This allows the assumption that the device is efficient to the characterization of each subject, which favors more individualized approaches. On the other hand, no significant differences were found between the four domains investigated by the Quality of Life questionnaire (physical, psychological, social relationships and environment). Interestingly, the highest levels of dissatisfaction are related to the environment.

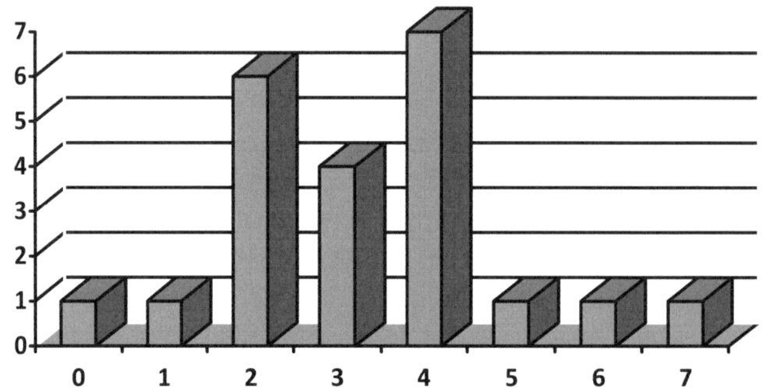

Fig. 2. Number of subjects and number of areas of progress in the Social Cognitive Performance

3.3 Discussion

The results concerning the qualitative analysis of the orientation sessions have important elements of consideration, and they also confirm of other previously reported results. The fact that it was possible to observe that some mothers find it easier to identify weaknesses and unpleasant than the reverse, reflects the need to focus on backward motion brought by the families spontaneously; that is, when the family only describes the problems, bring on about the skills; and when the family only describes the successes, remember about needs and difficulties.

The fact that most of the reported weaknesses refer to issues of communication and behavior and the unpleasant situations refer to times when children have behavioral disorders may be associated with issues such as noisy, unknown or confuse environments and stressful activities of daily living reinforces the suggestion of flexible, relaxed but predicable therapeutic settings. Since disruptive behaviors are frequently described as a source of stress for parents it is useful to help them determining this kind of environment around the child at home and other meaningful locations.

The importance of group situations to orientation activities for parents of autistic children also have been mentioned and confirmed by this study. Thus, it was interesting to note the mention of shared attention as one of the strengths observed in these patients by their mothers, because this is usually described as an element of difficulty for them. It may be useful, therefore, to try to identify the specific elements that facilitate the joint attention opportunities and replicate them in other scenarios.

Focus on the communication of the children allowed the identification of elements that may improve successful interaction during daily activities, such as:

- obtaining the child's attention,
- initiative of communication or any joint activity,
- latency for the response,
- use of materials and toys for the child's interest and
- identification of sources of communication breaks.

The ability to generate small changes in family routine that foster communication, responds to long-term goals for this type of intervention because it tends to generate more comprehensive, lasting and multiplied results. Regarding the results presented by patients in the analysis of

Functional Communicative Profile and on the Social Cognitive Performance, the data from this study can be compared what was obtained in other studies after longer periods of time (Cardoso & Fernandes, 2004; Fernandes 2000a; 2005; Fernandes & Ribeiro, 2002).
The results for the Quality of Life questionnaire can be compared to a recent survey of the same population, held the same service, but with other participants (Barbosa & Fernandes, 2009), that reported that the greatest difficulties reported by caregivers of autistic children also refer to environmental issues.

3.4 Conclusion

The first objective of this research was to study the interference of orientations offered to their mothers, on the processes of communication and language development of autistic children, in their communicative and social-cognitive performance was reached, although it requires the exercise of caution in generalizing the results.
It can be argued that all study participants showed progress on at least one of the assessment rates proposed in a general smaller period of time than in previous studies involving the same therapeutic procedures and the same evaluation criteria.
It is, however, a small difference, with a small set of data, which does not allow the complete determination of its causality. Unfortunately, practical difficulties make it hard to establish the procedures for more rigorous research, as would be required for this type of conclusion. Small studies, as presented here, are nevertheless useful because these data could be added to others, performed in other centers or with other groups, in order to provide clearer evidence of interference between the processes of therapy language and family orientation.
The second goal of the research, to determine the interference of orientation about the processes of communication and language of autistic children in the way mothers observe their child, according to criteria adapted from the Questionnaire of the World Health Organization Quality of Life was not fully reached. The answers provided by the mothers did not allow analysis related to the group. Apparently there was an unanticipated interference, possibly due to the fact that these questionnaires are being applied in the same department in which children receive the language therapy. That established a kind of "ceiling effect" in responses. The questionnaires reflect satisfied mothers, without big problems with their children (here the question of the difficulties of transport appears as an exception because there are systematic references to it). It is supposed that if the questionnaires were applied outside the environment of care, or at least by unidentified people with him could be obtained more realistic results. Anyway, even if it was not possible to determine the degree of infiltration of the advice given from the results of questionnaires on quality of life, this positive interference was evident in the qualitative analysis of intervention processes.
Thus, the hypothesis that "systematic and specific orientations, held for short periods of time and with the possibility of return may not only contribute to the communicative environment of the autistic child but also for the family to understand the capabilities and difficulties of each child " remains open. The need for major adjustments in research procedures that can measure more effectively the degree of interference should not obscure the fact that there was an undeniably positive impact of a systematic procedure of orientation, taken with the process of language therapy for children (and not replacing it), focused on issues of communication and language and that, although they have a script and running registration, permit adjustments to the needs and demands of each group.

4. Other intervening factors in language therapy with autistic children

Systematic reports about therapy processes may be another way to contribute to a body of evidence that can support informed decisions about intervention proposals with ASD children.

This was the aim of this study: to describe three years of individual speech and language therapy with 3 children with ASD, with different developmental characteristics, different environmental situations and different responses to the therapeutic process. The children received speech and language therapy once a week, for 45 minutes, in a specialized service and the parents signed the approved consent form allowing the descriptions of their clinical development. The speech and language therapy started approximately 6 months prior to the first reports presented here.

4.1 Case reports

Case 1 is a girl with diagnosis of autism, 6 years of age at the onset of the speech and language therapy, attending regular public preschool. She is brought to the therapy by her mother but her absence index is about 50%. The main features of development during the 3 years of intervention can be described as:

Behaviour, socialization and interests:

- 2007: manipulates magazines and books; brings sheets of paper to the therapy but just leafs through them. Very agitated, stays for just few minutes in each place of the room or with any toy. During the second semester she starts to show some interest in miniature household items. The teacher reports some aggression episodes.
- 2008: maintains the interest in paper items but starts to play with miniatures, performing seriating task and differed imitation; during the second semester starts to play with puzzles and is less agitated but with reduced attention span. Sometimes, in the beginning of the year, refuses to leave the room by the end of the session, throwing herself on the floor, but by the second semester is more adapted to the routine and social markers (kisses when saying goodbye). She engages in interactive exchanges during the year, accepting and demanding physical contact.
- 2009: makes systematic eye contact, maintains the short attention span and little interest in any activity. Plays with puzzles and performs symbolic games with themes related to every-day life activities. During these activities engages in joint attention activities with the therapist's initiative.

Language and communication:

- 2007: uses mainly the gestural means of communication in regulation and interaction activities. Exchanges communicative turns but her utterances characterize as vocalizations due to the large articulation distortions that hinder the speech intelligibility.
- 2008: continues to use mainly the gestural communicative mean but starts to use vocal and verbal means more frequently. Despite the articulation problems the vocabulary limitations become evident. Starts to show more communication intent.
- 2009: some articulation problems continue to exist and the preference order of the use of communicative means is gestural and vocal. There was a clear increase in the proportion of communication addressed toward the other and in joint play.

Figure 3 shows the evolution of the functional communicative aspects of occupation of the communicative space, communicative acts produced per minute and proportion of interpersonal communication observed in the three years of language therapy with the child of Case 1.

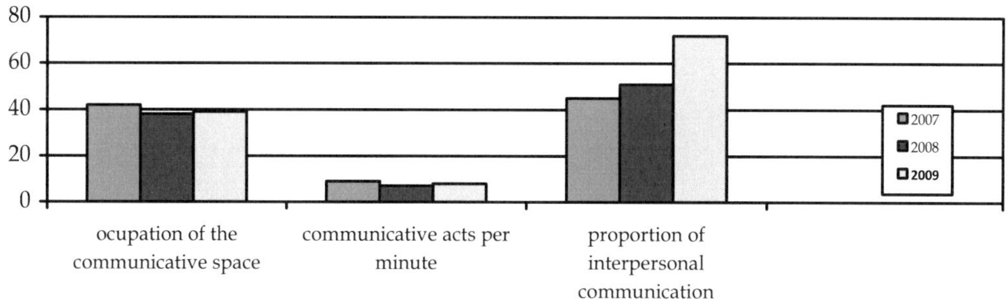

Fig. 3. Functional communicative aspects (case 1)

Case 2 is a boy with diagnostic of autism, 8 years of age at the onset of speech and language therapy, well adapted to the second year of a regular public school. He is brought to the therapy by his mother and has less than 5% of absences. His reported main features of development in the 3 years of intervention are:

Behaviour, socialization and interests:

- 2007: a talkative child that initiates communicative turns with unknown adults but do not holds a dialogue with several conversational turns. Performs complex symbolic plays and keeps the same activity for long periods of time in self-centered games, rarely engaging in joint attention activities. Manifestations that aren't adequate to the context, like singing and dancing in inappropriate situations, are eventually observed.
- 2008: maintains a good contact with the therapist and accepts the participation of others in several situations, is less self-centered and stays in the same activity for smaller periods of time but do not proposes other alternatives. When he is very involved with an activity, doesn't allow the therapist's participation. These situations frequently involve complex and detailed symbolic play.
- 2009: continues attentive and focused but starts to ask for the therapist's help when meets any difficulties and verbally communicates his intentions and desires. His favorite activities now include dolls and he engages in cooperative activities with the therapist, participating in long dialogues with the intermediation of dolls.

Language and communication:

- 2007: presents frequent delayed echolalia in situations of self-centered play. The preferred communicative mean is the verbal, which he uses in socially appropriate ways in superficial contacts, generally politeness and recognition of others markers, which are basically the sole spontaneous communication initiatives. Although he usually responds to the therapist's initiations, he generally does it with one-word phrases.
- 2008: seems to present better understanding of gestures and facial expressions but still makes very little eye contact. Continues to present some delayed echolalia that seems to

be related to communicative initiation, as requests for social routines. Presents more communicative initiatives related to his interests with short phrases or isolated words.
- 2009 – continues to present some delayed echolalia in moments of less interaction but initiates communicative turns, identifies and corrects communication failures, identify breaks and uses strategies to maintain the communication partner's attention. He uses some gestures, mainly as support to communicative acts with protest expression function.

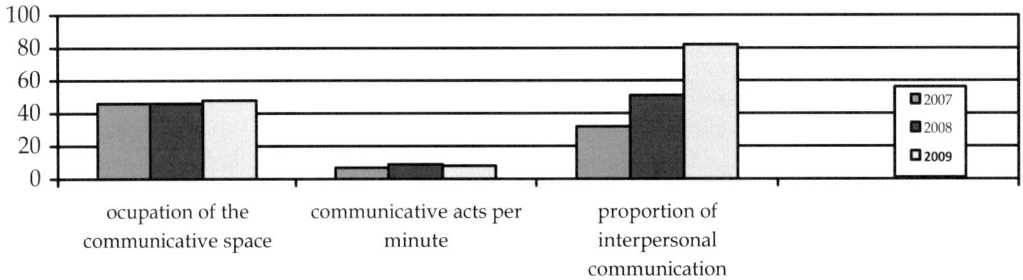

Fig. 4. Functional communicative aspects (case 2)

It is possible to observe the similarities between Figures 3 and 4, although the described children are very different form each-other.

Case 3 is a boy with diagnosis of autism, 4 years of age at the onset of the speech and language therapy, attending regular public preschool with reports of good performance and a special interest in reading. He is brought to the therapy by her mother and almost never fails to be present.

Behavior, socialization and interests:

- 2007: recognizes the therapist, maintains eye contact and uses it as a strategy to get the communication partner's attention. He always refuses changes in routine or activities. Sometimes presents tantrum crises, throwing himself on the floor at the end of the therapeutic session, refusing to go home and crying very much. Engages in symbolic play and joint games. Performs logographic reading and is interested in reading but doesn't say the names of colors, although recognizes them.
- 2008: maintains eye contact and shows better adaptation to the routine and duration of the therapy do not presenting disruptive behaviors at the end of the sessions. Engages in complex symbolic games but do not proposes new situations during the game. Reads some words.
- 2009: asks for physical contact and exchanges communicative turns, but his eye contact is less systematic and there is little attention to the therapist's facial expression. Develops some routines as to step over the red parts of the floor. Shows a great interest in the computer but accepts proposals of other activities.

Language and communication:

- 2007: communicates mainly using verbal and vocal means with the support of gestures. Has some articulation imprecision but agrees in repeating or rephrasing his utterances when is asked to do so. He doesn't present evidences of difficulties in understanding language.

- 2008: presents longer phrases and repairs communicative failures when the therapist requests but do not recognizes the failures without this support. His utterances are better articulated what contributes to the increase in the proportion of the use of the verbal communicative mean.
- 2009: shows communicative intention, produces phrases with adequate syntax and understands simple and complex orders. Initiate turns, introduces topics and engages in dialogues when interested. Uses gestures as support in a more consistent form, what contributes to the increase in the use of this mean. But he doesn't make coherent narratives.

Figure 5 Figure 3 shows the evolution of the functional communicative aspects of occupation of the communicative space, communicative acts produced per minute and proportion of interpersonal communication observed in the three years of language therapy with the child of Case 3.

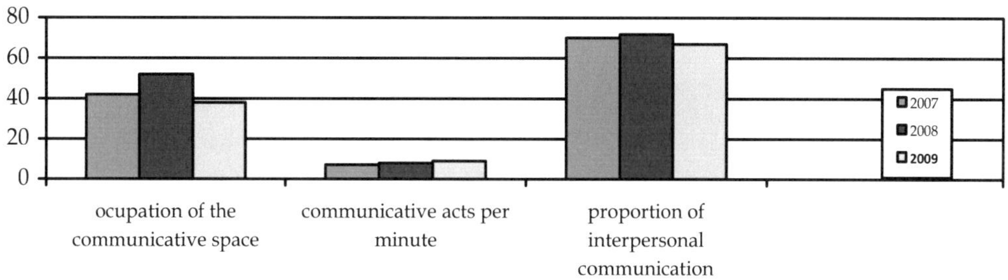

Fig. 5. Functional communicative aspects (case 3)

Table 4 shows the results observed in the different areas of the Social-Cognitive Performance of the three children during the three years. It should be remembered that to the areas of gestural and vocal communicative intent and of combinatory and symbolic play, the scores vary from 1 to 6 while in the areas of gestural and vocal imitation and tool use it varies from 1 to 4.

Tested areas	2007			2008			2009		
	C1	C2	C3	C1	C2	C3	C1	C2	C3
Gestural communicative intent	4	6	3	6	6	6	6	6	6
Vocal communicative intent	4	6	3	5	6	6	5	6	6
Tool use	3	3	3	4	4	3	4	4	4
Gestural imitation	3	4	3	4	4	4	4	4	4
Vocal imitation	4	3	-	3	4	2	3	4	4
Combinatory play	6	5	-	5	5	3	5	6	5
Symbolic Play	6	6	-	6	6	6	6	6	-

Table 4. Social-cognitive performance tested in 2007, 2008 and 2009 in the 3 children

4.2 Discussion

The 3 children received individual language therapy once a week during the whole period of this study. In each year there are 2 vacation periods with duration of 2 weeks in July and 3 weeks by the end of December and beginning of January.

The cases presented highlight the diversity of the phenotype of autism since we have a six-year old girl with important behavior problems, very few intelligible utterances and a very restrict range of non-functional interests. The first boy described has eight years of age, good performance in a regular school to which he is well adapted but with empathy impairments, few communicative initiatives, out of context behaviors and echolalia. The second boy presented is four-year old, presents cognitive performance above the expected for his age, has interests that are not age-appropriate and good abilities with the formal aspects of language.

Although this was not the aim of this study, the reference to the three different diagnosis included in the autism spectrum is clear (i.e., low functioning autism, high functioning autism and Asperger syndrome). This way, the intervention processes were subjected to subtle changes adjusting them to the needs and possibilities of each child along the 3 year period.

It is interesting to note that all children had important progresses in their performances. The girl started to engage in joint attention and symbolic play activities and increased the proportion of interpersonal communication. The first boy started to engage in joint play, dialogues and interpersonal exchanges; initiates communicative turns, makes adequately use of the discursive resources and uses non-verbal communication as support. The second boy is interested in computers but agrees to alternate its use with more interactive initiatives; consistently uses support of gestures, has adequate syntactic and discursive abilities although he doesn't present productive narratives.

These results demand the consideration of the intervening factors of each process. As observed before the girl was absent from almost half of the planned therapeutic sessions and even so her progress was significant. It poses the question of what would have happened if she had attended to all sessions and of what may be the managing alternatives to cases like this. It is common that the absences to the therapeutic sessions are justified by objective and real factors, especially in complex environments such as big cities. However, the consideration of the resources allocated in the frequency, even when not systematic, and by the reservation of therapeutic time for a not frequent patient demand objective data to support any decision. The observed in this case is that, even with a large proportion of absences, the therapeutic process was productive to the child.

The first boy presents a virtually opposed situation. The family and school are collaborative and interested and the possibility of offering therapy just once a week demands efforts to allow the increase of this offer. Probably due to the kind of disorder presented this child was brought to a specialized service with more than six years of age, when there are consistent reports of better results with children that receive earlier adequate intervention. On way to compensate this delay would be a more intensive intervention program, what has not been accessible to all children in our reality.

The second boy, on the other hand, raises the interest of family members as well as school personal due to his interest in reading and in the formal aspects of language that creates the impression of an above-average functioning. It has lead to the increase in the availability of activities and materials that reinforce the interests and the maintenance of systematization activities, decreasing the ones that include empathy. This reinforces the need for more investments in actions directed towards family and school orientation.

4.3 Comments

The longitudinal individual analysis of the therapeutic intervention processes brings the focus to associated aspects that may be determinant of the results and that demand a consistent approach.

The analysis of individual experiences in such a way that they can be significant to an evidence-based practice depends on the systematic record of these therapeutic processes.

In what refer to the autism spectrum, considering the incidence now determined, it is essential that individual and small-group experiences are systematized in a way to provide alternatives to a much larger group of children that probably present the same needs but that haven't been diagnosed or didn't reach specialized services.

5. Conclusion

Recent studies point out that the occurrence of Autism Spectrum Disorders (ASD) is up to 1%. Such a high incidence places the demand if the urgent identification of efficient intervention models and of factors that may have a positive impact in these processes.

Understanding that there is not one single therapeutic proposal that will be equally successful with all autistic children doesn't mean that all the efforts to improve efficiency and economic available alternatives should not be undertaken.

The studies presented indicate that there are some points that can be considered applicable at least to a significant proportion of the autistic children and their families:

- Focus on the individual profile.
- The communication interactivity must always receive careful attention.
- Symmetric communicative situation allow useful challenging experiences.
- The attention to all communicative means will contribute to more effective and personal exchanges.
- The therapeutic setting must be flexible and offer opportunities to problem solving while also being organized enough to avoid producing stress and anxiety.
- Naturalistic communicative situations favor the practice of discursive abilities.
- The inclusion of families allows the multiplication of opportunities for exercising newly acquired abilities and identifying important focus of interest.

Issues about educational management, early access to specialized intervention and adequate follow-up, must be included as some of the aspects considered in the overall process of treating children and adolescents of the autism spectrum.

Decisions about whether the individual with autism should attend to a normal or a specialized school must also take into account the individual characteristics and needs. Both alternatives should be considered according to the individual's present performance and reassessed periodically to obtain the best possible results.

Although it is now clear that early intervention generally results in better results, recent studies have shown that even individuals that only started to get some specialized treatment during adolescence also show progress after relatively short periods of time (six month periods). It clearly indicates that these individuals should not be excluded from intervention programs.

Language therapy with autistic individuals are generally long term processes that must be periodically and systematically re-evaluated in order to guarantee constant attention to the evolution patterns of each individual and therefore the best management of specific needs and opportunities.
In any case, language therapy with children of the autism spectrum is an activity that presents daily challenges, demands constant adjustments and offers constant development opportunities for everyone involved.

6. References

Baltaxe, C.A.M. & D'Angiola, N. 1996. Referencing skills in children with autism and specific language impairment. *Euro J Disord Communic,* Vol. 31, No.2, (June, 1996), pp. 245-258. ISSN 0963-7273

Barbosa, M.R.P. & Fernandes, F.D.M. 2009. Quality of life of autistic children's caretakers. *Rev Soc Bras Fonoaudiol,* Vol.14, No.4, (December, 2009), pp. 482-486, ISSN 1516-8034

Bates, E. 1976. *Language and Context : The Acquisition of pragmatics (language, though and culture).* New York: Academic Press, ISBN 0120815508, New York, USA

Bates, E. 1979. On The Evolution and development of symbols. In: *The Emergence of Symbols: cognition and communication in infancy.*Bates E, Benigni D, Bretherton C, Camaioni L, Volterra V, editores. pp. 1-32, New York: Academic Press, ISBN 0120815400, New York, USA

Bernard-Opitz,V.,Ing, S. & Kong, T.Y. 2004. Comparison of behavioural and natural play interventions for young children with autism. *Autism,*Vol.8, No.3, (September, 2004), pp.319-332, ISSN 1362-3613

Bruckner, C.T. & Yoder, P. 2007. Restricted object use in young children with autism. *Autism*, Vol.11, No.2, (April, 2007), pp.161-171, ISSN 1362-3613

Cardoso, C. & Fernandes, F.D.M. 2006. Relation between social cognitive aspects and functional communicative profile in a group of adolescents of the autistic spectrum. *Pró-Fono Rev Atual Cient*, Vol.18, No.1, (April, 2006), pp.89-98, ISSN 0104-5687

Cardoso, C. & Fernandes, F.D.M. 2004. The communication of autistic dpectrum children in group activities. *Pró-Fono Rev Atual Cient*, Vol.16, No.1, (April, 2004), p.67-74, ISSN 0104-5687

DiLala, D.L. & Rogers, S.J. 1994. Domains of the Childhood Autism Rating Scale: Relevance for diagnosis and treatment. *J Autism Develop Disord* , Vol.24, No.1, (March, 1994), pp.2-13, ISSN 0162-3257

Dominguez, A., Ziviani, J. & Rodger, S. 2006. Play behaviours and play object preferences of young children with autistic disorder in a clinical play environment. *Autism,* Vol. 10, No.1,(March, 2006), pp. 53-69, ISSN 1362-3613

Eigsti, I.M., Bennetto, L. & Dadlani, M.B. 2007. Beyond Pragmatics: Morphosyntactic Development in autism. *J Autism Develop Disord,* Vol.37, No.3,(September, 2007), pp.1007-1023. ISSN 0162-3257

Fernandes, F.D.M. 2000a. Objective data about speech and language procedures on an infantile psychiatric day-care center - communicative profile as a performance indicator. *Pró-Fono Rev Atual Cient, Vol.*12, No.1, (March, 2000), pp.1-9, ISSN 0104-5687

Fernandes, F.D.M. 2000b. Objective data about speech and language procedures on an infantile psychiatric day-care center - socio-cognitive performance. *Pró-Fono Rev Atual Cient,* Vol.12, No.1, (March, 2000), pp.10-16, ISSN 0104-5687

Fernandes, F.D.M. & Ribeiro, S.L. 2002. Relations between functional aspects of communication, lexical development and social-cognitive performance of children with pervasive developmental disorder. *Rev Soc Bras Fonoaudiol,* Vol.7, No.2, (June, 2002), PP.60-65, ISSN 1516-8034

Fernandes, F.D.M. 2005.Language therapy results with adolescents of the autistic spectrum. *Pró-Fono Rev Atual Cient,* Vol.17, No.1, (March,2005), pp.67-76, ISSN 0104-5687

Fernandes, F.D.M. 2009. Families with autistic children: international literature. *Rev Soc Bras Fonoaudiol,* Vol.14, No.3, (September, 2009),pp. 427-432, ISSN 1516-8034

Giddan, J.J., Wahl, J. & Brogan, M. 1995. Importance of communication training for psychiatric and residents and mental health trainees. *Child Psychiat Human Develop,* Vol.26, No.1, (March, 1995), pp.128-135, ISSN 0009-398X

Gothem, K., Risi, S., Pickles, A. & Lord, C. 2007. The autism diagnostic observation schedule: revised algorithms for improved diagnostic validity. *J Autism Dev Disord,* Vol.37, No.4, (December, 2007), pp. 613-627, ISSN 0162-3257

Grela, B.G. & Mclaughlin, K.S. 2006. Focused stimulation for a child with autism spectrum disorder: a treatment study. *J Autism Dev Disord,* Vol.36, No.2, (June, 2006), pp.753-756, ISSN 0162-3257

Grindle, C.F., Kovshoff, H., Hastings, R.P. & Remington, B. 2009. Parents' Experiences of Home-Based Applied Behavior Analysis Programs for Young Children with Autism. *J Autism Dev Disord,* Vol.39, No.1, (March, 2009), pp. 42–56, ISSN 0162-3257

Halliday, M.A.K. 1978. *Language as Social Semiotic - the social interpretation of language and meaning,* University Park Press, ISBN 0839111835, Maryland, USA

Ingersoll, B. & Schreibman, L. 2006. Teaching reciprocal imitation skills to young children with autism using a naturalistic behavioral approach: effects on language, pretend play and joint attention. *J Autism Dev Disord,* Vol.36, No.4, (December, 2006), pp.487- 505, ISSN 0162-3257

Keen, D., Rodger, S., Doussin, K. & Waite, M.B. 2007. A pilot study of the effects of a social-pragmatic intervention on the communication and symbolic play of children with autism. *Autism,* Vol.11, No.1, (March, 2007), pp.63-71, ISSN 1362-3613

Koegel, L.K. 2000. Interventions to facilitate communication in autism. *J Autism Develop Disord,* Vol.30, No.5, (October, 2000), pp.383-291, ISSN 0162-3257

Kuschner, E.S., Bennetto, L. & Yost, K. 2007. Patterns of nonverbal cognitive functioning in young children with autism spectrum disorders. *J. Autism Develop Disord,* Vol.37, No.3, (July, 2007), pp.795-807, ISSN 0162-3257

Laugeson, E.A., Frankel. F., Mogil, C. & Dillon, A. R. 2009. Parent-Assisted Social Skills Training to Improve Friendships in Teens with Autism Spectrum

Disorders. *J Autism Dev Disord,* Vol.39, No.4, (August, 2009), pp.596–606, ISSN 0162-3257

Mandell, D. S. & Salzer, M. S. 2007. Who joins support groups among parents of children with autism. *Autism,* Vol.11, No.2, (June, 2007) pp.111-122, ISSN 1362-3613

Mesibov, G., Fuentes, J., Prior M. & Wing, L. 2007. The past decade. *Autism,* Vol.10, No.1, (March, 2007), pp.7-10, ISSN 1362-3613

Mesibov, G, Shea, V. 2011. The TEACCH Program in the Era of Evidence-Based Practice. *J Autism Dev Disord,* Vol.40, No.5, (May,2010), pp. 570-579, ISSN 0162-3257

Miilher, L.P. & Fernandes, F.D.M. 2006. Communicative functions expressed by language therapists with children of the autism spectrum. *Pró-Fono Rev Atual Cient,* Vol.18, No.3, (September 2006), pp.239-248, ISSN 0104-5687

Mundy, P. & Stella, J. 2001. Joint attention, social orienting, and nonverbal communication in autism. In: *Autism Spectrum Disorders – A Transactional Developmental Perspective,* A.Wetherby, B.Prizant, (Eds.), 55-77, Paul Brooks, ISBN – 1-5576-6445-5, Baltimore, USA

Partington, J.W. & Sundberg, M.L. 1998. *The Assessment of Basic Language and Learning Skills (ABLLS),* Pleasant Hill: Behavior Analysts, ASIN B0006RMKGY, Massachussets, USA

Perkins, M.R., Dobbinson, S., Boucher, J., Bol, S. & Bloom, P. 2006. Lexical knowledge and lexical use in autism. *J Autism Dev Disord,* Vol.36, No.6, (December, 2006), pp.795-805, ISSN 0162-3257

Prizant, B. 1996. Brief report: communication, language, social and emotional development. *J Autism Develop Disord,* Vol.6, No.2, (June, 1996), pp.173-179, ISSN 0162-3257

Prizant,B.&Rubin,E.1999.Contemporary issues in interventions for autism spectrum disorders: A commentary. *J Associat Persons Sev Hadic,* Vol.24, No.3 (September, 1999), pp.199-208, ISSN0274-9483

Reed, P., Osborne, L.A. & Corness, M. 2007. Brief Report: Relative Effectiveness of Different Home-based Behavioral Approaches to Early Teaching Intervention. *J Autism Dev Disord,* Vol.37, No. 8, (December, 2007), pp.1815–1821, ISSN 0162-3257

Rogers, S.J. & Benetto, L. Intersubjectivity in autism – the roles of imitation and executive function. In: *Autism Spectrum Disorders – A Transactional Developmental Perspective,* A. Wetherby & B. Prizant, (Eds.),79-107, Paul Brooks ISBN - 1-5576-6445-5, Baltimore, USA

Rogers, S.J., Hayedn, D., Hepburn, S., Charlifue-Smith, R., Hall, T. & Hayes, A. 2006. Teaching Young Nonverbal Children with autism Useful Speech: a Pilot Study of the Denver Model and PROMPT Interventions. *J Autism Develop Disord,* Vol.36, No.6, (October, 2006), pp.1007-1024, ISSN 0162-3257

Rutter, M. 1983. Cognitive deficits in the pathogenesis of autism. *J Child Psychol Psychiat,* Vol.24, No.4, (December, 1983), pp.513-531, ISSN 0009-398X

Rutherford, M.D., Young, G.S., Hepburn, S. & Rogers, S.J. 2007 A longitudinal study of pretend play in autism. *J Autism Dev Disord*, Vol.37, No.8, (December, 2007), pp.1024-1039, ISSN 0162-3257

Sigafoos, J., Roberts, P., Kerr, M., Couzens, D. & Baglioni, G. 1994. Opportunities for Communication in Classrooms serving Children with Developmental Disabilities. *J Autism Develop Disord*, Vol.24, Vol.3, (September, 1994), pp.237-246, ISSN 0162-3257

Solomon, R., Necheles, J., Ferch, C. & Bruckman, D. 2007. Pilot study of a parent training program for young children with autism. *Autism*, Vol.11, No.3, (September, 2007), pp.205-224, ISSN 1362-3613

Solomon, M., Ono, M., Timmer, S. & Goodlin-Jones, B. 2008. The Effectiveness of Parent–Child Interaction Therapy for Families of Children on the Autism Spectrum. *J Autism Dev Disord*, Vol.38, No.6 (October, 2008), pp.1767–1776, ISSN 0162-3257

Sutera, A., Pandely, J., Esser, E.L., Rosenthal, M.A., Wilson, L.B., Barton, M., Green, J., Hodgson, S., Robins, D.L., Dumont-Matieu, T. & Fein, D. 2007. Predictors of optimal outcome in toddlers diagnosed with autism spectrum disorders. *J Autism Develop Disord*, Vol.37, No.1, (February, 2007), pp.98-107, ISSN 0162-3257

Tanguay, P.E., Robertson, J. & Derrick A. 1998. A dimensional classification of autism spectrum disorder by social communication domains. *J Am Acad Child Adoles Psychiat*, Vol.37, No. 2, (April, 1998), pp. 271-277, ISSN 0980-8567

Tomasello, M., Striano, T. & Rochat, P. 1999. Do young children use objects as symbols? *British J Develop Psychol*, Vol.17, No.3, (September, 1999), pp.563-584, ISSN 2044-835X

Toth, K., Munson, J., Meltzoff, A.N. & Dawson, G. 2006. Early predictors of communication development in young children with autism spectrum disorder: joint attention, imitation and toy play. *J. Autism Develop Disord*, Vol.36, No.5, (August, 2006), pp.993-1005, ISSN 0162-3257

Turner, L.M., Stone, W.L., Pozdol, S.L. & Coonrod, E.E. 2006. Follow-up of children with autism spectrum disorders from age 2 to age 9. *Autism*, Vol.10, No.3, (September, 2006), pp. 243-265, ISSN 1362-3613

Vismara LA, Rogers SJ. 2010. Behavioral treatments in autism spectrum disorder: what do we know? *Annu Rev Clin Psychol*, Vol.27. No.6, (April, 2010), pp. 447-68, ISSN 1548-5943

Wetherby, A., Prizant, B. & Schuler, A.L. 2001. Understanding the nature of communication and language impairment. In: *Autism Spectrum Disorders – A Transactional Developmental Perspective*, A.Wetherby & B. Prizant, (Eds), 109-141, Paul Brooks ISBN - 1-5576-6445-5, Baltimore, USA

Wetherby,A. & Prutting, C. 1984. Profiles of communicative and cognitive-social abilities in autistic children. *J.Speech Hear Res*, Vol.27, N.2, (April, 1981), pp.364-377, ISSN 1092-4388

Whalen, C., Schreibman, L. & Ingersoll, B. 2006. The collateral effects of joint attention training on social initiations, positive affect, imitation and spontaneous speech for young children with autism. *J Autism Dev Disord,* Vol.36, No.5, (October, 2006), pp.655-664, ISSN 0162-3257

Wollner, S. & Geller, E. 1982 Methods of assessing pragmatic abilities. In: *Pragmatics: the role in language development,* J. Irwin, (Ed), 135-159, Fox Point Publishing, ISBN 091170700X, La Verne, California, USA

3

Repetetive Extralinguistic, Prosodic and Linguistic Behavior in Autism Spectrum Disorders-High Functioning (ASD-HF)

Hila Green and Yishai Tobin
Ben-Gurion University of the Negev, Israel

1. Introduction

Restricted repetitive behavior has been a defining feature of the Autism Spectrum Disorders (ASD) since the original description of autism (Kanner, 1943), and by diagnostic convention, all individuals with ASD display some form of these "restricted repetitive and stereotyped patterns of behavior, interests, and activities" (Diagnostic and Statistical Manual for Mental Disorders-Forth Edition [DSM-IV], American Psychiatric, [APA], 1994:71). Although ASD is associated with a wide range of specific forms of atypical repetition, this issue received far less research attention than social and communication deficits. Indeed, it was not our original attention to examine the prosody of ASD high functioning (ASD-HF) children from the perspective of the presence or the absence of repetitive behavior, we were concentrating on "prosody" within the context of linguistic behavior - whether or not the manifestation of the "different" prosody by ASD-HF individuals may reflect "delays and deficits in language and communication", which is another core feature of ASD. However, the data we collected in our research brought this issue into focus and raised new questions regarding the centrality of the restricted repetitive behaviors in ASD.

This chapter is based on results and insights from linguistic research. This research (Green, 2010) comparing and contrasting the prosodic features of 20 peer-matched 9-13 year old male Israeli Hebrew-speaking participants (10 ASD-HF subjects and 10 controls without developmental disorders (WDD) strongly indicated that the prosodic features that were examined exhibited a limited and repetitive repertoire in the ASD-HF population compared with the prosodic features of the WDD control population (Green, 2005; Green & Tobin 2008a, b, 2009 a, b, c; Green, 2010). Furthermore, this significant limited repetitive repertoire of behavior patterns was also exhibited in the extra-linguistic and the linguistic (lexical) domains of the ASD-HF participants.

2. The experimental research

As already noted, this chapter is based on experimental research and deals with the "restricted repetitive behavior" phenomenon. In the original linguistic-oriented research there were four major goals:

1. To describe, compare and contrast the phonetic realization of the fundamental frequency and the prosodic features of intonation in the language of children with ASD-HF and WDD children,
2. To establish a methodology which allows the analysis of more than one feature of prosody simultaneously,
3. To make use of instrumental measurements, (using recently developed speech technology tools) as well as perceptual analysis, and
4. To explain the results within the context of the theory of Phonology as Human Behavior (PHB) (e.g. Diver, 1979, 1995; Tobin, 1997, 2009), a linguistic theory which declares that: (a) Language is a symbolic tool, whose structure is shaped both by its communicative function and the characteristics of its users (Tobin, 1990, 1993, 1994, 2009), and (b) Language represents a compromise in the struggle to achieve maximum communication using minimal effort as presented in the theory of Phonology as Human Behavior (PHB) (Diver, 1979,1995; Tobin, 1997, 2009).

Our empirical data were drawn from the speech samples of 20 children between the ages 9-13 years, in two main groups:

a. Research group: subjects diagnosed clinically with ASD-HF (N=10)
b. Control group: participants without developmental disorders (WDD, N=10)

The research group includes ten children with ASD aged 9-13 years. They were recruited from mainstream schools that have special education classes for children with ASD. The ASD diagnosis was made by a child psychiatrist who determined that the child met the DSM-IV, APA (1994) criteria for autism. Each child's special needs were discussed and defined by an "Evaluation Committee", entrusted with the placement of special needs pupils in appropriate class settings. For all of the children in this group the committee determined that a special class for children within the ASD spectrum is required. IQ scores were re-assessed by the school psychologist within the current year using the Wechsler Intelligence Scale for Children - a Revised Edition [WISC-R]. For the purposes of this research, High Functioning is defined by an IQ 85 and above. All ASD subject's have typical, within the average, school performance in the mainstream class in language and reading, as reported by their teachers.

The control group was composed of children without developmental disorders (WDD) and was drawn from the same schools as the research group. Similar to the research group subjects, in their teachers' judgment, all the children are average students and do not exhibit any particular academic difficulties or exceptional abilities. The group members have not been tested to determine their IQ scores, but from the information received in interviews with the teachers and parents it can be assumed that they have intelligence in normal range. Their parents report that they have not been referred to a specialist for any developmental reasons. In our study, two language measures were used for peer matching. In addition to similar chronological ages (within two month), the peers were matched on the basis of (a) language fluency in spontaneous-speech sample as measured in MLU-W (within the minimal linguistic unit of one word) and (b) the standardized score of the verbal part in the IQ test within the norm or above. Match between subjects and controls are presented in Table 1.

The analysis of the speech samples of this group provides the basis for the characterization of the prosodic features of Israeli Hebrew (Green, 2009a; Green & Tobin 2009b, c; Green, 2010). All participants were male and at least second generation Israeli-born, and were monolingual speakers of Israeli Hebrew (IH). All participants were from comparable socioeconomic backgrounds and attend mainstream schools. Their mothers all have at least 12 years of education, an indication of socioeconomic status, since maternal education level is the most significant predictor of language functioning in children (Dollaghan et al., 1999). None of the members of the participants' immediate families has learning or other known disabilities.

ASD-HF subjects						WDD control group			
Research Group ASD-HF	Mo	VIQ	PIQ	Age	MLU -W	Control Group WDD	Mo	Age	MLU-W
1-ADR	13	109	94	9:0	5.62	11-AVY	13	9:0	5.28
2-ITE	17	121	91	9:2	5.34	12-NIS	15	9:3	4.04
3-UDX	15	108	94	10:8	7.86	13-IDR	17	10:7	6.94
4-YOL	17	111	101	11:1	5.77	14-YVO	16	10:11	5.16
5-RAE	12	86	97	11:6	5.68	15-ITS	17	11:6	4.04
6-BAB	17	109	97	11:11	7.42	16-AVS	16	11:9	7.18
7-ETR	16	100	102	12:5	5.14	17-LIS	13	12:3	5.22
8-TOB	15	108	99	12:8	6.42	18-IDW	16	12:6	6.20
9-NOR	14	90	99	13:0	6.5	19-OMX	14	12:11	5.86
10-OMG(*)	14	89	85	13:0	4.8	20-IDS	17	12:11	6.1

Mo=Mother's years of Education, VIQ/PIQ= verbal/performance Intelligence score (WISC-R) (*) Participants 10 and 20 do not meet the requirements of the definitions used for peer matching, and are consequently excluded from comparison between the groups. Their results are, however, included when the discussion is about differences within the group.

Table 1. Matched peers and subject's characteristics

The speech samples were collected at the participant's house, in his own room. There were three types of elicitation tasks: (a) Repetition: this task comprised four sentence pairs, a WH-Question and its answer, (b) Reading Aloud: participants were asked to read a short story, and (c) Spontaneous speech: these were elicited spontaneous speech sequences in response to open questions, relevant to the child's daily life.

In order to conduct acoustic analyses the speech files were digitized at a rate of 44.1KHz with 16-bit resolution, directly into a laptop computer (Hp Compaq 6710b), using the speech-recording software Audacity (a software package for recording and editing sound files) and a small microphone. The data were subsequently analyzed using the speech analysis program Pratt, version 5.0.30 (Computer program, from http://www.praat.org/). Scripts were written to extract data from the transcriptions. Script is a short program that is used to automate Pratt activities and enables the analysis of large data sets, quick processing of information and results, preparation for the use of simple statistics tools, and generation of summary information for control purposes, i.e. to identify errors in the manual transcription process.

3. Restricted repetitive behavior

Restricted repetitive behaviors are a heterogeneous group of behaviors and a wide range of specific forms of atypical repetition that have been identified and described with relation to

ASD (e.g. APA, 1994; Bodfish et al., 2000; Esbensen et al., 2009; Kanner 1943; Lewis & Bodfish, 1998; Militerni et al., 2002; Richler et al., 2007; Rutter, 1996; Szatmari et al., 2006; Turner, 1999). This restricted repetitive behavior can be observed across individuals with ASD, and multiple categories of abnormal repetition can occur within the individual with autism (e.g. Lewis & Bodfish, 1998; Wing & Gould, 1979). These behaviors can be socially inappropriate, increase the plausibility of living in a more restricted environment, and stigmatizing (Bonadonna, 1981; Durand & Carr 1987, Varni et al., 1979).

Several researchers who examined age related aspects of repetitive behavior patterns in ASD suggested that age and level of functioning are associated with variation in the manifestation of restricted repetitive behaviors in individuals with ASD (e.g. Esbensen et al., 2009; Militerni et al., 2002; Lam & Aman, 2007). The overall severity of the ASD has been shown to be significantly positively correlated with the overall severity of repetitive behaviors (e.g. Campbell et al., 1990; Prior & MacMillan, 1973). Esbensen et al. (2009) examined the restricted repetitive behaviors among a large group of children and adults with ASD in order to describe age related patterns of symptom expression and examine if age related patterns are different for the various types of restricted repetitive behaviors. In this research, they combined data from several previous studies to have a large sample size (n = 712), spanning a broad age range (age 2–62), and they measured restricted repetitive behaviors using a single instrument, the Repetitive Behavior Scale-Revised (RBS-R: Bodfish et al., 2000) with the modification of the subscales (Lam & Aman, 2007). The empirically derived subscales include: Stereotyped Behavior (movements with no obvious purpose that are repeated in a similar manner), Self-injurious Behavior (actions that cause or have the potential to cause redness, bruising, or other injury to the body), Compulsive Behavior (behavior that is repeated and performed according to a rule or involves things being done "just so"), Ritualistic/sameness Behavior (performing activities of daily living in a similar manner; resistance to change, insisting that things stay the same), and Restricted Interests (limited range of focus, interest, or activity). Their analyses suggest that repetitive behaviors are less frequent and less severe among older individuals than among younger individuals regardless of whether examining total display of restricted repetitive behaviors, or whether examining each of the various subtypes. One may ask whether restricted repetitive behaviors decrease with age or whether they merely take a different form. A thought previously arise by Piven et al. (1996). Piven's idea was that manifestation of ASD changes as the individual develops.

Other research has suggested that the expression of restricted repetitive behaviors may be influenced by level of functioning (e.g. Bartak & Rutter, 1976; Campbell et al., 1990; Gabriels et al., 2005; Le Couteur et al., 2003; Turner, 1999). Low IQ or presence of mental retardation has been shown to be associated with increased occurrence of repetitive behaviors in autism including stereotypy and self-injury (Bartak & Rutter 1976; Campbell et al., 1990).

Turner (1997) proposed a taxonomy of repetitive behavior; consisting of eleven categories and in a later review (Turner, 1999) suggested that human repetitive behaviors can be divided into (a) lower-level and (b) higher-level categories. Lower-level repetitive behaviors include dyskinesia (involuntary, repetitive movements), tics, repetitive manipulation of objects, repetitive forms of self-injurious behavior and stereotyped movements. Turner's review indicates that although some stereotyped movements and repetitive manipulation of objects might be differentiating features of autism, there are some lower-level repetitive behaviors that may rather be related to ability level or the presence of organic pathology (e.g. Bishop et al., 2006; Bodfish et al., 2000; Cuccaro et al., 2003; Esbensen et al., 2009; Fecteau et al., 2003; Militerni et al., 2002; Lam & Aman, 2007; Szatmari et al., 2006). Irrespective of whether these low-level repetitive behavioral characteristics are unique to ASD or exist in a wider range of organic pathological conditions, they are all repetitive extra-linguistic behaviors.

The high-level repetitive behaviors include circumscribed interests, attachments to objects, insistence on maintenance of sameness and repetitive language. Turner (1999) suggested that certain types of higher-level behavior may be characteristic of and restricted to individuals with ASD once a certain level of development has been achieved.

3.1 Repetitive language behavior

During the data analysis phase we could not ignore the proliferation of word repetition and repetition of contents. Repetitive language behavior has been reported in the literature (e.g. Perkins et al., 2006), but as far as we can determine there has not been a comprehensive study of questions raised by this phenomenon.

The following is an example of the lexical repetition found in the spontaneous speech of BAB-ASD (age 11:11) regarding his "interest" (*hitanyenut*) in the "sciences" (*mada'im*). The data are taken from sequential utterances in the same short conversation:

U3:	[ani mi# *hahit'anyenut* sheli be'ika(r) *mada'im*] I from my INTEREST ESPECIALLY LIKE SCIENCE
U4:	[*hit'anyenti bemada'im* kvar begil ca'r] I was INTERESTED in SCIENCE since I was young
U5:	[meod ahavti *mada'im*] I LIKED very much SCIENCE
U6:	[*mada'im* # shama'ati *shemada'im* # ze ha'olam shemisvivenu] SCIENCE—I heard that SCIENCE is the world around us
U13:	[ani ohev et kol hamikco'ot aval be'iqar *mada'im*] I LIKE all the subjects BUT ESPECIALLY SCIENCE
U14:	[be'iqar *mada'im*] ESPECIALLY SCIENCE
U15:	[ani yoter beqeTa shel *mada'im*] I am more into SCIENCE

3.2 Repetitive prosodic behavior

The term 'prosody' is derived from the Greek '*prosodia* ', which is a musical term. Metaphorically, in linguistic contexts, it is implied that prosody is the musical accompaniment to the words themselves. The term "prosody" describes the way one says a particular utterance and covers a wide range of phenomena including: intonation patterns, stress and accent, and pauses and junctions, etc. in speech.

Atypical prosody have been reported in a wide range of developmental conditions including dysarthria (e.g. Brewester, 1989; Crystal, 1979; Vance, 1994), aphasia (e.g. Bryan, 1989; Cooper & Klouda, 1987; Moen 2009), in hearing impairment (e.g. Parkhurst & levitt, 1978; Monsen, 1983; Most & Peled, 2007), in developmental speech and language disorders and/or learning disabilities (e.g. Garken & McGregor, 1989; Hargrove, 1997; Hargrove &

McGarr, 1994; Wells & Peppé, 2003), in Williams Syndrome e.g. Setter et al., 2007; Stjanovik et al., 2007), and in ASD.
In ASD the atypical prosody has been identified as core feature and since the initial description, by Kanner (1943) and Asperger (1944, as cited in Frith 1991), the "unnatural" prosody was marked using different narrations such as "monotonous", "odd", "sing-song", "exaggerated", and more. Asperger, translated in Frith (1991) wrote: "*Sometimes the voice is soft and far way, sometimes it sounds refined and nasal but sometimes it is too shrill and ear-splitting. In yet other cases, the voice drones on in a sing-song and does not even go down at the end of sentence. However many possibilities there are, they all have one thing in common: the language feels unnatural*" (Frith, 1991:70)
Research on prosody within the ASD population, has shown that even when other aspects of language improve, prosodic deficits tend to be persistent and show little change over time (e.g. Kanner, 1971; Simmons & Baltaxe, 1975). This persistence of prosodic deficits seems to limit the social acceptance of children with ASD-HF mainstreamed into the larger community since they sound strange to their peers (McCann & Peppé, 2003; Paul et al., 2001).
Adapting Fujisaki's definition, "Prosody is the systematic organization of various linguistic units into an utterance or coherent group of utterances in the process of speech production. Its realization involves both segmental and suprasegmental feature of speech and serves to convey not only linguistic information, but also paralinguistic and non-linguistic information" (Fujisaki, 1997:28). By this definition, Fujisaki established the prosodic features by two major components that can be measured: (a) the word accent, (b) the intonation, and they are both manifested by the contour of the voice F0 (the frequency of the vibration of the vocal folds). Hence, in order to understand the results and the insights from the presented research, we will first explore the nature of these two components from both a conceptual and operative view.

3.2.1 Word accent and the intonation

Bolinger (1958) formulates the relations of stress-accent. He argues that the main means to express stress is pitch and proposed the term accent for prominence in the utterance. Following Bolinger, Pierrehumbert (1980) represents the F0 contour as a linear sequence of phonologically distinctive units - pitch accents and edge tones. The occurrence of these features within the sequence can be described linguistically as a grammar, within the Autosegmental-Metrical (AM) theory (Ladd, 1996; Liberman & Pierrehumbert, 1984; Pierrehumbert, 1980; Pierrehumbert & Hirschberg, 1990).
The AM theory is a generative phonological framework in which the tone is specified using an independent string of tonal segments and the prosody of an utterance is viewed as a hierarchically organized structure of phonologically defined features. Following the AM theory, Pierrehumbert (1980) proposes a description of intonation that consists of three parts:

1. The grammar of phrasal tones,
2. The metrical representation of the text,
3. The rules of assigning association lines.

Pierrehumbert assumes that the tonal units are morphemes of different kinds and those phonetic rules translate the abstract representations into concrete F0 contours. Thus, phonological aspects of intonation can be categorized according to the inventory of the phonological tones, and to the meanings assigned to phonological tones of a specific language. However it is the ToBI (Tones and Break Indices: Beckman & Hirshberg, 1994;

Beckman & Ayers 1997) transcription that was designed for this presentation, of the phonological tones, within the AM theory.
ToBI was first designed for Mainstream American English and then expanded into a general framework for the development of prosodic annotation systems of different typological languages (Jun, 2005). ToBI has been applied to a wide variety of languages that vary geographically, typologically and according to their degree of lexical specifications, and to tone languages. For the purpose of the present research, an IH-ToBI was established in order to create a systematic procedure for transcribing data for Israeli Hebrew (Green, 2009a, 2010; Green & Tobin, 2008a).

3.2.2 The inventory of the IH prosodic features of Intonation (IH-ToBI)

The starting point for the analysis of the prosodic pitch contour i.e. intonation, is the notion of an *intonation unit*. This unit can be defined by its phonetic-phonological characteristics: (a) there is a "unity of pattern" within the intonation unit i.e. the intonation unit has a distinct intonation pitch pattern, and (b) the intonation unit is delimited by a boundary tone.
In IH-ToBI, the intonational structure of the utterance is represented by a "Tone Tier" and three types of tonal events can be identified: (a) pitch accents, the event that associates with stressed syllables and two types of phrasal tones; (b) phrase accents and (c) boundary tones. Therefore, on the "Tone Tier" the perceived pitch contour is transcribed in terms of: (1) Pitch Accents (PAs) (2) Phrase Accents, and (3) Edge Tones (the last phrase accent and the final boundary tone).
In IH-ToBI every intonational phrase contains at least one *Pitch Accent* (PA). PAs are localized pitch events that associate with the stressed syllable but in contrast to stress (which is lexically determined), in the tone domain it is not expected that every stressed syllable will be accented. In the AM theory, PAs are perceptually significant changes in F0 aligned with particular words in an utterance, and give them prominence. IH-ToBI identified five PAs: two mono-tonal: high (H) and low (L) tonal patterns: H* and L*, and three bi-tonal: L+H*, H*+L and L*+H. As in other language's descriptions, the H and L tones are described as high or low relative to each speaker's pitch range. The H*- a high pitch accent starting from the speaker's middle range and realized as a F0 peak preceded by a small rise is by far the most frequently used pitch accent in IH.
Phrase accents and Boundary tones: IH-ToBI identifies two levels of phrasing: (a) the intermediate phrase and (b) the intonation unit. Each intonation unit contains at least one intermediate phrase. The edge tones for these phrases determine the contour from the last tone of the last pitch accent until the end of the phrase. There are two types of phrase accents in IH: (a) 'Hp' and (b) 'Lp'. Hp has roughly the same F0 value as the peak corresponding to the most recent H tone, which creates a plateau at the end of the phrase. Lp can either be a F0 minimum low in the range, or be down-stepped in relation to a previous tone.
Concerning the boundary tones, IH-ToBI identified three types: (a) an initial boundary tone '%', (b) a high boundary tone 'H%', and (c) a low boundary tone 'L%'. The two final boundary tones combine with the phrase accents in four different combinations i.e. the last intermediate phrase accent (Hp or Lp) combines with the intonational boundary tones to yield the configuration of LpL%, LpH%, HpL% or HpH%. These boundaries appear to have specific pragmatic functions. By analyzing the distribution of these configurations appearing in the spontaneous speech and the reading aloud corpus of our data, it was evident that

LpL% is the most frequently used boundary tone in IH and the L-boundary tone signals finality. The absence of finality i.e. signaling a continuation, is marked by a high (H) boundary tone or high phrase accent (Hp) with a L-boundary tone i.e., LpH%, HpH%, HpL%.

To conclude, the richness within the prosodic features (five pitch accents, two phrase accents three boundary tones and all their possible combinations) serve as the basis for the comparing and contrasting of the speech prosody of the ASD-HF subjects with their peers - the WDD controls.

Regarding our investigation of the realization of pitch accents in the speech of children with ASD-HF, our research concentrated on three variables to be analyzed: (1) frequency of high PAs occurrences, (2) distribution of the different IH PAs, and (3) PAs per word (PAs/W), followed by a case investigation of one subject and his matched peer, in order to explore the differences found at the lexical word level.

We found that the children with ASD-HF produced more high PAs than the control group of WDD children in both the reading aloud and spontaneous speech elicitation tasks, without statistical significance, but with high standard deviation within the research group. This high standard deviation shows that the variability within the ASD-HF research group is much greater than that within the WDD control group. In a comparison of peers within the groups, in seven of the nine matched peers, the ASD-HF participant showed a greater use of high PAs in the spontaneous speech task and in six matched peers, the ASD-HF participant shows a greater use of high PAs in the reading aloud task.

In the WDD control group only two participants demonstrate above 80% use of high PAs, while in the ASD-HF research group four participants produced above 80% use of high PAs. No participants in the ASD-HF research group produced less than 70% high PAs while in the WDD control group there are three participants with less than 70% high PAs. The differences arise when comparing the research group and the controls as a group in contrast with a comparison of peers – as a "group of case-studies". These intergroup differences lead to the conclusion that the characteristic of heterogeneity (e.g. Beglinger, 2001; Firth, 2004; Happe' & Frith, 1996a) within the ASD classification has methodological implications for research procedure in general and in the present research in particular: i.e. it was the aggregation of peer comparisons that motivated the exploration of the prosodic behavioral features in the group of subjects diagnosed with ASD-HF.

Concerning the PA prosodic feature, the most prominent results deal with PAs/W and the placement of PAs. In a peer-case-investigation it was evident that the ASD-HF subject produced almost twice as often, more PAs in function words than his mach-peer did, and in particular more than one PA per word, while his WDD peer hardly ever adds more than one PA in a word (15.69% of the words in the ASD-HF speech sample and 1.96% of the words in his WDD peer speech sample). These results are illustrated in the following example

This example is a sentence from the reading aloud elicitation task: yom `exad yac'a `orit lesaxek ba-xacer lefet'a ra'ata kadur Qatan umuzar munax ba-gina. (Translation: One day Orit went to play in the yard and suddenly saw a small, strange ball in the garden). In this example, the ASD-HF subject (1a below) produced the sentence with three intonation units. Every word has a PA. Function words (FW) are emphasized with a PA as well as content words (CW). The words /baxacer/ (yard) and /qatan/ (small) have two PAs each. In contrast, the matched pair (1b below) produced the same sentence with only two intonation units. Not every word has a PA and none of the words has more than one PA.

(1a) 1-ADR-ASD

IU-1:	/yom `exad	yac'a	`Orit	lesaxeq /			
Gloss:	day one	to go out	(name)	to play			
	FW	CW	CW	CW			
IU-2:	/ ba- xacer/						
Gloss:	in+yard						
	FW+CW						
IU-3:	/lefet'a	ra`ata	Kadur qa-Tan	umuzar	munax	ba- gina/	
Gloss:	suddenly	to see	ball small	and+strange	placed	in+garden	
	FW	CW	CW CW	FW+CW	CW	FW+CW	

(1b) 11-AVY-WDD

IU-1: /yom `exad yac'a `Orit lesaxek ba-xacer/

IU-2: /lefet'a ra`ata kadur qatan umuzar munax ba-gina/

As was previously found (e.g. Baltaxe, 1984; Balataxe & Guthrie, 1987; Fosnot & Jun, 1999; MacCaleb & Prizant, 1985), and extending over in the current research, it can be concluded that within the ASD individuals that exhibited atypicality in prosody 'accents' are likely to be affected.

Regarding the investigation of boundary tones and phrase accents, a variation in the distribution of edge contour patterns arises when comparing the edge contours of the matched peers within the groups. The research group subjects may be divided into two sub-groups:

a. ASD-HF subjects that produced a **full repertoire of edge contour patterns**, similar to the control group (4 subjects). Figure 2 is an example of the full repertoire prosodic behavior by the ASD-HF subject compared with his matched peer in the spontaneous speech elicitation task.

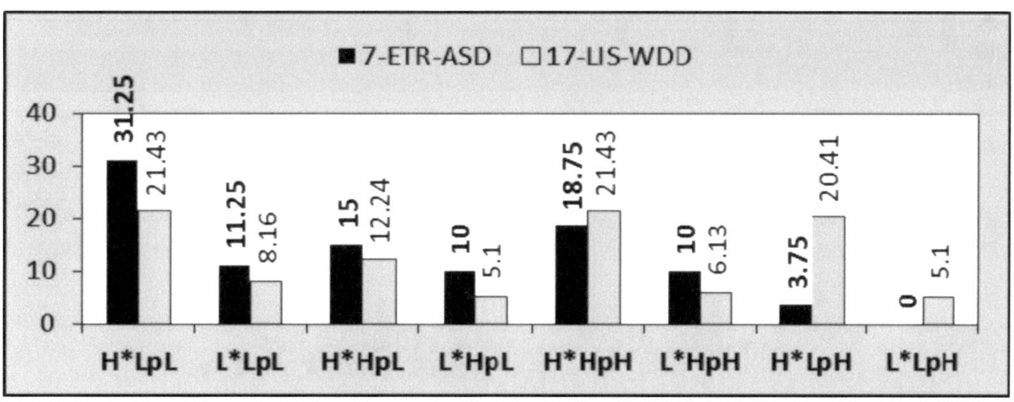

Fig. 2. Full repertoire of edge contour patterns. This figure shows the comparison between the edge contour patterns of 7-ETR-ASD, age: (12:5) and his matched peer LIS-WDD, age: (12:3) in the spontaneous speech task. The ASD-HF subject uses the same patterns as his peer and has the full repertoire of edge contour patterns (Green, 2010:106)

b. Of the nine matched peers, in the spontaneous elicitation task five of the subjects produced **a varied limited repeatedly used repertoire of the edge contour patterns.** Figure 3 presents the distribution of the edge contour patterns of two subjects in the reading aloud elicitation task and Figure 4 presents the results of five subjects in the spontaneous speech elicitation task.

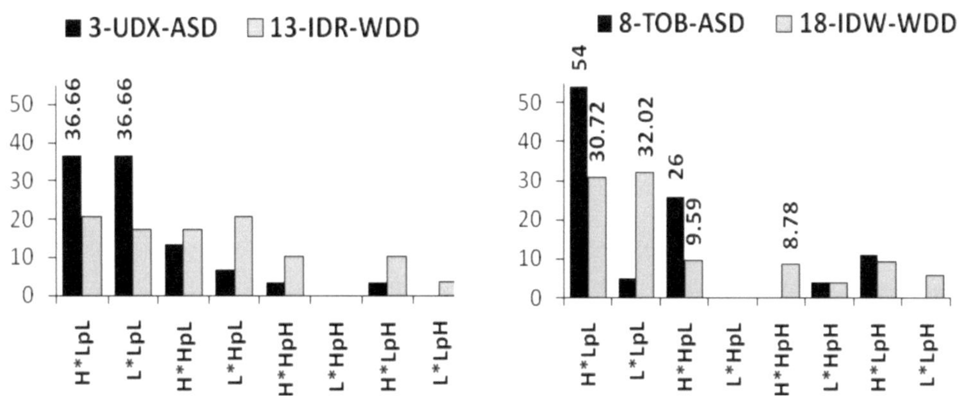

Fig. 3. Limited repeatedly used repertoire in the reading aloud elicitation task (Green, 2010:106)

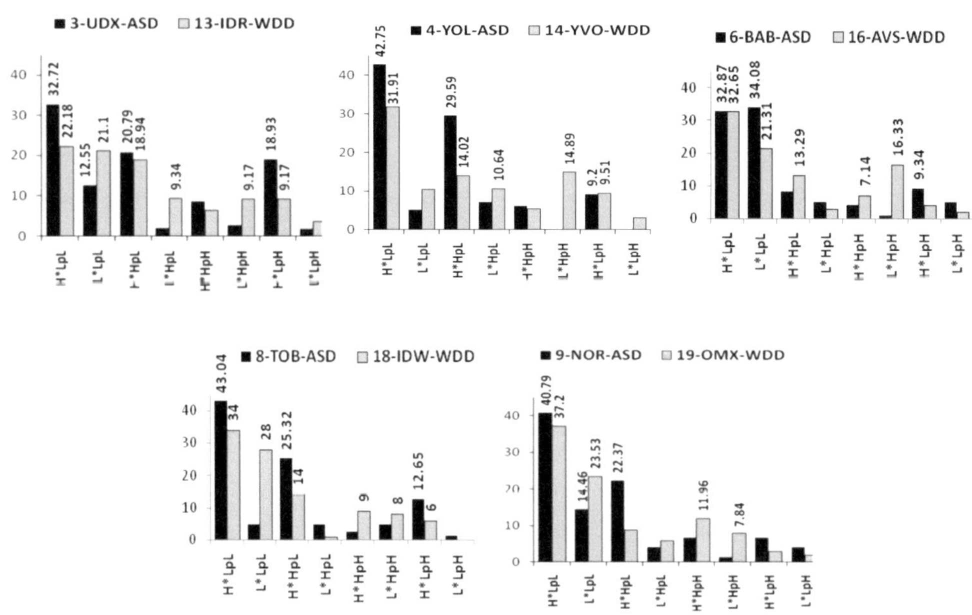

Fig. 4. Limited repeatedly used repertoire in the Spontaneous speech ellicitation task (Green, 2010:107)

In conclusion we will emphasize certain aspects that were manifested in the present study. The starting point in our study was the need to characterize the prosodic features of children diagnosed with ASD-HF who mainstreamed in regular schools. The research established methodology, which allows the analysis of more than one feature of prosody simultaneously and described, compared and contrasted the phonetic realization of the fundamental frequency and the prosodic features of intonation in the language of 10 children with ASD-HF and 10 children WDD. By using recently developed speech technology tools, we performed an extensive investigation of thc prosody of children with ASD-HF between the ages of 9-13 years. The speech sample analysis yielded quantitative results, of group comparison, peer comparison and of subjects within the ASD-HF group. The peer comparison highlights the greater variations within the ASD-HF subjects, as compared with their peers and between themselves. From this study we can conclude that not all ASD-HF subjects present an a-typicality in each of the different prosodic features examined, but no subject performed in the same way as his WDD peer.

It was found that ASD-HF subjects produce more high PAs and less low PAs. If the variations in intonation are a result of differences in the kinds of PAs and transitions between the prominent components, then when the prominence in the ASD-HF subjects exists in a more frequent single high PA and there are consequently fewer transitions, a monotonous accent is created. The ASD-HF present repetitive behavior expressed over the use of pitch accents within a word - a repetitiveness that did not observed in the control group.

One of the most significant founding is concern with the use of edge tone i.e., the tonal events at the edge of prosodic domains. The ASD-HF subjects primarily use three different edge tone patterns, although they do make a very limited use of all the other patterns. Thus, the problem is not the absence of patterns due to lack of competence to produce them, rather it is the nature of the behavior that the ASD-HF exhibited. Although the ASD-HF subjects are capable of producing a wide range of prosodic patterns, they concentrate on a limited repertoire of the most basic prosodic patterns. Both the monotonous accent and the repetitiveness of edge tones create a stiff sounding prosody in subjects within the ASD-HF group.

Our claim based on all the data collected and results from our research indicates that the restricted repetitive behavior of the ASD-HF subjects, appears in a parallel way across the board in the extralinguistic, paralinguistic (prosody) and linguistic (lexical choice) domains. Then, Turner's distinction between higher and lower level behavioral categories may only reflect the observable symptoms of ASD behavior rather than their fundamental motivation. We suggest that the concept of limited and repetitive behavior found on all levels of extralinguistic, paralinguistic and linguistic behaviors in a parallel way among different populations with ASD should play a more central role in research to help us better understand ASD.

4. References

American Psychiatric Association. (1994). *Diagnostic and statistical manual of mental disorders* (4th ed.). Washington, DC: American Psychiatric Association.

Baltaxe, C. A., (1984). Use of contrastive stress in normal, aphasic, and autistic children. *Journal of speech and Hearing Research*, 27, 97-105.

Baltaxe, C. A., & Guthrie, D. (1987). The use of primary sentence stress by normal, aphasic and autistic children. *Journal of Autism and Developmental Disorders*, 17, 255-271.

Bartak L, Rutter M. (1996). Differences between mentally retarded and normally intelligent autistic children. *Journal of Autism Childhood Schizophrenia*, 6, 109-120.

Beglinger, L. G., & Smith, T. H. (2001). A review of subtyping in autism and proposed dimensional classification model. *Journal of Autism and Developmental Disorders*, 31, 411-422.

Bishop, S., Richler, J., & Lord, C. (2006). Association between restricted and repetitive behavior and nonverbal IQ in children with autism spectrum disorders. *Child Neuropsychology*, 12, 247-267.

Bodfish, J. W., Symons, F. J., Parker D. E., & Lewis, M. H. (2000). Varieties of repetitive behavior in autism: comparisons to mental retardation. *Journal of Autism and Developmental Disorders*, 30, 237-243.

Bonadonna, P. (1981). Effects of a vestibular stimulation program on stereotypic rocking behaviour. *The American Journal of Occupational Therapy*, 35(12), 775-781.

Boersma, P. & Weenink, D. (2009). Praat: doing phonetics by computer (Version 5.1.05). Retrieved May 1, 2009, from http://www.praat.org

Campbell M, Locascio J, Choroco B, et al. (1990). Stereotypies and tardive dyskinesia: Abnormal movements in autistic children. *Psychopharmacol Bull*, 26, 260-266.

Cuccaro, M. L., Shao, Y., Grubber, J., Slifer, M., Wolpert, C. M., Donnelly, S. L., et al. (2003). Factor analysis of restricted and repetitive behaviors in autism using the Autism Diagnostic Interview-R. *Child Psychiatry and Human Development*, 34, 3–17.

Diver, W. (1979). Phonology as human behaviour. In D. Aaronson & P. Reiber (Eds.), *Psycholinguistic research: Implications and applications* (pp. 161-186). Hillside, NJ: Lawrence Erlbaum.

Diver, W. (1995). The theory. In E. Contini-Morava & B. S. Goldberg (Eds.), *Meaning as explanation: Advances in linguistic sign theory* (pp. 43-114). Berlin: Mouton de Gruyter.

Dollaghan, Ch. A., Campbell, T. F, Paradise, J. L., Feldman, H. M., Janosky, J. E., Pitcairn, D. N., & Kurs-Lasky, M. (1999). Maternal education and measures of early speech and language. *Journal of Speech, Language, and Hearing Research*, 42, 1432-1443.

Durand, V. M., & Carr, E. G. (1987). Social Influences on "selfstimulatory" behavior: Analysis and treatment applications. *Journal of Applied Behavior Analysis*, 20(2), 119-132.

Esbensen, A. J., Seltzer, M. M., Kristen S., Lam, L., & Bodfish, J. W. (2009). Age-related differences in restricted repetitive behaviors in autism spectrum disorders. *Journal of Autism and Developmental Disorders*, 39, 57-66.

Fecteau, S., Mottron, L., Berthiaume, C., & Burack, J. A. (2003). Developmental changes of autistic symptoms. *Autism*, 7, 255-268.

Fosnot, S., & Jun, S. A. (1999). Prosodic characteristics in children with stuttering or autism during reading and imitation. *Proceedings of 14th International Congress of Phonetic Sciences* (pp.1925-1928).

Frith, U. (2004). Emanuel Miller lecture: confusions and controversies about Asperger syndrome, *Journal of Child Psychology and Psychiatry*, 45, 672-686.

Fujisaki, H. (1997). Prosody, models, and spontaneous speech, In Y. Sagisaka., N. Campbell & N. Higuchi (Eds.), *Computing prosody: Computational models for processing spontaneous speech* (pp. 27-40). New York: Springer.

Gabriels, R. L., Cuccaro, M. L., Hill, D. E., Ivers, B. J., & Goldson, E. (2005). Repetitive behaviors in autism: Relationships with associated clinical features. Research in Developmental Disabilities, 26, 169–181.

Green, H. (2005). *The contour of the prosodic intonation in the spoken language of children with high functioning autism according to the theory of phonology as human behavior.* M.A. Thesis, Ben-Gurion University of the Negev, Be'er-Sheva: Israel.

Green, H., & Tobin, Y. (2008a). A phonetic analysis of the prosody of Hebrew-speaking children with high functioning autism. *Proceedings of the 18th International Congress of Linguists.* Seoul, Korea. (CD ROM).

Green, H., & Tobin, Y. (2008b). Intonation in Hebrew speaking children with high-functioning autism: A case study. In A. B. Plinio., S. Madureira & C. Reis (Eds.), *Proceedings of the fourth conference on speech prosody SP2008* (pp.237-240). Campinas, Brazil.

Green, H. (2009a). Intonation in Hebrew-speaking children with high functioning autism. *Asian-Pacific Journal of Speech, Language and Hearing,* 12, 187-198.

Green, H., & Tobin, Y. (2009b). Prosodic analysis is difficult…but worth it: A study in high functioning autism. *International Journal of Speech-Language Pathology,* 11, 308-316.

Green, H., & Tobin, Y. (2009c). Phonology as human behavior: A prosodic study of high functioning autism. In: Victoria Marrero Idaira Pineda (eds.). *La Lingüística ante el reto de la aplicación clínica/Linguistics: The Challenge of Clinical Application: Actas del II Congreso Internacional de Lingüística Clínica/Proceedings of the 2nd International Clinical Linguistics Conference,* Madrid November 11-13, 2009. Madrid: Universidad de Nacional Educación a Distancia and Euphonia Ediciones, pp. 378-382.

Green, H. (2010). Prosodic features in the spoken language of children with autism spectrum disorders high-functioning (ASD-HF) according to the theory of phonology as human behavior. PhD. Thesis, Ben-Gurion University of the Negev, Be'er-Sheva: Israel.

Happé, F. G., & Frith, U. (1996). The neuropsychology of autism. *Brain,* 119, 1377-1400.

Jun, S. A. (Ed.) (2005). Prosodic typology: The phonology of intonation and phrasing. Oxford: Oxford University Press.

Kanner, L. (1943). Autistic disturbances of affective contact. *Nervous Child,* 2, 217-250.

Kanner, L. (1971). Follow-up study of eleven autistic children originally reported in 1943. *Journal of Autism and Childhood Schizophrenia, 1,* 119-145.

Ladd, R. R. (1996). *Intonational phonology.* Cambridge: Cambridge University Press.

Lam, K. S. L., & Aman, M. G. (2007). The Repetitive Behavior Scale-Revised: Independent validation in individuals with autism spectrum disorders. *Journal of Autism and Developmental Disorders,* 37, 855–866.

Lecavalier, L., Aman, M. G., Scahill, L., McDougle, C. J., McCracken, J. T., Vitiello, B., et al. (2006). Validity of the autism diagnostic interview-revised. *American Journal of Mental Retardation,* 111, 199-215.

Lewis, M. H., & Bodfish, J. W. (1998). Repetitive behavior disorders in autism. *Mental Retardation and Developmental Disabilities Research Reviews,* 4, 80-89.

McCaleb, P., & Prizant, B. M. (1985). Encoding of new versus old information by autistic children. *Journal of Speech and Hearing Disorders,* 50, 230-240.

McCann, J. & Peppé, S. (2003). Prosody in autism spectrum disorders: a critical review. *International Journal of Language and Communication Disorders,* 38, 325-350.

Militerni, R., Bravaccio, C., Falco, C., Fico, C., & Palermo, M. T. (2002). Repetitive behaviors in autistic disorder. *European Child & Adolescent Psychiatry,* 11, 210-218.

Paul, R., Shriberg, L. D., McSweeny, J. L, Cicchetti, D., Klin, A., & Volkmar, F. (2005). Brief report: Relations between prosodic performance and communication and socialization ratings in high functioning speakers with autism spectrum disorders. *Journal of Autism and Developmental Disorders*, 35, 861-869.

Perkins, M. R., Dobbinson, S., Boucher, J., Bol, S., & Bloom, P. (2006). Lexical knowledge and lexical use in autism. *Journal of Autism and Developmental Disorders, 36,* 795-805.

Pierrehumbert, J. B. (1980). *The phonology and phonetics of English intonation.* Unpublished PhD dissertation, MIT. Reproduced by Indiana University Linguistics Club, Bloomington, IN.

Pierrehumbert, J. & Hirschberg, J. (1990). The meaning of intonation in the interpretation of discourse. In P. Cohen., J. Morgan & M. Pollack (Eds.), *Intentions in communication* (pp. 271-311). Cambridge: MIT Press.

Piven, J., Harper, J., Palmer, P., & Arndt, S. (1996). Course of behavioral change in autism: A retrospective study of high-IQ adolescents and adults. *Journal of the American Academy of Child and Adolescent Psychiatry,* 35, 523–529.

Prior, M., MacMillan, M. (1973). Maintenance of sameness in children with Kanner's Syndrome. *Journal of Autism and Childhood Schizophrenia*, 3, 154-167.

Richler, J., Bishop, S. L., Kleinke, J. R., & Lord, C. (2007). Restricted and repetitive behaviors in young children with autism spectrum disorders. *Journal of Autism and Developmental Disorders*, 37, 73-85.

Rutter, M. (1996). Autism research: Prospects and progress. *Journal of Autism and Developmental Disorders*, 26, 257-275.

Simmons, J. Q., & Baltaxe, C. (1975). Language patterns in adolescent autistics. *Journal of Autism and Childhood Schizophrenia, 5,* 333-351.

Szatmari, P., Georgiades, S., Bryson, S., Zwaigenbaum, L., Roberts, W., Mahoney, W., et al. (2006). Investigating the structure of the restricted, repetitive behaviours and interests domain of autism. *Journal of Child Psychology and Psychiatry*, 47, 582-590.

Tobin, Y. (1990). *Semiotics and linguistics.* London: Longman.

Tobin, Y. (1993). *Aspect in the English verb: Process and result in language.* London: Longman.

Tobin, Y. (1994). *Invariance, markedness and distinctive feature analysis: A contrastive study of sign systems in English and Hebrew.* Amsterdam and Philadelphia: John Benjamins.

Tobin, Y. (1997). *Phonology as human behaviour: Theoretical implications and clinical applications.* Durham, NC: Duke University Press.

Tobin, Y. (2009). Phonology as human behaviour: Applying theory to the clinic. *Asian-Pacific Journal of Speech, Language and Hearing, 12,* 81-100.

Turner, M. (1997). Towards an executive dysfunction account for repetitive behaviour in autism. In J. Russell (Ed.), *Autism as an executive disorder* (pp. 57–100). New York: Oxford University Press.

Turner, M. (1999). Annotation repetitive behaviors in autism: A review of psychological research. *Journal of Child Psychology and Psychiatry and Allied Disciplines*, 40, 839-849.

Varni, J. W., Lovaas, O. I., Koegel, R. L., & Everett, N. L. (1979). An analysis of observational learning in autistic and normal children. *Journal of Abnormal Child Psychology*, 7, 31-43.

Wing, L., & Gould, J. (1979). Severe impairments of social interaction and associated abnormalities in children: epidemiology and classification, *Journal of Autism and Developmental Disorders*, 9, 11-29.

4

Variability in Language and Reading in High-Functioning Autism

Cheryl Smith Gabig
Lehman College, The City University of New York
USA

1. Introduction

Autism is a complex developmental disorder characterized by a triad of core deficits in verbal communication, reciprocal social interaction, and cognitive flexibility reflected in restrictive and repetitive patterns of behavior and poor symbolic play. Poor verbal communication is a defining feature of ASD, but a high degree of variability exists in the clinical manifestation of the disorder, especially within the communication and language domains. Some children with autism never develop functional speech or language and remain nonverbal; others use well-developed speech (Tager-Flusberg, Paul, & Lord, 2005; Kjelgaard & Tager-Flusberg, 2001; Wilkinson, 1998). A significant developmental milestone in children diagnosed with autism in the preschool years is whether the child acquires useful speech and language skills by the age of 5 years, a developmental marker shown to be an indicator of a better prognosis for long-term outcome and is characteristic of those who are *higher-functioning* (Howlin, 2002).

Although the classifications systems and the diagnostic categories applied to the differential diagnosis of Autism Spectrum Disorders (ASD) are well recognized, verbal children with autism are often referred to as *high-functioning autism* (HFA), a term not included in the classification of autism spectrum disorders in the DSM-IV. Rather, HFA is a clinical description used for children who meet three criteria: a) a clinical history and behavioral manifestation of the diagnostic criteria for a diagnosis of autism (DSM-IV, APA, 1994; ICD-10, WHO, 1992), including a history of delay in acquiring speech and language, difficulty in reciprocal social interaction, and odd or repetitive behaviors, b) have functional verbal behavior, and c) an IQ criterion, absent mental retardation. Individuals with autism are considered as high-functioning if the IQ is above 70, the psychometric point of demarcation for mental retardation. Currently there is little consensus in the literature concerning which domain of intellectual functioning to use for the application of the IQ criterion in defining HFA for research purposes. For example, should the Full Scale IQ composite score be used, or would either the Verbal or Nonverbal Performance score suffice? This is a situation that may contribute to difficulty in comparing results among different studies focusing on children with HFA. Recent research suggests that there may be subgroups of children with HFA based on differing cognitive profiles. For example, children showing a profile of a higher Verbal IQ than Nonverbal IQ score higher on a measure of adaptive communication skills , have fewer social symptoms, and demonstrate better overall functioning than children showing the reverse cognitive profile (e.g. NVIQ > VIQ) (Black, Wallace, Sokoloff & Kentworthy, 2009). Yet, when the IQ criterion is investigated across studies on children or adults with HFA, differing IQ criterion are noted. Some investigators set the cognitive criterion for HFA to be a Full Scale IQ $\geq$ 70 (Asarnow, Tanguay, Bott, Freeman, 1987; Mayes & Calhoun, 2008; Minshew, Goldstein & Siegel, 1995), or a Full Scale IQ $\geq$ 80 (Landa & Goldberg, 2005). Other researchers have chosen to use only the Verbal IQ score (Losh & Capps, 2003) or the Nonverbal IQ ($\geq$ 70) (Freeman, Lucas, Forness, Ritvo, 1985; Smith Gabig, 2008; 2010) as the cognitive criterion. Still, others do not rely on an IQ criterion, rather they use a measure of receptive vocabulary > 70 as an index of overall verbal ability and verbal intelligence (Emerich, Creaghead, Grether, Murray, and Grasha, 2003), or a combination of an expressive vocabulary standard score > 70, and educational placement in the general education classroom, as the criteria for classification as *high-functioning* (Jones & Schwartz, 2009).

The term HFA is used to characterize children with autism who are verbal and have higher intellectual functioning, yet no single language profile has been identified in the group. Some of the children show normal language function and others range from mild language impairment to significant language impairment independent of intellectual functioning. However, deficits in the pragmatic use of language are a defining feature (Kjelgaard & Tager-Flusberg, 2001; Tager-Flusberg, Paul, & Lord, 2005). Children with autism will demonstrate impairments in pragmatic aspects of language use even if other aspects of language, such as morphosyntactic or lexical-semantic ability, are well developed (Stone & Caro-Martinez, 1990; Tager-Flusberg, 2003). Deficits in the pragmatic function of language are so pervasive in the clinical population of autism that it distinguishes between children with autism from other developmental language delays (Rice, Warren, & Betz, 2005; Wilkinson, 1998).

Beyond anticipated impairments in the pragmatic aspect of language functioning, investigators of language profiles of subgroups of children with ASD focus on patterns of performance in the areas of syntax and semantics that may distinguish groups of children with autism. There is accumulating evidence that some children with HFA present with deficits in syntax, similar to children with Specific Language Impairment (SLI). For example, Kjelgaard & Tager-Flusberg, (2001) found significant language and communication differences in the verbal behavior of HFA children with some of the children scoring in the normal range and others, in the profoundly language impaired range, even in the presence of a Full Scale IQ > 85. High-functioning individuals with autism are often referred to having *fluent autism*. The spontaneous speech and language characteristics reported include fluent narrative speech, frequently with grammatically correct sentences, the use of repetitive topics reflecting a narrow range of interests, odd phrasing and word choices, and abnormalities in prosody (Rice et al., 2005).

Currently, two theoretical perspectives on the nature and cause of language impairment in individuals with HFA appear in the literature. One perspective is that the abnormalities in communication and language functioning can be explained by the presence or absence of syntactic deficits; those with impairments in syntax are more likely to also demonstrate additional language difficulty in other linguistic domains, principally semantics (Condouris, Meyer, & Tager-Flusberg , 2003; Kjelgaard & Tager-Flusberg, 2001). The other perspective is that the language and communication characteristics seen in HFA are consistent with a generalized deficit in complex information processing abilities that preserve basic speech and language functioning, yet impact higher level propositional language (Minshew & Goldstein, 1998; Minshew, Goldstein, & Siegel, 1995; Minshew, Goldstein, Taylor & Siegel, 1994). These separate viewpoints have generated research investigating the nature of and causal linkages to the profile of language variability and impairment of individuals with HFA, each with compelling findings to support the separate theoretical framework (Condouris, Meyer, & Tager-Flusberg, 2003; Landa and Goldberg, 2005; McGregor, Berns, Owen, Michels, Duff, Bahnsen & Lloyd, 2011; Minshew, Goldstein, & Siegel, 1995; Minshew, Goldstein, Taylor & Siegel, 1994) .

In addition to variability in oral language functioning, significant variation is also seen in reading ability in verbal children with HFA . Some individuals with HFA present with excellent phonetic decoding ability yet poor comprehension, while others struggle with phonetic decoding of unfamiliar words , perhaps contributing to difficulties with reading comprehension (Nation, Clarke, Wright & Williams, 2006). Variability in the comprehension and use of spoken language and reading has compelling implications for the academic success of school-age children with HFA. Children with HFA are often included within the regular classroom to facilitate access to the general education curriculum and to gain social interaction with peers. High-Functioning children with autism are faced with increasingly more complex discourse processing demands as each grade progresses (Cazden, 1988). The language of the curriculum often is complex and abstractly removed from the language used in social control and interaction placing additional cognitive -linguistic demands on the child with HFA in the classroom (Loveland & Tunali-Kotoski, 2005).

The purpose of this chapter is: 1) to review the research on HFA from the two theoretical perspectives on the nature of and possible causal explanations to language impairment and variability in *fluent autism* and , 2) to examine the current research on literacy in school-age children and adolescents who meet the clinical and psychometric profile of HFA. A third goal is examine the association between oral language and literacy in children and adolescents with HFA in order to better understand the language functioning in HFA across these domains, and to gain insight into why many children with HFA demonstrate reading comprehension difficulty . It is important to consider both the oral language and literacy ability in individuals with HFA for two reasons. First, by definition, children with HFA have a history of speech and language delay and impaired communication seen in the preschool years. Even if the child has achieved well developed verbal ability by 5- years of age, deficits in oral language ability initially seen in the preschool years may contribute to uneven performance in later academic functioning, such as reading ability, reported in children with HFA. Second, there is a strong relationship between oral language competence and reading in typically developing and in non-autistic language-impaired populations. Aspects of oral language ability, including, phonology, syntax, narrative ability, metalinguistic awareness, and vocabulary have been shown to be critical predictors of reading acquisition and literacy achievement (Catts, Fey, Zhang, & Tomblin, 1999; Nation, Clarke, Marshall & Durand, 2004; Roth, Speece, Cooper, De La Paz, 1996; Snyder & Downey, 1991). Therefore, it is seems likely that children with HFA will demonstrate significant variability in literacy as well as reported variability in oral language and communication.

In order to meet the objective of this review, literature was reviewed that examined either oral language or literacy functioning in school-age children or adolescents with HFA. Studies were included if the participants met the specific inclusionary criteria of a diagnosis of autism and an IQ criterion > 70 (either Full-Scale, Verbal, or Performance IQ) , or if high-functioning autism could be extrapolated from psychometric data reported for any group of children with ASD included in a study on language or literacy functioning. Careful attention was paid to studies on spoken or written language ability in children with autism that included direct assessment using standardized tests assessing aspects of receptive and expressive language particularly in the lexical/semantic and syntactic domains of language. This decision is in keeping with the recently proposed and recommended assessment framework for younger children with ASD by experts on language disorders in autism convened by the National Institute on Deafness and Other Communication Disorders (NIDCD) (Tager-Flusberg, Rogers, Cooper, Landa, Lord, Paul, et al., 2009). Likewise, studies on literacy functioning and achievement in children with HFA were carefully screened for an emphasis on critical aspects of reading competency identified by the Report of the National Reading Panel (NIH, 2000), including phonological awareness, word reading accuracy, and reading comprehension.

2. Language abilities of children with high-functioning autism: Lexical–semantic and morphosyntactic abilities

There is a general consensus in the literature on language profiles of verbal children with autism that aspects of language form, including phonology and basic grammar and sentence structure syntax, are often areas of relative strength, followed by lexical- semantic abilities reflected in receptive and expressive single-word vocabulary measures of language content. Higher order morphosyntactic skill, narrative discourse, and pragmatic competence are more profoundly impaired (Rice, Warren, & Betz, 2005; Tager-Flusberg, 1999; 1981). Speech articulation is essentially spared (Kjelgaard & Tager-Flusberg, 2001; Tager-Flusberg, 2003) with the exception of prosody, phrasing, and consonant distortions on later acquired phonemes (Shriberg et al., 2001). There is recent compelling evidence that many verbal, high-functioning children with *fluent autism* also have significant deficits in complex morphosyntactic ability as well as higher level lexical semantic processing, and that the relative strengths or weaknesses in these language domains contribute to each other, effecting overall language competence (Condouris, Meyer, & Tager-Flusberg, 2003; Kjelgaard & Tager-Flusberg, 2001).

Kjelgaard & Tager-Flusberg, (2001) identified a subgroup (N = 44) of children as high-functioning autism in their study of a larger heterogeneous group of 89 children, between the ages of 4-14 years (M = 7.4). The diagnosis of autism was validated using the *Autism Diagnostic Interview-Revised* (Lord, Rutter, & LeCouteur, 1994) and the *Autistic Diagnostic Observation Schedule-Generic* (Lord, Risi, et al., 2000). The majority of the children in the sample were school-age into young adolescence (M (*age*) = 7.4 ; range 4-14 years). Intelligence was assessed using the *Differential Abilities Scale* (Eliott, 1983). All the children were given a battery of standardized tests including the *Goldman-Fristoe Test of Articulation* (GFTA), (Goldman & Fristoe, 1986), the *Clinical Evaluation of Language Fundamentals* (CELF-III, Semel, Wiig & Secord, 1995), or, depending on the age, the *Clinical Evaluation of Language Fundamentals* - Preschool (CELF-P; Wiig & Semel, 1992), the *Peabody Picture Vocabulary Test-III* (PPVT) (Dunn & Dunn, 1997), the *Expressive Vocabulary Test* (EVT) (Williams, 1997). Overall, the children scored highest in the areas of speech articulation, receptive vocabulary, and expressive vocabulary , indicating that these speech-language areas are not as impaired for the ASD group. Speech articulation and single-word vocabulary ability are considered by some researchers as basic mechanical aspects of language functioning, and not reflective of higher -language processing (McGregor, Berns, Owen, Michaels, duff, Bahnsen & Lloyd, 2011). Amend: (McGregor, Berns, Owen, Michaels, Duff, Bahnsen & Lloyd, 2011). Only 49 % (N= 44) of the children were able to complete the CELF, a standardized language measure considered to assess more complex aspects of lexical-semantic and morphosyntactic processing and production. For example, one of the core measures of language content on the CELF for children 5-12 years is a task that requires the child to follow increasingly more complex directions requiring logical operations. Older children (e.g. 9-12 years) complete a task that measures the ability to understand and explain the relationships between words based on semantic class or word meaning, and analyze or define words. Similarly, the syntactic domain is measured by tasks of sentence imitation and sentence formulation that taps the ability to formulate grammatically and semantically complete sentences.

The cognitive profile of children completing the CELF indicated significantly higher Full-Scale IQ scores (M = 85, D= 17.3) than for the children who could not complete the CELF (M= 50; SD 16.8). This pattern of higher FS IQ scores for the CELF completers also held for the standard scores on the two vocabulary measures, the PPVT, measuring receptive vocabulary, and the EVT, measuring expressive vocabulary, with higher performance in these as well. Based on the Full Score IQ in the average range (M = 85) and the cognitive-linguistic ability to complete the CELF, Kjelgaard & Tager-Flusberg, (2001) considered this group of ASD children to be the *high-functioning* children with autism.

Kjelgaard & Tager-Flusberg, (2001) examined the performance by the children with HFA on the CELF and noted that the composite score for Expressive Language was better than the Receptive Language Composite Score, suggesting that the fluent speech and language observed in many children with HFA may mask difficulty in understanding and processing more complex aspects of language. Kjelgaard & Tager-Flusberg, (2001) also divided the HFA group into three subgroups by overall standard score performance on the CELF: *normal* language learners with an overall language quotient in the normal range (SS $\geq$ 85), *borderline* language learners (SS = 70-84), and *impaired* language learners (SS < 70). The group identified as *normal* language learners (SS = $\geq$ 85) scored within the average range on all speech and language areas measured, including receptive vocabulary (PPVT), expressive vocabulary (EVT), speech articulation (GFTA), and higher-order semantic and morphosyntactic abilities measured by the CELF. In addition, the normal language group demonstrated average ability to repeat novel phonological sequences as measured by the Nonword Repetition Test (NWRT). These normal language learners also had the highest Full Scale IQ as a group (FSIQ Mean = 93; SD = 16.52) 85). The group identified as *borderline* in language learning (SS = 70-84) had deficits in all aspects of language including receptive and expressive vocabulary, higher order semantic and morphosyntactic measures , and below average performance in phonological working memory, measured by the NWRT. However, speech articulation ability was within the average range of performance for age for the borderline language group. The Full Scale IQ for the *borderline* language learning group was in the low end of the normal range (FSIQ Mean = 85; SD = 13.86). Finally, the group identified as most language impaired (SS < 70) showed significant language deficits across lexical-semantic and morphosyntactic domains with accompanying deficits in NWRT. This group also had the lowest IQ (FSIQ = 58; SD = 18.76).

According to the IQ criterion for a diagnosis of HFA, this final language impaired group cannot be considered as HFA since their FSIQ mean is < 70; although some of the children in this impaired group may have had a FSIQ of 70 or greater, given the standard deviation. If we exclude the most impaired language group because of the IQ criterion, we are left with two subgroups of children with *fluent autism* who meet the IQ criterion for HFA, *normal* language learners, and *borderline* language learners. Therefore, two subgroups of HFA children can be identified via the IQ criterion in this study: a group that has a higher IQ and normal language learning, and a group with borderline language and low average IQ (M = 85). The *borderline* language group with low average FSIQ (M = 85; SD = 13.86) may also contain some children who score well within the average range for IQ (>90). The *borderline* language group of children with HFA displayed language impairments in both lexical-semantic and morphosyntactic domains, despite the appearance of fluent verbal ability and the ability to attend to a complete standardized measures of language functioning.

2.1 Differences in standardized testing versus spontaneous language function

In a follow-up study of the identified cohort group of 44 high-functioning children from the original Kjelgaard and Tager-Flusberg (2001) study , Condouris, Meyer, & Tager-Flusberg (2003) further investigated the lexical-semantic and grammatical domains of language functioning using both standardized measures and spontaneous language sampling . The 44 children with ASD in this study were the group initially described by Kjelgaard and Tager-Flusberg (2001) as the children with ASD who were able to complete the language testing. Recall that, as a group, the 44 children ranged in age from 4-to-14 years (M = 7;3), with IQ functioning above 80, although a wide range in scores was noted for both cognitive domains (VIQ: *M* = 84, range = 53-133; NVIQ: *M* = 90, range = 49-153). The purpose of the Condouris, et al. (2003) study was to compare the use of standardized measures of language with spontaneous language measures, since both types of assessment practices are widely used with children with developmental language delay. Higher level lexical-semantic and morphosyntactic knowledge was assessed using either the CELF-P for children younger than 6 years, or the CELF-III for children age 6 years and above. Natural language samples were also included in order to compare the results from the use of standardized measures of language function with spontaneous speech measures. Spontaneous language sampling was measured for MLU and number of differing word roots used (NDWR). Both spontaneous language measures (MLU and NDWR) demonstrated significantly below average performance for age, with children scoring 2 *SDs* below the reference database. Partial correlations, controlling for the effects of age and Nonverbal IQ, between standardized measures of lexical-semantic processing and morphosyntactic ability with natural spontaneous language measures of MLU and NDWR revealed that all correlations were positive, indicating that the majority of the verbal children with HFA have broad language deficits affecting lexical-semantic processing and morpho-syntactic ability, and that these two domains of language interact and predict language function.

2.2 Interaction between syntactic impairment and lexical-semantic functioning

Following the proposed linkages and associations between lexical-semantic processing and morphosyntactic processing, McGregor, Berns, Owen, Michels, Duff, Bahnsen & Lloyd (2011) sought to move beyond the descriptions of strengths and weaknesses in lexical-semantic and morphosyntactic domains and explore the interactive relationship between syntactic competence and breadth and depth of the semantic lexicon in two groups of children with HFA, one with syntactic deficits, and one group of HFA children without syntactic deficits (McGregor, Berns, Owen, Michels, Duff, Bahnsen & Lloyd, 2011). The study also included a group of non-autistic children with developmental language impairment (e.g. *specific language impairment,* SLI) in order to explore the overlap of language functioning in the two phenotypes. There were two control groups; one an age-matched , typically developing group (AM), and a younger syntactic-matched group (SM). All the children were between 9-to-14 yeas old and all had a Nonverbal IQ > 85, based on the matrices subtest of the *Kaufman Brief Intelligence Test*-2 (Kaufman & Kaufman, 2004). No Verbal IQ score was reported. Children with autism were identified as ASD language impaired (ASDLI) if they scored < 8 (e.g. at least 1 *SD* below the M) on the syntactic subtests (Formulated Sentences and Recalling Sentences) of the CELF−4 (Semel et al., 2003). Likewise, the group of children with SLI, also language impaired, scored more than 1 SD below the mean (e.g. < 8) on the syntactic subtests of the CELF-4. The non-syntactic impaired ASD group scored > 7 on the syntactic subtests of the CELF-4. Breadth and depth of lexical knowledge was assessed using two experimental semantic activities and standardized vocabulary tests, specifically the PPVT-III (Dunn & Dunn, 1997) and the Expressive Vocabulary Test (EVT) (Williams, 2007). The two experimental lexical-semantic tasks were verbal definitions and verbal association tasks. In addition, each participant completed an experimental measure of sentence production, using a sentence formulation format. Each of the three experimental measures used the same 40 concrete and abstract noun and verb stimuli that varied in frequency of occurrence. For the sentence production task, children were asked to produce a sentence for each of the 40 stimuli words; sentences were analyzed for syntactic complexity. The definition task required the child to generate a definition for each of the 40 word stimuli, while the association task asked the child to provide a word association for each word. Children's responses on both the definition and word association tasks were scored using scales from 0-3 for level of completeness, thus generating sensitive measures of depth of word knowledge.

Results showed that the ASDLI group produced fewer clauses during the sentence production task, similar to the SLI group, than the non-language impaired group of children with ASD . This finding was not surprising since the ASDLI and the SLI children were identified as having deficits in syntax prior to the experimental procedures. When breadth and depth of the semantic lexicon was considered, the children with ASDLI and SLI scored below average on the receptive vocabulary measure (PPVT-III), but showed greater deficits for expressive vocabulary, scoring more than one-standard deviation below average on the expressive vocabulary test (EVT) . The non-language impaired ASD group scored within the expected average range for age, much like the typically developing children. Likewise, the ASDLI and SLI groups showed shallow depth of word knowledge producing more incomplete or partially complete word definitions and less mature word associations than the ASD and age-matched typically developing children. A positive correlation was also found between expressive syntax as measured by the sentence formulation and sentence repetition tasks on the CELF-4 and depth of lexical knowledge as measured by the definition and word association tasks. The researchers concluded that the presence or absence of syntactic deficits in verbal, HFA children with ASD predict the breadth and depth of inherent lexical knowledge of the child. Not all children with HFA have syntactic deficits, but when they do, language impaired HFA perform similarly to SLI children and demonstrate sparse lexical semantic knowledge.

3. Language abilities of children with high-functioning autism: Executive function

Impairments in Executive Function (EF) in individuals with idiopathic autism have been hypothesized to be a causal link to the variability in language functioning seen in HFA. Executive function is evident in cognitive behaviors such as planning and cognitive flexibility, referred to as set-shifting; children with autism have been shown to demonstrate impairments in both aspects of EF (cf. Landa and Goldberg, 2005). Working memory, another feature of EF, has also been reported as impaired in individuals with autism (Bennetto, Pennington, & Rogers, 1996; Smith Gabig, 2008). Researchers hypothesize that impairments in EF are mirrored in specific aspects of language, such as complex syntactic and lexical-semantic processing , and that language variability and language competence can be predicted from executive functioning (Landa & Goldberg ; 2005).

A recent study by Landa & Goldberg (2005) examined language functioning relative to social functioning and executive functioning (EF) in 19 school-age children with idiopathic autism (*Mean Age* = 11; range 7.3-17.3), and a Full-Scale IQ in the average range (M = 109.7; range 81-139). Notably, there was a 9 - point difference between the Verbal IQ (M = 113.5; range 90-142) and the Nonverbal IQ scores (M = 104.6; range = 74-135), a difference considered to be indicative of discrepant cognitive functioning between domains for the group, as a whole, in the study (Black, Wallace, Sokoloff & Kentworthy, 2009). Landa & Goldberg (2005) studied two aspects of language function, expressive syntax and comprehension of figurative language , and three areas of EF:, *spatial working memory, planning*, and *cognitive flexibility* in children with HFA and two control groups, one age-matched group, and one IQ matched group. The researchers chose to examine expressive syntax through a sentence formulation task, hypothesizing that complex sentence formulation would be impaired in the HFA children and that compromised syntactic ability would be related to poor performance on EF tasks of spatial memory, planning and cognitive-flexibility. Likewise, a task of figurative language was chosen to evaluate abstract language processing and cognitive flexibility in EF, the ability to shift from one meaning of a word or phrase to another meaning. In addition, the researchers hypothesized that social functioning would also be related to language competence. The researchers hypothesized that children with HFA would perform less well than age-matched, typically developing counterparts on the language and the EF measures , and that specific aspects of language would be correlated with EF and social function.

The Formulated Sentences subtest of the Clinical Evaluation of Language Fundamentals-Revised (CELF-R; Semel, Wiig, & Secord, 1987) was administered to assess the ability to form grammatically and semantically correct sentences. The Test of Language Competence (TLC; Wiig & Secord, 1989) was used to assed the comprehension and interpretation of metaphors and figures-of-speech. Executive function was assessed using selected tasks from the *Cambridge Neuropsychological Test Automated Battery* (CANTAB, Cambridge Cognition, 1996). The subtests used were spatial working memory (SWM), the *Stockings of Cambridge* test, (a measure of spatial planning), and the *Intra-Dimensional/Extra-Dimensional Shift* task to assess cognitive flexibility (set-shifting). All three EF tasks were administered electronically using a PC with a LCD flat panel display touchscreen (cf. Landa & Goldberg , 2005, for a complete description of tasks and procedures). Social functioning was examined using the Social Domain summary score of the Autism Diagnostic Interview (ADI) or the Autism Diagnostic Observation Scale (ADOS).

Results were mixed; the children with HFA showed variable performance on both language measures and measures of EF, ranging from unimpaired to impaired functioning in both domains. The HFA group, as a whole, scored significantly below age and IQ matched controls on the measures of expressive grammar/syntax and understanding and use of figurative language. The investigators noted that, despite having intact IQ (Full Scale, Verbal, and Performance IQ), the majority of the children in the HFA group were impaired in both these areas of language function. The authors suggest that the integrity of the grammar system of children with HFA may be compromised even in the face of fluent verbal ability and the use of full sentences in spontaneous speech. Likewise, impaired abstract language processing, evident in difficulty understanding and interpreting non-literal metaphors and figures-of-speech, is also compromised and may contribute to social dysfunction and poor reading comprehension often seen in children with HFA.

As stated, the HF group also demonstrated more difficulty on all aspects of EF measured in this study including spatial working memory (SWM) , planning, and cognitive flexibility. On the SWM task, children needed to search for a blue token in boxes and to collect enough blue tokens to fill a container on the right-side of the screen. Children with HFA made more within-search and between -search errors, often returning to a previously searched box, a form of perseveration and poor search strategy. Similarly, the children with HFA had more difficulty with the planning task than the typically developing age-matched and IQ-matched groups of children. However, no significant difference between children with HFA and the age-matched or IQ control groups was noted on the cognitive flexibility task. Contrary to the original hypothesis by the researchers, that aspects of EF would be correlated with grammaticality and abstract language processing, no significant correlations were found between aspects of EF and the language measures. Nevertheless, the observed EF difficulty seen in children with HFA for planning and spatial working memory suggests that they have difficulty with frontally mediated task performance relative to age peers.

4. Language abilities of children with high-functioning autism: Neuropsychological perspective

In addition to examining the role of EF, other investigators explore language variability in HFA via a neuropsychological model of language that makes a distinction between basic, mechanical use of language and more complex language skills that require the application of procedural knowledge to complete, such as the language used while reasoning, analyzing, and inferencing (Minshew, Goldstein, Taylor, & Siegel, 1994; Minshew, Goldstein, Siegel, 1995). Minshew et al. (1995) hypothesized that the variability and scatter in language profiles seen in individuals with HFA is characterized by a distinction between intact mechanical versus impaired procedural language abilities that require more complex information processing. The investigators examined 62 individuals with HFA and 50 neurologically and psychiatrically healthy control subjects who met the same distribution of age and IQ as the HFA group. Individuals were included in the study if they had a Verbal and Full Scale IQ of at least 70, and showed academic achievement at the 2nd grade level in reading, spelling, and mathematical skills. The diagnosis of HFA was verified through evaluation of clinical history and current symptoms by a clinical expert using either the ADOS (Lord, et al., 1989) or the ADI-R (LeCouteur et al., 1989). The mean age for the autistic group was 17.79 (SD = 10), and the mean age for the control group was 16.91 (SD =

9.96). The mean Verbal IQ and Full Scale IQ for the HFA group was > 90 (VIQ = 94; SD = 16.9; Mean FSIQ = 93 , SD = 14.4), similar to the control group.
Tests requiring basic mechanical or procedural language versus complex information processing were chosen to test the hypothesis that individuals with HFA would perform differently between these two distinctive types of language function. Five language tasks were used to assess basic procedural use of language: Animal Naming (Goodglass & Kaplan, 1972), Controlled Oral-Word Association (Benton & Hamsher, 1976), and three basic reading subtests (Word Attack, Word Identification, Visual-Auditory Learning) of the Woodcock Reading Mastery Test-Revised (WRMT-R) (Woodcock, 1987). More complex propositional language functioning was assessed by two reading comprehension subtests of the WRMT-R (Word Comprehension, Passage Comprehension), four measures of inferencing and figurative language from the Test of Language Competence (TLC; Wiig & Secord, 1985), and two measures of attention and working memory from the *Detroit Test of Learning Aptitude-2* (DTLA-2; Hammill, 1985) , the Oral Directions and Word Repetition subtests. Table 1 contains the list of tests used to tap basic/mechanical language versus complex propositional language. Results of the study confirmed the hypothesis that individuals with HFA are unimpaired in basic, procedural language, yet demonstrate significant impairment in more complex, propositional language observed in impaired expressive formulation, verbal reasoning, and figurative language. Minshew and colleagues attribute the deficits seen in language and reading comprehension and in the understanding and use of complex language as reflective of broad deficits in information processing for individuals with HFA.

Mechanical or Procedural Language Skills	Complex Language Skills
Animal Naming	Test of Language Competence (TLC) • Ambiguous Sentences • Making Inferences • Recreating Sentences • Metaphoric Expressions
Controlled Oral Word Reading Association	Detroit Test of Learning Aptitude (DTLA) • Oral Directions • Word Recall
WRMT-R • Word-Attack • Word Identification • Visual-auditory Learning	WRMT-R • Word Comprehension • Passage Comprehension

Table 1. Tests Used to Assess Mechanical/Procedural Basic Language and Complex Language Skills (adapted from Minshew, Goldstein, & Siegel, 1995).

4.1 Summary of language abilities in HFA

In summary, children with HFA vary considerably in language functioning with some children demonstrating normal language abilities, and some exhibiting impaired language functioning, scoring one or two standard deviations below expected standard scores for chronological age on language tasks measuring complex language processing. Severe or profound language impairment is not found in the profile of language performance in high-functioning, verbal, fluent autism. Based on the studies reviewed, a number of trends can me seen in the research about language functioning in *fluent autism*:

- Children with HFA are more likely to be able to attend to and complete standardized language and academic achievement testing.
- Intact verbal ability is often associated with a Higher Full Scale and /or Verbal IQ. Children with HFA and a FSIQ > 90 may present with language abilities in the normal range on standardized testing , including the areas of lexical-semantic processing and morphosyntactic abilities
- A FSIQ between 70-84 is often accompanied by borderline to impaired language functioning in both lexical-semantic and morphosyntactic domains.
- A pattern of better expressive language composite scores over receptive composite scores may be seen on the CELF, suggesting that the overall fluent verbal ability of children with HFA appears better than the ability to understand and process language. This trend may be reversed when performance on receptive/expressive vocabulary tests is examined. When comparing the PPVT and the EVT standard scores, language impaired HFA children score significantly poorer on the expressive measure than the receptive measure suggesting that naming and retrieving labels for objects/actions is more difficult for language impaired children with HFA.
- The presence or absence of syntactic deficits predicts overall language competence. Children with HFA who are display syntactic ability in the normal range, evidenced by the ability to formulate grammatically and semantically correct sentences, also demonstrate adequate lexical-semantic processing for vocabulary, word associations, and definitions. Children with HFA who have deficits in syntax usually demonstrate difficulty in the lexical-semantic aspects of language competence as well, including shallow breadth and depth of word knowledge.
- Language ability may be intact for basic, procedural language function, yet impaired for more complex language abilities such as understanding and using figurative language, completing complex oral directions, recalling words, and reading comprehension.

5. Variability in word reading accuracy and reading comprehension in children with HFA

Two skills are necessary for children to become independent readers: they must be able to decode the individual words on the page and they must be able to comprehend the text. The Simple View of Reading (Gough & Tunmer, 1986; Hoover & Gough, 1990) defines reading ability as a function of decoding and language comprehension skills. Word reading accuracy refers to single word reading in general, either by sight word recognition, word reading via the phonetic decoding of graphemes to phonemes, (e.g. sounding-out the printed word to its phonological corollary), or by determining the word pronunciation through structural analogy (Ehri, 1998). Text comprehension refers to the cognitive processes involved in transforming print into meaning. (Coltheart, 2006). Although intricately related, there is evidence that skill in word reading recognition is necessary, but not sufficient, for reading comprehension. Individuals may demonstrate adequate and fluent word recognition yet have poor reading comprehension referred to as a specific comprehension deficit (Cain & Oakhill, 2007). Despite the importance of literacy to academic functioning and social achievement, relatively few studies focus on reading ability in children with HFA.

5.1 Word reading accuracy

Research is beginning to emerge in the literature that shows word reading ability is quite variable within the ASD population (Nation, Clarke, Wright, & Williams, 2006; Smith Gabig, 2010). There is a common belief in educational settings and clinical practice that children and adolescents with ASD have advanced word reading, referred to as *hyperlexia*, yet have significant difficulty in reading comprehension. However, recent research challenges this notion of advance word reading skill in ASD (Nation et al, 2006; Smith Gabig, 2010). A recent investigation by Nation, et al. (2006) focused on patterns of component reading skills (e.g. single word identification, nonword decoding, reading text accuracy, and text comprehension) in 41 children with ASD between 6 and 15 years (Mean age = 10.8). Intellectual functioning was measured via the *Block Design* subtest from the *Wechsler Intelligence Scale for Children* (WISC-III; Wechsler, 1992), a measure of nonverbal intelligence. The Block Design mean score for the group was 8.4 (SD = 5.58) , based on a subtest mean of 10, SD +/- 3, indicating that , as a group, the participants scored in the normal range of nonverbal intelligence. However, there is a large standard deviation, so some of the children scored in the mentally retarded range for nonverbal intelligence, other scores in the normal range or above for nonverbal intelligence. Although a HFA subgroup of children cannot be extrapolated from this study, it is included here as a general discussion of overall patterns of reading ability in a heterogeneous group of children with ASD, and nonverbal intellectual ability in the average range. Sixteen of the subjects with ASD met the diagnostic criteria for autism, while 13 met the diagnostic criteria for atypical autism. The remaining children with ASD were considered as Asperger's syndrome. The investigators measured word reading, nonword decoding ability, reading connected text, and reading comprehension. There were two measures of oral language: a receptive vocabulary measure and an oral language comprehension task taken from the WISC-III. Nine (22%) of the children were completely unable to read at all; these children were excluded from further analyses. The 32 participants who were able to complete the reading assessment battery showed word reading accuracy (e.g. word reading, nonword decoding, text reading) in the normal range , although significant variability in performance was noted in the range of scores and in behavioral observation. Some children with ASD show accurate word reading yet were poor comprehenders, other children showed poor word reading ability for real words and nonwords, and some were able to read real words adequately, but could not apply phonetic decoding skills for nonwords (Nation, et al., 2006). Nation and her colleagues speculated that children with autism may have difficulty applying phonological coding strategies when faced with unfamiliar letter sequences as in a nonsense word reading , and may be relying on a visual association or visual memory when asked to read aloud words in a word identification reading task.

Discrepancies in word reading accuracy and weak phonetic decoding have also been reported for children with HFA (Smith Gabig, 2010). Fourteen school-age children with autism, and 10 age-matched, typically developing (TD) children between 5-7 years, were given two measures of single word recognition during reading, the word identification (WID) subtest and the phonetic decoding of nonwords, or word attack (WATTK) subtest from the Woodcock Reading Mastery Test-Revised (Woodcock, 1987). The children with HFA demonstrated nonverbal intelligence in the average range (M = 96; SD = 8), measured using the short nonverbal cognitive composite from the *Differential Abilities Scale (DAS)*, (Elliot, 1983). Two measures of phonological awareness ability were also given to the two groups of children, the *elision* task (ELI) and a *sound blending* task (BLW) from the *Comprehensive Test of Phonological Processing* (CTOPP; Wagner, Torgesen, & Rashotte, 1999). Receptive vocabulary and speech articulation skill was also measured using the *Peabody Picture Vocabulary Test-Revised,* (PPVT-R, Dunn & Dunn, 1997) and the articulation subtest of the *Test of Language Development –Primary* (TOLD-P; Newcomer & Hammill, 1997).

Word reading accuracy scores for WID and WATTK were in the average range for both groups of children, and no significant difference was seen for word reading accuracy between the HFA and the TD groups. However, children with HFA showed a statistical performance bias for single real word reading over phonetic decoding in nonword reading, a pattern not seen in the typically developing children. Although scoring within the average range of expected performance for age, clinical observation of nonword reading indicated that the children with autism struggled more with reading nonwords than real words, suggesting a divergence in ability between the direct lexical route to reading words and the indirect, non-lexical route involving a phonological recoding of an unfamiliar, written word (Coltheart, 2006; Coltheart, Rastle, Perry, Langdon, & Ziegler, 2001). A closer investigation of the individual word recognition profiles of each child with autism by Smith Gabig (2010) revealed that 60% (n = 9) struggled while reading nonwords, characterized by slow and labored decoding attempts that often were not accurate. Two of the children (22%) attempted to parse the individual graphemes/phoneme relationship and sound-out the nonword but could not blend the individual phonemes into a whole. The remaining two children (22%) were able to decode the nonwords rapidly and efficiently.

Adequate word recognition has also been demonstrated in older, high-functioning adolescents with autism. Minshew et al. (1994) examined academic achievement, including reading ability, in 54 high-functioning (FSIQ Mean = 95; SD 15.5) adolescent males and an age, gender, and cognitively-matched control group of 41 typically developing males. Reading ability was evaluated using the *Woodcock Reading Mastery Test-Revised* (Woodcock, 1987) and subtests from the *Kaufman Test of Educational Achievement* (Kaufman & Kaufman, 1995). They also included measures of complex oral language processing including the Oral Directions and Word Sequences subtests form the *Detroit Test of Learning Aprtitude-2* (Hammill, 1985). Results indicated that the HFA adolescents performed similarly to their age-matched counterparts in both word identification (sight-word vocabulary reading) and word attack (decoding of nonwords). However, contrary to the results reported by Nation et al. (2006) , and Smith Gabig, (2010) Minshew and colleagues found that nonword reading was slightly better than sight-word identification in the HFA adolescents, suggesting a heightened ability to apply phonetic analysis skills to decode nonwords. As expected, performance on the passage comprehension measure was significantly different between the two groups, with the adolescents with autism scoring significantly lower than the age-matched, typically developing cohorts. The HFA group also scored lower and statistically different on the oral language measures (e.g. Oral Directions ; Word Sequences *DTLA-2*). As noted previously , Minshew and colleagues found significant differences for composite scores that contrasted basic, mechanic/procedural skills versus more complex language comprehension skills. Both oral and reading composite comprehension scores were lower for the HFA group relative to composite scores for basic mechanical skill, exemplified in word identification and word decoding in reading.

5.2 Phonological awareness

Research over the past 30 years has shown that to be a good and accurate word reader or decoder, one must have a strong conceptualization of the underlying phonological structure of words (cf. National Reading Panel, 2000). Conscious awareness of the discrete sounds in words and the ability to manipulate sounds in words is critically tied to the development of word recognition and decoding ability in reading (Bradley & Bryant, 1983; Fox. & Routh , 1975; Liberman, Shankweiler, et al., 1974; Stanovich, 1986; Swank & Catts, 1994; Wagner & Torgesen, 1987). In order to acquire accuracy and speed in word recognition while reading, a child must apply knowledge of the sound structure represented by letters and letter combinations seen in print. Phonological awareness has been shown to play a critical role in both the decoding of unfamiliar words but also in the expansion of a sight-word vocabulary that can be easily recognized orthographically and transformed into its spoken form (Ehri, 1998; Share & Stanovich, 1995). Although phonological awareness plays a central role in development and accuracy of word reading ability little direct evidence exists on the emergence of phonological awareness ability and its relationship to word reach development and accuracy in children with ASD.

Children with HFA have also been shown to score below age-matched, typically developing children on tasks of phonological awareness (Smith Gabig , 2010). Fourteen children with high-functioning autism were given two measures of phonological awareness, a sound blending task and an elision task, which required the child to segment words into smaller parts. The children were also given two word reading measures from the WRMT-R (Woodcock, 1987) single word reading (Word Identification) and the phonetic decoding of nonwords (Word Attack). All participants were also tested for receptive vocabulary, using the PPVT-R (Dunn & Dunn, 1997), and speech articulation.

Dunn & Dunn, 1997), and speech articulation. The children with HFA scored significantly below their age-matched counterparts for phonological awareness and receptive vocabulary. There was no difference between the HFA group and the TD children on the word reading measures, or speech articulation. Also, no correlation was found between measures of phonological awareness and measures of word reading for the children with HFA, unlike the TD group who demonstrated a strong relationship between phoneme segmentation ability on the elision task and phonetic decoding of unfamiliar nonwords. Research on typically developing children has shown a strong and predictive relationship between phoneme awareness and word reading ability (Liberman, et al., 1974; Vellutino & Scanlon, 1987; Wagner & Torgesen, 1987).

Phonological awareness is a metalinguistic skill that may be inhibited in development for children with autism. Perhaps there are linguistic factors that may influence the development of phonological awareness. In the Smith Gabig (2010) study, a measure of receptive vocabulary (PPVT-R; Dunn & Dunn, 1997), was significantly related to performance on the elision task of phonological awareness for the children with HFA ($r = .62$, $p < .01$). The positive relationship between receptive vocabulary score and performance on the elision task for the HFA children suggests that reduced vocabulary size may hinder and delay the development of more cognitively demanding phonological analysis skills by the children with autism. There is increasing evidence that vocabulary size and phonological similarity among words in the lexicon helps to explain individual differences in aspects of phonological awareness, in typically developing children (Metsala, 1997; Metsala, 1999; Metsala & Walley, 1998; Rvaachew, 2006; Service, 2006). Evidence for this theoretical framework is seen in studies that demonstrate that typically developing children are sensitive to the phonotactic probability of nonwords (Edwards, Beckman, & Munson, 2004). Phonotactic probability refers to the likelihood that sublexical sequences of sounds may occur in a lexical item and is related to stored phonological representations and abstractions of lexemes in the lexicon. As children's vocabulary increases, their stored representations of possible phonetic sequences become more robust and defined, facilitating the phonological parsing words. In this study, the children with autism had lower overall receptive vocabulary scores than the typically developing children, consistent with the extant research demonstrating reduced vocabulary size for age (Kjelgaard, & Tager-Flusberg, 2001; Tager-Flusberg, 2003). This limitation in oral language functioning may have a significant impact on the development of phonological awareness ability in the children.

5.3 Reading comprehension

Reading comprehension is the cognitive ability in which meaning is assigned to written text. It is often described as an interactive process between the reader, the text, and the context (Cain & Oakhill, 2007; Whittaker, Gambrell, & Morrow, 2004). In order to comprehend written text, one must construct meaning of individual words, phrases, and sentences and integrate smaller aspects of meaning into the whole, constructing the larger meaning contained within the connected text. As one reads, one draws upon general knowledge to help process text and construct meaning. Children with autism often demonstrate reading comprehension difficulty, despite adequate word reading ability (Nation et al., 2006). Two factors may influence reading comprehension and literacy in children with autism. One factor is oral language competence, especially competence in the structural aspects of language (phonology, morphology, and syntax). The other factor as a possible source of variability in literacy achievement and reading comprehension is cognitive deficits (Norbury & Nation, 2010). Nation et al. (2006) reported significant variability in reading comprehension in 32 high-functioning children with autism, with the majority of the children (65%; N = 20) showing moderately impaired reading comprehension scores 1 SD below the expected mean, while the remaining 12 children (N = 38%) demonstrating significantly impaired reading comprehension, scoring more than 2 SD's below expected norms for age. Nation et al. divided the group of children into two groups, those scoring more than 2 SD below the mean (*Poor Comprehenders* ; SS < 85) and a group scoring 1 SD below expected performance for age (*Skilled Comprehenders* ; SS > 85. *Poor Comprehenders* showed adequate word reading accuracy, yet displayed significant impairments in oral language measures, (e.g. receptive vocabulary, oral comprehension) and low average nonverbal ability (Mean = 7.7; SD = 6.6) compared to the *Skilled Comprehenders* who demonstrated accurate word reading ability, as well receptive vocabulary and nonverbal ability in the average range. Thus, it appears that oral language competence and average cognitive ability bodes better for reading comprehension ability in children with HFA.

5.4 Influence of oral language competence and literacy

A recent study by Norbury & Nation (2010) directly addressed the question of the influence of oral language competence to reading comprehension and word reading accuracy in children with HFA. The researchers examined two phenotypes of individuals with HFA: one group with age-appropriate structural language (ALN), and a group with structural language deficits (ALI). Twenty-seven adolescent males were recruited for the study.

Thirteen adolescents with HFA were identified as language impaired via clinical history and current testing, scoring at least -1.25 SD on the Recalling Sentences subtest of the CELF (Semel, et al., 2003). The remaining 14 HFA adolescents demonstrated normal language functioning. Nonverbal ability was in the average range for both groups of adolescents with HFA. Nineteen age-matched and cognitive-matched typically developing adolescents were also recruited. The researches measured word reading ability, text reading accuracy, and reading comprehension using standardized test. Experimental measures were used to explore the adolescents' ability to use integrative and inferential comprehension monitoring processes while reading. Oral language competence was assessed for receptive vocabulary, nonword repetition, and oral language comprehension. Results revealed that language status was related to accuracy in word reading. The ALI group showed lower word reading and decoding ability than the ALN group, yet the ALN group also scored lower than the TD control group, suggesting that in addition to language status, group status influences word reading ability. In addition, language status also influenced comprehension monitoring and inferencing with the ALI group scoring significantly lower than the ALN and TD groups. Further analysis revealed that oral language competence uniquely influenced reading comprehension, beyond any variance accounted for word-reading accuracy alone. It appears that oral language competence uniquely contributes to reading comprehension.

5.5 Summary of variability in word reading and reading comprehension

High-functioning children with autism demonstrate variability in reading skill with some individuals able to read and decode words accurately with good passage comprehension, while others demonstrate a discrepancy between the domains of word reading accuracy and comprehension, with poor comprehension for connected text. Although word reading accuracy for sight words and for phonetic decoding of nonwords appears average for age in the HFA children, several studies have noted that phonetic decoding of nonwords is weaker, or less developed, than single word reading (Nation et al., 2006; Smith Gabig, 2010), although one study (Minshew et al., 1994) reported the reverse finding, that nonword reading had an advantage over real word reading. From a neuropsychological perspective, word reading accuracy is considered a basic/mechanical, procedural skill (Minshew et al., 1994; 1995) while text comprehension is considered as complex information processing. The significant contribution of oral language competence to reading comprehension cannot be ignored. HFA adolescents with structural language impairment are at high risk for impaired reading comprehension and its component skills, such as comprehension monitoring and inferencing.

6. Overall conclusions: Variability in language and reading

Significant variability is seen in language and literacy functioning in children with HFA, influenced by intellectual ability and oral language competence. Verbal children meeting the IQ criterion to be considered as having HFA demonstrate one of two oral language profiles: intact oral language ability or mild to moderate oral language difficulty in the domains of lexical -semantic and morphosyntactic processing. Those children with HFA and intact oral language functioning also score in the average to above average range for intellectual functioning. Lower intellectual achievement, in the low average or below average range (yet absent mental retardation), is associated with language deficits. Likewise, oral language competence and cognitive ability influence word reading accuracy and reading comprehension in HFA. It appears that deficits in receptive vocabulary and complex oral language processing, as well as below average nonverbal cognitive ability (absent mental retardation), are associated with variable performance on word reading accuracy, phonological processing, and poor reading comprehension. Skilled reading comprehenders demonstrate the opposite profile: accurate word reading ability, oral language in the average range, and average nonverbal intellectual achievement. What is not fully known is the relationship between the clinical history of the scope and severity of the symptom of speech language delay in the preschool years, later resolved or recovered, and language and reading functioning in the school-age child or adolescent with HFA. Do those children with HFA, with a clinical history of mild to moderate oral language delay and nonverbal intelligence in the average to above average range , go on to achieve adequate reading competence when oral language issues are recovered or resolved? Future research should address the trajectory of language development, overall language competence, and reading achievement associated with average to below average (absent mental retardation) intellectual functioning in children with HFA. Such research may inform us regarding those variables that most likely predict later average oral language and literacy functioning in children with HFA, and influence the intervention practices for children with HFA.

7. References

American Psychiatric Association. (APA), (1994). *Diagnostic and statistical manual of mental disorders* (4th ed.), Washington, DC: Author

Asarnow, r.F., Tanguay, P.E., bott, L., & Freeman, B.J. (1987). Patterns of intellectual functioning in non- retarded autistic and schizophrenic children. Journal of Child Psychology and psychiatry, 28, 273- 280.

Bradley, L., & Bryant, P. (1983). Categorizing sounds and learning to read: A causal connection. *Nature*, 301, 419-421.

Bartak, L. & Rutter, M. (1976). Differences between mentally retarded and normally intelligent autistic children. *Journal of Autism and Childhood Schizophrenia*, 6, 109-120.

Bennetto, L., Pennington, B.F., & Rogers, S. J. (1996). Intact and impaired memory function in autism. Child Development, 67, 1816-1835.

Benton, A. L. & Hamsher, K. deS. 91976). *Multilingual aphasia examination.* Iowa city: University of Iowa.

Black, d. O., Wallace, G.L., Sokoloff, J. L., Kenworthy, L. (2009). Brief report: IQ split predicts social symptoms and communication abilities in High-functioning children with autism spectrum disorders. *Journal of Autism and Developmental Disorders*, 39, 1613-1619.

Cain, K., & Oakhill, J. V. (2007). Reading comprehension difficulties: Correlates, causes, and consequences. In K. Cain & J.V.Oakhill, (Eds.), *Children's comprehension problems in oral and written language: A cognitive perspective.* New York: Guildford Press.

Cambridge Cognition. (1996). CANTAB. Cambridge, England: Cambridge Cognition Limited.

Catts, H.W., Fey, M.E., Zhang, X., & Tomblin, J.B. (1999). Language basis of reading and reading disabilities: Evidence from a longitudinal investigation. *Scientific Studies of Reading*, 3, 331-361.

Cazden, C. 91988). Cazden, C. (1988). *Classroom Discourse*. Portsmouth, NH: Heinemann.

Coltheart, M. (2006). Dual route and connectionist models of reading: An overview. *London Review of Education, 4*, (1), 5-17.

Coltheart M., Rastle, K., Perry, C., Langdon, R., & Ziegler, J. (2001). DRC: A dual route cascaded model of visual word recognition and reading aloud. *Psychological Review*, 108, 204-256.

Condouris, K., Meyer, E., & Tager-Flusberg, H. (2003). The relationship between standardized measures of language and measures of spontaneous speech in children with autism. *American Journal of Speech-Language Pathology*, 12, 349-358.

Dunn, L.M. & Dunn, L.M. (1997). *Peabody Picture Vocabulary Test-Revised*. Circle Pines, MN: American Guidance Service.

Edwards, J., Beckman, M.E., & Munson, B. (2004). The interaction between vocabulary size and phonotactic probability effects on children's production accuracy and fluency in nonword repetition. *Journal of Speech, Language, and Hearing Research*, 47, 421-436.

Ehri, L. C. (1998).Grapheme-phoneme knowledge is essential for learning to read words in English. In J. L. Metsala & L. C. Ehri (Eds.), *Word recognition in beginning reading* (pp. 3-40). Hillsdale, NJ: Lawrence Erlbaum.

Elliot, C. D. (1983). *Differential Ability Scale*. San Antonia, TX: The Psychological Corporation.

Fox, B. & Routh, D. K. (1975). Analyzing spoken language into words, syllables, and phonemes: A developmental study. *Journal of Psycholinguistic Research*, 4, 331-342.

Freeman, B. J., Lucas, J.C., Forness, S.R., & Ritvo, E.R. (1985). Cogntive processing of high-functioning autistic children: Comparing the K-ABC and the WISC-R. *Journal of Psychoeducational Assessment*, 4. 357-362.

Goldman, R. & Fristoe, M. (1986). The *Goldman-Fristoe Test of Articulation*. Circle Pines, MN: American Guidance Service.

Goodglass, H. & Kaplan, e. (1972). Assessment of aphasia and related disorders. Philadelphia: Lea & Febiger.

Hammill, d.D. (1985). *DTLA-2; Detroit Tests of Learning Aptitude*. Austin, TX: Pro-Ed.

Howlin, P. (2005). Outcomes in autism spectrum disorders. In Volkmar, F.R.; Paul, R; Klin, A; & Cohen, D.J., (Eds.), *Handbook Of Autism And Pervasive Developmental Disorders*, 3rd edition. New York: John Wiley and Sons, pp 201-220.

Jones, c.d. & Schwartz, I.S. (2009). When asking questions is not enough: An observational study of social communication differences in high functioning children with autism. *Journal of Autism and Developmental Disorders*, 39. 432-443.

Kaufman, A.S. & Kaufman,, N. L. (2004). *The Kaufman Brief Intelligence Test-2*. Circle pines, MN: American Guidance Services.

Kjelgaard, M.A. & Tager-Flusberg, H. (2001). An investigation of language profiles in autism: Implications for genetic subgroups. *Language and Cognitive Processes*, 15, 1-22.

Landa , R.J. & Goldberg, M. C. (2005). Language , social, and executive functions in high functioning autism: A continuum of performance. . *Journal of Autism and Developmental Disorders*, 35. 557-573.

LeCouteur, A., Rutter, M., Lord, C., Rios, P., Robertson, S., et al.. (1989). Autism diagnostic interview: A standardized investigaror-based instrument. *Journal of Autism and Developmental Disorders*, 19, 363- 387.

Liberman, I. Y., Shankweiler, D., Fischer, F.W., & Carter, B. (1974). Explicit syllable and phoneme segmentation in the young child. *Journal of Experimental Child Psychology*, 18, 201-212.

Lord, C., Risi, S., Lambrecht, L., Cook, E., Leventhal, B., DiLavore, P., Pickles, A., & Rutter; M. (2000). The autism diagnostic observation schedule-generic: A standard measure of social and communication deficits associated with the spectrum of autism. *Journal of Autism and Developmental Disorders*, 30, 205-223.

Lord, C., Rutter, M., & Le Couteur, A. (1994). Autism Diagnostic Interview-Revised. *Journal of Autism and Developmental Disorders*, 24, 659-685.

Losh, M. & Capps, L. (2003). Narrative ability in high-functioning children with autism or Asperger's syndrome. *Journal of Autism and Developmental Disorders*, 23, 239-251.

Loveland, K.A.& Tunali-Kotoski, B. (2005). The school-aged child with an autistic spectrum disorder. In F. Volkmar, A. Klin & R. Paul (eds.), *The Handbook of Autism and Pervasive Developmental Disorders* (3rd ed., pp. 247-287). New York : Wiley.

Mayes, S.D.; Calhoun, S. L. (2008). WISC-IV and WIAT-II profiles in children with high-functioning autism. Journal of Autism and Developmental Disorders, 38, 428-439.

McGregor, K.K., Berns, A.J., Owen, A.J., Michels, S.A., Duff, D., Bahnsen, A.J., & Lloyd, M. (2011). Associations between syntax and the lexicon among children with or without ASD and language impairment.

Metsala, J. L. (1997). Spoken word recognition in reading disabled children. *Journal of Educational Psychology, 89*, 159-169.

Metsala, J. L. (1999). Young children's phonological awareness and nonword repetition as a function of vocabulary development. *Journal of Educational Psychology, 91*, 3-19.

Metsala, J. L., & Walley, A. C. (1998). Spoken vocabulary growth and the segmental restructuring of lexical representations: Precursors to phonemic awareness and early reading ability. In J. L. Metsala & L. C. Ehri (Eds.), *Word recognition in beginning literacy* (pp. 89 -120). Mahwah, NJ: Lawrence Erlbaum Associates.

Minshew, N.J. & Goldstein, G. (1998). Autism as a disorder of complex information processing. *Mental Retardation and Developmental Disabilities Research Reviews* , 4: 129-136.

Minshew, N. J., Goldstein, G. & Siegel, D. J. (1995). Speech and language in high-functioning autistic individuals . *Neuropsychology*, 9, 225-261.

Minshew, N. J., Goldstein, G., Taylor, H. G., & Siegel, D. J. (1994). Academic achievement in high functioning autistic individuals. *Journal of Clinical and Experimental Neuropsychology, 16*, 261-270.

Nation, K., Clarke, P., Wright, B., & Williams, C. (2006). Patterns of reading ability in children with autism spectrum disorder. *Journal of Autism and Developmental Disorders, 36*, 911-919.

Nation, K., Clarke, P., Marshall, C..M., & Durand, M. (2004). Hidden language impairments in children: parallels between poor reading comprehension and specific language impairment? *Journal of Speech-Language-Hearing Research*, 47, 199-211.

National Institute of Child Health and Human Development. (2000). *Report of the National Reading Panel. Teaching children to read: An evidence-based assessment of the scientific research literature on reading and its implications for reading instruction* (NIH Publication No. 00-4769). Washington, DC: U.S. Government Printing Office.Newcomer, P.L. & Hammill, D.D. (1997). Test of Language Development: Primary. Austin: Pro-Ed.

Norbury, C. & Nation, K, (2010). Understanding variability in reading comprehension in adolescents with autism spectrum disorders: Interactions with language status and decoding skill. Scientific Studies of Reading, 1-20.

Rice, M.L., Warren, S. F., & Betz, S. K. (2005). Language symptoms of developmental language disorders: An overview of autism, Down syndrome, fragile X, specific language impairment, and Williams syndrome. *Applied Psycholinguistics*, 26, 7-27.

Roth, F.P., Speece, D.L., Cooper, D.H., & De La Paz, S. (1996). Unresolved mysteries: How do metalinguistic and narrative skills connect with early reading? *Journal of Special Education, 30*, 257-277.

Rvachew, S. (2007). Longitudinal predictors of implicit phonological awareness skills. *American Journal of Speech-Language Pathology*, 15, 165-176.

Service, E. (2006). Phonological networks and new word learning. *Applied Psycholinguistics*, 27, 581-584).

Semel, E., Wiig, E.H., & Secord, W.A. (2003). *Clinical Evaluation of Language Fundamentals*, Fourth Edition. San Antonio: Pearson Publishing.

Semel, E., Wiig, E.H., & Secord, W.A. (1995). *Clinical Evaluation of Language Fundamentals*, Third Edition. San Antonio: The Psychological Corporation, Harcourt Brace & Co.

Semel, E., Wiig, E.H., & Secord, W.A. (1987). *Clinical Evaluation of Language Fundamentals, Revised*. San Antonio: The Psychological Corporation, Harcourt Brace & Co.

Share, D. L. & Stanovich, K.E. (1995). Cognitive processing in early reading development: A model of acquisition and individual differences. *Issues in Education: Contributions from Educational Psychology*, 1, 1-57

Shriberg, L., Paul, R., McSweeny, J., Klin, A., Cohen, D., & Volkmar, F. (2001). Speech and prosody characteristics of adolescents and adults with high-functioning autism and Asperger syndrome. *Journal of Speech, Language, and Hearing Research*, 44, 1097-1115.

Smith Gabig, C. (2008). Verbal working memory and story-retelling in school-age children with autism. *Language, Speech, and Hearing Services in Schools*, 39, 498-511.

Smith Gabig, C. (2010). Phonological Awareness and Word Recognition in Reading by Children with Autism. Communication Disorders Quarterly, 31, 67-85.

Snyder, L.S. & Downey, D.M. (1991). The language-reading relationship in normal and reading disabled children. *Journal of Speech-Language-Hearing Research*. Vol.34 129-140.

Stanovich, K.E. (1986). Explaining the variance in reading ability in terms of psychological processes. What have we learned? *Annals of Dyslexia*, 35, 67-96.

Stone, W. L., & Caro-Martinez, L. M. (1990). Naturalistic observations of spontaneous communication in autistic children. *Journal of Autism and Developmental Disorders*, 20, 437-453.

Swank, L.K. & Catts, H.W. (1994). Phonological awareness and written word decoding. *Language, Speech, and Hearing Services in Schools*, 25, 9-14.

Tager-Flusberg, H. (2003). Language impairment in children with complex neurodevelopmental disorders: The case of autism. In Levy, Y. & Schaeffer, J. (Eds.), *Language Competence Across Populations*. New Jersey: Lawrence Erlbaum Associates.

Tager-Flusberg, H. (1999). A psychological approach to understanding the social and language impairments in autism. *International Review of Psychiatry*, 11, 325-334.Tager-Flusberg, H. (1996). Current theory and research on language and Communication in autism. *Journal of Autism and Developmental Disorders*,26, 169–172.

Tager-Flusberg, H., Paul, R., & Lord, C. (2005). Language and communication in autism. In D. J. Cohen & F. R. Volkmar (Eds.), Handbook of autism and pervasive developmental disorders (3rd ed., pp. 335– 364). New York: John Wiley and Sons.

Tager-Flusberg, H., Rogers, S., Cooper, J., Landa, R., Lord, C., Paul, R., Rice, M., Stoel-Gammon, C., Wetherby, A., Yoder, P. (2009). Defining spoken language benchmarks and selecting measures expressive language development for young children with autism spectrum disorders. *Journal of Speech-Language-Hearing Research*, 52, 643-652.

Vellutino, F.R. & Scanlon, D.M. (1991). The preeminence of phonologically based skills in learning to read. In S. A. Brady & D.P. Shankweiler (Eds.) *Phonological Processes in Literacy*. New Jersey: Lawrence Erlbaum Associates.

Wagner, R. K. & Torgesen, J.K. (1987). The nature of phonological processing and its causal role in the acquisition of reading skills. *Psychological Bulletin*, 101, 192- 212.

Wagner, R. K., Torgesen, J. K., & Rashotte, C. A. (1999). *Comprehensive Test of Phonological Processing*. Austin: Pro-Ed.

Wechsler, d. (1992). *Wechsler Intelligence scale for Children, 3rd Ed.* . London: The Psychological Press

Whittaker, C.P., Gambrell, L.B., Morrow,L. M. (2004). Reading comprehension instruction for all students. In E.R. Siliman & L.C. Wildonson (Eds.*), Language and Literacy Learning in Schools*. New York: The Guilford Press.

Wiig, e. H.., & Secord, W. 91985). *Test of Language Competence*. San Antonio, TX: Psychological Corp.

Wiig, E.H., & Semel, E.(1992). *Clinical Evaluation of Language- Preschool*. San Antonio: The Psychological Corporation, Harcourt Brace & Co.

Wilkinson, K.M. (1998). Profiles of language and communication in autism. Mental Retardation and Developmental Disabilities Research reviews, 4; 73-79.

Woodcock, R. (1987). *Woodcock Reading Mastery Tests, Revised*. Circle Pines, MN: American Guidance Service

World Health Organization , (1992). International Classification of Diseases, 10th Ed., Geneva, Switzerland.

Part 2

Parenting and Autism Spectrum Disorders

5

Parenting Stress in Mothers and Fathers of Children with Autism Spectrum Disorders

Ewa Pisula
University of Warsaw
Poland

1. Introduction

A number of studies have demonstrated that parents of children with developmental disabilities experience higher levels of stress than parents of typically developing children (e.g. Hodapp et al., 2003; Johnson et al., 2003). Webster and colleagues (2008) found that the scores in the Parenting Stress Index were above 85th percentile in over 40% of parents of children with developmental delay, indicating significant parenting stress.

Parental stress is viewed as a complex set of non-specific, persistent and significant challenges associated with one of parents' most important roles, i.e. taking care of their child. Despite a considerable amount of data on stress in parents of children with disabilities, there is still no consensus on the conceptualization of this phenomenon (Perry, 2004). The theoretical framework adopted in a number of studies is the transactional model of stress and coping (Lazarus & Folkman, 1984). In this approach, stress is a particular type of an individual's relationship with the environment, which the individual appraises as putting certain demands or overextending his/her resources, and thus threatening his/her well-being (Lazarus & Folkman, 1984).

Parental stress is associated with the type of disability present in the child (Gupta, 2007). A number of authors have reported higher levels of stress in mothers of children with autism compared with mothers of children with other developmental disabilities, e.g. Down syndrome, fragile X syndrome, severe intellectual disability (Abbeduto et al., 2004; Weiss, 2002; White & Hastings, 2004), parents of children with special health care needs without developmental problems (Schieve et al., 2007) or typically developing children (Baker-Ericzén et al., 2005; Smith et al., 2001; Yamada et al., 2007). Tomanik, Harris and Hawkins (2004) found that two-thirds of mothers of children with autism in their study demonstrated elevated stress levels. Another revealing fact is that parents themselves often use the word "stressful" when talking about raising a child with autism (e.g. Gray, 2002a).

The present review of research on stress in parents of children with autism covers two main issues. In the first part, the most significant sources of parental stress in this group of parents are discussed and the results of research on stress profiles in mothers and fathers are presented. The second part offers an outline of individual determinants of parental stress, associated with personal characteristics of the parent (e.g., their sense of coherence, coping styles and strategies). Conclusion contains a brief account of the consequences of parental stress and potential implications of studies on stress for clinical practice.

2. Causes of stress in parents of children with autism

There are three major groups of factors that contribute to elevated stress in parents of children with autism: (1) child characteristics, in particular behavioural symptoms associated with autism and behavioural problems; (2) lack of adequate professional support and unsatisfactory relationships between parents and professionals from the stage of autism diagnosis to limited access to medical and educational services for the child; (3) social attitudes towards individuals with autism and lack of understanding for problems they and their families experience.

2.1 Child characteristics as a source of parenting stress

According to the currently available information, autism is characterised by the coexistence of three groups of symptoms: impaired social relations and communication, and restricted and repetitive patterns of behaviour (American Psychiatric Association, 2000). All of the above mentioned developmental difficulties may be severely distressing for parents.

So far there is no consensus on the relation between severity of children's impairment and stress in parents of children with autism. Some researchers report the presence of this relationship (e.g. Hastings & Johnson, 2001; Hoffman et al., 2008). Not all authors, however, have confirmed their results (e.g. Tobing & Glenwick, 2002), and some have even suggested that the severity of the child's autism symptoms is a relatively poor predictor of parental stress (Konstantareas & Papageorgiu, 2006). It seems that the root cause of this disparity in research findings are methodological issues, such as sample size, selection criteria and internal differentiation in the groups of parents and children in the studies, as well as the tools used to measure the children's developmental problems.

Furthermore, the role of particular types of the child's developmental and behavioural problems in the aetiology of parental stress is still unclear. Certainly, the most typical signs and symptoms of autism are pervasive deficits in socio-emotional development. They are especially apparent in limited ability of people with autism to initiate and maintain interaction (Volkmar et al., 2004). These difficulties may vary in form and severity, but even people with high-functioning autism (HFA) experience significant problems in interpersonal relations. Studies on parents of children with non-autistic developmental disorders show that low levels of the child's pro-social behaviour are related with the severity of parental stress (Richman et al., 2009). As Davis and Carter (2008) demonstrated in their study on parents of newly-diagnosed children with autism spectrum disorders (ASD), deficits in social relatedness may be a significant burden to parents. Similar results were obtained by Kasari and Sigman (1997), who found a relationship between the level of parental stress and child's responsiveness when interacting with the experimenter.

An important area in which the development of children with autism is untypical is the formation of interpersonal relations with parents. Studies have shown that the majority of these children's mothers consider their child's sings of attachment to be insufficient and rate their emotional reciprocity lower than mothers of children with other disabilities (Abbeduto et al. 2004; Hoppes & Harris, 1990). Even though mothers report that they would like their children to show more signs of attachment, this aspect of the child's functioning appears to be less salient in the emergence of parental stress than other difficulties experienced by mothers. Hoffman and colleagues (2009) found no differences in Attachment Subscale in Parenting Stress Index (PSI) between mothers of children with autism and mothers of typically developing children. Mothers of children with autism in the study reported high levels of stress in all other PSI subscales (both in the Child Domain, and the Parent Domain); their scores in the assessment of demands resulting from relationships with the child were similar to those obtained by mothers of typically developing children. It should be mentioned that mothers of children with autism scored highest in the Child's Domain: their mean PSI scores in these subscales were in the 99th percentile.

Another potential child characteristic which may contribute to elevated parental stress is limited communication with the child. Communication deficits are seen across a range of verbal and nonverbal skills: gestures, intonation, melody, rhythm of utterance, facial expression and posture (Walenski et al., 2006). These children also have difficulties using communication to regulate social relations. Tomanik, Harris and Hawkins (2004) showed that in mothers of children with pervasive developmental disorders (mostly autism) aged 2-7 years, stress is associated with the child's ability to participate in interactions and communicate. Mothers of children with autism report higher stress when their children have poor communication skills (Konstantareas & Papageorgiu, 2006). It should also be mentioned that communication deficits are usually the primary reason why parents seek professional help (Charman & Baird, 2002).

Social relations and communication problems are associated with cognitive impairments affecting children with autism (e.g. Joseph et al., 2002). It appears, however, that intellectual development of the child is not a determinant of the level of parental stress. Parents of high-functioning children with autism or Asperger syndrome also experience elevated stress levels (Mori et al., 2009; Rao & Beidel, 2009).

Among the most important predictors of parents' stress are the child's behaviour problems (Bishop et al., 2007; Estes et al., 2009; Herring et al., 2006; Tomanik et al., 2004). Children with autism present with a number of such problems, including aggression and self-injury (Matson & Rivet, 2008). Self-injury, aggressive and otherwise destructive behaviour are the strongest predictors of parental stress (Dunlap & Robbins, 1994; Richman et al., 2009). The child's stereotyped and self-stimulating behaviours are also a source of distress for parents. The actual degree to which specific behaviour problems contribute to parental stress depends on the child's age. Parents of adolescents cite destructive behaviour and withdrawal from contact as the most significant causes of concern, while self-stimulation and tantrums are mentioned primarily by parents of preschool children (Dunlap & Robbins, 1994).

The child's challenging behaviours, apart from posing direct problems by endangering the safety of the child or others or causing material damage, may also lead to parents' community isolation (Worcester et al., 2008). In addition, parents often feel helpless, seeing that their child's responses to their attempts at calming him down are completely unpredictable and incomprehensible: "*What scared me the most was his crying, and I would do anything to prevent it. When he was crying, I felt lost, because I could not hold him or kiss him since he hated it*" (Grodzka, 1995, p. 217). Thus, the effect of challenging behaviours on parental stress can be complex. Better insight into the relationships between these phenomena would certainly help develop more effective ways of supporting parents.

Impaired adaptive functioning, including lower daily living skills, may also add to the burdens experienced by parents (Fitzgerald et al., 2002; Tomanik et al., 2004). Children with low level of self-care skills require more assistance in everyday tasks involved in getting dressed, eating and daily hygiene. With the accumulation of such demands along with other behavioural problems, it is no surprise that mothers evaluate taking care of a child with autism to be much harder than raising most children of the same age (Montes & Halterman,

2008). It should be noted, however, that although some authors have found a relationship between low adaptive functioning in children with autism and elevated parenting stress (Hall & Graff, 2011), other reports suggest that the child's adaptive skills' level is less significant than other factors in the context of parental stress (Beck et al., 2004). The longitudinal study by Lecavalier and colleagues (2006) demonstrated that the level of adaptive skills in children and adolescents with ASD is a weaker predictor of parental stress than, for example, externalizing behaviour.

Parental stress is also associated with the child's regulatory difficulties. These problems affect a number of areas, including emotional and affective regulation, and circadian rhythm. Studies have shown that, according to parents, children with autism demonstrate more negative emotions than children with mental disability and typically developing children (Capps et al., 1993). There is a relationship between such child characteristics as irritability, social withdrawal, hyperactivity and non-compliance, and the level of stress in mothers (Tomanik et al., 2004). In a study by Konstantareas and Papageorgiou (2006), the most powerful determinant of mothers' stress was the child's temperament, and in particular, the child's general level of activity, low flexibility and low mood.

One of the sources of problems experienced by parents are also the disturbances in the child's circadian rhythm. A number of children with autism have sleeping problems, such as excessively short sleep time, trouble falling asleep, waking up multiple times at night, problems getting out of bed in the morning and drowsiness during the day (e.g. Goodlin-Jones et al., 2008). These problems cause significant fatigue in parents, sometimes bordering on exhaustion, and are associated with parents' elevated stress and sleeping disorders (Hoffman et al., 2008).

Parents are also troubled by the child's untypical behaviour resulting from sensory problems, such as fixation on some and avoidance of other objects, paradoxical responses to stimulation and susceptibility to sensory overload (Ben-Sasson et al., 2007; Tomchek & Dunn, 2007). For parents who are not educated about autism-specific deficits in sensory processing, such behaviours may seem incomprehensible and lead to elevated levels of stress.

A contributing factor to behavioural unpredictability is the child's asymmetrical development in various areas: from relatively typical development, through regression, to severe developmental delay (cf. Marcus et al., 1997). An illustrative example is a girl described by Moreno and Donnellan (1991), who was able to define words such as "perigee" and "apogee" at the age of seven, but was unable to communicate her everyday needs.

The above developmental and behavioural problems illustrate how tough a challenge parents of children with autism are facing. Standing up to that challenge is impossible without professional support. Unfortunately, interactions with professionals can also be a major source of parental stress.

2.2 Problems with diagnosis, relations with professionals and parental stress

One of the most significant causes of stress experienced by parents of children with autism is lack of adequate professional support (Bishop et al. 2007; Sharpley et al., 1997). Parents face problems receiving help from healthcare professionals already at the stage of diagnosis of their child's developmental deficits. Suffice to say that, on average, the child is assessed by more than four professionals before diagnosis, with mean time to diagnosis being approximately 2-3 years (Siklos & Kerns, 2007). Among the multiple factors contributing to this situation, a major cause is the general lack of education about the course of young children's development and its disorders among professionals (including physicians and psychologists), and insufficient knowledge of symptoms indicating significant developmental difficulties. Another important issue is the small number of diagnostic and treatment institutions offering specialised services to individuals with ASD.

As noted by Norton and Drew (1994), autism is usually diagnosed only when parents insist on careful assessment of their child. This finding was confirmed by data from Canada, indicating the presence of a relationship between the mother's education and the child's diagnosis of autism (Croen et al., 2002). Information collected from parents suggest that they initially become concerned with their child's development in the first half of his/her second year of life (De Giacomo & Fombonne, 1998). They are usually worried by the child's communication difficulties, in particular the lack of speech, as well as unusual social behaviour and play patterns (Charman et al., 2001; Goin-Kochel & Myers, 2005).

Parents are frustrated by delayed and drawn-out diagnostic process and disappointed with the level of professionals' knowledge about autism spectrum disorders (Brogan & Knussen, 2003; Mansell & Morris, 2004; Osborne & Reed, 2008). Their stress associated with fear for their child may be further compounded by the way they are treated by professionals. They are forced to long waiting times at specialised institutions, and they receive conflicting information on how to help their child. Their problems are exacerbated by poor interpersonal skills of some professionals.

Support for parents is also inadequate during and immediately after the diagnostic process. Parents find it difficult to cope with their child's diagnosis of autism. Their responses range from relief that the situation is finally clear, through shock, disbelief or denial, to profound sadness and depressed mood (Avdi et al., 2000; Midence & O'Neill, 1999). Many are unable to deal with the situation on their own and require professional support (Wachtel & Carter, 2008).

It should also be emphasized that regardless of how parents respond initially, diagnosis is only the first step in their adaptive process. Siegel (1997) notes that coming to terms with the child's autism is a long-term process, due to, among other things, absence of any signs of disability in the child's appearance, which means that even after the diagnosis some parents remain sceptical as to its correctness. In the course of "arriving" at the final diagnosis, they live a life of uncertainty, which is made worse by the fact that they usually receive contradicting information about the nature of their child's problems and prognosis for further development. Even when the diagnosis is final, many parents are not aware of its consequences for the child and family. Lack of proper support significantly hampers their adaptation to the new situation.

Although autism has been diagnosed in children for many years, accessibility of autism-specific services and professional support is still unsatisfactory. This problem is present in many different countries, as demonstrated by research conducted e.g. in the USA (Wachtel & Carter, 2008), Belgium (Renty & Roeyers, 2004), and Poland (Rajner & Wroniszewski, 2000). Consequently, the task of arranging proper support, as well as medical, educational and other services for the child often falls to the parents (e.g. Renty & Roeyers, 2006; Sharpley et al., 1997; Weiss, 2002), who are left alone to coordinate, advocate for, and make decisions about treatment (Wachtel & Carter, 2008). As a result, they are overburdened with duties, sometimes feeling incompetent and anxious whether they have made the right chose of intervention for their child.

A significant cause of parents' dissatisfaction with professionals are problems in obtaining specific information about autism and instructions on how to take care of the child. A study by Rhoades and colleagues (2007) showed that as few as 40% of physicians who give the child the diagnosis of autism follow up with additional information about the disorder for parents, and only approximately 15-34% give advice on choosing a medical/educational program. The results of research by Hall and Graff (2011) suggest that parents expect professionals to have up-to-date knowledge on available sources of support and to be able to direct the family so as to save it from being overloaded with unnecessary and unneeded activities. However, the results of studies on professionals show that they are uncertain about the aetiology of autism, diagnosis and the best types of intervention for affected children (e.g. Mavropoulou & Padeliadu, 2001). Additionally, they often lack qualifications when it comes to working with children with autism (Cascella & Colella, 2004).

When analysing issues in the relationships of parents of children with autism with professionals, one must mention another aspect of those relations, associated with dated and unproven concepts of parental contribution in the aetiology of their child's autism. According to current consensus, autism belongs to neurodevelopmental disorders, and its aetiology is determined by neurobiological mechanisms (see: Moldin & Rubenstein, 2006). Thus, our knowledge about the causes of this disorder has progressed a long way since the "refrigerator mother" hypothesis, popular in the 1950's (cf. Marcus et al., 1997). However, as Schreibman (2005) observes, theories of psychogenic aetiology of autism have left a climate full of suspicion and distrust in the relationship between parents and professionals. This remark was confirmed by the findings of Avdi, Griffin and Brough (2000), who demonstrated that parents suspected professionals of withholding information, being judgemental and controlling.

Another challenge for parents is the lack of adequate respite services. Additional demands over typical childcare duties mean that parents are tired and lack time for other tasks and for satisfying their own and their family's needs. This also has direct effects on employment choices. In the Montes and Halterman study (2008), nearly 40% of parents of children with ASD reported claimed that problems associated with childcare significantly affected their employment decisions and careers. The proportion was much lower in the case of parents of high risk and typically developing children.

Another source of stress for parents related to lack of adequate support is the sense of neglecting other children by not spending enough time with them. Here is an excerpt from a letter written by a mother of Janek, published in Grodzka (1995): *"As parents of two sons – the older one healthy, and the younger who is sick – for ten years we were so focussed on the younger one that our healthy boy, although only two years older, had anything but a rosy childhood. Only now are we starting to realize that. Can we ever make it up to him? I don't know. Our older son loves his brother very much, and it shows. But he is also fighting for equal treatment"* (p. 223).

As the above review suggests, not only are parents faced with inadequate support, but their relationship with healthcare professionals may actually place additional burden on them. In order to avoid painting a one-sided picture of the parents-professionals relationship, it should be pointed out that studies conducted in Great Britain show that over 60% of parents whose children with autism benefit from educational services at schools express their satisfaction with those services (Whitaker, 2007). Their positive assessment involves the belief that school staff understands their child's difficulties and responds to them with empathy and from their perception that the school is able to respond flexibly to the child's needs. The level of satisfaction is also related with the quality of communication between the family and school.

A number of difficult experiences of parents are caused by attitudes and behaviour towards their child demonstrated by others.

2.3 Social attitudes towards people with autism as a source of parental stress

There is no doubt that parents of children with autism must cope not only with problems resulting from their child's developmental disability and challenging behaviours, but also with distressing responses of others to the child's behaviour, as well as general lack of knowledge about autism.

The contrast between the child's appearance, which betrays no signs of disability, and his behaviour, which is perceived as abnormal and "strange", frequently puts parents in very unpleasant situations (e.g. Gray, 2002b; Portway & Johnson, 2005). The child's behaviour is often taken to be a symptom of poor upbringing: "*You're being a bad mother. He's behaving like that because you don't discipline him. If you did it this way you wouldn't have problems.' That kind of stuff...you know, it doesn't help*" (Farrugia, 2009, p. 1018). Social disapproval for the child's behaviour often leads to stigmatization, experience of shame for parents, and their exclusion from normal social activities (Farrugia, 2009).

One of the aspects that determine the attitudes and behaviour towards people with autism is lack of awareness about the disorder. Autism still remains an unknown condition (e.g. Huws & Jones, 2010). There is plenty to be done in this area in order to change negative attitudes towards people with autism, especially since it has already been demonstrated that the scope and manner of providing information about the disorder significantly affects the attitudes and the level of acceptance for people with this disability (Iobst et al., 2009).

Boyd (2002) found that informal support plays a particularly important role in the adaptation of mothers of children with autism. Unfortunately, availability of this type of help also tends to be limited. Problems with the child's functioning often mean that parents are left to care for their children alone, deprived of help even from close family members. The burden of childcare often takes its toll on their relationships with friends and acquaintances. Their social circle is usually significantly reduced (Farrugia, 2009).

Still, it should be noted that professionals declare positive attitudes towards people with autism (e.g. Weil et al., 2011), as suggested by the results of the study conducted by Horrocks et al. (2008), in which principals of public schools in Pennsylvania were asked about their views on placing a child with autism at their schools. In one study, people training for various health and social professions were asked about their opinions on working with individuals with autism. It was assessed as difficult, challenging, and frustrating but also rewarding, important and an opportunity for personal and professional growth (Werner, 2011).

Some stressors listed in this section are unique to parents of children with autism (e.g. burdens associated with their child's difficulties in social relatedness, atypical attachment behaviour), while others are also experienced by parents of children with other developmental problems (e.g. behavioural problems or negative social attitudes towards the child and its family members). The list of challenges faced by parents presented here is by no means exhaustive. It leaves out a number of important issues which are not specific to autism, such as the parents' sense of guilt or anxiety about the child's future, which are shared by parents of children with various developmental disabilities. However, the exceptional circumstances of parents of children with autism are present in these issues as well. Parental self-blame for their child's autism may be rooted in certain aetiological concepts, such as the "refrigerator mother" hypothesis mentioned above. On the other hand, anxiety about the child's future is related to the fact that problems in social interaction put people with autism at increased risk of isolation and lack of support from friends to a much greater degree than individuals with other disorders. With time, the question of their child's social relations and having even a small circle of friends become increasingly important for the parents.

As it has already been mentioned, parental stress is a multifaceted phenomenon. It is influenced by many factors which may affect its profile and severity, as well as its implications for the parents' and child's well-being and family life. The factors that determine the level of stress in parents of children with autism have been the focus of research for over 30 years. The following section of the article looks at some of those factors.

3. Individual determinants of parental stress

Important factors determining the stress of parents of children with autism include parent's sex and a number of individual characteristics (such as coping strategies and style, and sense of coherence). The role of these factors in the context of stress experienced by parents is discussed below.

3.1 Parental stress in mothers and fathers of children with autism

The majority of studies on parental stress associated with raising a child with autism have focused on mothers. The idea was to find a stable, and at the same time group-specific stress profile. In one of the first investigations on the topic, Holroyd and McArthur (1976) compared stress experienced by mothers of children with autism and mothers of children with Down syndrome. Apart from common problems related to health, depressive mood, sense of being overburdened, pessimistic view of the future and limited family opportunity, mothers of children with autism reported stress associated with taking the child to public places, the child's almost complete dependence on care and lack of access to specialised services. Later research also showed that mothers of children with autism have a less positive future perspective than mothers of children with Down syndrome (Abbeduto et al. 2004).

Similar results were obtained by Bouma and Schweitzer (1990) in their comparison of mothers of children with autism and children with a physical disability and healthy children. Mothers of children with autism experienced more strain from problems related to the child's cognitive development, the need for constant supervision, and the perspective of their child's continued dependence on care. Behaviour problems of their child with autism also featured as a significant contributor to stress.

Koegel et al. (1992) described a fairly stable pattern of difficulties experienced by mothers of children with autism, independent from the child's age, intellectual development, geographical region or cultural background. The core stress was associated with the child's future, his/her cognitive development, dependence on care and social exclusion.

In another study (Pisula, 2007), mothers of children with autism showed higher stress levels than did mothers of children with Down syndrome on seven of the 15 subscales of the Questionnaire of Resources and Stress (Holroyd, 1987). The largest differences between groups were found for overprotection / dependency of the child and child's difficult personality characteristics. Mothers of children with autism were also more concerned about their child's dependence on external care. Similar results were obtained by Dale, Jahoda and Knott (2006).

There is no doubt that bringing up a child with autism may also be a significant challenge to fathers. However, our knowledge of how they experience problems related with the child's developmental deficits is still limited. In a study dating back almost twenty years, Rodrigue et al. (1992) demonstrated that fathers noticed the child's effect on family members' opportunities to satisfy their own needs and on overall family activity. Later studies found that the level of stress in fathers of children with autism is higher than in fathers of typically developing children (Baker-Ericzén et al., 2005).

Very few research projects to date have compared the stress profiles of mothers and fathers. Tehee et al. (2009) found that mothers were significantly more stressed than fathers. As stated Moes et al. (1992), mothers experienced more stress in four areas: parenting problems, the child's self-sufficiency, behaviour, and physical development. Other findings suggest that stress in mothers is interrelated with their child's social skills, while no such relationship was found in fathers (Baker-Ericzén et al., 2005). Hastings (2003) showed that stress level in mothers was associated with the child's behavioural problems and the father's mental health, while the stress in fathers was not related to either the child's behaviour or mother's mental health. Other researchers (Knusen & Sloper, 1992) have also shown that mothers were particularly affected by behavioural problems demonstrated by the child, as well as his/her dependency, anxiety and poor communicative skills, while fathers, apart from communication problems, were most affected by the child's physical disability and presence of other stressful life events (e.g. career-related or associated with family finances). As for behavioural problems, fathers were mostly distressed by the child's externalizing problems, while mothers were more affected by the child's regulatory problems (Davis & Carter, 2008). A supplement to these findings is the information that mothers perceived significantly more stigmatizing behaviours of other people than did fathers (Gray, 2002b). Thus, it would seem that mothers are more sensitive to hostile behaviour of others towards the child than are fathers.

In the light of the above account, it is clear that we still know very little about the differences between mothers and fathers of children with autism in terms of parental stress they experience. Research has shown that mothers experience more stress and that their stress is more pervasive than stress experienced by fathers: scores are elevated in more domains measured in these studies.

3.2 Individual personal characteristics of parents and parental stress

Stress experienced by parents may significantly affect their adaptability to the demands of bringing up a child with developmental disability. Successful adaptation of parents depends on a range of factors, including their coping strategies and styles (McCubbin & Petterson, 1983).

The nature of challanges resulting from the child's developmental deficits affects the type of coping strategies used by parents. Some results indicate that parents of children with ASD employ more strategies that involve distancing and escape than parents of non-autistic children, and that they are less likely to use strategies involving self-control, seeking social support, and problem solving (Sivberg et al., 2002). Twoy et al. (2007) found that parents of children with autism aged ≤ 12 often resorted to strategies that included reframing and seeking social support.

The way parents cope with stress is correlated with their stress level (Hastings & Johnson, 2001). It should be noted, however, that the interrelations between parental stress in parents of children with autism and their stress coping in general have not been sufficiently researched. In one of only a handful of studies on the subject, Lyons and colleagues (2010) analysed the effect of autism severity and parents' coping strategies on parental stress. The most powerful predictor of stress was the child's autism severity. However, coping strategies also play an important role for the well-being of parents of children with autism. Smith et al. (2008) concluded that the well-being of mothers of toddlers with autism correlated with using less emotion-focused coping and more problem-focused coping, regardless of the severity of the child's deficits.

In a study on coping strategies in parents of preschool and school-aged children with autism, Hastings et al. (2005) distinguished four main coping dimensions: active-avoidance coping, problem focused coping, positive coping, and religious/denial coping. Out of those dimensions, active-avoidance coping was associated with a high level of stress and psychopathology in both mothers and fathers.

Some data also suggest that elevated level of parental stress is associated with religious coping (Tarakeswahr & Pargament, 2001). Lower stress, in turn, is associated with using coping strategies that involve reformulation and seeking informal support (Hastings & Johnson, 2001), problem-oriented coping (Lustig, 2002), as well as coping by focusing on family integration and co-operation (Jones & Passey, 2005). It has also been shown that adaptation of mothers of children with autism is facilitated by active coping patterns, while self-blame for the handicap is associated with poorer adaptation (Bristol, 1987).

Most studies on coping with stress in parents of children with autism focus on coping strategies. Much less is known about coping styles defined as a dispositional variable which refers to relatively stable characteristics of an individual (Endler & Parker, 1990). In a study on parents of high functioning children with autism, Lee (2009) found that they demonstrated lower adaptive coping skills than parents of typically developing children. Any analysis of stress coping in this group of subjects should take into account findings about a certain typical characteristics in their functioning. They suggest that there is a similarity in psychological functioning of the child and parents. Parents demonstrate higher rates of social difficulties (e.g. impaired friendships, aloofness, shyness, impairments in confiding relationships, social phobia) (e.g. Murphy et al., 2000; Piven, 1999), higher scores in aloof personality, rigid personality, and pragmatic language difficulties (Hurley et al., 2007). In addition, some of them show some cognitive features similar to the cognitive functioning of their children (e.g. Briskman et al., 2001). These characteristics may affect their ability to cope with the difficulties associated with the child's developmental problems.

Individual characteristics important in the context of parental stress and how parents cope with it also include sense of coherence (SOC), defined as "a global orientation that expresses the extent to which one has a pervasive, enduring though dynamic feeling of confidence that (a) the stimuli deriving from one's internal and external environments in the course of living and structured, predictable, and explicable (*comprehensibility*); (b) the resources are available to one to meet the demands posed by these stimuli (*manageability*); (c) these demands are challenges worthy of investment and engagement (*meaningfulness*)" (Antonovsky, 1987, p. 19). SOC has been shown to be closely associated with individual's health and psychological distress (e.g. Antonovsky, 1998; Olsson et al., 2008). Very few studies so far focused on the sense of coherence in parents of children with autism. From the few that have been conducted, is appears that they have weaker SOC than parents of children with other disabilities and parents of typically developing children (Olsson & Hwang, 2002; Pisula & Kossakowska, 2010; Sivberg, 2002). In the context of these findings, the results of the study by Mak, Ho and Law (2007), who analysed the relationship between SOC and parental stress in mothers of children with autism are particularly interesting. The study showed that mothers with stronger SOC perceived lower stress, regardless of the severity of their child's developmental difficulties.

Other factors that may potentially be related to parental stress include parents' lower control locus, lower levels of self-esteem, and vulnerability to mental health problems. However, the results of studies on the relationship between these variables and parental stress conducted so far are inconclusive. For example, Hamlyn-Wright et al. (2007) did not find locus of control to mediate the relationship between stress and anxiety or depression in parents of children with autism. Dunn et al. (2001) also failed to obtain a relationship between locus of control and parental stress. In addition, the level of stress in parents of children with autism is also determined by the factors mentioned in the first part of this section, i.e. availability of social support, social attitudes towards the child with autism, family's financial standing, family cohesiveness and marital satisfaction.

4. Conclusion

To summarize the present review of research on stress in parents of children with autism, significant sources of stress include, among others, lateness and difficulty in obtaining diagnosis, untypical and inconsistent development of the child, and behavioural problems, with particular emphasis of challenging behaviour in public. Parents are also hampered by the lack of systemic solutions for people with autism, ignorance of professionals, and general lack of understanding for their problems. The situation is further complicated by the fact that people with autism require considerable and wide-ranging support for a significant portion of their lives, and that currently used intervention methods fall short of expectations. These problems affect various individuals to different degrees and may actually be untypical in a particular case, which is why the experiences of different families can be so divergent.

Severe stress experienced by parents of children with autism has profound consequences for their health, well-being, interactions with the child and family life. Nevertheless, it is still difficult to pinpoint the exact mechanism behind these consequences. It has been demonstrated that parents of these children have poorer health and lower sense of psychological well-being than parents of children with other dysfunctions (e.g. Abbeduto et al., 2004; Kasari & Sigman, 1997). Phetrasuwan and Miles (2009) have also shown that mothers of children with ASD who reported higher stress, presented with more symptoms of depression and lower levels of well-being than mothers with lower stress. It is not clear, however, whether autism is unique in that respect, or if other disorders affect parents' well-being similarly. Greenberg and colleagues (2004) found no differences in terms of depression, well-being and health between mothers of adults with autism, Down syndrome and schizophrenia.

Studies have also shown that parental stress affects such aspects of family life as spending time together, capacity for spontaneous and flexible planning and marital relationship

(Hutton & Caron, 2005), and lower the efficacy of early interventions in children with ASD (Osborne et al., 2008).

Richard Hastings (2002) put forward a theoretical model combining the child's behaviour problems with developmental disability, parental stress and parenting behaviour. The model proposes the following chain of relations: (1) child's behaviour problems lead to parent's stress, (2) parental stress affects the way parent acts toward the child, (3) the parent's behaviour towards the child reinforces the development and persistence of behaviour problems. The model has not been fully tested yet, but some data partially support its validity (e.g. Estes et al., 2009). Kasari and Sigman (1997) proposed a similar model for interpreting the interrelations between the behaviour of a child with autism and parental stress, supplementing it with the shape of parent-child interactions. They suggest that elevated stress in the parent affects her behaviour toward the child, and, as a result, the course of their interactions.

There is no doubt that the application of the stress-coping paradigm in research on the circumstances of parents of children with autism has yielded a lot of interesting and important results, improving our understanding of the difficulties they must face. These findings help develop better methods of supporting families of children with autism. However, data in this field are often inconsistent, most likely due to methodological issues. Adequate tools for assessing parental stress still need to be designed, as shown by validity analyses of existing questionnaires (e.g. Zaidman-Zait et al., 2010).

The present article offers a comprehensive analysis of information about the challenges faced by parents who raise a child with autism. It should be noted, however, that parents also report positive aspects of their parenting experience. What's more, with time, as they adapt to the situation, their sense of well-being improves. Gray (2002a) analysed parents at two instances, 8-10 years apart. In the second study, parents reported better mood, fewer health problems and lower stress levels than at the initial assessment. They also notices improvement in their relationship with extended family and significant reduction in stigmatizing towards the child. Similar results were obtained by King et al. (2006), who found that with time parents achieved better sense of coherence and control. Their values and goals changed, which facilitated adaptation to the demands resulting from the child's developmental difficulties. Research on the factors that facilitate parents' adaptation to the unique challenges posed before them by their child's autism is still an important branch of scientific inquiry.

5. Acknowledgments

This paper was supported by a Grant BST 154536 from the Faculty of Psychology, University of Warsaw

6. References

Abbeduto, L., Seltzer, M. M., Shattuck, P., Krauss, M. W., Orsmond, G., Murphy, M. M. (2004). Psychological well-being and coping in mothers of youths with autism, Down syndrome, or fragile X syndrome. *American Journal on Mental Retardation,* 109, 3, 237-254.

American Psychiatric Association (2000). *Diagnostic And Statistical Manual Of Mental Disorders* (4th ed., revised). Washington, D.C.: Author.

Antonovsky, A. (1987). *Unravelling the Mystery of Health: How People Manage Stress and Stay Well.* San Francisco, CA: Jossey-Bass.

Avdi, E., Griffin, C., Brough, S. (2000). 'Parents' constructions of the "problem" during assessment and diagnosis of their child for an autistic spectrum disorder'. *Journal of Health Psychology,* 5, 2, 241–254.

Bakér-Ericzen, M. J., Brookman-Frazee, L., Stahmer, L. (2005). Stress levels and adaptability in parents of toddlers with and without autism spectrum disorders. *Research & Practice for Persons with Severe Disabilities,* 30, 4, 194-204.

Beck, A., Hastings, R., Daley, D. (2004). Pro-social behaviour and behaviour problems independently predict maternal stress. *Journal of Intellectual and Developmental Disability,* 29, 4, 339–349.

Ben-Sasson, A., Cermak, S. A., Orsmond, G. I., Tager-Flusberg, H., Carter, A. S., Kadlec, M. B., Dunn, W. (2007). Extreme sensory modulation behaviors in toddlers with autism spectrum disorders. *The American Journal of Occupational Therapy,* 61, 5, 584-592.

Bishop, S. L., Richler, J., Cain, A. C., Lord, C. (2007). Predictors of perceived negative impact in mothers of children with autism spectrum disorder. *American Journal on Mental Retardation,* 112, *6,* 450-461.

Bouma, R., Schweitzer, R. (1990). The impact of chronic childhood illness on family stress: A comparative study between autism and cystic fibrosis. *Journal of Clinical Psychology,* 46, 6, 722-730.

Boyd, B. A. (2002). Examining the relationship between stress and lack of social support in mothers of children with autism. *Focus on Autism & Other Developmental Disabilities,* 17, 4, 208-215.

Briskman, J., Happe, F., Frith, U. (2001). Exploring the cognitive phenotype of autism: Weak ``central coherence'' in parents and siblings of children with autism: II. Real-life skills and preferences. *Journal of Child Psychology & Psychiatry & Allied Disciplines,* 42, 3, 309-316.

Bristol, M. M. (1987). Mothers of children with autism or communication disorders: successful adaptation and double ABCX model. *Journal of Autism and Developmental Disorders,* 17, 4, 469-486.

Brogan, C. A., Knussen, Ch. (2003). The disclosure of a diagnosis of an autistic spectrum disorder. *Autism,* 7, 1, 31- 46.

Capps, L., Kasari, C., Yirmiya, N., Sigman, M. (1993). Parental perception of emotional expressiveness in children with autism. *Journal of Consulting and Clinical Psychology,* 61, 3, 475-484.

Cascella, P. W., Colella, C. S. (2004). Knowledge of autism spectrum disorders among connecticut school speech-language pathologists. *Focus on Autism and Other Developmental Disabilities,* 19, 4, 245-252.

Charman, T., Baird, G. (2002). Practitioner review: Diagnosis of autism spectrum disorder in 2- and 3-year-old children. *Journal of Child Psychology and Psychiatry,* 43, *3,* 289–305.

Charman T., Baron-Cohen S., Baird G., Cox A., Wheelwright S., Swettenham J., Drew A. (2001). Commentary: The Modified Checklist for Autism in Toddlers. *Journal of Autism and Developmental Disorders,* 31, 2, 145–148.

Croen, L. A., Grether, J. K., Hoogstrate, J., Selvin, S. (2002). The changing prevalence of autism in California. *Journal of Autism and Developmental Disorders,* 32, 3, 207-215.

Dale, E., Jahoda, A., Knott, F. (2006). Mothers' attributions following their child's diagnosis of autistic spectrum disorder. *Autism: The International Journal of Research & Practice,* 10, 5, 463-479.

Davis, N. O., Carter, A. S. (2008). Parenting stress in mothers and fathers of toddlers with autism spectrum disorders: Associations with child characteristics. *Journal of Autism and Developmental Disorders,* 38, 7, 1278–1291.

De Giacomo, A., Fombonne, E. (1998). Parental recognition of developmental abnormalities in autism. *European Child & Adolescent Psychiatry,* 7, 3, 131-136.

Dunlap, G., Robbins, F. R. (1994). Parents' reports of their children's challenging behaviors: Results of a statewide survey. *Mental Retardation,* 32, 3, 206-212.

Dunn, M. E., Burbine, T., Bowers, C. A., Tantleff-Dunn, S. (2001). Moderators of stress in parents of children with autism. *Community Mental Health Journal,* 37, 1, 39-52.

Endler, N. S., Parker, J. D. A. (1990). *Coping Inventory for Stressful Situation. Manual.* Toronto: Multi-Health Systems.

Estes, A., Munson, J., Dawson, G., Koehler, E., Zhou X-H., Abbott, R. (2009). Parenting stress and psychological functioning among mothers of preschool children with autism and developmental delay. *Autism,* 13, 4, 375–387.

Farrugia, D. (2009). Exploring stigma: medical knowledge and the stigmatisation of parents of children diagnosed with autism spectrum disorder. *Sociology of Health & Illness,* 31, 7, 1011–1027.

Fitzgerald, M., Birkbeck, G., Matthews, P. (2002). Maternal burden in families with children with autistic spectrum disorder. *The Irish Journal of Psychology,* 33, 1–2, 17.

Goin-Kochel, R. P., Mackintosh, V. H., Myers, B. J. (2006). 'How many doctors does it take to make an autism spectrum diagnosis?', *Autism,* 10, 5, 439–451.

Goodlin-Jones, B. L., Tang, K., Liu, J., Anders, T. F. (2008). Sleep patterns in preschool-age children with *autism*, developmental delay, and typical development. *Journal of the American Academy of Child and Adolescent Psychiatry,* 47, 8, 930-938.

Gray, D. E. (2002a). Ten years on: a longitudinal study of families of children with autism. *Journal of Intellectual and Developmental Disability,* 27, 3, 215-222.

Gray, D. E. (2002b). 'Everybody just freezes. Everybody is just embarrassed': felt and enacted stigma among parents of children with high functioning autism. *Sociology of Health & Illness,* 24, 6, 734–749.

Greenberg, J. S., Seltzer, M. M., Wyngaarden-Krauss, M., Jing-Ann Ch. R., Jinkuk H. (2004). The effect of quality of the relationship between mothers and adult children with schizophrenia, autism, or Down syndrome on maternal well-being: The mediating role of optimism. *American Journal of Orthopsychiatry,* 74, 1, 14-25.

Grodzka, M. (1995). Płacz bez łez. Listy rodziców dzieci autystycznych [A Tearless Cry. The letters from parents of children with autism]. Gdańsk: Wydawnictwo Medyczne MAKmed s.c.

Gupta, V. B. (2007). Comparison of parenting stress in different developmental disabilities. *Journal of Developmental and Physical Disabilities,* 19, 4, 417–425.

Hall, H. R., Graff, J. C. (2011). The relationships among adaptive behaviors of children with autism, family support, parenting stress, and coping. *Issues in Comprehensive Pediatric Nursing,* 34, 1, 4-25.

Hamlyn-Wright, S., Draghi-Lorenz, R., Ellis, J. (2007). Locus of control fails to mediate between stress and anxiety and depression in parents of children with a developmental disorder. *Autism*, 11, 6, 489-501.

Hastings, R. P. (2002). Parental stress and behaviour problems of children with developmental disability. *Journal of Intellectual & Developmental Disability*, 27, 3, 149-160.

Hastings, R. P. (2003). Child behaviour problems and partner mental health as correlates of stress in mothers and fathers of children with autism. *Journal of Intellectual Disability Research*, 47, 4/5, 231-237.

Hastings, R. P., Johnson, E. (2001). Stress in UK families conducting intensive home-based behavioral intervention for their young child with autism. *Journal of Autism and Developmental Disorders*, 31, 3, 327–336.

Hastings, R. P., Kovshoff, H., Ward, N. J., Espinosa, F., Brown, T., Remington, B. (2005). Systems analysis of stress and positive perceptions in mothers and fathers of pre-school children with autism. *Journal of Autism and Developmental Disorders*, 35, 5, 635-644.

Herring, S., Gray, K., Taffe, J., Tonge, B., Seeney, D., Einfeld, S. (2006). Behaviour and emotional problems in toddlers with pervasive developmental disorders and developmental delay: associations with parental mental health and family functioning. *Journal of Intellectual Disability Research*, 50, 12, 874-882.

Hodapp, R.M., Ricci, L.A., Ly,T.M., Fidler, D.J. (2003). The effects of the child with Down syndrome on maternal stress. *British Journal of Developmental Psychology*, 21, 1, 137–151.

Hoffman, Ch. D., Sweeney, D. P., Hodge, D., Lopez-Wagner, M. C., Looney, L. (2009). Parenting stress and closeness mothers of typically developing children and mothers of children with autism. *Focus on Autism and Other Developmental Disabilities*, 24, 3, 178-187.

Hoffman, Ch. D., Sweeney, D. P., Lopez-Wagner, M. C. (2008). Children with autism: Sleep problems and mothers' stress. *Focus on Autism and Other Developmental Disabilities*, 23, 3, 155-165.

Holroyd, J. (1987). *Questionnaire on Resources and Stress for Families with Chronically Ill or Handicapped Members (Manual)*. Brandon, VT: Clinical Psychology Publishing Co., Inc.

Holroyd, J., McArthur, D. (1976). Mental retardation and stress on the parents: A contrast between Down's syndrome and childhood autism. *American Journal of Mental Deficiency*, 80, 4, 431-436.

Hoppes, K., Harris, S. L. (1990). Perceptions of child attachment and maternal gratification in mothers of children with autism and Down syndrome. *Journal of Clinical Child Psychology*, 19, 4, 365-370.

Horrocks, J. L., White, G., Roberts, L. (2008). Principals' attitudes regarding inclusion of children with autism in Pennsylvania public schools. *Journal of Autism and Developmental Disorders*, 38, 8, 1462–1473.

Hurley, R., Losh, M., Parlier, M., Reznick, J., Piven, J. (2007). The Broad Autism Phenotype Questionnaire. *Journal of Autism & Developmental Disorders*, 37, 9, 1679-1690.

Hutton, A. M.; Caron, S. L. (2005). Experiences of families with children with autism in rural New England. *Focus on Autism & Other Developmental Disabilities*, 20, 3, 180-189.

Huws, J. C., Jones, R. S. P. (2010). "They just seem to live their lives in their own little world": Lay perceptions of autism. *Disability & Society*, 25, 3, 331-344.

Iobst, E., Nabors, L., Rosenzweig, K. (2009). Adults' perceptions of a child with autism. *Research in Autism Spectrum Disorders*, 3, 2, 401-408.

Johnston, C., Hessl, D., Blasey, C., Eliez, S., Erba, H., Dyer-Friedman, J., Glaser, B., Reiss, A. L. (2003). Factors associated with parenting stress in mothers of children with fragile X syndrome. *Journal of Developmental and Behavioral Pediatrics*, 24, 4, 267–275.

Jones, J., Passey, J. (2005). Family adaptation, coping and resources: Parents of children with developmental disabilities and behaviour problems. Preview. *Journal on Developmental Disabilities*, 11. Special issue: Special Issue on Families of Individuals with DD, 31-46.

Joseph, R. M., Tager-Flusberg, H., Lord, C. (2002). Cognitive profiles and social-communicative functioning in children with autism spectrum disorder. *Journal of Child Psychology & Psychiatry & Allied Disciplines*, 43, 6, 807-821.

Kasari, C., Sigman, M. (1997). Linking parental perceptions to interactions in young children with autism. *Journal of Autism & Developmental Disorders*, 27, 1, 39-57.

King, G. A., Zwaigenbaum, L., King, S., Baxter, D., Rosenbaum, P., Bates, A. (2006). A qualitative investigation of changes in the belief systems of families of children with autism or Down syndrome. *Child: Care, Health & Development*, 32, 3, 353–369.

Koegel R. L., Schreibman L., Loos L. M., Dirlich-Wilhelm H., Dunlap G., Robbins F. R., Plienis A. J. (1992). Consistent stress profiles in mothers of children with autism. *Journal of Autism and Developmental Disorders*, 22, 2, 205-216.

Konstantareas, M.M., Papageorgiou, V. (2006). Effects of temperament, symptom severity and level of functioning on maternal stress in Greek children and youth with ASD. *Autism*, 10, 6, 593-607.

Knussen, C., Sloper, P. (1992). Stress in families of children with disability: A review of risk and resistance factors. *Journal of Mental Health*, 1, 3, 241-256.

Lazarus, R. S. i Folkman, S. (1984). *Stress, appraisal, and coping*. New York: Springer.

Lecavalier, L., Leone, S., Wiltz, J. (2006). The impact of behaviour problems on caregiver stress in young people with autism spectrum disorders. *Journal of Intellectual Disability Research*, 50, 3, 172–183.

Lee, G. K. (2009). Parents of children with high functioning autism: How well do they cope and adjust? *Journal of Developmental & Physical Disabilities*, 21, 2, 93-114.

Lustig, D. C. (2002). Family coping in families with a child with a disability. *Education & Training in Mental Retardation & Developmental Disabilities*, 37, 1, 14-22.

Lyons A. M., Leon, S. C., Roecker Phelps, C. E. (2010). The impact of child symptom severity on stress among parents of children with ASD: The moderating role of coping styles. *Journal of Child and Family Studies*, 19, 4, 516-524.

Mak, W. W. S., Ho, A. H. Y., Law, R. W. (2007). Sense of coherence, parenting attitudes and stress among mothers of children with autism in Hong Kong. *Journal of Applied Research in Intellectual Disabilities*, 20, 2, 157–167.

Mansell, W., Morris, K. (2004). A survey of parents' reactions to the diagnosis of an autistic spectrum disorder by a local service. Access to information and use of services. *Autism*, 8, 4, 387-407.

Marcus, L. M., Kunce, L. J., Schopler, E. (1997). Working with families. In: *Handbook of Autism and Pervasive Developmental Disorders,* D. J. Cohen, F. R. Volkmar (eds), pp. 631-649. New York: John Wiley & Sons, Inc.

Matson, J. L., LoVullo, S. V., Boisjole, J. A., Gonzalez, M. L. (2008). The behavioral treatment of an 11-year-old girl with autism and aggressive behaviors. *Clinical Case Studies, 7,* 4, 313-326.

Mavropoulou, S., Padeliadu, S. (2000). Greek teachers' perceptions of autism and implications for educational practice: A preliminary analysis. *Autism,* 4, 2, 173–183.

McCubbin, H., Patterson, J. (1983). Family stress adaptation to crises: A double ABCX model of family behavior. In: *Social stresses and the family: Advances and developments in family stress thery and research,* H. McCubbin, M. Sussman, J. Patterson (eds.), pp. 7-37. New York: The Haworth Press.

Midence, K., O'Neill, M. (1999). The experience of parents in the diagnosis of autism. A pilot study. *Autism,* 3, 3, 273–285.

Moes, D., Koegel, R. L., Schreibman, L., & Loos, L. M. (1992). Stress profiles for mothers and fathers of children with autism. *Psychological Reports,* 71, 3, 1272-1274.

Moldin, S. O., Rubenstein, J. L. R. (2006) (eds.). *Understanding autism. From basic neuroscience to treatment.* Tayloy and Francis Group: Boca Raton, FL.

Montes, G., Halterman, J.S. (2008). Child care problems and employment among families with preschool-aged children with autism in the United States. *Pediatrics,* 122 (1), e202-208.

Moreno, S. J., Donnellan, A. M. (1991). *High-functionning individuals with autism: Advice and information for parents and others who care.* Crown Point, IN: Maap Services.

Mori, K., Ujiie, T., Smith, A., Howlin, P. (2009). Parental stress associated with caring for children with Asperger's syndrome or autism. *Pediatrics International,* 51, 3, 364–370.

Murphy, M., Bolton, P., Pickles, A., Fombonne, E., Piven, J., Rutter, M. (2000). Personality traits of the relatives of autistic probands. *Psychological Medicine,* 30, 6, 1411–1424.

Norton, P., Drew, C. (1994). Autism and potential family stressors. *The American Journal of Family Therapy,* 22, 1, 67-75.

Olsson, M. B., Hwang, C. P. (2002). Sense of coherence in parents of children with different developmental disabilities. *Journal of Intellectual Disabilities Research,* 46, 7, 548–559.

Olsson, M. B., Larsman, P., Hwang, P. C. (2008). Relationships among risk, sense of coherence, and well-being in parents of children with and without intellectual disabilities. *Journal of Policy & Practice in Intellectual Disabilities,* 5, 4, 227-236.

Osborne, L. A., McHugh, L., Saunders, J., Reed, P. (2008). Parenting stress reduces the effectiveness of early teaching interventions for autistic spectrum disorders. *Journal of Autism and Developmental Disorders,* 38, 6, 1092-1103.

Osborne, L. A., Reed, P. (2008). Parents' perceptions of communication with professionals during the diagnosis of autism. *Autism,* 12, 3, 309–324.

Perry, A. (2004). A model of stress in families of children with developmental disabilities: Clinical and research applications. *Journal on Developmental Disabilities,* 11, 1, 1-16.

Pisula, E. (2007). A comparative study of stress profiles in mothers of children with autism and those of children with Down's syndrome. *Journal of Applied Research in Intellectual Disabilities,* 20, 3, 274-278.

Pisula, E., Kossakowska, Z. (2010). Sense of coherence and coping with stress among mothers and fathers of children with autism. *Journal of Autism and Developmental Disorders*, 40, 12, 1485–1494.

Piven, J. (1999). Genetic liability for autism: the behavioural expression in relatives. *International Review of Psychiatry*, 11, 4, 299-308.

Phetrasuwan, S., Miles, M. S. (2009). Parenting stress in mothers of children with autism spectrum disorders. *Journal for Specialists in Pediatric Nursing*, 188, 3, 157-165.

Portway, S. M., Johnson, B. (2005). Do you know I have Asperger Syndrome? Risks of a non-obvious disability. *Health, Risk, and Society*, 7, 1, 73-83.

Rao, P. A., Beidel, D. C. (2009). Stress, sibling adjustment, and family functioning. The impact of children with high-functioning autism on parental stress, sibling adjustment, and family functioning. *Behavior Modification*, 33, 4, 437-451.

Rajner A, Wroniszewski M (2000). *Raport 2000* [Report 2000]. Warsaw: „Synapsis".

Renty, J., Roeyers, H. (2006). Satisfaction with formal support and education for children with autism spectrum disorder: the voices of the parents. *Child: Care, Health & Development*, 32, 3, 371–385.

Rhoades, R. A., Scarpa, A., Salley, B. (2007). The importance of physician knowledge of autism spectrum disorder: results of a parent survey. *BMC Pediatrics*, 7, 37; http://www.biomedcentral.com/1471-2431/7/37.

Richman, D. M., Belmont, J. M., Kim, M., Slavin, C. B., Hayner, A. K. (2009). Parenting stress in families of children with Cornelia de Lange syndrome and Down syndrome. *Journal of Developmental & Physical Disabilities*, 21, 6, 537-553.

Rodrigue, J. R., Morgan, S. B., Geffken, G. R. (1992). Psychosocial adaptation of fathers of children with autism, Down syndrome, and normal development. *Journal of Autism and Developmental Disorders*, 22, 2, 249-263.

Schieve, L. A., Blumberg, S. J., Rice, C., Visser, S. N., Boyle, C. (2007). The relationship between autism and parenting stress. *Pediatrics*, 119, Suppl. 1, 114-121.

Schreibman, L. (2005). *The science and fiction of autism*. Cambridge, MA, US: Harvard University Press.

Sharpley, C. F., Bitsika, V., Efremidis, B. (1997). Influence of gender, parental health, and perceived expertise of assistance upon stress, anxiety, and depression among parents of children with autism. *Journal of Intellectual and Developmental Disability*, 22, 1, 19–28.

Siklos, S., Kerns, K. A. (2007). Assessing the diagnostic experiences of a small sample of parents of children with autism spectrum disorders. *Research in Developmental Disabilities*, 28, 1, 9–22.

Siegel, B. (1997). Coping with the diagnosis of autism. In: *Handbook of Autism and Developmental Disorders*, F. Volkmar & D. Cohen (eds.), pp. 745–766. New York: Wiley.

Sivberg, B. (2002). Coping strategies and parental attitudes. A comparison of parents with children with autistic spectrum disorders and parents with non-autistic children. *International Journal of Circumpolar Health*, 61, Suppl. 2, 36-50.

Smith, T. B., Oliver, M. N. I., Innocenti, M. S. (2001). Parenting stress in families of children with disabilities. *American Journal of Orthopsychiatry*, 71, 2, 257–261.

Smith, L. E., Seltzer, M. M., Tager-Flusberg, H., Greenberg, J.S., Carter, A. S. (2008). A comparative analysis of well-being and coping among mothers of toddlers and mothers of adolescents with ASD. *Journal of Autism and Developmental Disorders*, 38, 5, 876-889.

Tarakeswahr, N., Pargament, K. I. (2001). Religious coping in families of children with autism. *Focus on Autism and Other Developmental Disabilities, 16, 4, 247-260.*

Tehee, E., Honan, R., Hevey, D. (2009). Factors contributing to stress in parents of individuals with autistic spectrum disorders. *Journal of Applied Research in Intellectual Disabilities*, 22, 1, 34–42.

Tobing, L. E., Glenwick, D. S. (2002). Relation of the Childhood Autism Rating Scale–Parent Version to diagnosis, stress, and age. *Research in Developmental Disabilities*, 23, 3, 211–223.

Tomanik, S., Harris, G. E., Hawkins, J. (2004). The relationship between behaviors exhibited by children with autism and maternal stress. *Journal of Intellectual & Developmental Disability*, 29, 1, 16–26.

Tomchek, S. D., Dunn, W. (2007). Sensory processing in children with and without autism: a comparative study using the short sensory profile. *The American Journal of Occupational Therapy*, 61, 2, 190-200.

Twoy, R., Connolly, P. M., Novak, J. M. (2007). Coping strategies used by parents of children with autism. *Journal of the American Academy of Nurse Practitioners*, 19, 5, 251-260.

Volkmar, F. R., Lord, C., Bailey, A., Schultz, R., Klin, A. (2004). Autism and pervasive developmental disorders. *Journal of Child Psychology and Psychiatry*, 45, 1, 135-170.

Wachtel, K., Carter, A. S. (2008). Reaction to diagnosis and parenting styles among mothers of young children with ASDs. *Autism*, 12, 5, 575–594.

Walenski, M., Tager-Flusberg, H., Ullman, M. T. (2006). Language in autism. In: *Understanding autism. From basic neuroscience to treatment*, Moldin S. O., Rubenstein, J. L. R. (eds), pp. 175-203. Boca Raton, FL: Taylor & Francic Group.

Webster, R. I., Majnemer, A., Platt, R. W., Shevell, M. I. (2008). Child health and parental stress in school-age children with a preschool diagnosis of developmental delay. *Journal of Child Neurology*, 23, 1, 32-38.

Weil, T. N., Bagramian, R. A., Inglehart, M. R. (2011). Treating patients with Autism Spectrum Disorder - SCDA members' attitudes and behavior. *Special Care In Dentistry*, 31, 1, 8-17.

Weiss, M. J. (2002). Hardiness and social support as predictors of stress in mothers of typical children, children with autism and children with mental retardation. *Autism*, 6, 1, 115-130.

Werner, S. (2011). Assessing female students' attitudes in various health and social professions toward working with people with autism: A preliminary study. *Journal of Interprofessional Care*, 25, 2, 131-137.

Whitaker, P. (2007). Provision for youngsters with autistic spectrum disorders in mainstream schools: what parents say - and what parents want. *British Journal of Special Education*, 34, 3, 170-178.

White, N., Hastings, R. P. (2004). Social and professional support for parents of adolescents with severe intellectual disabilities. *Journal of Applied Research in Intellectual Disabilities*, 17, 3, 181–190.

Worcester, J. A., Nesman, T. M., Mendez, L. M. R., Keller, H. R. (2008). Giving voice to parents of of young children with challenging behaviour. *Exceptional Children*, 74, 4, 509-525.

Yamada, A., Suzuki, M., Kato, M., Suzuki, M., Tanaka, S., Shindo, T., Taketani, K., Akechi, T., Furukawa, T. (2007). Emotional distress and its correlates among parents of children with pervasive developmental disorders. *Psychiatry & Clinical Neurosciences,* 61, 6, 651-657.

Zaidman-Zait, A., Mirenda, P., Zumbo, B. D. (2010). An item response theory analysis of the Parenting Stress Index-Short Form with parents of children with autism spectrum disorders. *Journal of Child Psychology and Psychiatry*, 51, 11, 1269-1277.

6

Psychological Adaptation in Parents of Children with Autism Spectrum Disorders

Pilar Pozo, Encarnación Sarriá and Ángeles Brioso
Universidad Nacional de Educación a Distancia, UNED
Spain

1. Introduction

Autism and Autism Spectrum Disorders (ASD) are among the most enigmatic and restricting disorders, given that affected individuals demonstrate alterations in three basic areas of development: reciprocal social interaction, verbal and non-verbal communication, and flexibility in their selection of interests and behaviours. The peculiar characteristics that define ASD cause major disturbances in the family dynamics and generate needs in all areas and contexts of development (Altiere, 2006; Baker et al., 2005; Shu, 2009; Smith, Hong et al., 2010).

Other problems are frequently associated with the nuclear characteristics of autism. These include mental retardation (Sigman & Caps, 1997) and behaviour problems such as stereotyped, self-injurious or aggressive conduct (Bryson, 1996; Hastings, 2003) that persist in the long term (Einfeld, Tonge & Rees, 2001). These problems, depending on the severity and frequency with which they occur, will affect the development of individuals with autism and the well-being and adaptation of their parents to a greater or lesser extent (Herring, et al., 2006; Lecavalier et al., 2006; Pozo et al., 2006; Tomanik et al., 2004).

Many studies have examined the emotional adjustment of parents of children with ASD. These studies have systematically documented that --compared to parents of children with other disorders or with parents of normally developing children-- parents of ASD children have higher levels of stress (Baker et al., 2005; Baker et al., 2003; Belchic, 1996; Cuxart, 1995), anxiety (Baxter et al., 2000; Hastings, 2003; Hastings et al., 2005a; Konstantareas & Homatidis, 1989), and depression (Feldman et al., 2007; Olsson & Hwang, 2002; Phetrasuwan, 2003; Singer, 2006; Smith et al., 2008).

Many studies also suggest that the concomitant behaviour problems in ASD, compared to the severity of the disorder itself, are most strongly associated with stress (Baker et al., 2002; Donenberg & Baker, 1993; Herring et al., 2006; Lecavalier et al., 2006; Tomanik et al., 2004) and with anxiety and depression (Baxter et al., 2000; Blacher, Shapiro et al., 1997; Quine & Pahl, 1991).

Nevertheless, some families, despite having children with severe ASD, have still managed successful psychological adaptation. From this we can infer that the characteristics of autistic children may not be the only factors that influence adaptation. Other types of variables are also involved, including social support, perception of problems and coping strategies. In the next section, we will describe the results of studies that have analysed the influences of these factors on adaptation.

Most of these studies have been carried out using partial analysis of variables. However, it is necessary to adopt a multidimensional and holistic approach to examine the influences of multiple variables simultaneously. In the third section of this chapter, we describe the characteristics of the Double ABCX model of adaptation. This theoretical model has proven to be effective for multi-dimensional analysis of stress and adaptation in families of children with ASD. This is also the theoretical model that our research group has used in the multidimensional analysis of adaptation in parents of children with ASD in the Spanish population, so we also explain the most relevant results of our own investigations.

One factor that has been shown to play a main role in adaptation is the "perception of the problem", evaluated by the variable sense of coherence (SOC). In our research, as in the studies reviewed, SOC plays a protective role against stress and promotes successful adaptation in parents of children with ASD. Given its influence on the outcome of adaptation, we will devote the fourth section of this chapter to describing the SOC and its components, as well as the role it plays in adaptation.

Continuing with the factor "perception of the problem", there has been increasing recognition of the importance of asking more positive questions about the perceptions and experiences of families of children with developmental disabilities (Hastings & Taunt, 2002). This perspective proposes that positive perceptions function as strategies that help families to adapt to or cope with the experiences of raising a child with developmental disabilities. The fifth section of the chapter will present our research on the positive contributions that children with ASD make to the family and the results that we have achieved in this area of research.

In the last section, we reflect on the findings that a positive perspective provides that are relevant to understanding the complexity of the adaptation of families of children with ASD. We also propose possible practical applications of the findings for professionals who work with families of children with ASD.

2. Factors involved in adaptation

In research on families of children with ASD, four factors have been shown to be significantly involved in the adaptation of parents: a) characteristics of the child with ASD – namely, the *severity of disorders and behaviour problems;* b) *social support*; c) *perception of problems;* and d) *coping strategies*. Here, we review the most relevant studies that have examined each of these factors and their influences on parent adaptation.

2.1 Characteristics of the child

With regard to the *characteristics of the child,* we must note that children with ASD vary greatly in the severity of the core symptoms of the disorders. The *severity of the disorder* varies on a continuum, where some people with ASD are severely affected (e.g., lack interest in others, have no language skills and show a very restricted repertoire of interests), whereas others have only slight impairment (e.g., show concern for others but have no social skills, have formal communication skills but not at a pragmatic level, have good cognitive function but may have specific skills in an area that becomes a stereotyped interest).

Several studies have found that the *severity of the disorder* is positively related to parenting stress (Bebko et al., 1987; Bravo, 2006; Hastings & Johnson, 2001; Kasari & Sigman, 1997;

Konstantareas & Homatidis, 1989; Pozo et al., 2006; Szatmari et al., 1994). That is, a more severe form of ASD is associated with higher levels of parenting stress. One possible explanation for these results is that a child with a severe form of the disorder has less personal autonomy and is more dependent on his or her parents to perform the tasks of daily life (e.g., eating, getting dressed and attending school). Parents of these children say that they have to spend much of their time and energy caring for their child. This makes ASD a potential source of parental stress.

However, the results identify the behavioural problems characteristic of children with ASD - namely, aggressive and self-injurious behaviour - as having more influence on parental stress and family adaptation (Herring et al., 2006; Lecavalier et al., 2006; Tomanik et al., 2004). These behaviours can become threatening to the physical integrity of family members, making home life difficult. Parents need to be constantly alert to try to maintain control of the situation. This constant vigilance can result in a high level of parental stress. This explains the high relevance of behaviour problems to family adaptation.

2.2 Social support

As we have seen, the families of children with ASD have to respond to multiple demands. These needs extend to different contexts -family, school and community- and change over time. One factor that has been shown to alleviate parental stress and improve response to the child's needs is *social support* (Bristol, 1984; Dyson, 1997; Sharpley et al., 1997). Dunst et al. (1986) define social support as a multidimensional construct that includes physical and instrumental assistance, attitude transmission, resource and information sharing, and emotional and psychological support. Social support may also refer to formal services one receives from professional-based organisations and/or services provided by more loosely structured organisations.

Boyd (2002) presents a critical review of the literature on the relationship between stress and social support in mothers of children with autism. Four groups of studies exist. One group investigates the characteristics of users of social support and of their children that lead parents to seek that support. One of the precursors that lead mothers to seek support is the amount of stress they experience as a result of rearing their child (Sharpley et al., 1997). When mothers are embedded in high-stress situations, they tend to seek social support as a strategy to help them cope. Other studies find an association between challenging child characteristics and a mother's inclination to seek social support (Bristol & Schopler, 1983; Koegel et al., 1992; Sharpley & Bitsika, 1997).

The second group of studies examines the negative effects on mothers of a lack of social support (Gray & Holden, 1992; Konstantareas & Homatidis, 1989; Sanders & Morgan, 1997). The results show that a scarcity of social support is related to higher levels of stress, anxiety, depression and pessimism and less social participation.

A third group of studies analyses the differential effects of two types of support on stress: *informal* and *formal support*. Bristol and Schopler (1983) defined *informal support* as a network that may include the immediate and extended family, friends, neighbours, and other parents of children with disabilities. They defined *formal support* as assistance that is social, psychological, physical, or financial and is provided either for free or in exchange for a fee through an organised group or agency. The results revealed that for mothers of children with autism, informal support appears to be a more effective stress buffer than formal support is.

Finally, the fourth group of studies examines the influence of support on parenting. Dunst et al. (1986) found that parental satisfaction with social support networks was associated with better personal well-being, more positive attitudes about the child, more positive interactions during parent–child play opportunities, and higher scores of their children on developmental tests. In the same way, the work of Raif and Rimmerman (1993) shows that parents who receive social support relate better emotionally to their children and engage in more positive interactions with them.

In summary, social support is a protective factor for the adaptation of parents of children with autism. Families that explain their experience with social support indicate that both the quantity and the quality of social support available to them are important. However, informal support is the more critical source of social support. This form of support provides invaluable emotional and instrumental help to the family. The community and professional support are important too, especially when the service includes family-oriented counselling and educational intervention for the child (Lounds, 2004).

2.3 Perception of the problem

The *perception of the problem* is another important factor involved in adaptation. Bristol (1987) assessed mothers' definitions of the stressful situation resulting from their child's disability through a *self-blame* variable – i.e., the degree to which the mother blames herself for her child's disability - and a *catastrophe* variable – i.e., the degree to which the mother perceives her child's disability as a family catastrophe-. The results demonstrated that these two variables are the best predictors of depression and marital satisfaction. Similarly, Saloviita et al. (2003) showed that the most important predictor of parental stress is a negative definition of the situation.

However, other studies have measured positive aspects that protect the family from stress and reduce the impact of the disability, such as: a) *hardiness* (Ben-Zur et al., 2005; Gill & Harris, 1991; Weiss, 2002); b) *self-efficacy* (Hastings & Brown, 2002); c) *ambiguous loss* (Boss, 1988, 1999); and d) *sense of coherence* (Olsson & Hwang, 2002). The *sense of coherence (SOC)* has been shown to be a protective factor in stress research in studies focused on family resilience across different contexts and disorders (McCubbin et al., 1998).

The origin of the *SOC* concept can be found in the theory of salutogenesis proposed by Antonovsky (1979, 1987). *SOC* is conceptualised as a "global orientation that expresses the extent to which one has a pervasive, enduring though dynamic feeling of confidence that: 1) the stimuli deriving from one's internal and external environments in the course of living are structured, predictable, and explicable (comprehensibility); 2) the resources are available to meet the demands posed by these stimuli (manageability); and 3) these demands are challenges worthy of investment and engagement and that life make sense emotionally" (1987, p.19).

The *SOC* is used in our research to assess the perception of the problem. The results indicate that it is a very significant variable in the adaptation of parents. Given its importance, we will devote a specific section of this chapter to SOC, explaining its characteristics and role in adaptation.

2.4 Coping strategies

Coping, or ways in which people respond to stress, is another factor that influences parental adaptation. Based on general theories of stress and coping (Lazarus & Folkman, 1984) as well as specific models of family adaptation (Crnic et al., 1983; McCubbin & Patterson, 1983), many studies show the important role played by coping in reducing stress. Folkman and Lazarus (1980) propose that there are two types of coping strategies: a) *problem-focused coping,* which includes cognitive and behavioural problem-solving efforts to alter or manage the source of stress, and b) *emotion-focused coping* strategies that attempt to reduce or manage emotional distress. Individuals usually access more than one coping strategy in managing challenging events and circumstances, and these can involve behavioural as well as cognitive approaches (Nolan et al. 1995).

Different studies have explored the types of strategies that are used by the parents of children with intellectual disabilities. Grant and Whittell (2000) interviewed family members to determine which problem-solving, cognitive and stress reduction coping strategies family they found useful. They found that *problem-solving* strategies are generally considered to be most effective when events and challenges are amenable to change and the person can accomplish the change. "The ability to build on personal experience and expertise" was the most relevant problem-solving strategy mentioned by the interviews. On the other hand, when problem-solving strategies do not work or are perceived to be irrelevant, caregivers may turn to *cognitive coping* in the form of managing meaning. The two most helpful strategies for coping in this category were realising that "there is always someone worse off than yourself" and that "the person you care for is not to blame". The last group of strategies that these authors found was *managing* or *alleviating stress.* Circumstances can arise when neither problem solving nor cognitive reappraisal work, so caregivers have to rely on dealing with the consequences of challenges and the associated stresses.

Coping is theoretically context dependent (Carver et al., 1989). Therefore, both the nature of the stress and the interaction between stressors and the environment should affect the development of coping efforts. Brown (1993) noted that the developmental stages of coping need to be better understood; for example, an initial response involving escape or withdrawal might be a necessary first step toward solving the problem.

Parents of children with ASD are faced with a variety of stressful situations, but many families are able to cope successfully. Some research has examined what kinds of strategies parents use to cope with the demands that accompany raising a child with ASD (Dunn et al., 2001; Hastings et al., 2005b). The findings of this line of research show that parents who adopt *escape-avoidance strategies* to cope with the stresses of raising children with ASD report more stress and mental health problems; in contrast, those using positive reframing strategies report less stress.

In summary, the specific types of coping strategies used by parents of children with ASD affect parental stress and adaptation. Professionals who work with families of children with ASD need to be aware of the coping strategies that parents use to deal with the demands of parenting. The studies show that active avoidance coping appears to be maladaptive and that positive approaches to coping may be adaptive. In this sense, intervention with parents might focus on reducing parents' use of avoidant coping strategies and increasing their use of positive strategies.

Most of the studies cited above carried out only partial analyses of the relations between variables. Only a few studies have examined in a global way the adaptation of parents of children with ASD (Bristol, 1987; Jones & Passey, 2005; Pakenham et al., 2005) or intellectual disabilities (Orr et al., 1991; Saloviita et al., 2003). These studies are based on the Double ABCX model of stress and adaptation (McCubbin & Patterson, 1983) and demonstrate the model's effectiveness in predicting adaptation. In the next section, we describe the characteristics of the Double ABCX model, the results of research using a multidimensional perspective to study parental adaptation, and our multidimensional studies on stress and family quality of life.

3. A multidimensional perspective: The double ABCX model

The Double ABCX model proposes that the adaptation outcome (factor xX) depends on interrelations between several factors: *stressors or characteristics of children* (factor aA); *social support or resources* (factor bB); *perception or definition of the stressor* (factor cC); and *coping strategies* (factor BC). The model postulates that the last three factors could reduce the negative impact of the characteristics of the child on parental adaptation.

Bristol (1987) assessed the factors of the model using the following variables: the severity of the child's handicap and other family stressors; family resources supporting cohesion; social support; the family's definition of the child's handicap; and coping patterns. This author conducted a canonical correlation analysis of data and multiple regressions, and the results showed that informal support and a negative definition of the child's handicap were the strongest predictors of adaptation.

The multiple regression analysis technique has also been used by Jones and Passey (2005) and Pakenham et al. (2005). Coping style and parental locus of control relating to control by the child were the most significant predictors of parental stress in the study by Jones and Passey. Likewise, Pakenham et al. (2005) found that, in support of their predictions, better maternal adjustment was related to higher levels of qualitative social support and emotional approach coping (i.e., positive reinterpretation and seeking social support) and lower levels of child behaviour problems, stress appraisals, and passive avoidant coping.

The multiple regression equations tested by Salovitta et al. (2003) confirm the importance of intervening factors in explaining the stress felt by parents of children with intellectual disabilities. The single most important predictor of parental stress was the definition of the situation. In mothers, this definition was associated with the behavioural problems of the child, whereas in fathers it was connected with the experienced social acceptance of the child.

These studies based on the ABCX model pose a system of data analysis to identify factors that are most predictive of adaptation but fail to analyse the interrelations of these factors in the adaptation model. A more advanced step toward a multidimensional analysis of adaptation is performed by Orr et al. (1991). These authors also discuss the adaptation of parents of children with mental retardation using the Double ABCX model, but, in this case, they use path analysis to examine the relations among the variables in the model. Path analysis allows researchers to make statements about patterns of causation and to identify the direct and indirect effects among the set of variables. Based on the results of their study, these researchers suggest that the actual order of the model could be viewed as a linear chain following an ACBX pattern. That is, the "perception of the problem" is the first step in coping with an event like the birth of a child with mental retardation.

This analysis of the state of the art demonstrates the need to take further steps in the study of the psychological adjustment of parents of children with ASD. Multidimensional analysis allows us to achieve a deeper understanding of the adaptation process by evaluating both the factors themselves and their interrelations. We carry out a study based on the Double ABCX model to analyse maternal stress in a sample of 39 Spanish mothers of children with

ASD (Pozo et al., 2006). We assessed the following variables: *characteristics of child (severity of disorders* and *behaviour problems); social support; the perception of the problem* (evaluate by *sense of coherence);* and *stress.* Path analysis was performed using the statistics program AMOS 5 Graphic. This method offers the possibility of providing a global interpretation of the information.

The empirical results of this study (see Fig. 1) demonstrate the utility of the theoretical model for the analysis of stress in mothers of children with ASD.

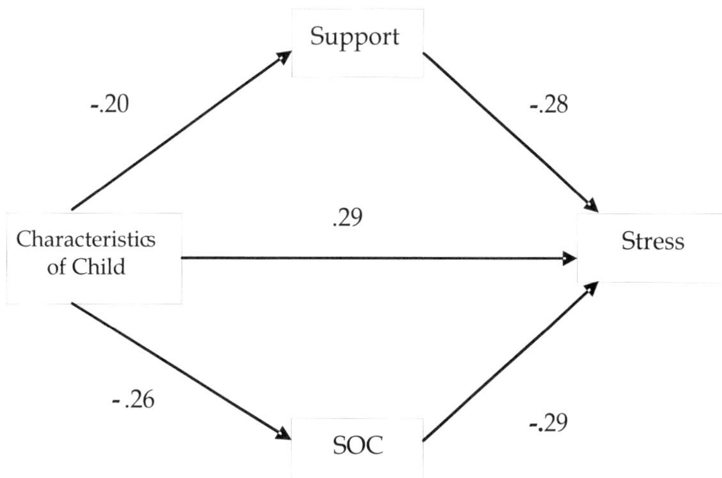

Fig. 1. Stress empirical model and standardized β coefficients

As shown in the figure, the characteristics of the child (*severity of disorder* and *behaviour problems)* direct and positively affect the level of *maternal stress.* Additionally, the model reveals two indirect ways of influence on stress: 1) the perception of the utility of *social support* in the family; and 2) the perception of the problem, evaluated by a *sense of coherence* (SOC). These variables—*social support* and *sense of coherence*—have a mediating role in the relation between characteristics of children with ASD and parental stress. This result might explain why there are families that despite having children with more *severe autism* and *behaviour problems* still exhibit better adaptation compared to other families in which the children are less severely affected.

On the other hand, most studies have used negative outcomes, such as stress, anxiety, and depression, to assess adaptation. We consider a positive perspective fundamental to advancing knowledge of adaptation in parents of children with ASD. It is necessary to know what variables are implicated in positive adaptation and to understand their effects on successful adaptation to account for them in designing family interventions to improve adaptation.

Recently, we carried out a multidimensional study to analyse the adaptation model using *family quality of life* as the dependent variable (Pozo, 2010). The participants were 59 mothers of children with ASD aged between 28 and 69 years (M = 44.6, δ = 7.9). The children were aged between 4 and 38 years (M = 14.2, δ = 7.9); 47 were boys and 12 girls. The distribution frequency in terms of diagnosis was: Autistic Disorder, 43; Asperger's Syndrome, 1; Rett Syndrome, 5; and PDD-NOS, 10.

Based on the Double ABCX model, we designed a theoretical model of the relations between the variables, which is represented in Figure 2.

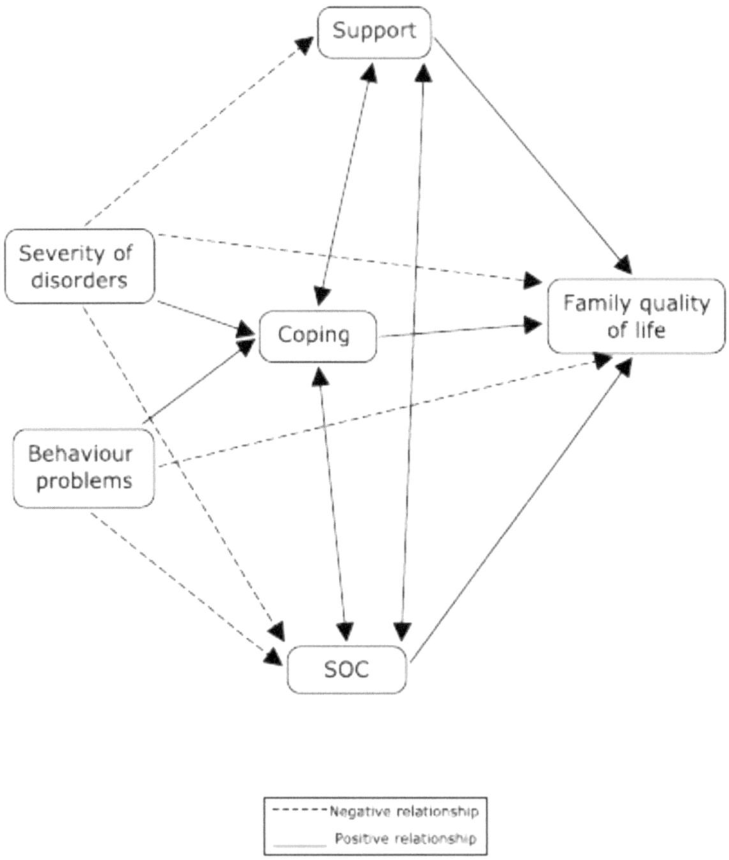

Fig. 2. Theoretical model of family quality of life and interrelationships between variables

Information about the factors and variables was obtained through the following questionnaires:

- Childhood Autism Rating Scale (CARS) (Schopler et al., 1988; adapted to Spanish by García Villamisar and Polaino Llorente, 1992; reliability: α = .92)
- The Behaviour Problems Inventory (BPI) (Rojahn et al., 2001; reliability: α = .89)
- Checklist of Supports for Parents of the Handicapped (CSPH) (Bristol, 1979; reliability: α = .89)
- Sense of Coherence Questionnaire (SOC) (Antonowsky, 1987; reliability: α = .90)
- Brief Coping Orientation of Problems Experienced (COPE) (Carver, 1997; adapted to Spanish by Crespo & Cruzado, 1997; reliability: α = .77)
- Family Quality of Life (FQL) (Poston *et al.*, 2003; adapted to Spanish by Sainz et al.,, 2005; reliability: α = .94)

Path analysis was carried out with the statistical program AMOS 5 Graphics. In the following figure, we present the empirical model of quality of life in mothers of children with ASD.

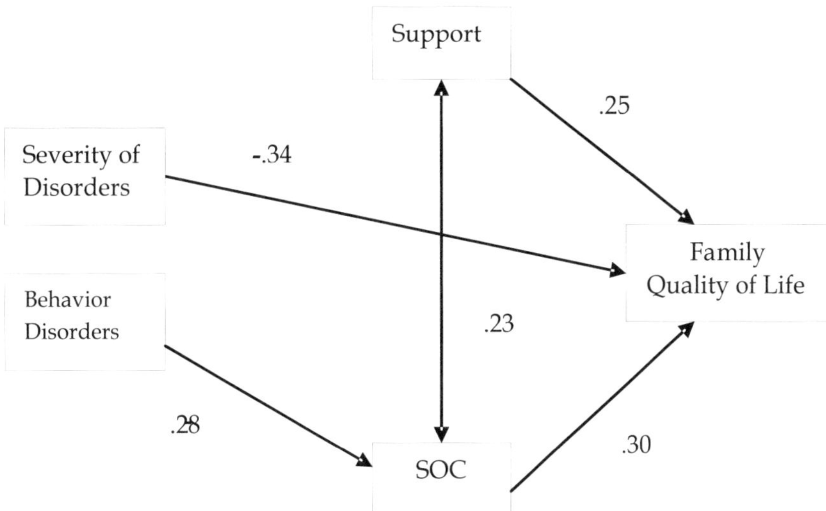

Fig. 3. Family quality of life empirical model and standardized β coefficients

The results show that the empirical models adequately fit the theoretical model, but in a peculiar way. As we can see in Figure 3, *severity of disorders* has a direct and negative relation with family quality of life. That is, mothers who have a child who is more severely affected perceive lower quality of life in the family. More specifically, they might feel fewer positive feeling regarding their family life, and the resources that are readily available to satisfy their needs remain insufficient (i.e., two dimensions of *family quality of life*).

On the other hand, behaviour *problems* show an indirect effect on quality of life, specifically through the *sense of coherence* (SOC). Thus, the effects of behaviour problems on adaptation are moderated by the level of SOC in mothers. Mothers with a high level of SOC probably perceive that the *behaviour problems* of the child are more controllable and less threatening than would a mother with lower levels of SOC.

With regard to *social support*, mothers who perceive that they have adequate social support to cope with the demands of caring for their children are likely to report a better family quality of life.

In summary, in all of the existing studies of adaptation in parents of children with autism, the perception of the problem is the most relevant predictor of adaptation. Our studies demonstrate that SOC plays a fundamental role in adaptation as a mediator of the effects of stress and family quality of life. The next section describes the SOC and explains its influence on adaptation.

4. The sense of coherence as a mediator and predictor variable

Antonowsky (1979) sought to explain the relation between life stresses and health in the theory of salutogenesis by what he calls the *sense of coherence (SOC)*. SOC was defined as: "a global orientation that expresses the extent to which one has a pervasive, enduring, though dynamic, feeling of confidence that one's internal and external environments are predictable and that there is a high probability that things will work out as well as can reasonably be expected" (p. 132).

The salutogenetic perspective proposed by Antonowsky (1987) suggests that SOC enables people to resolve tension in a health-promoting manner, to reflect about their external and internal resources, to identify and mobilise them, and to promote effective coping by finding solutions.

SOC is conceived as a personality characteristic or coping style, an enduring tendency to see one's life space as more or less orderly, predictable, and manageable. This theoretical model suggests that individuals develop a generalised way of looking at the world as more or less coherent. This sense of coherence tentatively appears in childhood; it becomes more definitive during adolescence, becoming fully developed around age 30 (Antonowsky & Sagy, 1986).

The SOC consists of three components. The first component is a cognitive aspect called comprehensibility. It is defined as the ability of the family or the individual to understand life situations and give them some order and structure. The second component is manageability, which emphasises the emotional aspect. It refers to the ability to handle or respond to situational demands or the feeling that one is capable of obtaining the necessary resources to do so. Finally, the component that corresponds to the motivational aspect is the meaning, or sense, which refers to the extent that one feels that life makes sense. People with high scores on this component see problems as challenges and commitments that are worth the effort necessary to address them.

A significant amount of research has investigated the SOC, especially its contribution to the development and maintenance of health from salutogenesis theory. Eriksson and Lindström (2006) review 25 years of research (458 scientific publications) on the relation between the SOC and health. Their analysis and conclusions show that SOC is strongly related to health, especially mental health. In general, stronger SOC is related to better perceived health. This relation is manifested in study populations regardless of age, sex, ethnicity or nationality. SOC alone does not explain overall health but is an important contributor to the development and maintenance of health. SOC seems to play a main, mediating role in the explanation of health. Furthermore, the SOC seems to be able to predict health. From a psychological perspective, research has characterised its relation to psychological well-being (Cohen & Dekel, 2000; Pallant & Lae, 2002; Sagy et al., 1990) and its inverse relation with anxiety (Antonovsky & Sagy, 1986).

SOC is conceptualised as a coping mechanism characterised by the tendency to see life as predictable and manageable. Thus, a person with a high SOC is less likely to perceive a situation as threatening and anxiety arousing compared to a person with a weak SOC. Family life is filled with stressors, even more so for the parents of a child with ASD, but some parents adjust well and become empowered.

Stressors can be either acute or chronic, and the two forms have different relations with the SOC (Antonowsky, 1987). An acute stressor is discrete and time limited. Individual differences in SOC levels predict individual differences in coping with acute stressors. A person with a weak SOC is more vulnerable to the stressor. Knowledge of the diagnosis that one's child has ASD can be characterised as an acute stressor. Therefore, the SOC level of the parent prior to the diagnosis may determine how he or she deals with the impact of the news and adjusts to life with the child. High-SOC parents of children with ASD may perceive their situation as a challenge and assume that they can adapt to the demands. The underlying confidence that things will work out and that one has the resources to cope is a relevant strength.

The results of studies show that SOC acts as a mediator in the relation between autistic symptom severity and parenting stress (Mak et al., 2007; Pozo et al., 2006) and in the relation between children's behavioural problems and parents' perceptions of family quality of life (Pozo, 2010).

A chronic stressor is a generalised and long-lasting life condition or characteristic that is embedded in the life of a person. Antonowsky (1993) found evidence that women with certain chronic illnesses have very low levels of SOC. Olsson & Hwang (2002) raised the interesting question of whether parenting a child with autism could become a chronic stressor that influences the parent's SOC level negatively over time. The birth or the diagnosis of a child with disabilities can be considered an acute stressor, but an acute stressor can alter a family's life in such a way that it becomes a chronic stressor. They found that mothers of children with autism have lower SOC levels than mothers of children with intellectual disability but without autism, who, in turn, had lower SOC levels than control mothers. Fathers' SOC scores did not differ significantly among the three groups. Their hypothesis, i.e., that the presence in a family of a child with an intellectual disability is a chronic stressor that influences the parents' SOC level negatively over time, was only partly supported, since no relation was found between the age of the child and SOC levels in parents of children with intellectual disability or autism.

The SOC, as a stable trait, may be adversely affected by crisis situations, but over time it can be reset and restored to its previous values (Antonowsky, 1987). The impact of a child's diagnosis of autism and the first and most difficult experiences of facing life with a child with intellectual disabilities and behavioural problems are inevitably acute stressors that can adversely affect the SOC. However, we also think that the passage of time and the progressive increase in control of the situation may allow improved SOC. The parents improve the perception that the course of life is structured, predictable, and explicable, that resources are available to meet the demands, and that these demands are challenges worthy of investment and engagement. Data from a longitudinal study of 21 mothers of children with ASD support this hypothesis (Pozo, 2010). The scores for this group of mothers on the SOC scale (Antonowsky, 1987) in two times of measurement, with an interval of four and half years, reflected a statistically significant increase due to improvements in two of the components of SOC: comprehensibility and manageability. The meaning or significance dimension is stable between the two measurement points. These results support not only the mediating or modulating role of SOC (Pozo et al., 2006; Pozo, 2010) but also the possibility of regaining higher levels of manageability and comprehensibility perception and their protective benefits

In summary, studies on the SOC in the broad health context and specifically in parents of children with ASD and the results of empirical studies suggest that the concept of SOC, its theoretical framework and the body of related research are valuable tools for understanding the psychological adjustment of parents of children with ASD.

5. Positive contributions to the family

Until the late 1980s, family and disability studies focused on the analysis of the negative effects of a child's disorder and its consequences in the family. Empirical research on the positive contributions of a disabled child to the family was very rare. However, parents' narratives about their relationships with their disabled children have always included positive aspects. Thus, Mullins (1987), in a review of 60 books written by parents of disabled children, found that parents inevitably mention negative aspects of their lives (e.g., demands, needs, anxiety, stress), but also appear to be positive (e.g., positive feelings, personal growth, family strength).

One of the most significant studies on the positive contributions of children with disabilities in the family was conducted by Behr et al. (1992). This research served as the basis for the construction of the four scales that constitute the Kansas Inventory of Parental Perceptions (KIPP). One of the four scales is the "Scale of Positive Contributions". Interviews were conducted with 28 families in which parents asked to describe explicitly the positive contributions of living with a disabled child. The aim of this study was to identify the categories that define the positive contributions that parents report. A qualitative analysis of the interviews revealed 16 categories of positive perceptions that, after conducting a factor analysis, were finally grouped into 5 factors. Further validation in a sample of 1,262 families of children with disabilities revealed four additional factors that were not identified in the previous phase. Thus, the "Positive Contributions" Scale is composed of 50 items corresponding to 9 dimensions. A more recent study (Hastings, Allen, McDemontt and Still, 2002) applying this scale found only 3 different factors describing disabled children's positive contributions: a) Happiness and Fulfilment; b) Strength and Family Closeness; and c) Personal Growth and Maturity. The factor structure was reduced, but the positive perceptions that parents reported in the different studies showed a pattern of systematic categories.

A few interesting studies explore the possible influence of positive perceptions of family adaptation through their relation with variables such as stress and family well-being. These studies show that positive perceptions reduce the negative impact that disability can have on the family and that these relationships can be modulated further by individual variables, such as gender of the parents (Hastings and Taunt, 2002).

Most studies have focused on disability in general. Targeted research is needed on the perception of positive contributions by parents of children with ASD and the influence of these contributions on the parents' psychological adjustment. With this objective in mind, we conducted an empirical study in a sample of Spanish families with a child affected by ASD. We wanted to study the influence of *perceptions of positive contributions* on family adaptation to the problems posed by ASD through its relations with *family quality of life, anxiety, depression* and *stress*. We were also interested in determining whether there were significant differences between mothers and fathers in positive perceptions as a contributor to adjustment.

Although there is no explicit theory on positive perceptions, both stress and coping theory and the theory of cognitive adaptation propose that positive perceptions function as resources and strategies that help families to adapt to the challenge of caring for a disabled child. Therefore, we formulated the hypothesis that the parents' perception of positive contributions would have inverse correlations with depression, anxiety and stress and a positive correlation with quality of family life (Pozo et al, 2010).

The study involved 24 fathers and 33 mothers aged between 36 and 78 years ($M = 45.79$, $\delta = 8.39$). The children were aged between 6 and 32 years ($M = 13.85$, $\delta = 7.83$); 24 were boys and 11 girls. The distribution in terms of diagnosis was: Autistic Disorder, 24; Asperger's Syndrome, 2; Rett Syndrome, 1; disintegrative disorder, 1; and PDD-NOS, 7.

The Positive Contribution Scale (Behr et al., 1992), discussed earlier, was used for the evaluation of the perception of positive contributions. This is a 50-item scale with 9 subscales, although our study used only 3 dimensions, as proposed by Hastings et al. (2002).

The scales used to assess the variables related to family adaptation and reliability results obtained in the study were as follows:

- Family Quality of Life (FQL) (Poston *et al.*, 2003; adapted to Spanish by Sainz et al,, 2005). Reliability (α = .95).
- The Hospital Anxiety and Depression Scale (HADS) (Zigmon & Snaith, 1983; adapted to Spanish by Tejero et al.,, 1986). Reliability (α = .75).
- Parenting Stress Index (PSI) (Abidin, 1995; adapted to Spanish by Pozo, 2010). Reliability (α = .82).

T-tests were applied to compare the means both of the adjustment variables and of the measures of positive perceptions between mothers and fathers. The results are shown in Table I

		N	M	t
Total Positive Contribution (PC)	father	24	123.83	2.01*
	mother	33	131.64	
PC Happiness	father	24	16.71	.95
	mother	33	17.49	
PC Strength	father	24	19.62	3.01*
	mother	33	21.93	
PC Growth	father	24	17.45	.32
	mother	33	17.75	
Family Quality of Life Satisfaction	father	24	88.16	.53
	mother	33	85.84	
Family Quality of Life Importance	father	24	96.29	.59
	mother	33	98.93	
Anxiety	father	24	6.08	2.03*
	mother	33	7.51	
Depression	father	24	4.66	.92
	mother	33	5.39	
Stress	father	24	105.75	.64
	mother	33	108.36	

Table 1. Positive contributions and adaptation: mean differences between mothers and fathers

The first notable result is that the degree of *stress* in both fathers (M = 105.75) and mothers (M = 108.36) achieved clinically significant levels (values above 90), although there were no significant differences between mothers and fathers in this variable. The only adaptation variable in which there are significant gender differences is anxiety ($t = 2.03$, $p < 0.05$). The mothers have higher levels of anxiety compared to the fathers. With regard to positive perceptions, there are significant differences in the Positive Contribution Scale Total ($t = 2.01$, $p < 0.05$) and the subscale of Strength and Family Closeness ($t = 3.01$, $p < 0.05$), with the mothers scoring higher on both measures.

To accomplish the second objective, namely, to ascertain the relation of the positive contributions to family adaptation, we proceeded to an analysis of correlations using the Pearson coefficient (see Table 2).

The results show that, for the fathers, the subscale of Strength and Family Closeness is positively and significantly related to Quality of Family Life in two dimensions: Satisfaction (r = .43, p <0.01) and Importance (r = .47, p <0.01). In mothers, only the Personal Growth and Maturity subscale shows a significant relationship with the *anxiety* variable (r = -.55, p <0.01), with a negative sign. That is, those mothers who believe that caring for their child will bring them feelings of personal growth and maturity will face situations more calmly, thus reducing their level of anxiety about the demands and challenges posed by their situation.

	Total		**Happiness**		**Strenght**		**Growth**	
	father	**mother**	**father**	**mother**	**father**	**mother**	**father**	**mother**
FQL Satisfaction	.18	.33	-.02	.16	**.43****	.26	-.29	.24
FQL Importance	.27	.10	-.03	.05	**.47****	.27	-.19	-.22
Anxiety	.29	-.23	.22	-.25	.21	.04	.23	**-.55****
Depression	-.09	-.16	-.15	.12	-.15	-.17	-.07	-.27
Stress	-.08	-.31	-.23	-.26	-.19	-.18	.28	-.33

Table 2. Matrix correlations between Positive Contributions scales and adaptation variables

In summary, these data show that the perception of positive contributions is relevant to the psychological adjustment of parents. Parental perception of Strength and Family Closeness shows a close relation with perception of Quality of Family Life in the two dimensions of Satisfaction and Importance. The fathers' perception of positive contributions does not affect their mental health, as manifested by depression, stress or anxiety. However, the level of perceived positive contributions and the role that perceived positive contributions play in the process of adaptation are different for fathers and mothers. Mothers perceive more positive contributions compared to fathers. The mothers also have higher levels of anxiety. At the same time, their capacity for the perception of positive contributions, particularly their perception of Personal Growth and Maturity, is negatively related to their levels of anxiety (r = -. 55, p <0.01). These results are not contradictory.

In general, mothers are more involved than fathers are in the care of a child with ASD. In that sense, mothers are more exposed to the challenges and demands of raising the child and show higher levels of anxiety. At the same time, mothers may have more opportunities to observe positive changes in the child and to experience personal growth associated with overcoming the daily challenges of organising the child's life and responding to the needs of the child. We could also say that the perception of the positive contributions plays a protective role that is especially relevant to psychological adaptation in the case of mothers.

The study results reflect the relevance of research on the positive aspects of raising a child with ASD and underline the need for further research. The findings also show that the Positive Contribution Scale can be a useful tool to explore positive perceptions in families of children with ASD and to identify specific actions to increase positive perceptions.

6. Implications for intervention

Despite their limitations, we believe that these studies, especially the multidimensional perspective, provide new data that will help researchers and clinicians to better understand the complexity of the adaptation of families of children with ASD. These findings may be directly applicable to the planning of objectives and strategies for professionals working with families of children with ASD. Two major aspects stand out as possible points for intervention: the importance of the perception of positive contributions and the protective role of the SOC and its resilience to chronic stress.

When the adjustment of families of children with ASD is studied, the focus is often on negative effects, while the positive effects are ignored. From a prevention and intervention perspective, it is important to understand what the negative effects are to provide family members with adequate strategies and techniques for reducing or counteracting them. However, the positive aspects of having a child with ASD are equally important to consider. Some parents who are initially depressed with their child's diagnosis of autism recover and cope effectively with the situation. Why are some families insulated from the more adverse effects of stress and able to grow and become empowered?

The results of these empirical studies support the important role other authors have proposed for protective factors in their models of family adaptation. The family adaptation model described by Lounds (2004) proposes that three groups of factors exert important influences on family functioning: historical factors, family coping resources and family social support. She places special emphasis on family coping resources as protective factors. Protective factors can serve to increase family resiliency and to reduce the potential adverse effects of the challenges on the family. These protective factors may be improved with appropriate intervention. These resources include, among others, parenting knowledge and skills, problem-solving skills, organisational skills and optimism.

The challenges confronting families of children with ASD are quite varied, and in the long term, so are the organisational abilities, priorities and routines, and problem-solving skills that will be critical to family survival and a feeling of control of their lives. Psychologists and counsellors often teach these skills to their clients. Families that do not have well-developed organisational skills can acquire them with counselling and practice. However, what about optimism? What about positive perceptions?

Family members' attitudes about the situation may be more important than the concrete challenges that the family faces. Positive attitudes lead to hope and other positive emotions. Hasting and Johnson (2001) found that parents of children with autism who were able to positively reframe challenging events were less likely to report being depressed. We found that the mothers of children with ASD who reported experiencing personal growth and maturity as a result of their life with a child with autism experience lower anxiety levels. Parents' reports of their children's positive contributions are also related to their adaptation, particularly to the perception of quality of family life.

Can psychologists, teachers, medical personnel, and service providers help parents to discover and appreciate the positive contributions that their children with autism bring to their lives?

The work that accompanies the development of a child with ASD will always include goals to achieve, but parents must learn to value milestones that have already been reached. Communication educators, service providers, and psychologists should not focus only on problems and difficulties when interacting with parents but should always leave time to highlight the positive aspects of the child's development, including his or her strengths and improvements. For example, consider the dynamics of communication between the parents and the child's school. The communication system is based on requests for meetings with parents when there are problems or difficulties in inclusive education. This system will surely help solve the problems, but it will not encourage the development of positive perceptions among parents. On the contrary, if the school has a good communication protocol that feeds positive information back to parents, trains teachers on the importance of communication with parents and seeks balance in the parent meetings between a summary of the child's progress and a discussion of his or her challenges, great benefits to parents will result. Parents whose children attend such schools report higher perceived school support and less anxiety about their decisions on the education of their children (Babío, 2009).

It should be kept in mind that the perception of positive contributions to the psychological adjustment of parents can lead clinicians, teachers, and others who interact with children with ASD modulate their strategies and forms of communication to provide opportunities and content that promote positive perceptions.

As we have seen in previous sections, one of the factors that are relevant to the explanation of psychological adaptation in parents is the perception of the problem. Both the literature review and the results of the studies presented here emphasise the protective role of SOC. The SOC works as a global mechanism that modulates the impact of child behaviour problems and facilitates the selection of the best coping strategies. .The SOC protects the psychological and social well-being of parents. This demonstrated importance raises the question of how professionals can strengthen parents' SOC.

Antonowsky (1993), who first developed the concept of SOC, raises the same question and another that is no less important: do we have a criterion for avoiding strategies that may weaken the SOC? To answer these questions, the author lays out some key principles:

1. It is important to understand that "to optimize the chances of successful coping with a stressor one must believe that one *understands* the problem and that one has at one's disposal the *resources* that are needed, and one must *wish* to cope with the problem" (p. 117).
2. It is essential to understand that a strong SOC is not a particular coping style. Potential stressors in life are so many and so varied that there is no pattern of coping that fits all of them: "What the person with a strong SOC does is to select the particular coping strategy that seems most appropriate to deal with the stressor being confronted" (Antonowsky, 1987, p. 138). For coping to be successful, it is important to respond appropriately given the nature of the stressor. It is therefore crucial that parents have a wide repertoire of coping strategies and the flexibility to choose and implement the most appropriate strategy for each challenge at a given time.
3. The SOC has three components: comprehensibility, manageability and meaningfulness. Antonowsky sees meaningfulness as primary. Do the parents see their child's developmental disability as a burden or challenge? This is the motivational core of the matter. Do they wish to cope? This is a critical question. Without motivation, providing information or support is unlikely to be useful. If parents start by seeing coping as possible and desirable, increasing comprehensibility and manageability is more likely.

In conclusion, our first challenge as professionals should be to help parents of children with ASD to overcome their hopelessness and maintain the motivation and desire to cope with the challenges of parenting a child with ASD. On this basis, we can help strengthen the comprehensibility and the manageability of the situation for parents.

Providing parents with the necessary information about the disorder has always made sense, but the present results on the role of SOC as a protective variable argue for even more attention to be paid to this need. Adequate and well-managed information helps parents to understand the problem and to have a perception of greater control and ability to manage the situation. Parents who know more about autism and its treatment and, overall, how to parent a child with autism, will be better able to adjust their expectations about the development of the child as well as their own feelings of well-being and competency. Professionals can help to strengthen parents' SOC by identifying strengths and internal and external resources at their disposal. They can help parents to make use of these resources despite difficult circumstances. Social support from family, friends, institutions, associations or support groups can make life more manageable and understandable. Social participation by parents is important and should be a goal in itself.

As stated by Meyer (1993), a natural response to a crisis in the family is the desire to do something to improve the situation. Early intervention programs usually involve mothers, but other family members may not be included. Without opportunities to contribute to ameliorating the crisis, family members may feel powerless. By contrast, programs that provide family members with concrete ways of improving the family's situation may promote mental well-being. By providing family members with opportunities for support and information, fathers, siblings and grandparents can increase their sense of control over the crisis. Moreover, the involvement of those members of the family, especially fathers, will have reverberating positive effects on mothers.

Providing parents with a wide repertoire of coping strategies -cognitive, emotional and instrumental - and developing the flexibility and the understanding needed to choose and implement the most appropriate strategy to tackle each challenge are also important objectives of professional interventions to help families of children with ASD.

7. Conclusions

In conclusion, we want to emphasise that the families of children with ASD can be helped to meet the child's needs in appropriate ways. Moreover, in this process of adaptation, some parents have an experience of growth and maturity that empowers them. Research on adaptation processes can help to identify risks and protective factors. In this sense, the multidimensional perspective has proven particularly suitable to allow analysis not only of the weights of the various factors but also of the relationship dynamics that explain the psychological adjustment of parents. It is important to identify the needs and difficulties involved in caring for children with ASD to provide or develop the actions necessary for support. However, it is equally important to identify the positive contributions to family life of a person affected by ASD and to study family adaptation from a positive perspective, looking for factors promoting psychological well-being and enhancing the perceived quality of family life. Research in this area is only beginning, and much future work is needed.

8. Acknowledgements

We thank professor Richard Hastings and his team for their contributions in the design of this research during the stay of the first author at the University of Bangor.

9. References

Abidin, R. R. (1995). *Parenting Stress Index Manual.* Odessa, FL: Psychological Assesment Resources.

Altiere, M. J. (2006). *Family functioning and coping behaviours in parents of children with autism. Unpublished doctoral dissertation*, University of Eastern Michigan, EE. UU.

Antonovsky, A. (1979). *Health, stress and coping.* Jossey-Bass, ISBN: 0875894127, San Francisco.

Antonovsky,A. (1987). Unravelling the mystery of health: How people manage stress and stay well (1ª.ed.), Jossey-Bass, ISBN: 1555420281, San Francisco.

Antonovsky, A. (1993). The structure and properties of the sense of coherence scale. *Social Science and Medicine, 36,* (725–733), ISSN: 0277-9536.

Antonovsky, A., & Sagy, S. (1986). The development of a sense of coherence and its impact on responses to stress situations. *Journal of Social Psychology 126,* (213–225), ISSN: 1099-0992.

Babío, M. (2009). La percepción de apoyo escolar Equipo de Orientación Educativa y Psicopedagógica de la Comunidad de Madrid, Spain. Unpublished report.

Baker, B. L., Brookman L., & Stahmer, A. (2005). Stress level and adaptability in parents of toddlers with and without autism spectrum disorders. *Research and Practice for Persons with Severe Disabilities, 30 (4),* (194-204), ISSN: 0274-9483.

Baker, B. L., McIntyre, L. L., Blacher, J., Crnic, K. A., Edelbrock C., & Low C. (2003). Preschool children with and without developmental delay: Behaviour problems and parenting stress over time. *Journal of Intellectual Disability Research, 47,* (217-230), ISSN: 0964-2633.

Baxter, C., Cummins, R. A., & Yiolitis, L. (2000). Parental stress attributed to family members with and without disability: A longitudinal study. *Journal of Intellectual and Developmental Disability, 25(2),* (105-118), ISSN: 1366-8250.

Bebko, J. M., Konstantareas, M. M., & Springer, J. (1987). Parent and professional evaluations of family stress associated with characteristics of autism. *Journal of Autism and Developmental Disorders, 17 (4),* (565-576), ISSN: 0162-3257.

Behr, S. K., Murphy, D. L., & Summers, J. A. (1992). *User's Manual: Kansas Inventory of Parental Perceptions (KIPP).* Lawrence, KS: Beach Center on Families and Disability.

Belchic, J.K. (1996). Stress, social support and sense of parenting competence: A comparison of mothers and fathers of children with autism, Down syndrome and normal development across the family life cycle. *Dissertation Abstracts International: Section A: The Humanities and Social Sciences, 57* (2-A), p. 574.

Ben-zur, H., Duvdevany, I., & Lury, L. (2005). Associations of social support and hardiness with mental health among mothers of adult children with intellectual disability. *Journal of Intellectual Disability Research, 49 (1),* (54-62), ISSN: 0964-2633.

Blacher, J., Shapiro, J., Lopez, S., Diaz, L., & Fusco, J. (1997). Depression in Latina mothers of children with mental retardation: A neglected concern. *American Journal on Mental Retardation, 101,* (483-496), ISSN: 0002-9351.

Boss, P. G. (1988). *Family stress management.* Sage Publications, ISBN: 0-916174-58-1. Newbury Park, CA.

Boss, P. G. (1999). *Ambiguous loss.* Harvard University Press, ISBN: 0674003810, Cambridge.

Boyd, B. A. (2002). Examining the relationship between stress and lack of social support in mothers of children with autism. *Focus on Autism and Other Developmental Disabilities, 17(4),* (208-215), ISSN: 1088-3576.

Bravo, K. (2006). Severity of autism and parental stress: The mediating role of family environment. *Dissertation Abstracts International: Section A: The Humanities and Social Sciences, 66 (10),* 3.821.

Bristol, M. (1984). Family resources and successful adaptation to autistic children, In: *The effects of autism on the family,* E. Schopler & G. Mesibov (Eds.), (289-319), Plenum Press, ISBN: 8449301173, New York, EE. UU.

Bristol, M., & Schopler, E. (1983). Stress and coping in families of autistic adolescents, In: *Autism in adolescents and adults,* E. Schopler y G. B. Mesibov (Eds.), (251–276), Plenum Press, ISBN: 1557661715, New York.

Brown, J. D. (1993). Coping with stress: The beneficial role of positive illusions. In: *Cognitive coping, families and disability,* A. Turnbull, J.M. Patterson, S. Behr, D. Murphy, J. Marquis y M. Blue-Banning (Eds.), (123-133), Paul H. Brookes Publishing Co, ISBN 0 86758 4998, Baltimore, EE. UU.

Bryson, S. (1996). Brief report: Epidemiology of autism. *Journal of Autism and Developmental Disorders, 26, (2),* (115-281), ISSN: 0162-3257.

Carver, C. S. (1997). You want to measure coping but your protocol's too long: Consider de brief COPE. *International Journal of Behavioural Medicine, 4(1),* (92-100), ISSN: 0883-6612.

Carver, C. S., Scheier, M. F., & Weintraub, J. K. (1989). Assessing coping strategies: A theoretically based approach. *Journal of Personality and Social Psychology, 56,* (267–283), ISSN: 0022-3514.

Cohen, O., & Dekel, R. (2000). Sense of coherence, ways of coping and well-being of married and divorced mothers. *Contemporary Family Therapy: An International Journal 22,* (467–486), ISSN: 0892-2764.

Crespo, M., & Cruzado, J. A. (1997). La evaluación del afrontamiento: Adaptación española del cuestionario COPE con una muestra de estudiantes universitarios. *Análisis y Modificación de conducta,* 23, (797-830), ISSN: 0211-7339.

Crnic, K. A., Friedrich, W. N., & Greenberg, M. T. (1983). Adaptation of families with mentally retarded children: A model of stress, coping, and family ecology. *American Journal of Mental Deficiency, 88,* (125–138), ISSN: 0162-3257.

Donenberg, G., & Baker, B. L. (1993). The impact of young children with externalizing behaviours on their families. *Journal of Abnormal Child Psychology, 21,* (179–198), ISSN: 1573-2835.

Dunn, M. E., Burbine, T., Bowers, C. A., & Tantleff-Dunn, S. (2001). Moderators of stress in parents of children with autism. *Community Mental Health Journal, 37,* (39–52), ISSN: 1573-2789.

Dunst, C. J., & Trivette, C. M. (1990). Assessment of social support in early intervention programs. In: *Handbook of early childhood intervention,* S. Meisels & S. J. Shonkoff (Eds.), (326-349), Cambridge University Press, ISBN: 0521585732, New York.

Dunst, C. J., Trivette, C. M., & Cross, A. H. (1986). Mediating influences of social support: Personal, family, and child outcomes. *American Journal of Mental Deficiency, 90(4),* (403-417), ISSN: 0002-9351.

Dyson, L. L. (1997). Fathers and mothers of school age children with developmental disabilities: Parental stress, family functioning and social support. *American Journal on Mental Retardation, 102, (3),* (267-279), ISSN: 0895-8017.

Einfeld, S. L., Tonge, B. J., & Rees, V. W. (2001). Longitudinal course of behavioral and emotional problems in Williams syndrome. *American Journal on Mental Retardation, 106,* (73–81), ISSN: 0895-8017.

Ericksson, M., & Lindtröm, B. (2006). Antonovsky's sense of coherence scale and the relations with health: A systematic review. *Journal of Epidemiology and Community Health, 60, (5),* (376-381), ISSN: 1470-2738.

Feldman, M., McDonal, L., Servin, L., Stack, D. Secco, M. D., & Yu, C. T. (2007). Predictors of depressive symptoms in primary caregivers of young children with or at risk for developmental delay. *Journal of Intellectual Disability Research, 51(8),* (606-619), ISSN: 0964-2633.

Folkman, S., & Lazarus, R. S. (1980). An analysis of coping in a middle-aged community sample. *Journal of Health and Social Behavior, 21,* (219-239), ISSN: 0022-1465.

García-Villamisar, D., & Polaino-Lorente, A. (1992). Evaluación del autismo infantil: Una revisión de los instrumentos escalares y observacionales. *Acta Pediátrica Española, 50(6),* (383-388), ISSN: 0001-6640.

Gill, M. J., & Harris, S. L. (1991). Hardiness and social support as predictors of Psychological discomfort in mothers of children with autism. *Journal of Autism and Developmental Disorders, 21(4),* (407-416), ISSN: 0162-3257.

Grant, G., & Whittell, B. (2000). Differentiated coping strategies in families with children or adults with intellectual disabilities: the relevance of gender, family composition and the life span. *Journal of Applied Research in Intellectual Disabilities* 13, (256-275), ISSN: 1468-3148.

Gray, D. E., & Holden, W. J. (1992). Psycho-social well-being among the parents of children with autism. *Australia and New Zealand Journal of Developmental Disabilities, 18,* (83–93), ISSN: 07263864.

Hastings, R. P., Kovshoff, H., Brown, T., Ward, N. J., degli Espinosa, F., & Remington, B. (2005b). Coping strategies in mothers and fathers of preschool and school-age children with autism. *Autism, 9,* (377–391), ISSN: 1362-3613.

Hastings, R. P. (2003). Child behaviour problems and partner mental health as correlates of stress in mothers and fathers of children with autism. *Journal of Intellectual Disability Research, 47,* (231–237), ISSN: 0964-2633.

Hastings, R. P., Allen, R., McDermott, K., & Still, D. (2002). Factors related to positive perceptions in parents of children with intellectual disabilities. *Journal of Applied Research in Intellectual Disabilities, 15,* (269-275), ISSN: 1360-2322.

Hastings, R. P., & Brown, T. (2002). Behavior problems of autistic children, parental self-efficacy and mental health. *American Journal on Mental Retardation, 107,* (222-232), ISSN: 0895-8017.

Hastings, R. P., & Johnson, E. (2001). Stress in UK families conducting intensive home-based behavioral intervention for their young child with autism. *Journal of Autism and Developmental Disorders, 31, (*327–336), ISSN: 0162-3257.

Hastings, R. P., Kovshoff, H., Ward, N. J., degli Espinosa, F., Brown, T., & Remington, B. (2005a). Systems analysis of stress and positive perceptions in mothers and fathers of pre-school children with autism. *Journal of Autism and Developmental Disorders, 35,* (635–644), ISSN: 0162-3257.

Hastings, R. P., & Taunt, H. M. (2002). Positive perceptions in families of children with developmental disabilities. *American Journal on Mental Retardation, 107,* (116-127), ISSN: 0895-8017.

Herring, S., Gray, K., Taffe, J., Tonge, B., Sweeney, D., & Einfeld, S. (2006). Behaviour and emotional problems in toddlers with pervasive developmental disorders and developmental delay: Associations with parental mental health and family functioning. *Journal of Intellectual Disability Research, 50 (12),* (874–882), ISSN: 0964-2633.

Jones, J., & Passey, J. (2005). Family adaptation, coping and resources: Parents of children with developmental disabilities and behaviour problems. *Journal on Developmental Disabilities, 11(1), (*31-46), ISSN: 118-9136.

Kasari, C., & Sigman, M. (1997). Linking parental perception to interaction in young children with autism. *Journal of Autism and Developmental Disorders, 27,* (39-57), ISSN: 0162-3257.

Koegel, R. L., Schreiban, L., Loos, L. M., Dirlich-Wilhelm, H., Dunlap, G., Robbins, F. R., et al. (1992). Consistent stress profiles in mothers of children with autism. *Journal of Autism and Developmental Disorders, 22, (2*05-216), ISSN: 0162-3257.

Konstantareas, M. M., & Homatidis, S. (1989). Assessing child symptom severity and stress in parents of autistic children. *Journal of Child Psychology and Psychiatry, 30,* (459–470), ISSN: 1469-7610.

Lazarus, R., & Folkman, S. (1984). *Stress, appraisal and coping,* Springer, New York.

Lecavalier, L., Leone, S., & Wiltz, J. (2006). The impact of behaviour problems on caregiver stress in young people with autism spectrum disorders. *Journal of Intellectual Disability Research 50 (3),* (172–183), ISSN: 0964-2633.

Lounds, J. (2004). Family Stress and Coping, In: *The development of autism: A self–regulatory perspective* T. L. Whitman (Ed), (233-278), Jessica Kingsley Publishers, ISBN: 184310735X, London.

Mak, W., Ho, A., & Law, R. (2007). Sense of coherence, parenting attitudes and stress in mothers of children with autism in Hong Kong. *Journal of Applied Research in Intellectual Disabilities, 20,* (157–167). ISSN: 1360-2322.

McCubbin, H. I., & Patterson, J. M. (1983). The family stress process: The Double ABCX model of adjustment and adaptation, In: *Social stress and the family: Advances and developments in family stress theory and research,* H.I. McCubbin, M.B. Sussman y J. M. Patterson (Eds.), (7-37), The Haworth Press, ISBN: 0866561631, New York.

McCubbin, H.I., Thompson, E. A., Thompson, A. I., & Fromer, J. E. (1998). *Stress, coping and health in families: sense of coherence and resiliency.* SAGE Publications, Inc., ISBN: 0-7619-1396-3, EE.UU.

Meyer, D. J. (1993). Lessons Learned. Cognitive Coping Strategies of Overlooked Family Members, In: *Cognitive Coping, Families, and Disabilities,* A. P. Turnbull, J. M. Patterson, S.K. Behr, D. L. Murphy, J. G. Marquis & M. J. Blue-Banning (Eds.), (pp. 81-93), P. H. Brookes, ISBN: 1557661146, Baltimore.

Mullins, J. B. (1987). Authentic voices from parents of exceptional children. *Family Relations, 36,* (30–43), ISSN: 0197-6664.

Nolan M., Keady J., & Grant G. (1995). CAMI: a basis for assessment and support with family carers. *British Journal of Nursing, 4(14),* (822-826), ISSN: 0966-0461.

Olsson, M. B., & Hwang, C.P. (2002). Sense of Coherence in parents of children with different developmental disabilities. *Journal of Intellectual Disability Research, 46(7),* (548-559), ISSN: 0964-2633.

Orr, R. R., Cameron, S., & Day, D. (1991). Coping with stress in families with children who have mental retardation: An evaluation of the Double ABCX model. *American Journal on Mental Retardation, 95(4),* (444-450), ISSN: 0895-8017.

Pakenham, K. I., Sofronoff, K., & Samios, C. (2005). Finding meaning in parenting a child with Asperger syndrome: Correlates of sense making and benefit finding. *Research in Developmental Disabilities, 25(3),* (245-264), ISSN: 0891-4222.

Pallant, J., & Lae, L. (2002). Sense of coherence, well-being, coping and personality factors: Further evaluation of the sense of coherence scale. *Personality and Individual Differences, 33(1),* (39-48), ISSN: 0191-8869.

Phetrasuwan, S. (2003). Psychological adjustment in mother of children with autism spectrum disorders. *Dissertation Abstracts International: Section B: The Sciences and Engineering, 64(11B),* 5452.

Poston D., Turnbull A. P., Park J., Mannan H., Marquis J. & Wang M. (2003). Family quality of life: A qualitative inquiry. *Mental Retardation, 41,* (313-328), ISSN: 1934-9556.

Pozo, P. (2010). Adaptación psicológica en madres y padres de personas con trastornos del espectro autista: Un estudio multidimensional. Unpublished doctoral dissertation. UNED, Spain

Pozo, P., Sarriá, E., & Brioso, A. (2010). Contribuciones positivas que las personas con trastornos del espectro autista (TEA) aportan a la familia. In *Investigaciones sobre autismo en español: Problemas y perspectivas,* M. Belinchón (Ed.), (pp. 319-324). CPA-UAM, ISBN: 978-84-614-1786-5, Madrid.

Pozo, P., Sarriá, E., & Méndez, L. (2006). Estrés en madres de personas con autismo. *Psicothema, 18(3),* 342-347, ISSN: 0214-9915.

Quine, L., & Pahl, J. (1991). Stress and coping in mothers caring for a child with severe learning difficulties: A test of Lazarus' transactional model of coping. *Journal of Community and Applied Social Psychology, 1,* (57–70), ISSN: *Journal of Community and Applied Social Psychology.*

Raif, R., & Rimmerman, A. (1993). Parental attitudes to out-of-home placement of young children with developmental disabilities. *International Journal of Rehabilitation Research, 16,* (97–105), ISSN: 0962-9343.

Rojahn, J., Matson, J.L., Lott, D., Svensen, A., & Smalls, Y. (2001). The *Behavior Problems Inventory:* An instrument for the assessment of self-Injury, stereotyped behavior, and aggression/destruction in individuals with developmental disabilities. *Journal of Autism and Developmental Disorders, 31(6),* (577-588), ISSN: 0162-3257.

Sagy, S., Antonovsky, A., & Adler, I. (1990). Explaining life satisfaction in later life: The sense of coherence model and activity theory. *Behavioral Health and Aging 1,* (11–25), ISSN: 1049-085X.

Sainz, F. Verdugo, M. A., & Delgado, A. (2005). *Escalas de calidad de vida familiar.* Spanish adaptation to the scale Family Quality of Life Survey. INICO: Universidad de Salamanca, Spain.

Saloviita, T., Itaelinna, M., & Leinonen, E. (2003). Explaining the parental stress of fathers and mothers caring for a child with intellectual disability: A Double ABCX Model. *Journal of Intellectual Disability Research 47,* (300–312), ISSN: 0964-2633.

Sanders, J. L., & Morgan, S. B. (1997). Family stress and adjustment as perceived by parents of children with autism or Down syndrome: Implications for intervention. *Child and Family Behavior Therapy, 19(4),* (15-32), ISSN: 0731-7107.

Sharpley, C. F., Bitsika, V., & Efremidis, B. (1997). Influence of gender, parental health, and perceived expertise of assistance upon stress, anxiety, and depression among parents of children with autism. *Journal of Intellectual and Developmental Disability, 22,* (19-28), ISSN: 1366-8250.

Schopler, E., Reichler, R. J., & Reisner (1988). *The Childhood Autism Rating Scale (CARS).* Los Angeles: Western Psychological Services.

Shu, B. (2009). Quality of life of family caregivers of children with autism: A mother's perspective. *Autism, 13,* (81-92), ISSN: 1362-3613.

Sigman, M., & Capps, L. (1997). *Children with autism: A develomental perspective.* Harvard University Press, ISBN: 978-0674053137, Cambridge, MA.

Singer, G. H. (2006). Meta-analysis of comparative studies of depression in mothers of children with and without developmental disabilities. *American Journal on Mental Retardation, 111,* (155–169), ISSN: 0895-8017.

Smith, L., Hong A., Seltzer M., Greenberg J., Almeida D., & Bishop, S. (2010). Daily experiences among mothers of adolescents and adults with ASD. *Journal of Autism and Developmental Disorders, 40(2),* (167-178), ISSN: 0162-3257.

Smith, L., Seltzer, M., Tager-Flusberg, H., Greenberg, J., & Carter, A. (2008). A comparative analysis of well-being and coping among mothers of toddlers and mothers of adolescents with ASD. *Journal of Autism and Developmental Disorders, 38,* (876-889), ISSN: 0162-3257.

Szatmari, P., Archer, L., Fisman, S., & Streiner, D. L. (1994). Parent and teacher agreement in the assessment of pervasive developmental disorders. *Journal of Autism and Developmental Disorders, 24,* (703-717), ISSN: 0162-3257.

Tejero. A., Guimerá, E. M., & Farré, J. (1986). Uso clínico del HAD (Hospital Anxiety and Depression Scale) en población psiquiátrica: Un estudio de su sensibilidad, fiabilidad y validez. *Revista del Departamento de Psiquiatría de la Facultad de Medicina de Barcelona, 13,* (233-238), ISSN: 0213-7429.

Tomanik, S., Harris, G. E., & Hawkins, J. (2004). The relationship between behaviours exhibited by children with autism and maternal stress. *Journal of Intellectual and Developmental Disability, 29(1),* (6-26), ISSN: 1366-8250.

Weiss, M. J. (2002). Hardiness and social support as predictors of stress in mothers of typical children, children with autism and children with mental retardation. *Autism, 6(1),* (115-130), ISSN: 1362-3613.

Zigmond, A. S., & Snaith, R. P. (1983). The Hospital Anxiety and Depression Scale (HADS). *Acta Psychiatrica Scandinavica, 67,* (361–370), ISSN : 0001-690X.

7

A Comparative Study on Self Perceived Health and Quality of Life of Parents of Children with Autism Spectrum Disorders and Parents of Non Disabled Children in Croatia

Tomislav Benjak[1], Gorka Vuletić Mavrinac[2],
Ivana Pavić Šimetin[1] and Branko Kolarić[3]
[1]*Croatian National Institute of Public Health*
[2]*University J.J.Strossmayer in Osijek, Faculty of Philosophy, Department of Psychology*
[3]*Department of Public Health, Zagreb County*
Croatia

1. Introduction

Autism is defined as an organic developmental brain disorder that is manifested in difficulties in social interactions and communication, as well as unusual behaviors (Volkmar& Pauls, 2003; Gillham et al., 2000). Epidemiological report by the *Centers for Disease Control* (CDC) in Atlanta, USA, about autism spectrum disorders states the rate at 6.6 per 1000 births (Centers for Disease Control and Prevention [CDC], 2000). One of the leading experts in autism epidemiology, E. Fombonne, performed a meta-analysis of 32 epidemiological studies of autism spectrum disorders conducted between 1966 and 1991. Data was collected on the prevalence of autism spectrum disorders in 13 different countries on a sample of nearly five million inhabitants. According to this research, of 10,000 live births, 13 people are born with autism and 3 people are born with Asperger's syndrome. Another study found that 60 people of 10,000 live births have autism spectrum disorders (Fombonne, 2005). The term autism spectrum disorders (ASD) was officially used in Croatia, according to the International classification of diseases, Tenth Revision (ICD-10) published by World Health Organization. Global report of health status in European Union for 2007, underlines the diverse criteria for the diagnostic of ASD and the methodology which produces different prevalence. For example in Cambridgeshire (United Kingdom) total rate, in the age group 5-11, was 57 per 10, 000 while in Nord-Trondelag (Norway) whit same used criteria (DSM-IV) total rate, in the age group 3-14, was 3,8 per 10, 000 (European commision health&consumer protection directorate, 2005). Consequently, harmonization of the above segments is needed. In the Global report data for Croatia are not included, but they are available from the Croatian Disabilities Registry. Croatia regulates the collection of data on persons with ASD via the Croatian Disabilities Registry Act, according to which ASD are distinguished as a separate disability category. The prevalence of ASD in child population (0-18) in Croatia is approx. 1 in 1000, three times more common in boys (Croatian Public Health Institute, 2008).

While caregiving is a normal part of being the parent, providing the high level care required by a child with long-term functional limitations can become burdensome and may impact upon both the physical and mental health of the parents. A series of studies has been published about subjective health and health-related quality of life of family caregivers. Previous studies on family caregivers of people with chronic health problems reviled higher level of burden, stress, and depression (Canam & Acorn, 1999). Although it has been argued that all chronic illnesses and disabilities of children can negatively affect health-related quality of life of the parents; each disease present unique challenges (Epstein et al., 2005; Raina et al., 2005). According to some authors (Blanchard et al., 2006; Olsson& Hwang, 2001), parents of children with ASD are a particularly vulnerable group as they take over practically the entire burden of family care for their severely disabled child. Parenting children who have ASD was related to the impaired wellbeing of the parents themselves (Allik et al., 2006), their higher morbidity of anxiety, depression (Olsson& Hwang, 2001; Bailey et al., 2007) and obsessive compulsive symptoms (Abramson et al., 2005). Caregivers also reported somewhat lower marital happiness, disturb family cohesion, and family adaptability (Higgins et al., 2005). Moreover, an analysis of both qualitative and quantitative data indicate that primary carers report substantially low subjective quality of life (SQoL) (Cummins, 2001).

In the process of deinstitutionalization persons with intellectual disorders, parents of children with ASD become, also a key factor for improving the functioning of their children (Early et al., 2002). According to the latest guidelines on therapy and rehabilitation of children with ASD (daily lifetime therapy), and from the standpoint of harmony in all life aspects of the child, parents assume to have a very important role in the care and rearing (Olsson& Hwang, 2008; Welch, 1997). For parents to be able to care for their child with ASD and contribute to the quality of their child's rehabilitation procedure, they need, more than anything else, to be of good health themselves, as this care will exert great psychological and physical efforts (Kelly& Hewson, 2000). Because the parents are in the centre of support for the needs of the child with intellectual disability and ASD (Turnbull et al., 2004), preserving parents' good health and well being is precondition for optimal care for child. Poor caregiver health may contribute to recurrent hospitalizations (Kelly& Hewson, 2000) and out-of-home placements for children with chronic conditions and disabilities (Bromley& Blacher, 1991; Llewellyn et al.,1999; Duvdevany& Vudinsky, 2005). The therapy and rehabilitation of persons with ASD in Croatia is mostly administered in the Zagreb Autism Center, which conducted this study. The Center has its branch offices in Split, Rijeka and Nova Gradiška. The same institution administers rehabilitation and therapeutic measures for 333 persons. The inpatient unit accommodates 89 patients, 37 of whom never come into contact with their parents. This mode of care, which includes persons who have ASD into day therapeutic rehabilitation programs while being placed in the care of the family, is in line with the global trends of care and social inclusion of persons with ASD (Hare et al., 2004; Hastings& Johnson, 2001). According to these facts and data that over 80% of persons with ASD in Croatia live with their families (Croatian Public Health Institute, 2008) we think that is necessary to assess health and quality of life of parents who are at the same time caregiver for their disabled children. The purpose of this study was to examine self-assessed health, quality of life and chronic medical conditions in parents of children with ASD, and compare with parents of non-disabled children in Croatia. The starting hypothesis was that parents of children with ASD, due to required child care, have a lower self-assessed health with lower quality of life and higher chronic medical conditions' load, which may contribute to more frequent chronic diseases in comparison with parents of non-disabled children. This is one of the aspects of community efforts to provide social support which are one of the important factors for these families (Whitaker, 2002; Brown et al., 2003).

2. Participants and methods

2.1 Participants

The study included 178 parents of children with ASD (diagnosed under code F84 of ICD-10) median age 43 yrs (27-83yrs), of which 105 were mothers (59%) and 73 were fathers (41%). The control group was 172 parents of non-disabled children, median age 42 yrs (24-82 yrs), of which 101 were mothers (58.7%) and 71 were fathers (41.3%). A majority of respondents in both groups were married, though a higher number of single parent families existed in the group of parents of children with autism spectrum disorders (11.2%), as compared with 9.3% of parents of non-disabled children. About third of respondents had a university education (37.1%), with a distribution over all educational fields (Table 1).

	No. (%) of parents of		
	child with autism spectrum disorders (ASD) (n=178)	non-disabled child (n=172)	*P*
Characteristic			
Mother / Father	105 (59) / 73 (41)	101 (58.7) / 71 (41.3)	0.886 *
Family status:			
both parents	158 (88.7)	156 (90.7)	0.675 *
single parent	20 (11.2)	16 (9.3)	
Education level:			
primary	17 (9.6)	13 (7.6)	
secondary	96 (53.9)	91 (52.9)	0.729 *
university	65 (36.5)	68 (39.5)	
Median age (min-max. years)	43 (27-83)	42 (24-82)	0.822**

* χ^2
** Man Whitney U-test

Table 1. Demographic data of the study participants

There was no difference between groups in respect to family status, education level, and age. The sample included 83.7% parents of male children with autism spectrum disorders and 16.3% parents of female children with autism spectrum disorders. Parents of children with ASD were contacted through the Croatian Autism Center in Zagreb and its branch offices in Rijeka, Split and Nova Gradiška, and educational centers for children with disability in Pula and Osijek. The Centres database of users was basis for sample frame. Targeted sample were the parents whose children were at the time clients of the above centers. The research was conducted in 29 Croatian municipalities. Parents were approached at the Parents meetings at the Centres and individually when they came to Center (if they didn't attend the meetings). The purpose of the study was presented to parents by project leader at the Parents' meetings. Questionnaires were distributed personally by Centers staff and project leader to parents (both mothers and fathers) who agree to participate in the study. All together 250 questionnaires distributed to parents. Each questionnaire has a cover letter with information about research. 178 of them responded with correctly filled questionnaire within the given deadline. The original plan was to have both of the parents fill out the questionnaire. However some 20% less fathers responded. The matching control group of parents was based on the following characteristics of the collected group of parents with children with ASD: sex and age of children (+/- 5 yrs), parent age group (+/- 5 yrs), and educational background of parents and municipality of residence. Data collection for the control group was organized as part of the primary health care and primary schools in municipalities of residence of parents with children with ASD. Participants for the matching control group were searched one by one according to list of participants in already collected first group. Family doctors and school administration were provided with the list of first group participants and their key characteristics according to which they selected matching parent from their client database.

This research was conducted under the Croatian National Strategy of Equalization of Possibilities for Persons with disabilities with the written approval of the Ministry of Family Affairs, War Veterans and Intergenerational Solidarity as a coordinator of the Strategy.

2.1.1 Measures

Parents' self-perceived health was assessed using the health status questionnaire SF-36 - Croatian version (Ware et al., 1993; Maslić Seršić & Vuletić, 2006). SF-36 is a multi-purpose, short-form health survey that consists of 36 questions (Ware et al., 1993). It represents a theoretically based and empirically verified operationalization of two general health concepts, physical and psychological, and their two general manifestations, functioning and well-being. Accordingly, the questionnaire contains four types of scales, or four conceptually different measures of health. They refer to the following assessments or indicators of health: a) functioning at the behavioral level, b) perceived well-being, c) limitations connected with social life and the realization of central life roles, and d) direct personal perception of total health. At the manifested level, each of the questionnaire items refers to one of the following eight different health indicators (24): physical functioning (10 items); role-physical, referring to the limitations in performing important life roles due to physical health (4 items); bodily pain (2 items); general health (5 items); vitality and energy (4 items); social functioning (2 items); role-emotional, referring to the limitations in performing important life roles due to emotional problems (3 items); mental health, referring to the absence of anxiety and depression (5 items); and one final self-evaluated health transition item (five levels from "much better than a year ago" to "much worse than a year ago"), which is not used in the score of any of the scales but is useful in estimating average change in health status over a year before its administration. Five questionnaire scales - physical functioning, role-physical, bodily pain, social functioning, and role-emotional - define health as the absence of limitations and inability, so they represent continual and one-dimensional health measures. The three remaining scales - general health, vitality, and mental health - are bipolar, meaning they measure a much wider range of negative and positive aspects of health. The physical functioning, role-physical, and bodily pain scales refer to the general factor of physical health, and social functioning, role-emotional, and mental health scales measure psychological health. Scales vitality and general health are moderately connected with both factors. The total result is shown in the

form of the profile defined with eight points that represent the measure of individual aspects of health transformed into a standardized score from 0 (minimum) to 100 (maximum). On all scales, higher results indicate better subjective health. Psychometric validation revealed good psychometric properties of the Croatian version of the SF-36 (Maslić Seršić & Vuletić, 2006). The Croatian version of SF-36 questionnaire was licensed to Andrija Štampar School of Public Health and using permission was obtained.
In this research, a multidimensional approach was used to measure QoL (Cummins, 1996). Parents' subjective QoL was assessed using the Personal Wellbeing Index (PWI; International Wellbeing Group, 2006). The PWI scale contains seven items of satisfaction, each one corresponding to a quality of a life domain: standard of living, health, achievements in life, close relationships, personal safety, community connectedness, and future security. These seven domains theoretically represent the first level deconstruction of the global question: "How satisfied are you with your life as a whole?" The overall Personal Wellbeing Index score is an aggregate average score across the seven domains. Each domain is rated on a bipolar 11-point (0-10) end-defined scale where 0 means 'completely dissatisfied' and 10 is 'completely satisfied'. PWI has satisfactory metric characteristics; Cronbach alpha lies between .70 and .85. Inter-domain correlations are often moderate at around .30 to .55 and item-total correlations are at least .50. The index has also demonstrated good test-retest reliability across 1-2 week intervals with an intra-class correlation coefficient of 0.84 (International Wellbeing Group, 2006). Furthermore, parents filled out a general questionnaire containing three parts: demographic part (sex, age, marital status, parent educational background, as well as child's sex and age); health part including questions on self-reported chronic medical conditions, and the part on the needs and defining the type of help considered important by parents to advance their health and well-being.

2.1.2 Statistics

Descriptive statistics was used to present data on sex, age, family status and education level of study participants. Original results from health status questionnaire SF-36 and PWI were transformed according to authors' algorithm which results in 8 health dimensions and 7 domain of quality of life. The results from PWI domains and for the overall QoL index were transformed and presented in a standard form of the "percentage of scale maximum" (%SM), means original results were transformed to a 0–100 point scale. This conversion does not alter the statistical properties of the data, since the process is a simple linear conversion, with the advantage that the data from the PWI and other scales is compared directly in terms of mean and standard deviations. The differences self-perceived health between the two groups were assessed with Mann-Whitney U test since distributions were not normal. Difference in distributions of categorical data was tested with chi-square test. To assess the impact of the variables measured for the QoL in parents of children with autism spectrum disorders, bivarate and multiple logistic regression analysis were used. The dependent binary variable - quality of life - was defined as high (PWI≥60%SM) or low (PWI<60%SM). In determining the above values, data from the Croatian National Survey was used which was conducted on 9070 adult participants and revealed an average satisfaction with quality of life at 60% SM (Vuletić, 2006). Numerical variables were tested for linearity in logit, while all variables were tested for co-linearity. The level of statistical significance was chosen as $\alpha = 0.05$.
Statistical analysis was performed by statistical software Statistica, ver.7,1 (STATISTICA, 2005).

2.2 Results

2.2.1 Self perceived health and chronic medical condition

For all dimensions of health, except for physical health, there was a significant difference in self-assessed health between parents of children with ASD and parents of non- disabled children (Table 2).

	Score median (interquartile range) for the parents of		
Health dimension	child with autism spectrum disorders (ASD)	non-disabled child	*P**
Physical functioning	80.0 (40.0)	80.0 (30.0)	0.118
Role physical	75.0 (78.5)	100.0 (25.0)	0.000
Role emotional	66.7 (100)	100.0 (33.3)	0.000
Social functioning	55.6 (22.3)	77.8 (22.2)	0.000
Mental health	52.0 (22.0)	72.0 (20.0)	0.000
Vitality/Energy	50.0 (30.0)	60.0 (15.0)	0.000
Bodily pain	60.0 (40.0)	70.0 (30.0)	0.000
General health	57.0 (27.0)	67.0 (20.0)	0.000

* Man Whitney U-test

Table 2. Eight health status dimensions and significance of difference between two groups of study participants

The worst dimensions of health in parents of children with ASD are the energy, vitality and social functioning dimension. Thirty-five percent of parents of children with ASD reported their health deteriorated in the last year which is 18% higher than in parents of non-disabled children (Table 3). The difference between the groups were statistically significant (χ^2 = 17.500, df = 4, P = 0.002).

	No. (%) of parents of	
Change in health during the last year	child with autism spectrum disorders (ASD)	non-disabled child
much worse	10 (5.6)	2 (1.2)
somewhat worse	52 (29.4)	27 (15.7)
about the same	96 (54.2)	115 (66.8)
somewhat better	11 (6.2)	20 (11.6)
much better	8 (4.5)	8 (4.7)

Table 3. Frequency distribution for the item 'change in health during the last year' for two groups of study participants

Furthermore, 41% of parents of children with ASD stated that they suffered from a chronic medical condition, as well as 30.2% of parents of non-disabled children. Due to data distributions with small frequencies in several categories test statistics was not performed.

However, we could observe that most common chronic medical conditions listed by parents of children with ASD were those of the musculoskeletal system and connective tissue (21,2%), and circulatory system (17,3%), while parents of non-disabled children stated medical conditions of respiratory system (27,1%). Furthermore, it was noticeable in Table 4, that 11% parents of children with ASD suffered from psychological disorders (F00-F99 ICD-10 code group) what was 6,7% above frequency for parents of non-disabled children what was the largest difference in specified chronic medical conditions between the examination groups.

	No. (%) of parents of	
Group of disease according to ICD-10 (code)	child with autism spectrum disorders (ASD)	non-disabled child
Communicable and parasitic diseases (A00-B99)	2 (1.6)	1 (1.4)
Neoplasm's (C00-D48)	6 (4.7)	2 (2.9)
Endocrine, nutritional and metabolite diseases (E00-E90)	19 (15)	9 (12.8)
Mental and behavioral disorders (F00-F99)	14 (11)	3 (4.3)
Diseases of the nervous system (G00-G99)	8 (6.3)	3 (4.3)
Diseases of the eye and ear (H00-H95)	3 (2.4)	2 (2.9)
Diseases of the circulatory system (I00-I99)	22 (17.3)	10 (14.3)
Diseases of the respiratory system (J00-J99)	8 (6.3)	19 (27.1)
Diseases of the digestive system (K00-K93)	14 (11)	5 (7.1)
Diseases of the skin and subcutaneous tissue (L00-L99)	1 (0.8)	3 (4.3)
Diseases of the musculoskeletal system and connective tissue (M00-M99)	27 (21.2)	11 (15.7)
Diseases of the genitourinary system (N00-N99)	3 (2.4)	2 (2.9)
Total	127 (100)	70 (100)

Table 4. Chronic medical conditions reported by two groups of study participants according to International Classification of Diseases Tenth Revision (ICD-10) disease group

2.2.2 Quality of life

Descriptive statistics and difference statistics for PWI scores on seven QoL domains and overall index for the two sample groups are shown in Table 5. The results show that parents of children with ASD have statistically significantly lower subjective QoL ($p < 0.001$) as compared to parents of non-disabled children in all domains of QoL, as well as in overall PWI scores. Both groups were least satisfied with their future security, with a significantly low score in the group of parents of children with ASD, indicating strong dissatisfaction. In the domain of 'future security' a major difference is noticeable in the dominant answer, where parents of children with ASD were predominantly completely dissatisfied (mode = 0) and the control group of parents of non-disabled children was mostly highly satisfied (mode = 80). Parents in both groups were most satisfied with the 'close relationships' domain. Although parents of children with ASD were significantly less satisfied than parents of non-disabled children, this was the domain that contributed to lowering their total QoL.

	Parents - child with autism spectrum disorders			Parents - non-disabled child			
Domain	N	M	SD	N	M	SD	t-test
Standard of Living	177	48.6	26.5	169	63.7	21.9	-5,759**
Personal Health	177	58.5	26.9	169	70.7	20.7	-4,730**
Achievements	176	53.9	26.2	169	71.1	19.1	-6,965**
Close relationships	177	66.0	28.2	169	79.6	20.1	-5,189**
Personal safety	177	43.7	31.8	169	67.0	23.5	-7,785**
Community	177	49.3	30.7	169	70.9	24.5	-7,233**
Future security	177	35.3	28.3	169	55.3	25.5	-6,925**
PWI	176	50.67	23.02	169	68.33	16.93	-8,140**

** $p<0.01$

Table 5. Means and standard deviations (%SM) for seven domains and overall personal wellbeing (PWI) scores and test statistics for the two groups of parents

Bivariate logistic models found 10 variables to be significant (age of parent, age of disabled child, presence of chronic disease and all seven domains of PWI) and 4 insignificant (parent and child gender, level of education and marital status). Nevertheless, in the multiple logistic model, only 5 variables remained statistically significant (age of parent and disabled child, and these PWI domains: achievement in life, personal relationships and future security). The results of the multiple logistic regression analysis are shown in Table 6.

Variable	Odds ratio (OR)	Standard error for OR	p value	95% confidence interval for OR	
Parent age	0.693	0.094	0.007	0.531	0.905
Age of child	1.277	0.152	0.040	1.010	1.612
Achievement in life	3.762	1.508	0.001	1.716	8.253
Personal relationships	4.890	2.063	0.001	2.138	11.181
Future security	13.316	10.556	0.001	2.815	62.975

Table 6. Multiple logistic model for outcome achieving high quality of life (PWI≥60%SM)

2.3 Policy measures

When asked whether they felt that certain measures could improve their health and well-being 71% of parents of children with ASD thought that enhancing different policy measures which applied to them and their children with ASD (economic, social, educational, etc.) could advance their health and well-being. They defined over 60 different measures which could be undertaken or advanced to improve their quality of life. Three most commonly suggested measures were: financial aid to parents; a comprehensive system of diagnostics, therapy and rehabilitation to enable a better integration of individual in the community; and the need for more institutions and for advancing the quality of the existing ones (table 7).

Measures	N(%)
Financial assistance for parents	35 (20)
The complete system diagnostics, therapy and rehabilitation of ASD that will provide an opportunity to better integrate person into society	31 (17)
The need for more facilities and improving the quality of existing	26(15)
Improvement of health policy and health care for parents and children	20 (11)
Improvement of social policy	16 (9)
Sensitization of society	13 (7)
Creating the conditions for housing	11 (6)
Education for parents	11(6)
Psychological help for parents	10(6)
Provide non-institutional forms of care (playgroups, organized trips, etc.)	9 (5)

Table 7. Ten most common measures, which in the opinion of parents of child with autism spectrum disorders, could be undertaken or advanced to improve their quality of life

2.4 Discussion

Study results confirm the hypothesis regarding the difference in self-perceived health between parents of children with ASD and parents of non-disabled children in a sense of significantly poorer health for all dimensions, except for physical health, of parents of children with ASD. Energy and vitality and social functioning were particularly deteriorated dimensions. The only dimension of health in which there was no difference in relation to the parents of non-disabled children was physical health, which can be explained by the fact that 71% of surveyed parents with children with ASD were under 50 years of age. Especially important is the fact that even 35% of parents of children with ASD perceived their health as worse than last year, which was 18% higher in comparison to parents of non-disabled children. This discrepancy in self-perceived health between parents was confirmed by the finding that 41% of parents of children with ASD, in comparison with 30% of parents of non-disabled children, reported the existence of a chronic medical condition, with about three times higher frequency of psychological disturbances than the parents of non-disabled children, what was the largest difference in specified chronic medical conditions between the examination groups (Table 4). The research results also confirm the hypothesis regarding the difference in the SQoL between parents of children with ASD and parents of non-disabled children. The first group had lower SQoL. It was also confirmed that, despite the difficult situation of parents of children with ASD, there are parents who have SQoL levels in the normative range for the general population. Overall SQoL scores for parents of non-disabled children were within the range of expected values for the non-disabled adult population, while 62% of parents of children with ASD scored below 60%SM, with the average overall SQoL measured at 50.8%SM. This finding is of particular concern, as the latter value, according to references, is below the global normative range of the general population, which is 60-80%SM (Cummins 2000; Cummins et al. 2003), and the Croatian average of 60.1 %SM from a national health survey conducted in 2003 (Vuletic 2006). The fact that persons who suffer from a challenged homeostasis when their QoL falls below 60%SM develop symptoms of depression points to the significant vulnerability of this population (Cummins and Nistico 2002). Despite all of the above facts we identified parents of children with ASD who have the same level of QoL as the general population in Croatia (Vuletic 2006). Thirtyeight percent of parents of children with ASD, retain SQoL equal to, or even better than, the general Croatian population, which indicates that they may have developed resilience to the existing situation. Regression analysis shows that the ages of the parents and the disabled child, satisfaction with achievements in life, close relationships and future security are statistically significant in predicting a higher SQoL for the group of parents of children with ASD. These may, consequently, be deemed to be protective factors in maintaining a normal SQoL. The existence of parents who have a normal quality of life draws attention to community supports and services. All these facts are consistent with research conducted in the world (Blanchard et al., 2006; Olsson& Hwang, 2001; Allik et al., 2006; Bailey et al., 2007) which indicate that the parents of children with ASD are a particularly vulnerable and that the parenting disabled children who have ASD was related to the impaired their wellbeing. In order for the care of disabled family member to have a positive effect on the family according to world authors (Olsson& Hwang, 2008; Yau& Li-Tsang, 1999; Cummins, 2001) parameters are needed which enable the above hypothesis. These parameters are: harmonious family relationships, high socio-economic status and the community which supports such families. Unfortunately in Croatia all of the above is in disharmony with the parameters that should exist for the care for a disabled family member to have utterly positive impact on the family. The findings that in Croatia the percentage of divorce in families with children with ASD is higher by about 2% than in families with healthy children, that Croatia is a post-war country with a low GDP and one of the poorest countries in Europe (Eurostat, 2009), and that the poorest dimensions of health in parents of children with ASD are energy, vitality and social functioning dimensions, indicate possible deviations from the parameters that, according to Yau and Li-Tsang (Yau& Li-Tsang, 1999), guarantee the highest quality of parenthood to a disabled child, including children with ASD. All those findings, and especially the fact that the health of parents with children with ASD compromised, are the potential threat to optimal care for child (Kelly& Hewson, 2000; Bromley& Blacher, 1991; Llewellyn et al.,1999; Duvdevany& Vudinsky, 2005). All discussed facts have resulted in the finding that a great majority (71%) of parents of children with ASD believes that enhancing different political aspects would contribute to or improve their situation, quality of life and health, focusing of the social, economic and health policy, as well as streamlining the legislature, when it comes to parents of children with ASD. Parents from our study gave a series of proposals which may be summarized as measures for enhancing their, and by extension their children's, health and quality of life. These measures would include sensitization and education of the society on the issue of ASD, advancing the educational system and integration of children with ASD in the society, categorizing autism as 100% disability and claiming the pertaining rights, advancing the organizational aspects focusing on better service staffing and accommodation for children with ASD, introducing personal assistants, as well as a legal provision for mothers with the career status. All the above listed may directly or indirectly have a bearing on improving health for the group of parents of children with ASD.

However, there are some factors that limit the generalizability of our results and they are associated with the methodology used in our study. Sample of parents was not random from open population; in survey participated only parents with children in Autism Center, from them only those who voluntary answered the questionnaire. In that way group of parents of children with ASD was pre-selected comprise those who already receiving various support through Centres. We are aware that sample omits those parents who were, for example, dislocated and from whatever reason unable to use Centers. According to Croatian register (Croatian Public Health Institute, 2008) there are about 800 persons with diagnosed ASD living in Croatia, and Centers uses about 1/3 of them. So we may expect to find even more difficulties and health problems in the population of all parents of children with ASD. However, we try to overcome this limitation with the matching control group.

3. Conclusion

Parents of children with ASD had poorer health and quality of life than the control group in all components, except physical health. Because the parents are in the focus of support for the needs of the child with ASD, preserving parents' good health and well being is precondition for optimal care for child, so current system for treating children with ASD in Croatia should also include permanent improvements their health and well-being.With our findings and with the type of help what parents of children with ASD specified that is important to advance their health and well-being we want provide the basis for permanent improvements their health and well-being. In the world special attention is devoted to the improving caregiver well-being (Brown et al., 2003; Mittelman et al., 2006; Hebert et al., 2007). Organized support for family caregivers benefits the patient, but also the caregiver, and the healthcare team (Glajchen, 2004; Herring et al., 2006). Croatia has regulations on disabled persons, but these do not define or give enough significance to the disability in ASD persons and persons with other intellectual disorders. It should be pointed out that ASD, like other intellectual disorders, are not covered by a single legal provision to determine the degree of disability. Completing legal provisions, familiarizing parents with their rights, as well as interdepartmental cooperation, combined with empathy for disabled persons, will result in improving the position of persons with ASD and their families. In addition to streamlining the legislation, it is necessary to stress the importance of early diagnostic of pervasive developmental disorders, application of a suitable life-long approach, as well as giving support to the family and experts included in the treatment (Landa, 2008; Chawarska et al., 2007). Our results suggest that the current system for treating children with ASD in Croatia should also include close monitoring of parents' health and well-being. Appropriate treatment and psycho-social support should be provided before the health of parents becomes seriously compromised. Such measures, besides encouraging a positive attitude in the society, may improve the well being of autistic persons and their families. Additional attention should be focused on especially vulnerable groups of parents of children with ASD that we identified which needs for support and help are greater then needs of other. The National Strategy of Equalization of Possibilities for Persons with disabilities for 2007-2015 stresses the importance of interdepartmental collaboration for the improvement of well being of all disabled persons and their families, as well as persons with ASD. The strategy also points out that Croatia is among the first signatories of the Convention on the Rights of Persons with Disabilities. It is these two acts that serve as guidelines on how to improve the position of disabled persons in Croatia.

4. Acknowledgment

This work was conducted within The National Strategy of Equalization of Possibilities for Persons with disabilities for 2007-2015. The authors specially thanks Ministry of Family,

Veterans' Affairs and Intergenerational Solidarity, employees of Autism Center Zagreb, employees in primary schools around Croatia and all the parents whose support this research.

5. References

Abramson, R.; Ravan, S.; Wright, H.; Wieduwilt, K.; Wolpert, C.; Donnelly, S. et al. (2005). The relationship between restrictive and repetitive behaviours in individuals with autism and obsessive compulsive symptoms in parents. *Child Psychiatry Hum Dev.*, Vol.36, No.2, pp.155-65

Allik, H.; Larsson, J.; Smedje, H. (2006). Health-related quality of life in parents of schoolage children with Asperger Syndrome or High-Functioning Autism. *Health & Quality of Life Outcomes,* Vol.4, No.4, pp.1

Bailey, DB Jr.; Golden, RN.; Roberts, J.; Ford, A. (2007). Maternal depression and developmental disability: research critique. *Ment Retard Dev Disabil Res Rev.*, Vol.13, No.4, pp. 321-9

Blanchard, LT.; Gurka, MJ.; Blackman, JA. (2006). Emotional, developmental, and behavioral health of American children and their families: a report from the 2003 National Survey of Children's Health. *Pediatrics,* Vol.117, No.6, pp.1202-12

Bromley, BE.; Blache, J. (1991). Parental reasons for out-of-home placement of children with severe handicaps. *Ment Retard.,* Vol.29, No. 5, pp. 275-80

Brown, I.; Anand, S.; Fung, WLA.; Isaacs, B.; Baum, N. (2003). Family quality of life: Canadian results from an international study. *Journal of Developmental and Physical Disabilities,* Vol. 15, pp. 207-230

Canam, C.; Acorn, S. (1999). Quality of life for family caregivers of people with chronic health problems. *Rehabil Nurs.*, Vol.24, No.5, pp. 192-6, 200

Centers for Disease Control and Prevention. (2000). Prevalence of autism spectrum disorders-autism and developmental disabilities monitoring network, six sites, United States. *MMWR Surveill Summ. 2007,* Vol.56, No.1, pp.1-11

Chawarska, K.; Klin, A.; Paul, R.; Volkmar, F. (2007). Autism spectrum disorder in the second year: stability and change in syndrome expression. *The Journal of Child Psychology and Psychiatry,* Vol. 48, No.2, pp. 128-38

Croatian Public Health Institute. (2008). Report about persons with disabilities in Croatia, 14 March 2011., Available from: http://www.hzjz.hr/epidemiologija/kron_mas/invalidi08.pdf

Cummins, R. A. (1996). The domains of life satisfaction: An attempt to order chaos. *Social Indicators Research*, Vol. *38*, pp. 303–332

Cummins, R. A. (2000). Objective and Subjective Quality of Life: An Interactive Model. *Social Indicators Research*, Vol. *52*, pp. 55–72

Cummins, RA. (2001). The subjective wellbeing of people caring for a family member with a severe disability at home: A review. *Journal of Intellectual & Developmental Disability,* Vol. 26, No. 1, pp. 83-100

Cummins, R. A., & Nistico, H. (2002). Maintaining life satisfaction: The role of positive bias. *Journal of Happiness Studies*, Vol. *3*, pp. 37–69

Cummins, R. A., Eckersley, R., Pallant, J., Van Vugt, J., Misajon R. (2003). Developing a National Index of Subjective Wellbeing: The Australian Unity Wellbeing Index. *Social Indicators Research*, Vol. *64*, No. 2, pp. 159-190

Duvdevany, I.; Vudinsky, H. (2005). Out-of-home placement of children with intellctual disability:Israel-born parents vs. New immigrants from the ex-USSR. *Int J Rehabil Res.*, Vol. 28, No. 4, pp. 321-30

Early, TJ.; Gregoire, TK.; Mcdonald, TP. (2002). Child Functioning and Caregiver Well-being in Families of Children with Emotional Disorders. *Journal of Family Issues,* Vol.23, No.3, pp. 374-391

Epstein, I.; Stinson, J.; Stevens, B. (2005). The effects of camp on health-related quality of life in children with chronic illnesses: a review of the literature. *J Pediatr Oncol Nurs.*, Vol.22, No.2, pp. 89-103

European commision health&consumer protection directorate. (2005). Some elements about the prevalence of Autism Spectrum Disorders (ASD) in the European Union, 14 March 2011., Available from: http://ec.europa.eu/health/ph_information/dissemination/diseases/autism_1.pdf

Eurostat. *GDP per capita in Purchasing Power Standards,* 14 March 2011., Available from: http://epp.eurostat.ec.europa.eu/tgm/table.do?tab=table&init=1&plugin=1&language=en&pcode=tsieb010

Fombonne, E. (2005). Epidemiology of autistic disorder and other pervasive developmental disorders. *Journal of Clinical Psychiatry*, 66(10), pp. 3-8

Gillham, JE.; Carter, AS.; Volkmar, FR.; Sparrow, SS. (2000). Toward a developmental operational definition of autism. *Journal of Autism & Developmental Disorders*, Vol.30, No. 4, pp. 269-78

Glajchen, M. (2004). The emerging role and needs of family caregivers in cancer care. *J Support Oncol.*, Vol. 2, No. 2, pp.145-55

Hare, D.; Pratt, C.; Burton, M.; Bromley. J.; Emerson, E. (2004).The health and social care needs of family carers supporting adults with autistic spectrum disorders. *Autism,* Vol. 8, No. 4, pp. 425–444

Hastings, R.; Johnson, E. (2001). Stress in UK families conducting intensive home-based behavioral intervention for their young child with autism. *Journal of Autism and Developmental Disability,* Vol. 31, No. 3, pp. 327–336

Hebert, R.; Arnold, R.; Schulz, R. (2007). Improving Well-Being in Caregivers of Terminally Ill Patients. Making the Case for Patient Suffering as a Focus for Intervention Research. *Journal of Pain and Symptom Management,* Vol.34, No. 5, pp. 539-546

Herring, S.; Gray, K.; Taffe, J.; Tonge, B.; Sweeney, D.; Einfeld, S. (2006). Behaviour and emotional problems in toddlers with pervasive developmental disorders and developmental delay: associations with parental mental health and family functioning. *J Intellect Disabil Res.,* Vol. 50, No. 12, pp. 874-82

Higgins, DJ.; Bailey, SR.; Pearce, JC. (2005). Factors associated with functioning style and coping strategies of families with a child with an autism spectrum disorder. *Autism,* Vol.9, No.2, pp.125-37

International Wellbeing Group. (2006). Personal Wellbeing Index. Melbourne: Australian Centre on Quality of Life, Deakin University, 14 March 2011., Available from: http://www.deakin.edu.au/research/acqol/instruments/wellbeing_index.htm

Kelly, AF.; Hewson, PH. (2000). Factors associated with recurrent hospitalization in chronically ill children and adolescents. *J Paediatr Child Health.*, Vol.36, No.1, pp. 13-8

Landa, RJ. (2008). Diagnosis of autism spectrum disorders in the first 3 years of life. *Nature Clinical Practice Neurology*, Vol. 4, No. 3, pp. 138-47

Llewellyn, G.; Dunn, P.; Fante, M.; Turnbull, L.; Grace, R. (1999). Family factors influencing out-of-home placement decisions. *J Intellect Disabil Res.*, Vol. 43, No. 3, pp. 219-33

Maslić Seršić, D.; Vuletić, G. (2006). Psychometric Evaluation and Establishing Norms of Croatian SF-36 Health Survey: Framework for Subjective Health Research. *Croat Med J.*, Vol. 47, pp. 95-102

Mittelman, MS.; Haley, WE.; Clay, OJ.; Roth, DL. (2006). Improving caregiver well-being delays nursing home placement of patients with Alzheimer disease. *Neurology*, Vol. 67, No. 9, pp. 1592-9

Olsson, MB.; Hwang, CP. (2001). Depression in mothers and fathers of children with intellectual disability.*Journal of Intellectual Disability Research*, Vol. 45, pp. 535-43

Olsson, MB.; Hwang, CP. (2008). Socioeconomic and psychological variables as risk and protective factors for parental wellbeing in families of children with intellectual disabilities. Journal of Intellectual Disability Research, Vol.52, No.12, pp. 1102-1113

Raina, P.; O'Donnell, M.; Rosenbaum, P.; Brehaut, J.; Walter, SD.; Russell, D. et al. (2005). The health and well-being of caregivers of children with cerebral palsy. *Pediatrics*, Vol.115, No.6, pp.626-36

STATISTICA, wer.7,1; StatSoft, Inc. (2005)

Turnbull, A. P., Brown, I., Turnbull III, H. R., Turnbull, H. R. (2004). Families and Persons With Mental Retardation and Quality of Life: International Perspectives (pp 4). Washington, CT: American Association on Mental Retardation

Volkmar, FR.; Pauls, D. (2003). Autism. *Lancet*, Vol.362, No.9390, pp.1133-41

Vuletić, G. (2006). Health related quality of life and satisfaction with life in Croatia. Proceedings of the 8th Australian Conference on Quality of Life. Deakin University, Melbourne, Australija, 12 October 2009., Available from: http://acqol.deakin.edu.au/Conferences/abstracts_papers/2006/index.htm

Ware, JE.; Kosinski, M.; Gandek, B. (1993). *SF-36 Health Survey.Manual and interpretation guide.* Lincoln (RI), Quality Metric Inc

Welch, W. (1997). *Approaches to autism* (3rd ed), The National Autistic Society, London

Whitaker, P. (2002). Supporting Families of Preschool Children with Autism: What Parents Want and what Helps. *Autism*, Vol. 6, pp. 411-426

Yau, MKS.; Li-Tsang, CWP. (1999). Adjustment and adaptation in parents of children with developmental disability in two-parent families: a review of the characteristic and attributes. *British Journal of Developmental Disabilities*, Vol. 45, pp. 38-52

Part 3

Cross Culture and Autism Spectrum Disorders

8

Cross Cultural Variation in the Neurodevelopmental Assessment of Children - The Cultural and Neurological to 2nd Language Acquisition and Children with Autism

Karen Mendez[1], Karen M, Levy[2], Marley Nelms[2], Dayna Hoff[2], Jean M. Novak[3] and Michael L. Levy[1]
[1]*University of California San Diego – Rady Children's Hospital of San Diego, Division of Pediatric Neurosurgery*
[2]*Autism Tree Project Foundation – San Diego*
[3]*Department of Communicative Disorders and Sciences, San Jose State University, USA*

1. Introduction

With the increased incidence of autism on an international level (1), early detection and diagnosis of children with autism is of paramount importance and key to providing early intervention. Research indicates the outcome for academic success is significantly enhanced by early identification and intervention (2). Researchers have identified that early identification and intervention of communicative disorders have given children the opportunity to decrease later academic and literacy difficulties, and experience success in the school setting (3). Many times children see various health providers that do not provide the appropriate diagnosis of a child with autism, thus delaying the process of that child to receive appropriate services. Consequently, a significant lag between the parents' first concerns regarding their child and the eventual diagnosis exists, which in turn postpones the onset of appropriate treatment and as a result precious time is lost.

Screening toddlers represents the first level of evaluation for early detection of autism. However, very few screenings exist that tap into the early identification of children with autism. The value of identifying children with autism utilizing the M-CHAT by neurodevelopmental pediatricians in Poland and the US has recently been reported by us. The efficacy of the M-CHAT screener has been documented as an adequate standard in identifying 18 month old toddlers who are at risk for autism. Results obtained in Krakow, Poland have been compared with those obtained in San Diego, California, USA. The M-CHAT has been found to be an adequate tool in screening 18 month old toddlers, as it was able to retrospectively identify children who already received a diagnosis of autism with statistical significance (4). This tool has value on the international level allowing comparisons of both similarities and differences in the results in different countries that may be important in identifying children with autism at an early age. In addition to the communicative behaviors screened by the M-CHAT, neurobiological and socio-cultural variables and "red-flags" should be carefully considered before giving a child definitive diagnosis of autism.

Neurological aspects related to brain development both in-utero and after-birth play an important role in children with autism also known as a 'disconnected syndrome', related to neuronal migration, synaptogenesis, mirror neurons, myelination, and epigenetic effects (5). Biological variations include differences in the areas of motor processes (motor maturity, tone, head control, defensive movements, and vigor of movement), and regulation of states (habituation, irritability, consolability, and self-quieting), and motor-sensory skills (6).

Cross-cultural factors also need to be taken into consideration in order that a missed diagnosis or mis-diagnosis does not occur. One of the most significant considerations is the importance of ethnographic interviewing (7) highlighting social and cultural differences and the utilization of parent interviewing and parental input into their child's behavior (8).

In a world where more than one language may be spoken in the home, second language development studies have revealed that a child that is exposed to a second language may go through a normal developmental "silent period" in language development that may be labeled as a disorder or an autistic behavior. This and other factors related to second language development should also be taken into consideration before looking at specific behaviors exhibited by a child before a definitive diagnosis is given to the child.

This chapter will identify the important factors that need to be taken into consideration for the early identification and diagnosis of children with autism, addressing early neuro-biological development and socio-cultural variables. Utilization of developmental testing, behavioral observations, along with parental input can provide an accurate profile of the child's abilities and disabilities. The use of ethnographic interviewing strategies using culturally relevant questions and the importance of parental input for an accurate and early diagnosis of autism will also be discussed.

Autism is a developmental disorder likely caused by a central nervous system abnormality or injury during initial stages of brain growth and development. It results in lifelong impairments, of social interaction and communication, in addition to restricted and repetitive patterns of behavior and concentration. Behaviors manifest usually include problems with poor or limited eye contact and facial expressions, repetitive behaviors, repetitive motor mannerisms (flapping and/or rocking) which likely result in reinforcing self-stimulatory behaviors. They also can manifest preoccupation with parts of objects or the alignment of objects, and adherence to nonfunctional routine. Development of speech is usually delayed with a paucity of words until after 24 months of age and usually phraseology until after 36 months which tends to develop as monotone and tangential. A majority of children with ASD never achieve language capabilities. Up to 75% of children with ASD have associated developmental delay. Children with ASD tend to have minimal interest in other children and a higher frequency of parallel play. Of the interaction that does occur it is most often related to behaviors that will result in specific needs being met as opposed to actual interaction with peers or others.

The incidence of ASD has now exceeded that of diabetes, cancer, spina bifida, and Down syndrome in children (9). In 2002, the incidence of autism was 10-12 people per 10,000 (10). With the increase also related to the changes in how autism is diagnosed. According to the Center for Disease Control, an average of 1 in 110 children in the United States has an Autism Spectrum Disorder (ASD). While the median age for earliest diagnosis is between 4.5 and 5.5 years, developmental concerns have been recorded for children younger than three years for

51-91 percent of children diagnosed with ASD (11). Early identification is critical for early treatment. The American Academy of Pediatrics is a strong advocate for early and continuous surveillance and screening for ASD in children to increase the likelihood of early identification and intervention (12). Although there is a rising awareness of ASD, caution must be taken in diagnosis. The M-CHAT is a valuable screening tool but it is important to note the many factors that can contribute to a positive diagnosis in order to be aware of the potential for false positive and false negative diagnosis. Since the primary goal of the M-CHAT was to maximize sensitivity, there is a high false positive rate and not all children who score at risk for ASD will be diagnosed with ASD. (13) In fact, the M-CHAT also identifies children with language and developmental delays who do not have an ASD. (14) Socio-cultural factors that can contribute to a false positive diagnosis with the M-CHAT screening tool include: multilingualism, shared cultural beliefs, and parental interpretation of the child's behavior. Because the M-CHAT has language assessment components, a child who is exposed to multiple languages may not be equally developed in all languages. If the child is being assessed for English language understanding but the primary language spoken at home is something other than English, then the child may be labeled "at risk." Children raised in a multilingual environment may develop skills in one language at a different rate than the other language, putting them in a unique situation for ASD screening. Despite the distinct circumstance, they are expected to develop language skills in a similar rate as their monolingual peers (15). Additionally, there is great room for interpretation of the child's behavior and the responses to the M-CHAT questionnaire can vary depending on which parent completes the survey. Cultural beliefs play a role in the interpretation of the child's behavior, and may influence the likelihood of excusing a child's lack of development as being normal. Even without having a clear understanding of the age that certain milestones are reached, a parent may notice that his or her child is unlike his or her peers. The culture may promote silence or it may promote a parent to voice his or her concerns to the physician during a routine visit. Many factors, including social, cultural, and biological, may influence ASD diagnosis. Boys are more likely to be diagnosed with an ASD than girls. A recent study also found that young mothers and mothers of first-born children were less likely to have a child diagnosed with an ASD. Additionally, maternal depression before and during the presentation of the child's autistic difficulties was found to inhibit ASD diagnosis (16).

Given the increased incidence of autism on an international level (Autism Society, 2010), (17–23), determining the prevalence of ASD outside of the US is problematic. There is a report from the EAIS that looks at Prevalence Data and Accessibility to Service in European Countries. However, because the diagnosis of ASD is based upon behavioral characteristics and, other than the DSM IV R and the WHO Classification Systems) there are a limited amount of appropriate diagnostic tools available, many of which are simply translations which may not reflect cultural relevance, determination of the prevalence remains an issue. In the United States, the rate of diagnosis varies with race. (United States Department of Education, 2003) and the percentage of Asian/Pacific (0.13%) children identified with autism is disproportionately high. This begs the question as to an actual difference in the rate of ASD based upon racial/cultural variables, which is unlikely, versus diagnostic error on the part of the therapists, their experience and skill sets, and the screening exams being utilized. Additionally, are certain behaviors which do not fit within the spectrum of ASD found to be abnormal amongst parents of differing cultures which may result in the increased referral of the children for evaluation.

2. Early detection and diagnosis

Early detection accompanied by early intervention provides the best scenario for improved long-term outcome in children with ASD (24, 25). Rapid detection must be based upon the implementation of specific, evidence-based batteries. Yet given that the significant experience in early detection has been in Caucasian children, the accuracy of low incidence of ASD in Peru, Argentina, Brazil, and Venezuela, Kenya, India, and Hungary (26 - 28) may represent more of a compromise in the actual testing as opposed to a true decrease in incidence. Additional, cultural variances in incidence of ASD are also well documented in the US.

In 1999 The Child Neurology Society and American Academy of Neurology proposed Practice Parameters for the Diagnosis and Evaluation of Autism by a multidisciplinary Consensus Panel and recommended a dual-level approach to improve the rate of early suspicion and diagnosis of autism (29, 30).

In the Report of the Quality Standards Subcommittee of the American Academy of Neurology and the Child Neurology Society it was noted that early identification of children with autism and intensive, early intervention during the toddler and preschool years improves outcome. They recommend a dual approach including 1) routine developmental surveillance and screening specifically for autism to be performed on all children to first identify those at risk for any type of atypical development, and to identify those specifically at risk for autism; and 2) to diagnose and evaluate autism, to differentiate autism from other develop- mental disorders (31).

Very few screenings exist that tap into the early identification of children with autism. It is well known that early evaluations by interventionists may not reflect the cultural and linguistic diversity of the population they work with (32).

The interaction or partnership between professionals and families in the evaluation and subsequent treatment of children with ASD is likely defined by the socio-cultural environment in which it exists. The impact of this environment may not only effect the therapeutic intervention and relationship itself, but also change over time. Iglesias and Quinn (33) state, "the challenge posed to early interventionists is how to provide intervention programs that are consistent with the research literature, based on professional knowledge, and at the same time respect the culture of the families who are served."

3. Cultural validity of the assessment instruments

Autism knows no racial, ethnic, or social boundaries (Autism Society of America, 2000). Given the significant cultural diversity of the United States, assessment tools utilized for the early detection of ASD are of both national and global importance (34-36). As the number of children from diverse cultural backgrounds increases, the need for culturally sensitive tools becomes more important. In a world where more than one language may be spoken in the home, second language development studies have revealed that a child that is exposed to a second language may go through a normal developmental "silent period" in language development that may be labeled as a disorder or an autistic behavior. This and other factors related to second language development should also be taken into consideration before looking at specific behaviors exhibited by a child before a definitive diagnosis is given to the child.

In February 2005, the European Commission for Health and Consumer Protection Directorate-General stated that due to methodological limitations, the high prevalence rates reported in the EU and USA cannot be used to derive absolute conclusions. Rather An ASD response policy was necessary in the EU and More complex monitoring systems were required to accurately reflect the prevalence of ASD. The European Autism Alliance (EAA), initiated the European Autism Information System Project (EAIS) to better understand those impacted with an ASD in the EU by better understanding the services related to public health, educational system, social service and the problems associated with determining prevalence in the participant countries of Bulgaria, Czech Republic, Denmark, England, France, Italy, Malta, Poland, Portugal, Scotland Highland Region and Spain) (37).

The EAIS is attempting to explore and measure the ASD prevalence in 11 European countries of which nearly 48 million are below 14 years old using a questionnaire focused on services and data access. The questionnaire (Q-EAIS) allows for the recording of the most common diagnostic criteria and subtypes used, existing registries and/or prevalence studies, services provided by health, educational and social systems in addition to parental organizations to children with ASD country. As expected, the results support the variability of the services provided by different countries and intra-country differences. Roughly there are 288,000 children with an ASD diagnosis in these eleven countries (prevalence rate of 6 cases per 1,000). The data also notes differences in socio-demographic characteristics and social organizations. Based upon the answers in the Q-EAIS certain summary data can be defined to address the question of whether the rising ASD prevalence represents a true increase or is the result of other explanations (38). Given the concern for diverse multicultural issues, future harmonized prevalence studies need to be designed to address these differences.

To date, prevalence studies are difficult given the paucity of services involved in ASD management, the complexity of the diagnosis, the variability or lack of services provided, and the lack of data. The collection of data from different service providers in each country is required as is the validation of the data. The Q-EAIS questionnaire is a relatively new epidemiological tool used to obtain preliminary data of the ASD services and accessibility in various countries. The Q-EAIS Modified facilitates aggregated data analysis.

The four most common Assessment Instruments include the Vineland Adaptive Behavior Scales (39), The Checklist for Autism in Toddlers, the Modified Checklist for Autism in Toddlers, and the Childhood Autism Rating Scale. The Vineland Adaptive Behavior Scales which are used for routine screening contain sections concerning social relationships and language which may help to establish a basic understanding of whether the child has delays or deviant behavior. The Checklist for Autism in Toddlers consists of 2 parts, with each assessing parallel functioning in three main areas including proto-declarative pointing, gaze monitoring, and pretend play . The Modified Checklist for Autism in Toddlers (M-CHAT) developed by Robins, Fein, Barton, and Green (40) in the United States, adds an additional 9 questions from the original CHAT and an additional 14 questions which address core symptoms present among young children with autism and may be more resistant to cultural bias. It is a simple screening tool for the identification of children with ASD up to 24 months of age. The parental questionnaire with has 23 yes/no questions, with 9 questions from the original CHAT and an additional 14 questions addressing core symptoms present among young children with autism. The M-CHAT addresses areas of social relatedness (interest in other children and imitation), joint attention (proto-declarative pointing and gaze monitoring), bringing objects to show parents, and responsiveness to name responses to calling. Joint attention was addressed in the original CHAT, whereas the other areas are addressed only in the M-CHAT. Another tool is the Childhood Autism Rating Scale (41). Some of these do not function as well as others in the screening of children with autism from a cultural standpoint.

4. Addressing early neuro-biological development and socio-cultural variables

Neurological aspects related to brain development both in-utero and after-birth play an important role in children with autism. Important factors that need to be taken into consideration for the early identification and diagnosis of children with autism, must address early neuro-biological development and socio-cultural variables. Utilization of developmental testing, behavioral observations, along with parental input can provide an accurate profile of the child's abilities and disabilities. We have found the use of the M-CHAT as a culturally sensitive screening tool which has been helpful in our experience (as noted above). This in addition to other ethnographic interviewing strategies using culturally relevant questions and parental input can potentially result in an accurate and early diagnosis of ASD. We emphasize the use of culture and ethnographic interviewing to get the most amount of information needed, as well as parental attitudes, and the importance of understanding how culture affects the way autism is perceived by the family.

Kliewer et al used ethnographic methods to examine literacy development in nine children with disabilities over two years. Teachers fostered the citizenship of all children in the literate communities of these classrooms (42, 43). The utilization of developmental testing, behavioral observations, along with parental input can provide an accurate profile of the child's abilities and disabilities. The variables of culture, values, belief, family units, and primary language contribute to a family's attitudes and beliefs about child rearing, disability, and assessment. While it is understood that a child and family, and/or communities' background with regard to methodologies of communication can impact how a child interacts with their peers, family, adults, or strangers. It can additionally impact the manner in which the child interprets or utilizes the process of communication itself. Additionally, the toys available to a child or resources available to a child and family can influence early cognitive and linguistic experiences (44). The primary issue in the U.S, and most European Countries is that the developers of the assessment tools and the therapists, and educators are for the most part White and middle class (45). This coupled with the fact that most research on the early identification of ASD has been in predominately Caucasian populations, cultural diversity represents a significant cofounding variable resulting in an increased false negative rate in the identification of children with ASD. It is important to note that cultural variables may not only impact the identification of children with ASD but also the initiation of resources to the children and their families. Of the utmost importance is that children are diagnosed appropriately (46). Testing must not only be modified or integrated differently based upon cultural diversity but the interpretation of the results must also be completed in a culturally competent. The goal is the accurate assessment and subsequent intervention to children with ASD and their families in a culturally competent way by therapists and professionals 'culturally proficient' in their understanding of the families' socio-cultural practices and values (47).

5. Culture vs. cross-cultural competence

There are Basic assumptions about culture influence exiting and potential cross-cultural models, approaches, methods, and strategies used in the therapeutic approach to children that we must expand upon (48).

Cross-cultural competence refers to the ability to relate and communicate effectively when the individuals involved in the interaction do not share the same culture, ethnicity, or language, Cross, Bazron, Dennis, and Isaacs (1989): stated that such competency is "a set of congruent behaviors, attitudes, and policies that come together in a system, agency, or amongst professionals and enables that system, agency, or those professionals to work effectively in cross-cultural situations" (49). Barrera and Kramer define cultural competence as "the ability of service providers to respond optimally to all children, understanding both the richness and the limitations of the socio-cultural contexts in which children and families, as well as the service providers themselves, may be operating" (50). Data on early interventionists implies that they do not reflect the cultural diversity of the population they serve which may impact not only their interaction with patients and families but also with other health care providers. The likely conclusion is that interactions that are culturally similar are more likely to be of benefit and reinforcing of one another in culturally and linguistically diverse children with special needs to maximize interactive and learning behaviors, socio-cultural experiences, and language usage and proficiency (51).

Harry (52) noted the challenge of early intervention in children and families whose cultural beliefs are different from that of the therapist. Five areas are addressed to maximize impact of therapy including the meaning of disability, concepts of family structure and identity, parenting style, goals of early childhood intervention, communication styles, and views of professionals' roles.

The video, Essential Connections: Ten Keys to Culturally Sensitive Care supports the concept of how the natural process of culture impacts feelings of belonging, family and personal history, and community in child development. It suggests ways to structure programs for infants and toddlers to strengthen their connections with family and home culture. It recommends that programs (a) provide cultural consistency, (b) work toward representative staffing, (c) create small groups, (d) use the home language, (e) make environments relevant, (f) uncover your cultural beliefs, (g) be open to the perspectives of others, (h) seek out cultural and family information, (i) clarify values, and (j) negotiate cultural conflicts (53).

Other approaches include strategies to develop cultural competence, and improve home/school relationships and encouraging greater participation of families who are not part of the mainstream culture (54). A primary goal of therapeutic intervention is the integration of children with disabilities with normal developing peers, developing collaborative relationships with families, and understanding the importance of diversity among children and their families. (55).

Conceptually, the approach to therapeutic interventions in culturally diverse environments must take into consideration family definitions, roles, relationships, and child-rearing techniques; health, illness, and disability beliefs and traditions; and communication and interactional styles. The publication Serving Culturally Diverse Families of Infants and Toddlers with Disabilities addresses how to maximize therapeutic interactions in effective, culturally sensitive, early intervention programs for infants and toddlers with disabilities and their families (56).

6. Maximizing the competence of testers

It is obvious that there is, to date, inadequate preparation for culturally and linguistically diverse children and families. Manoleas (57) noted that "the single most important factor involved in any practitioner's ability to effectively help clients from other cultural groups is prolonged exposure to people of that group" (58). Dyches has noted that "When students with ASDs are from culturally or linguistically diverse families, the professionals assessing and providing services to the students need the additional dimension of how cultural and linguistic differences may affect identification, assessment, and treatment strategies" (59). Cross et. al described a developmental continuum ranging from cultural destructiveness, cultural incapacity, cultural blindness, cultural precompetence, cultural competence, to cultural proficiency with each component representing the response of an individual to diversity. Whereas cultural competence represents the ability of the tester to accept and respect differences, cultural proficiency represents the goal of learning more about diverse groups through research (60). All stage-based models assume a continuum through which therapists improve their cross-cultural competence, which is ongoing.

Serving Culturally Diverse Families of Infants and Toddlers with Disabilities (61) was one of the initial publications to focus on the issue of unmet needs among families from diverse cultural and linguistic groups when considering programs of early identification and intervention. Sue's work is frequently referenced and the basis for many of the assessment tools in the field (62–64). Subsequently, cross-cultural sensitivity was suggested to be less sensitive to the changes required to enhance diagnosis and therapeutic interactions to children and families from diverse cultural and linguistic backgrounds (65). This resulted in broad systemic and programmatic changes which were more specific (66-68). In the long-term, how can one accurately assess cross-cultural competence in individual providers? (69). Tools to allow for such assessment include the CCCI-R; MCAS:B; MCI; and MAKS(counseling) and CSES (nursing) though all are limited in scope as a result of all but one (CCCI-R) being based upon self review (70, 71).

Established models utilized in multi/intercultural communication, counseling, and education in nursing (72), social work (73), and bilingual education (74) can be utilized to modify existing methodologies by which children are evaluated (75–82). Such models have been included as standards in numerous professional organizations (83–86). Surveys have also been used to assess students within the context of individual supervision and mentoring in clinical settings (87–93). These results also suggest that ongoing support for students in practicum situations is important (94). The validity of the model in which students have direct experiences with diverse populations has been verified graduates from counseling and clinical psychology programs (95), What remains problematic is the perception by students that their learning was neither meaningful nor adequate for them to really develop a practical approach for working with culturally diverse children..." (96).

In conclusion, numerous strategies have been proposed to increase the cultural competence of individuals despite the paucity of peer-reviewed literature. To date, impact has been measured as been self-reported changes in approach, by those receiving training, albeit over short durations. We still are unsure as to the impact of education on participants' education base, skills, or social interactions. While it is likely that stage-based and competency-based models are efficacious, more long-term follow-up is required to document efficacy. A potential solution is that the existing model needs to be modified so that the 'providers' embrace the culture of the recipients (97-99). The diagnostic and therapeutic approach must be consistent with increasingly diverse populations and integrate in a culturally consistent fashion. The development of such will likely be the result of increased education and/or the recommendations of relevant professional societies (100-101). Despite this, few universities have modified their curricula to adequately address multicultural course (102).

Preparing therapists and personnel to interact effectively with culturally and linguistically diverse populations remains a primary goal. To maximize efficacy, training of cultural awareness or sensitivity needs to be further developed. While transformation and activism approaches are potentially viable future approaches, there is little research to support which techniques work best in developing cross-cultural competence in individuals or institutions (103-104). Evaluation of individual training activities which is based upon self-report needs the support of long-term follow-up. The availability of individuals and organizations that have progressed from cultural competence to cultural proficiency is a primary goal. Especially in the setting of complex and developing cultures (105). Educational resources will likely require the interaction of universities and professional organizations in addition to communities and families. Better education and cultural immersion continue to improve early therapeutic detection and intervention for ASD (106-107). We now understand that not only the methodologies of education and determination of efficacy need to be improved but cultural immersion with continued and long-term exposure to backgrounds, traditions, and languages needs to be a continued goal.

7. Continued problems

Despite continued improvement in both the training of professionals involved in the diagnosis and early intervention in children with ASD and the instruments they use, even in culturally diverse groups completely integrated into the concept of society as a whole. Zhang has recently reported on cultural issues found when utilizing current assessment instruments (108) in Chinese children being evaluated in the U.S. They evaluated the diagnostic capabilities of four Assessment Instruments from a Chinese Cultural Perspective including The Vineland Adaptive Behavior Scales, The Checklist for Autism in Toddlers, the Modified Checklist for Autism in Toddlers, and the Childhood Autism Rating Scale. They noted that the Vineland Adaptive Behavior Scales which are used for routine screening contain sections concerning social relationships and language which may help to establish a basic understanding of whether the child has delays or deviant behavior but may result in an incomplete evaluation of a typical traditional Chinese child who may miss many culturally-based questions. The Checklist for Autism in Toddlers consists of 2 parts, with each assessing parallel functioning in three main areas including proto-declarative pointing, gaze monitoring, and pretend play. The CHAT can also result in spurious results based upon culturally distinct questions. The Modified Checklist for Autism in Toddlers adds an additional 9 questions from the original CHAT and an additional 14 questions which address core symptoms present among young children with autism and may be more resistant to cultural bias.

The Childhood Autism Rating Scale also may not be optimal as a screening indicator of children with autism. As Zhang notes "the child may avoid looking the adult in the eye to show his/her respect to the adult; or the child may be quiet because he/she is waiting politely for his/her turn." This may also be confounded by the fact that children with autism do not typically make eye contact. He elucidates that "question 18 from the communication domain (indicates preference when offered a choice), question 23 (opens and closes scissors with one hand), question 26 (cuts across a piece of paper with scissors), question 30 (cuts paper along a line with scissors), question 34 from motor skills domain (cuts out complex items with scissors), question 41 from the daily living skills domain (assists in food preparation requiring mixing and cooking), and question 38 from the daily living skills domain (clears table of breakable items)" may all be ineffective in discerning children with ASD given the potential cultural lability of the questions. The significance of such research is that it can only positively impact the approach and tools utilized to better evaluate children with ASD and further improve our understanding of such.

Dyches has noted that pertinent questions related to potential culturally based impact on diagnosis includes reluctance of families to pursue a diagnosis, advocacy for a preferential diagnosis of ASD as opposed to other potential diagnosis, cultural relevance of certain behaviors that normally would be indicative of ASD, and the lack of information of developmental milestones and symptoms, and economic capability to pursue an evaluation (109).

Racial, cultural and linguistic diversity can impact referral rate and clinical diagnosis and create additional challenges in the diagnosis of these children (110-111). The approach of multidisciplinary teams to the diagnosis of ASD likely strays from being culturally responsive given the demographics of team members (112). African American or Asian/Pacific Islanders are classified at approximately twice the rate as students who are American Indian/Alaskan or Hispanic (113). In addition, mis-diagnosis and delayed intervention may be the result of the patient receiving a symptom based diagnosis (developmental delay, mental retardation, speech-language impairment, emotional disorder) as opposed to a diagnosis that is more culturally relevant (114). One of ASHA's core principles for serving students with ASDs states that speech-language pathologists should "form partnerships with families of individuals with ASDs in assessment and intervention, while incorporating family preferences, honoring cultural differences, and respecting the challenges associated with limited resources." Valuing families as important members of multidisciplinary teams will facilitate the accurate identification of culturally or linguistically diverse—and, in fact, all—students with ASDs.

Broad-based screening of children for ASD is not universal across cultures. The detailed screening algorithm promoted by the American Academy of Pediatrics (115-116) is based more upon subjective than comprehensive evaluations which may result in a missed diagnosis of ASD if the deficits noted are considered to be culturally related. Additionally, limited access to health care services related to lack of parental recognition (117-118). Cultural or economic variables may also result in a missed diagnosis (119). Cultural awareness can only maximize diagnostic potential given that three primary diagnostic characteristics of autism, social interaction, communication, and restricted behavioral repertoire appear to be universal across cultures (120-121).

Comprehensive evaluations for ASD include an interview, period of observation, and testing. In current settings, cultural barriers such as language need to be minimized (123). Interviews should be conducted in the family's native language amongst members of the same cultural definitions. The use of social language should also be observed to identify deficiencies as opposed to differences. Observations should be made in a culturally consistent environment while utilizing both primary and secondary languages to assess for language impairment which will likely impact both languages. Multidisciplinary teams can then make a diagnosis and recommendations based upon testing that is technically sound, valid, and reliable using a variety of tools including dual language scoring. Tests must be free from racial/cultural bias (both on the part of the exam and examiner(s)) and administered in a format and language that will maximize efficacy (124). Tests must assess basic interpersonal communication skills and cognitive academic language proficiency. Expected disparities in learning second languages as noted between BICS (6 to 24 months) and CALP (> 60 months) may differ for children with ASD with more rapid CALP development (Aspergers), global delay in development (intellectual delay or culturally diverse student with ASD).

No single measure can be used to determine the presence of ASD. Level 1 screening measures are used by physicians to differentiate children with potential ASD from their peers. Level 2 tools are used in schools or developmental clinics to differentiate ASDs from developmental disabilities from their peers. Asperger Syndrome Diagnostic Scale (ASDS), Autism Behavior Checklist (ABC), Childhood Autism Rating Scale (CARS), Gilliam Autism Rating Scale - 2nd Edition (GARS-2), Autism Spectrum Quotient (AQ) - Adolescent Version, and Social Communication Questionnaire (SCQ). Only a paucity of screening measures have been documented to be applicable in the evaluation of bilingual children with disabilities (125), though some exiting instruments have been modified to more accurately assess to cultural differences (126-129). Despite this, any screening tool, including the M-CHAT, must be scrutinized for reliability when cross-cultural evaluations are being implemented in toddlers. Culturally relevant variables include responses related to pointing touch, vocalization, gestures, and/or eye contact among others.

8. Current roles

ASHA states that, "Speech and language professionals have the expertise to distinguish a language disorder from 'something else' (130) which can be related to 'cultural and linguistic differences, socioeconomic factors, lack of adequate prior instruction, and the process of acquiring the dialect of English used in the schools" (131). It also states that "speech-language pathologists should form partnerships with families of individuals with ASD in assessment and intervention, while incorporating family preferences, honoring cultural differences, and respecting the challenges associated with limited resources." A companion document, Guidelines for Speech-Language Pathologists in Diagnosis, Assessment, and Treatment of Autism Spectrum Disorders Across the Life Span notes that "Clinicians and educators need to determine which different strategies are effective with students/clients presenting varying developmental levels; social, linguistic, and cultural backgrounds; learning styles; behavior repertoires; and communication needs," while also considering family resources and cultural values.

In the setting of continuing cultural diversity, our approaches must be based upon methodologies that culturally competent in order to maximize our diagnostic capabilities for culturally distinct children with ASD. In addition to our understanding of the requisite approaches we must continue to educate both educators and students of how culturally distinct variables can impact both verbal and nonverbal communication, and which tests are most sensitive to discern ASD in culturally based nonverbal behavior.

9. Summary and conclusion

Given the significant socio-economic impact of ASD on families and society, in addition to the profound impact on children falling into the spectrum, early detection and early intervention remain primary goals in addressing this disease process. The corollary to this is not only the reliability of the testing tools utilized but also the individuals involved in the initial diagnosis and subsequent therapeutic interventions. High-quality, evidence-based interventions must be continuously developed, scrutinized, and improved to approach such a lofty goal. The consideration of the cultural diversity of the children and their families' backgrounds in addition to that of the therapists must be included in all discussions concerning the efficacy of diagnosis and intervention. Additionally, it is essential to take into consideration the various factors that may impede diagnosis or contribute to mis-diagnosis. As we have discussed, current research has shown that diagnosis rates vary by race and, thus, it is of value to explore factors that may play a role in such variance such as the effectiveness of exams and examiners. Suggestions for improved diagnosis rates are presented, such as minimizing cultural barriers and conducting interviews in the family's native language. Such measures will contribute to earlier diagnosis for individuals of any ethnic or cultural group. By pressing for the re-evaluation of culturally competency in ASD screening and assessment methods, we hope to increase the early diagnosis rates of ASD among all populations and subsequently the timeliness and impact of an earlier intervention.

10. Acknowledgement

This paper was supported entirely by a research grant from the Autism Tree Project Foundation in San Diego, California.

11. References

[1] Autism Society Website (2010). Incidence of Autism around the World. Bethesda, MD.
[2] National Research Council. (2001). Educating children with autism. Washington, DC:
[3] Reynolds, R., Want, M., and Wahlberg, H. (2003). Early childhood programs for a new century. Washington, DC: Child Welfare League of America, Inc.
[4] Novak, J., Levy, M., Wardega, L., & Usowicz, T. (2010). A retrospective study on the M-CHAT: A comparison of results between the USA and Poland. Presentation at International Conference on Child Neurology. Cairo, Egypt.
[5] Geschwind, D., & Levitt, P. (2007). Autism Spectrum Disorders: Developmental disconnection syndromes. Curr Opin Neurobiol., 17(1): 103-111.
[6] Brookes Freedman, D. (1979). Human sociobiology. New York: The Free Press.
[7] Barrera, I., & Kramer, L. (2009). Using skilled dialogue to transform challenging interactions. Baltimore, MD:
[8] Westby, C., Burda, A., & Mehta, Z. (2003, April 29). Asking the right questions in the right ways: Strategies for ethnographic interviewing. The ASHA Leader.
[9] Filipek PA, Accardo PJ, Baranek GT, Cook EH Jr, Dawson G, Gordon B, Gravel JS, Johnson CP, Kallen RJ, Levy SE, Minshew NJ, Ozonoff S, Prizant BM, Rapin I, Rogers SJ, Stone WL, Teplin S, Tuchman RF, Volkmar FR: The screening and diagnosis of autistic spectrum disorders. J Autism Dev Disord. 1999;29(6):439.

[10] Byrd, R. (2002). Report to the legislature on the principle findings from *The epidemiology of autism in California: a comprehensive pilot study.*
[11] Centers for Disease Control and Prevention, Division of Birth Defects, National Center on Birth Defects and Developmental Disabilities. (2010). Autism spectrum disorders (ASDS) data and statistics.
[12] American Academy of Pediatrics (AAP), children's health topics, autism.
[13] Robins, D., Fein, D., Barton, M. (1999). The Modified Checklist for Autism in Toddlers (M-CHAT). Storrs, CT: University of Connecticut.
[14] Weissman, L, Sices, L, & Augustyn, M. (2010). "He is just a little shy like me": screening for autism in a young child. Journal of Developmental & Behavioral Pediatrics, 31(8), 675-677.
[15] Bernard-Opitz, V., Kwook, K.-W., & Sapuan, S. (2001). Epidemiology of autism in Singapore: Findings of the first autism survey. *International Journal of Rehabilitation and Research, 24,* 1–6.
[16] Russell, G, Steer, C, & Golding, J. (2010). Social and demographic factors that influence the diagnosis of autistic spectrum disorders. *Soc Psychiatry Psychiatr Epidemiol.*
[17] Dyches, T. T., Hobbs, K., Wilder, L. K., Sudweeks, R. R., Obiakor, F. E., & Algozzine, B. (2005). Multicultural representation in autism. *Linking Research and Practice in Special Education: An International Perspective. 1*(1),1–15.
[18] Ellefsen, A., Kampmann, H., Billstedt, E., Gillberg, I. C., & Gillberg, C. (2007). Autism in the Faroe Islands: An epidemiological study. *Journal of Autism and Developmental Disorders, 37,* 437–444.
[19] Fombonne, E., Du Mazaubrun, C., Cans, C., & Grandjean, H. (1997). Autism and associated medical disorders in a French epidemiological survey. *Journal of the American Academy of Child and Adolescent Psychiatry, 36,* 1561–1569.
[20] Lauritsen, M. B., Mors, O., Mortensen, P. B., & Ewald, H. (2002). Medical disorders among inpatients with autism in Denmark according to ICD-8: A nationwide register-based study. *Journal of Autism and Developmental Disorders, 32*(2), 115–119.
[21] Keenan, M. (2004). Autism in Northern Ireland: The tragedy and the shame. *Psychologist, 17*(2), 72–75.
[22] Montiel-Nava, C., & Peña, J. A., (2008). Epidemiological findings of pervasive developmental disorders in a Venezuelan study. *Autism, 12,* 191–202.
[23] Dyches, T. T., Wilder, L. K., Sudweeks, R. R., Obiakor, F. E., & Algozzine, B. (2004). Multicultural Issues in Autism. *Journal of Autism and Developmental Disorders,* Vol. 34, No. 2, April 2004
[24] Rogers SJ (1998): Neuropsychology of autism in young children and its implications for early intervention. Mental Retardation and Developmental Disabilities Research Reviews. Special Issue Autism. Volum4 4:104- 112, 1998.
[25] Chakrabarti, Suniti; Haubus, Christine; Dugmore, Sally; Orgill, Gill; Devine, Frank: A Model of Early Detection and Diagnosis of Autism Spectrum Disorder in Young Children Infants & Young Children. 18(3):200-211, July/September 2005.
[26] Sanua, V. D. (1981a). Autism, childhood schizophrenia and culture: A critical review of the literature. *Transcultural Psychiatric Research Review,* 18, 165–181.
[27] Sanua, V. D. (1981b). Cultural changes and psychopathology in children: With special reference to infantile autism. *Acta Paedopsychiat,* 47, 133–142.

[28] Sanua, V. D. (1984). Is infantile autism a universal phenomenon? An open question. *International Journal of Social Psychiatry*, 30, 163–177.

[29] Pauline A. Filipek,2,17 Pasquale J. Accardo,3 Grace T. Baranek,4 Edwin H. Cook, Jr.,5 Geraldine Dawson,6 Barry Gordon,7 Judith S. Gravel,8 Chris P. Johnson,9 Ronald J. Kallen,5 Susan E. Levy,10 Nancy J. Minshew,11 Barry M. Prizant,12 Isabelle Rapin,8 Sally J. Rogers,13 Wendy L. Stone,14 Stuart Teplin,4 Roberto F. Tuchman,15 and Fred R. Volkmar16: The Screening and Diagnosis of Autistic Spectrum Disorders1. Journal of Autism and Developmental Disorders Vol. 29, No. 6, 1999)

[30] Edwards, D. R., & Bristol M. M. (1991). Autism: early identification and management in family practice. *American Family Physician, Nov 1991 v44 n5* p1755(10)

[31] P. A. Filipek, P. J. Accardo, S. Ashwal, G. T. Baranek, E. H. Cook, G. Dawson, B. Gordon, J. S. Gravel, C. P. Johnson, R. J. Kallen, S. E. Levy, N. J. Minshew, S. Ozonoff, B. M. Prizant, I. Rapin, S. J. Rogers, W. L. Stone, S. W. Teplin, R. F. Tuchman, F. R. Volkmar In the Report of the Quality Standards Subcommittee of the American Academy of Neurology and the Child Neurology Society. NEUROLOGY 2000;55:468–479

[32] Powell, T. H., Hecimovic, A., & Christensen, L. (1992). Meeting the unique needs of families. In D. E. Berkell (Ed.), *Autism: Identification, education and treatment* (pp. 187–224). Hillsdale, NJ: Erlbaum.

[33] Iglesias, A. & Quinn, R. (1997). Culture as a context for early intervention. In K. Thurman, J. Cornwell, & S. Gottwald, *The context of early intervention: Systems and settings,* (pp. 55-72). Baltimore, MD: Paul H. Brookes.

[34] Sparrow, S. S., Balla, D., & Cicchetti, D. (1984). Vineland Adaptive Behavior Scales—Survey form. *Circle Pines, MN: American Guidance Service* U.S. Census Bureau (1990). Census 1990. *Washington, DC: Author.*

[35] United States Department of Education (2002). Twenty-third annual report to Congress on the implementation of the Individuals with Disabilities Education Act. *Washington, DC: Author.*

[36] United States Census Bureau (2004). We the people: Asians in the United States. *Census 2000 special reports.*

[37] European Autism Information System (EAIS) Report on the 'Autism Spectrum Disorders Prevalence: Data and Accessibility to Services' Questionnaire (QEAIS). Manuel Posada, Patricia Garcia Primo, Maria José Ferrari and Maria Concepción Martín-Arribas Research Institute for Rare Diseases, Instituto de Salud. Carlos III, Madrid. 20 March 2007

[38] Fombonne, E. (2005). Epidemiology of autistic disorder and other pervasive developmental disorder. *Journal of Clinical Psychiatry, 66* (Suppl. 10), 3-8.

[39] Sparrow, S. S., Balla, D., & Cicchetti, D. (1984). Vineland Adaptive Behavior Scales Survey form. *Circle Pines, MN: American Guidance Service* U.S. Census Bureau (1990). Census 1990. *Washington, DC:.*

[40] Robins, D. L., Fein, D., Barton, M. L., & Green, J. A. (2001). The modified checklist for autism in toddlers: an initial study investigating the early detection of autism and pervasive developmental disorders. *Journal of Autism and Developmental Disorders,* 31:131-144

[41] Schopler, E., Reichler, R. J., & Renner, B. R. (1988). The childhood autism rating scale (CARS). Los Angeles: Western Psychological Services

[42] Kliewer, C., Fitzgerald, L. M., Meyer Mork, J., Hartman, P., English Sand, P., & Raschke, D.: Citizenship for all in the literate community: An ethnography of young children with significant disabilities in inclusive early childhood settings. Harvard Educational Review, 74(4), 373-403. 2004

[43] Ann H. Hains, Eleanor W. Lynch, Pamela J. Winton: CLAS Technical Report #3: Moving Towards Cross-Cultural Competence in Lifelong Personnel Development: A Review of the Literature. October 2000

[44] Crais, E. R., & Roberts, J. E. (2004). Assessing communication skills. *In McLean, M., Wolery, M. & Bailey, D. B., Assessing infants and preschoolers with special needs (3rd edition).* pp. 357-359. New Jersey: Pearson Education

[45] Ladson-Billings, G. (2001). *Crossing over to Canaan: The journey of new teachers in diverse classrooms.* San Francisco: Jossey-Bass

[46] Dyches, T. T., Wilder, L. K., Sudweeks, R. R., Obiakor, F. E., & Algozzine, B. (2004). Multicultural Issues in Autism. *Journal of Autism and Developmental Disorders,* Vol. 34, No. 2, April 2004

[47] Lynch, E. W. & Hanson, M. J. (2004). Family diversity, assessment, and cultural competence. *In McLean, M., Wolery, M. & Bailey, D. B., Assessing infants and preschoolers with special needs (3rd edition),* pp. 72-74. New Jersey: Pearson Education

[48] Carter, R. T., & Qureshi, A. (1995). A typology of philosophical assumptions in multicultural counseling and training. In J.G. Ponterroto, J.M. Casas, L. A. Suzuki, & C. M. Alexander (Eds.), *Handbook of multicultural counseling* (pp. 239-262). Thousand Oaks, CA: SAGE.

[49] Cross, T.L., Bazron, B.J., Dennis, K.W., & Isaacs, M.R. (1989). *Towards a culturally competent system of care,* (Volume 1). Washington, DC: National Center for Technical Assistance Center for Children's Mental Health, Georgetown University Child Development Center.

[50] Barrera, I., & Kramer, L. (1997). From monologues to skilled dialogues: Teaching the process of crafting culturally competent early childhood environments. In P.J. Winton, J. A. McCollum, & C. Catlett (Eds.), *Reforming personnel preparation in early intervention: Issues, models, and practical strategies* (pp. 217-251). Baltimore: Paul H. Brookes.

[51] Barrera, I. (1993). Effective and appropriate instruction for all children: The challenge of cultural/linguistic diversity and young children with special needs. *Topics in Early Childhood Special Education,* 13(4), 461-487.

[52] Harry, B. (1992). Developing cultural self-awareness: The first step in values clarification for early interventionists. *Topics in Early Childhood Special Education, 12* (3), 333-350.

[53] (The California Department of Education, Child Development Division, Center for Child and Family Studies, WestEd. Essential Connections. Ten Keys to Culturally Sensitive Care [Video] (1995). California Department of Education: Sacramento, CA.).

[54] Marilyn Sass-Lehrer, Barbara Gerner de Garcia, Michele Rovins. Creating a Multicultural School Climate for Deaf Children and Their Families (1997). PreCollege National Mission Programs/Gallaudet University: Washington, DC.

[55] Sally E. Pisarchick, Phillip Safford, Judith Stahlman, Lisa Barnhouse, Vivian Nutter, Arnie Henry, Becky Storer, Michele Beery. Project Prepare: Planning: Competency Based Personnel Preparation in Early Childhood Education (1995). Ohio Department of Education: Columbus, OH.)

[56] Penny P Anderson, Emily Fenichel. Serving Culturally Diverse Families of Infants and Toddlers with Disabilities (1989). National Center for Clinical Infant Programs: Washington, D.C.

[57] Manoleas, P. (1994). An outcome approach to assessing the cultural competence of MSW students. In P. Keys (Ed.), *School social workers in the multicultural environment: New roles, responsibilities, and educational enrichment,* (pp. 43-57). Binghamton, NY: The Haworth Press, Inc.

[58] Campinha-Bacote, J. (1995). The quest for cultural competence in nursing care. *Nursing Forum, 30*(4), 19-25.

[59] Dyches, T. T. (2011, January 18). Assessing Diverse Students With Autism Spectrum Disorders. The ASHA Leader.

[60] Cross, T.L., Bazron, B.J., Dennis, K.W., & Isaacs, M.R. (1989). *Towards a culturally competent system of care,* (Volume 1). Washington, DC: National Center for Technical Assistance Center for Children's Mental Health, Georgetown University Child Development Center.

[61] Anderson, P. P., & Fenichel, E. S. (1989). *Serving culturally diverse families of infants and toddlers with disabilities.* Washington, DC: National Center for Clinical Infant Programs.

[62] Sue, D. W., Bernier, J. B., Durran, M., Feinberg, L., Pedersen, P., Smith, E., & Vasquez-Nuttall, E. (1982). Position paper: Cross-cultural competencies. *The Counseling Psychologist, 10,* 45-52.

[63] Sue, D. W. (1997). Forward. In D.B. Pope-Davis & H.L.K. Coleman (Eds.), *Multicultural counseling competencies: Assessment, education and training, and supervision,* pp. ix-xi. Thousand Oaks, CA: Sage Publications.

[64] Sue, D.W., Arredondo, P., & McDavis, R.J. (1992). Multicultural counseling competencies and standards: A call to the profession. *Journal of Multicultural Counseling and Development, 20,* 64-88.

[65] Cross, T.L., Bazron, B.J., Dennis, K.W., & Isaacs, M.R. (1989). *Towards a culturally competent system of care,* (Volume 1). Washington, DC: National Center for Technical Assistance Center for Children's Mental Health, Georgetown University Child Development Center.

[66] Sleeter, C.E. (Ed.). (1991). *Empowerment through multicultural education.* Albany, NY: State University of New York.

[67] Isaacs, M.R., & Benjamin, M.P. (1991). *Towards a culturally competent system of care,* (Volume II). Washington, DC: National Technical Assistance Center for Children's Mental Health, Center for Child Health and Mental Health Policy, Georgetown University Child Development Center.

[68] Wayman, K.I., Lynch, E.W., & Hanson, M.J. (1991). Home-based early childhood services: Cultural sensitivity in a family systems approach. *Topics in Early Childhood Special Education, 10*(4), 56-75.

[69] Ponterotto, J.G., Alexander, C.M., & Grieger, I. (1995). A multicultural competency checklist for counseling training programs. *Journal of Multicultural Counseling and Development, 23,* 11-20.

[70] Pope-Davis, D.B., & Dings, J.G. (1995). The assessment of multicultural counseling competencies. In J.G. Ponterotto, J.M. Casas, L.A. Suzuki, & C.M. Alexander (Eds.). *Handbook of multicultural counseling* (pp. 287-311). Thousand Oaks, CA: SAGE.

[71] Ponterotto, J. G., Casas, J. M., Suzuki, L. A., & Alexander, C. M. (1995). *Handbook of multicultural counseling.* Thousand Oaks, CA: SAGE.

[72] Campinha-Bacote, J. (1995). The quest for cultural competence in nursing care. *Nursing Forum, 30*(4), 19-25.

[73] Manoleas, P. (1994). An outcome approach to assessing the cultural competence of MSW students. In P. Keys (Ed.), *School social workers in the multicultural environment: New roles, responsibilities, and educational enrichment,* (pp. 43-57). Binghamton, NY: The Haworth Press, Inc.

[74] Chu, H., & Levy, J. (1988). Multicultural skills for bilingual teachers: Training for competency development. *NABE Journal,* Winter, 153-169.

[75] Seelye, H. N. (1996). *Experiential activities for intercultural learning,* (Vol. 1). Yarmouth, ME: Intercultural Press.

[76] Ponterotto, J. G. (1996). Multicultural counseling in the twenty-first century. *The Counseling Psychologist, 24*(2), 259-268.

[77] Ponterotto, J. G., Casas, J. M., Suzuki, L. A., & Alexander, C. M. (1995). *Handbook of multicultural counseling.* Thousand Oaks, CA: SAGE.

[78] Pope-Davis D. B., & Coleman, H. L. K. (1997). *Multicultural counseling competencies: Assessment, education and training, and supervision.* Thousand Oaks, CA: SAGE.

[79] Sodowsky, G.R., Kuo-Jackson, P.Y., Loya, G.J. (1997). Outcome of training in the philosophy of assessment: Multicultural counseling competencies. In D.B. Pope-Davis & H.L.K. Coleman (Eds.), *Multicultural counseling competencies: Assessment, education and training, and supervision,* pp. 3-42. Thousand Oaks, CA: Sage Publications.

[80] Banks, J. A., & Banks, C.A.M. (1995). *Handbook of research on multicultural education.* New York: Macmillan.

[81] LaBelle, T. G., & Ward, C. R. (1994). *Multiculturalism and education.* Albany, NY: State University of New York Press.

[82] Sleeter , C. E., & Grant, C. A. (1994). *Making choices for multicultural education: Five approaches to race, class, & gender,* (2nd ed). New York: Macmillan.

[83] American Psychological Association (1986). Accreditation handbook (Rev. ed.). Washington, DC: APA Committee on Accreditation and Accreditation Office.

[84] Reston, VA: Council for Exceptional Children (CEC). (1996*). What every special educator must know: The international standards for the preparation and certification of special education teachers* (2nd ed.)

[85] NAEYC. (1996b). *Guidelines for preparation of early childhood professionals: Guidelines developed by the National Association for the Education of Young Children, Division for Early Childhood of the Council for Exceptional Children, & National Board for Professional Teaching Standards..* Washington, DC:

[86] National Council for Accreditation of Teacher Education. (1994). *Approved curriculum guidelines.* Washington, DC:.

[87] Brown, M. T., & Landrum-Brown, J. (1995). Counselor supervision: Cross-cultural perspectives. In J.G. Ponterroto, J.M. Casas, L. A. Suzuki, & C. M. Alexander (Eds.), *Handbook of multicultural counseling* (pp. 263-286). Thousand Oaks, CA: SAGE.,

[88] Fenichel, E. S. (1992). *Learning through supervision and mentorship to support infants, toddlers, and their families: A source book*. Arlington, VA: Zero to Three/The National Center for Clinical Infant Programs.

[89] Fong, M. L., & Lease, S. H. (1997). Cross-cultural supervision: Issues for the white supervisor. In D.B. Pope-Davis & H.L.K. Coleman (Eds.), *Multicultural counseling competencies: Assessment, education and training, and supervision*, pp. 387-405. Thousand Oaks, CA: Sage Publications.

[90] Krajewski-Jaime, E.R., Brown, K.S., Ziefert, M., & Kaufman. E. (1996). Utilizing international clinical practice to build inter-cultural sensitivity in social work students. *Journal of Multicultural Social Work, 4*(2), 15-29.

[91] Shanok, R. S., Gilkerson, L., Eggbeer, L., & Fenichel, E. (1995). *Reflective supervision: A relationship for learning: Discussion guide and videotape*. Arlington, VA: Zero to Three/The National Center for Clinical Infant Programs.

[92] Shanok, R. S., Gilkerson, L., Eggbeer, L., & Fenichel, E. (1995). *Reflective supervision: A relationship for learning: Discussion guide and videotape*. Arlington, VA: Zero to Three/The National Center for Clinical Infant Programs.

[93] Stone, G. L. (1997). Multiculturalism as a context for supervision: Perspectives, limitations, and implications. In D.B. Pope-Davis & H.L.K. Coleman (Eds.), *Multicultural counseling competencies: Assessment, education and training, and supervision,* pp. 263-289. Thousand Oaks, CA: Sage Publications.

[94] Alpers, R. R., & Zoucha, R. (1996). Comparison of cultural competence and cultural confidence in senior nursing students in a private southern university. *Journal of Cultural Diversity, 3*(1), 9-15.

[95] Allison, K. W., Crawford, I., Echemendia, R., Robinson, L., & Knepp, D. (1994). Human diversity and professional competence: Training in clinical and counseling psychology revisited. *American Psychologist, 49* (9), 792-796.

[96] Hyun, E. (1995). *Phenomena of early childhood pre-service teachers' sense making of developmentally and culturally appropriate practice (DCAP)*

[97] Focal Point. (1994). *Developing culturally competent organizations,* Vol. 8, No. 2. Portland OR: Bulletin of the Research and Training Center on Family Support and Children's Mental Health, Portland State University.

[98] Phillips, C.B. (1993*). Early childhood reform: Innovative approaches to cultural and racial diversity among families*. Alexandria, VA: National Association of State Boards of Education.

[99] Pang, V. O., Gay, G., & Stanley, W. B. (1995). Expanding conceptions of community and civic competence for a multicultural society. *Theory and Research in Social Education, 23*(4), 302-331.

[100] Pope-Davis D. B., & Coleman, H. L. K. (1997). *Multicultural counseling competencies: Assessment, education and training, and supervision*. Thousand Oaks, CA: SAGE.

[101] Sue, D. W. (1997). Forward. In D.B. Pope-Davis & H.L.K. Coleman (Eds.), *Multicultural counseling competencies: Assessment, education and training, and supervision*, pp. ix-xi. Thousand Oaks, CA: Sage Publications.

[102] Ponterotto, J.G. (1997). Multicultural counseling training: A competency model and national survey. In D.B. Pope-Davis & H.L.K. Coleman (Eds.), *Multicultural counseling competencies: Assessment, education and training, and supervision,* pp. 111-130. Thousand Oaks, CA: Sage Publications.

[103] Banks, J.A. (1993). Education and cultural diversity in the United States. In A. Fyfe & P. Figueroa (Eds.), *Education for cultural diversity: The challenge for a new era* (pp.49-68). New York: Routledge.

[104] Derman-Sparks, L., & Phillips, C. B. (1997). *Teaching/learning anti-racism: A developmental approach.* New York: Teachers College Press.

[105] National Black Child Development Institute (1993). *Paths to African American leadership positions in early childhood education: Constraints and opportunities.* Washington, DC:

[106] Bredekamp, S. (1992). The early childhood profession coming together. *Young Children, 47*(6), 36-39.

[107] Buysse, V., & Wesley, P. (1993). The identity crisis in early childhood special education: A call for professional role clarification. *Topics in early childhood special education, 13*(4), 418-429.

[108] Jie Zhang, John J. Wheeler, Dean Richey: Cultural validity in assessment instruments for children with Autism from a Chinese cultural perspective. Int J Spec Ed 21 (1), 2006

[109] Dyches, T. T. (2011, January 18). Assessing Diverse Students With Autism Spectrum Disorders. The ASHA Leader.

[110] Begeer, S., El Bouk, S., Boussaid, W., Terwogt, M. M., & Koot, H. M. (2009). Under diagnosis and referral bias of autism in ethnic minorities. *Journal of Autism and Developmental Disorders, 39,* 142–148.

[111] Mandell, D. S., Wiggins, L. D., Carpenter, L. A., Daniels, J., DiGuiseppi, C., Durkin, M. S., et al. (2009). Racial/ethnic disparities in the identification of children with autism spectrum disorders. *American Journal of Public Health, 99,* 493–498.

[112] Chabon, S., Brown , J. E. & Gildersleeve-Neumann, C. (August 3, 2010). Ethics, equity, and English-language learners: A decision-making framework. *The ASHA Leader.* Retrieved from www.asha.org/Publications/leader/2010/100803/Ethics-Equity-ELL.htm.

[113] Dyches, T. T., Wilder, L. K., Sudweeks, R. R, Obiakor, F. E., & Algozzine, B. (2004). Multicultural issues in autism. *Journal of Autism and Developmental Disorders,* 34, 211–222.

[114] Wilder, L. K., Dyches, T. T., Obiakor, F. E., & Algozzine, B. (2004). Multicultural perspectives on teaching students with autism. *Focus on Autism and Other Developmental Disabilities, 19,* 105–113.

[115] Johnson, C. P.., Myers, S. M., & the Council on Children with Disabilities (2007). Identification and evaluation of children with autism spectrum disorders. *Pediatrics, 120*(5), 1–33.

[116] Begeer, S., El Bouk, S., Boussaid, W., Terwogt, M. M., & Koot, H. M. (2009). Under diagnosis and referral bias of autism in ethnic minorities. *Journal of Autism and Developmental Disorders, 39,* 142–148.

[117] Dumont-Mathieu, T. & Fein, D. (2005). Screening for autism in young children: The Modified Checklist for Autism in Toddlers and other measures. *Mental Retardation and Developmental Disabilities Research Reviews, 11,* 253–262.

[118] Zhang, J., Wheeler, J. J., & Richey, D. (2006). Cultural validity in assessment instruments for children with autism from a Chinese cultural perspective. *International Journal of Special Education, 21*(1), 109-114.

[119] Durkin, M. S., Maenner, M. J., Meaney, J., Levy, S. E., DiGuiseppi, C., Nicholas, J. S. et al. (2010).Socioeconomic inequality in the prevalence of autism spectrum disorder: Evidence from a U.S. cross-sectional study. *PLoS ONE 5*(7): e11551. doi:10.1371/journal.pone.0011551.

[120] Ametepee, L., & Chitiyo, M. (2009). What we know about autism in Africa: A brief research synthesis. *Journal of the International Association of Special Education, 10*(1), 11-13.

[121] Papageorgiou, V., Georgiades, S., & Mavreas, V. (2008). Brief report: Cross-cultural evidence for the heterogeneity of the restricted, repetitive behaviours and interests domain of autism—A Greek study. *Journal of Autism and Developmental Disorders, 38*, 558-561.

[122] Wakabayashi, A., Baron-Cohen, S., Uchiyama, T., Yoshida, Y., Tojo, Y., Kuroda, M., et al. (2007). The Autism-Spectrum Quotient (AQ) Children's Version in Japan: A cross-cultural comparison. *Journal of Autism and Developmental Disorders, 37,* 491-500.

[123] Austin, L. B. (2007). Considerations of native language service provision in speech therapy for students with severe impairments from Spanish-speaking homes. *Texas Journal of Audiology and Speech-Language Pathology*, 30, 41-46.

[124] Gibb, G. S., & Dyches, T. T. (2007). *Guide to writing quality individualized education programs* (2nd ed.). Needham Heights, MA: Allyn & Bacon).

[125] Chabon, S., Brown , J. E. & Gildersleeve-Neumann, C. (August 3, 2010). Ethics, equity, and English-language learners: A decision-making framework. *The ASHA Leader.*

[126] Bolte, S., & Poustka, F. (2004). The German form of the Autism Diagnostic Observation Schedule (ADIOS): First results on reliability and validity. *Zeitschrift fur Kinder und Jugendpsychiatrie und Psychotherapie, 32*(1), 45-50.

[127] Hedley, D., Young, R., Gallegos, M. A. J., & Salazar, C. M. (2010). Cross-cultural evaluation of the Autism Detection in Early Childhood (ADEC) in Mexico. *Autism, 14*, 93-113.

[128] Wong, V., Hui, L. H., Lee, W. C., Leung, L. S., Ho, P. K., Lau, W. L., et al. (2004). A modified screening tool for autism (Checklist for Autism in Toddlers [CHAT-23]) for Chinese children. *Pediatrics, 114,* 166-76.

[129] Johnson, C. P.., Myers, S. M., & the Council on Children with Disabilities (2007). Identification and evaluation of children with autism spectrum disorders. *Pediatrics, 120*(5), 1-33.

[130] American Speech-Language-Hearing Association (2004). *Knowledge and Skills Needed by Speech-Language Pathologists and Audiologists to Provide Culturally and Linguistically Appropriate Services..*

[131] American Speech-Language-Hearing Association (2010). *Roles and Responsibilities of Speech-Language Pathologists in Schools* [Professional Issues Statement].

9

Autism Spectrum Disorders in Iran

Mohammad-Reza Mohammadi, Maryam Salmanian and Shahin Akhondzadeh
Tehran University of Medical Sciences, Psychiatry and Psychology Research Center, Iran

1. Introduction

Autism Spectrum Disorders (ASDs), which consist of Autistic Disorder, Asperger Syndrome and PDD Not Otherwise Specified (PDD-NOS), are subsets of Pervasive Developmental Disorders (PDD) (1, 2). Obviously, ASDs are characterized by abnormalities in social interaction and communication, as well as repetitive and stereotyped behaviors (3). Although various studies have been conducted in ASDs etiology across the world, it seems that they are still unknown in developing and developed countries. In fact, ASDs have been introduced as multifactorial disorders; from ascendancy of genetic to environmental factors are involved in causing them (4-7).

Although there are substantial biological bases for ASDs, no perspicuous symptoms exist for their diagnostic conditions. Therefore, behavioral criteria are mainly utilized to identify individuals with ASDs. Some assessment instruments are Autism Diagnostic Interview-Revised (ADI- R), Autism Diagnostic Observation Schedule (ADOS), Childhood Autism Rating Scale (CARS), Diagnostic Interview for Social and Communicative Disorders (DISCO), Developmental, Dimensional and Diagnostic Interview (3di), Autism Spectrum Disorders-Diagnostic for Children (ASD-DC), Autism Spectrum Disorders-Comorbidity for Children (ASD-CC) and Autism Spectrum Disorders-Behavior Problem for Children (ASD-BPC) (8-15). There is universal agreement in diagnostic criteria of ASDs; however, the cultural differences influence their diagnosis (16).

With regards to obscure etiology of ASDs, they have not been specifically treated up to now. Nevertheless, several treatments have been performed to improve ASDs including behavioral, medical, biological, sensory- motor and relationship development interventions (17-21).

Whereas cultural factors play an essential role in prevalence, diagnosis and treatment of ASDs, cross-cultural studies should be performed (22-24). Hence, some scientific researches have been conducted on ASDs in Iran. Several preliminary investigations have been done to evaluate ASDs prevalence and some risk factors and effective variables have also been studied in the field of etiology. Diagnostic evaluation of ASDs, especially based on EEG, and several pharmacological and behavioral interventions for ASDs treatment have been performed in Iran. In parental studies, mental health, stress levels and personality characteristics were investigated in parents of children with ASDs, with focus on mothers.

A systematic literature review was performed to identify the ASDs studies in Iran. Accordingly, PubMed, ISI web of Science, and four Iranian databases, including IranPsych, IranMedex, Irandoc and Scientific Information Database (SID) were searched to find Iranian studies in ASDs using combination of two groups of terms. The first group included the following terms: Autism Spectrum Disorders, Autism, Autistic disorder, PDD Not Otherwise Specified and Asperger, combined with OR; and the second group consisted of Iran or its major cities. The name of famous Iranian researchers in ASDs field and their curriculum vitae were also searched to find scientific studies on ASDs in Iran. Case reports were excluded. The results of 39 investigations including the original, review, editorial material and proceedings articles and available dissertations were separately assigned to prevalence, etiology, diagnosis and treatment divisions.

2. ASDs prevalence

Less attention has been paid to studying ASDs -especially about their epidemiology- in developing countries. In fact, most studies about ASDs prevalence have been done in the United States and Europe (25). Overall, recent scientific researches indicated more rates of ASDs. The study of ASDs prevalence in primary school children estimated the rate of 157 per 10,000 children in the United Kingdom (26). The only investigation on adults with ASDs evaluated the prevalence of these disorders to be 98 per 10,000 in England (27). Another study on 8 year-old children with ASDs estimated an average rate of 90 per 10,000 participants in the United States (28). In a comprehensive review article, the prevalence rate was around 20 per 10,000 for Autistic disorder, 30 per 10,000 for PDD-NOS, and 2 per 100,000 for Asperger syndrome (29). However, the rates of Asperger syndrome were estimated to be 36 out of 10,000 and 48 per 10,000 children in Sweden (30, 31). There were various results about ASDs prevalence across the world. Accordingly, diversity among prevalence estimations could be related to the age of participants, diagnostic criteria, and geographical locations.. In addition, less prevalence of ASDs can be explained by the less available services and lack of awareness about ASDs in developing countries (32).

While no advanced study have been conducted on the prevalence of ASDs in Iran (33), Ghanizadeh` s preliminary investigation on school children (2008) indicated the rate of 19 per 1000 for probable autistic disorder ,and 5 per 1000 for probable Asperger syndrome, which seem more than reported estimations of ASDs prevalence across the world (34). Also, Nejatisafa (2003) performed the first preliminary study to investigate the frequency of ASDs in university students ; while the scores were significantly higher for men than women, the results showed the frequency of 120 out of 1000 adult participants (35).

Another study showed the highest prevalence rate of ASDs for autistic disorder, then Asperger syndrome and PDD-NOS. It also indicated that boys were 4 times more likely than girls to have autistic and Asperger disorders (36). The prevalence rates of autistic students have been displayed 0.366% among exceptional students (37).

3. Etiology of ASDs

ASDs have multiple etiologies; genetic polymorphisms, epigenetics, convergent molecular abnormalities, mutations, chromosomal aberrations, disorders in mirror neuron system and central coherence, brain structure anomalies, cytogenetic abnormalities, and single-gene defects, toxic exposures, teratogens, measles-mumps-rubella vaccines, some prenatal, obstetric and neonatal factors and etc have been specified as the contributing factors in the etiologies of ASDs in the different researches across the world (7, 38-44).

The relationships between ASDs and some effective factors have been investigated in Iran. In a recent study, the theory of mind development was significantly affected by gender and IQ. so low functioning autistic children had the poorest performance in the theory of mind development compared to high functioning autistic children and normal group (45). In one study, IQ variable was an important factor to determine visual memory of meaningless shapes in children with ASDs. While a significant difference was observed in visual memory of meaningless shapes between children with ASDs and normal group by entering the IQ effect, the results were contradictory as the association was inversed by removing IQ. However, IQ variable was not correlated to face memory in children with ASDs. Overall, there was no significant difference in face memory between children with ASDs and normal group in this study (46).

In a clinical study, no significant correlation was observed between gender and age, diagnosis and severity of the symptoms in children with ASDs (47).

Sasanfar (2010) investigated the parental age and education level as risk factors and indicated that higher paternal age, but not maternal age, and higher education level increased the risk of autism. However, it seems that parents with high education usually seek the diagnostic and therapeutic services more than less educated parents (48).

In another Iranian study, no correlation was observed between autism and Celiac diseases in autistic children compared to age and sex matched normal group (49).

Since brain stem has a critical role in processing hearing inputs, its hearing function has been investigated by an auditory brain stem response tool in children with slight and severe autism compared to normal group. This research demonstrates brain stem abnormality in severe autistic children which may result in intensifying autism symptoms (50).

Social interaction and stereotyped behaviors were investigated between autistic and trainable mentally retarded children. The results showed higher mean scores of qualitative damage to social interaction and stereotyped behaviors in autistic children compared to trainable mentally retarded children (51).

4. Diagnosis of ASDs by EEG

Several studies have been administered to diagnose abnormalities using quantitative electroencephalography (qEEG) analysis in children with ASDs compared with normal children. Considering that the relaxed eye-opened condition in alpha band was the best condition to discriminate between children with ASDs and normal group, the ASDs had significant lower spectrogram criteria values ($p<0.01$) at Fp1, Fp2, F3 and T5 electrodes and lower values ($p<0.05$) at T3, P3 and O1 electrodes. Accordingly, spectrogram criteria had displayed more abnormalities in the left brain hemisphere and prefrontal lobe in children with ASDs compared to normal children (52).

Moreover, Magnitude Squared Coherence values at 171 pairs of EEG electrodes in the relaxed eye-opened condition illustrated more abnormalities in the connectivity of temporal lobes with other lobes in gamma frequency band in children with ASDs (54).

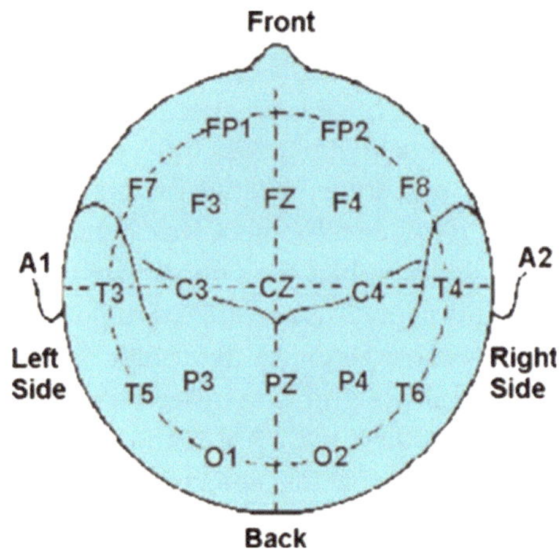

(From: Niedermeyer E, Lopes da Silva F. Electroencephalography: Basic principles, clinical applications, and related fields, 5th ed. Philadelphia: Lippincott Williams & Wilkins; 2005, p 140) (53)

Fig. 1. International EEG electrodes placement system

Electrodes	ASD children (Mean±SD)	Control children (Mean±SD)	p
Fp1*	0.238±0.156	0.381±0.131	0.018
Fp2	0.256±0.165	0.357±0.157	0.122
F7*	0.245±0.131	0.376±0.146	0.021
F3**	0.197±0.076	0.442±0.103	0.000
Fz	0.237±0.106	0.309±0.175	0.192
F4	0.270±0.174	0.309±0.137	0.529
F8	0.300±0.198	0.337±0.118	0.583
T3**	0.254±0.136	0.405±0.130	0.007
C3*	0.251±0.156	0.401±0.121	0.013
Cz*	0.267±0.146	0.407±0.173	0.030
C4	0.291±0.182	0.310±0.190	0.796
T4	0.313±0.175	0.391±0.219	0.308
T5*	0.238±0.156	0.396±0.150	0.014
P3	0.300±0.154	0.411±0.133	0.063
Pz	0.310±0.196	0.395±0.147	0.231
P4	0.340±0.194	0.407±0.179	0.373
T6	0.319±0.170	0.388±0.123	0.258
O1	0.304±0.169	0.381±0.151	0.234
O2	0.308±0.161	0.293±0.163	0.821

** $p<0.01$ and * $p<0.05$

(From: Sheikhani A, Behnam H, Mohammadi MR, Noroozian M, Mohammadi M. Detection of Abnormalities for Diagnosing of Children with Autism Disorders Using of Quantitative Electroencephalography Analysis. J Med Syst 2010) (54)

Table 1. The spectrogram criteria values of the EEG for the children with autism spectrum disorder (ASD) and control children for all electrodes in alpha band (8–13 Hz)

Notably, one research presented the gamma frequency band as the best discriminant in children with Asperger compared to normal group. Children with Asperger disorder had significant lower spectrogram criteria values (p<0.01) at Fp1 electrode and lower values (p<0.05) at Fp2 and T6 electrodes. Coherence values at 171 pairs of EEG electrodes displayed the connectivity at (T4, P4), (T4, Cz), (T4, C4) electrode pairs and (T4, O1) had significant differences (p<0.01) in the two groups in the gamma band. Accordingly, the prefrontal and right temporal lobes had more abnormalities based on using spectrogram, and coherence values showed more abnormalities in the connectivity of right temporal lobe with the other lobes in the gamma frequency band in children with Asperger Syndrome (55).

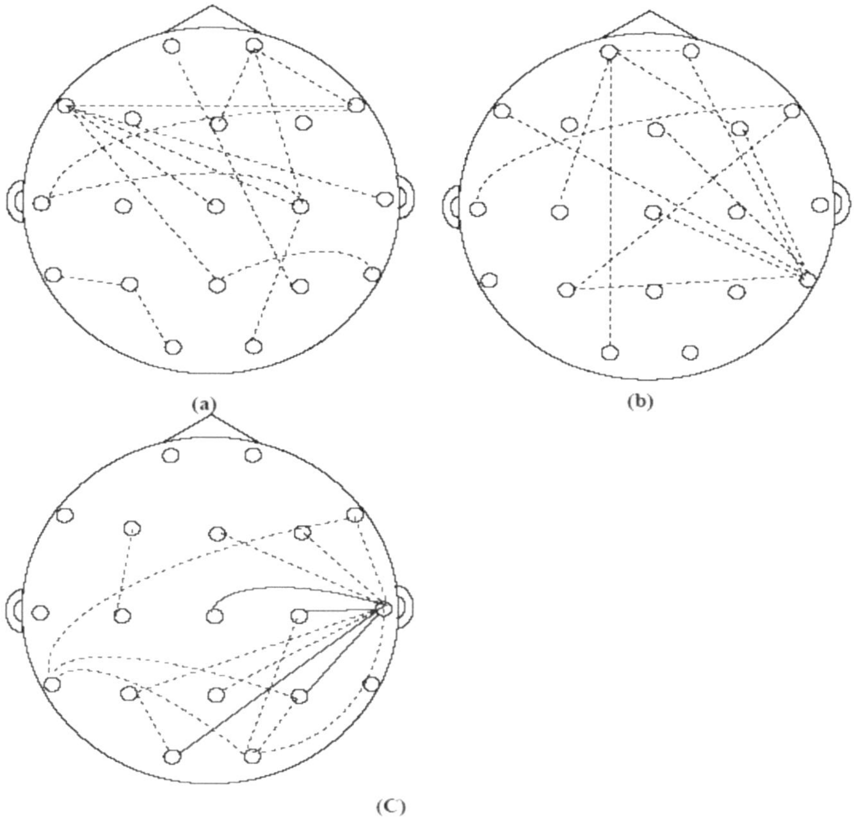

(From: Noroozian M, Sheikhani A, Behnam H, Mohammadi MR. Abnormalities of Quantitative Electroencephalography in Children with Asperger Disorder Using Spectrogram and Coherence Values. Iran J Psychiatry 2008; p 68) (55)

Fig. 2. Results of connectivity in 171 pairs of electrodes that had significant differences in frequency bands, Significantly differences with p<0.05 in two groups control subjects and Asperger disorder shown with dot lines and with p<0.01 shown with solid lines, a) alpha, b) beta and c) gamma frequency band.

In another study, a chaos theory was used to introduce a neural network model for EEG-based assessment of ASD ,and it appraised a precision of 90% (56).

5. Pharmacological therapy of ASDs

Although there is no strong evidence of dopamine involvement in autism, neuroleptics have been used for a long time to decrease aggressive behaviors, stereotypic behaviors, and impulsivity. Low-potency neuroleptics were soon abandoned due to their cognitive and sedative side effects. Among high-potency neuroleptics, haloperidol has been studied the most. Several controlled studies showed benefits over placebo among young children treated with dosages in the range of 1 to 2 mg daily to improve attention and to reduce hyperactivity, anger outbursts, and stereotypes (57, 58). However, problematic side effects in the form of acute dystonic reactions, withdrawal dyskinesias, and tardive dyskinesias were noted. Typical neuroleptics have been replaced with atypical antipsychotics that combine dopamine (D2) and serotonin (5-HT2) receptor antagonist actions (57-60). Following several open-label studies suggesting the efficacy of risperidone, a 12-week, double-blind, placebo-controlled trial was conducted with 31 adults (mean age 28 years) with autism and PDD NOS. Significantly, at a mean dosage of 2.9 mg daily, more responders (57% *vs.* 0%) were found in the risperidone than in the placebo group, and improvements were noted for irritability, anxiety or nervousness, aggression, repetitive behaviors, and depression. There were no improvements on objective measurements of social behavior and language, suggesting that the drug targets nonspecific behavioral problems associated with autism (61, 62). The drug was well tolerated. More recently, a multicentric, 8-week, double- blind, placebo-controlled trial of risperidone (dosage range 0.5 to 3.5 mg daily) was completed on 101 children with autism aged 5 to 17 years (mean age 8.8 years) presenting with clinical levels of tantrums, aggression, and self-injurious behavior. Significant benefits of the active medication were observed for the 2 primary outcome measures of reduced irritability scores (57% *vs.* 14%) and a rating of "much improved" or "very much improved" on a Clinical Global Improvement (CGI) scale (69% *vs.* 12%). Side effects such as fatigue, drowsiness, increased appetite, and drooling were more common in the risperidone group, as was a significantly higher weight gain (2.7 *vs.* 0.8 kgs). Promising open label studies have been conducted with olanzapine, quetiapine, clozapine, and ziprasidone. Several randomized studies are also under way. Atypical neuroleptics, therefore, appear to be promising agents in treating those behavioral symptoms which often occur among autism patients. Yet, despite their good tolerance, these drugs are associated with some undesirable adverse effects, such as tachycardia in young children taking risperidone and sedation for all atypicals, the most serious of which is substantial weight gain. There are no long-term studies of the drugs' efficacy and tolerability (60-64).

Several pharmacological interventions for children with ASDs have been performed in Iran. Akhondzadeh et al. (2010) administered a 10-week double-blind placebo-controlled trial to access the effects of pentoxifylline added to risperidone in comparison with placebo plus risperidone in the treatment of autistic disorder. The dose of risperidone was assayed up to 3 mg/day, and pentoxifylline was assayed 600 mg/day. The Aberrant Behavior Checklist-Community Rating Scale indicated lower scores for Irritability, Lethargy/Social Withdrawal, Stereotyped Behavior, Hyperactivity/Noncompliance and Inappropriate Speech in autistic children who used pentoxifylline plus risperidone as compared to the other group (65). In another study, Akhondzadeh examined the efficacy of piracetam added to risperidone in autistic disorder in a 10-week study. The dose of risperidone was assayed up to 2 mg/day for children between 10 and 40 kg and 3 mg/day for children weighting above 40 kg. The dose of piracetam was assayed up to 800 mg/day. The scores comparison of the Aberrant Behavior Checklist-Community Rating Scale between the autistic children who had received piracetam plus risperidone and the group who had received placebo plus risperidone in the baseline and week 10 revealed that a combination of atypical antipsychotic medications and a glutamate agent such as piracetam may increase synergistic effects in the treatment of autism (66). In addition, combination of topiramate with risperidone demonstrated reduced scores for irritability, stereotypic behavior and hyperactivity/noncompliance in comparison with using placebo plus risperidone in autistic children. In this 8-week, double-blind, placebo-controlled study, the dose of risperidone was assayed up to 2 mg/day for children between 10 and 40 kg and 3 mg/day for children weighting above 40 kg. The dose of topiramate was assayed up to 200 mg/day for children weighting above 40 kg, and 100 mg/day for children weighting less than 30 kg (67). In another double-blind placebo-controlled trial, cyproheptadine as a 5-HT2 antagonist plus haloperidol was evaluated in the treatment of autistic disorder. The results suggested that the combination of cyproheptadine with a conventional antipsychotic may be more effective than conventional antipsychotic alone for autistic children (68). In comparison of celecoxib added to risperidone with risperidone plus placebo, significant differences were observed between the two groups and the results showed reduced scores for Irritability, Lethargy and Stereotyped behavior in autistic children who used celecoxib plus risperidone (69). Ghanizadeh (2011) hypothesized that Glycine site on the N-methyl-D: -aspartic acid (NMDA) glutamate receptor can be tested as a new strategy for the treatment of autism (70). He also introduced neurotensin as a novel approach to treat autism (71).

6. Behavioral and social therapies of ASDs

There are various intervention approaches for training children with ASDs. For instance, Applied Behavioral Analysis (ABA), Eclectic-Developmental (ED), Training and Education of Autistic and other Communication Handicapped Children (TEACCH), Picture Exchange Communication System (PECS), Learning Experiences and Alternative Program for Preschoolers and Their Parents (LEAP), and Early Intensive Behavioral Intervention (EIBI). Several studies indicated that these behavioral and social interventions can improve non-verbal IQ, expressive IQ, receptive language, adaptive behavior, verbal cognitive abilities, socialization, communication adaptive skills, reciprocal social interaction, intellectual and educational gains in children with ASDs (72-80).

Applied Behavioral Analysis is a science that utilizes operant conditioning principles to increase desirable behaviors and decrease problematic behaviors; accordingly, reinforcement and punishment can be used to train individuals with ASDs. In ABA approach, firstly the baseline levels of target behaviors in individuals with ASDs should be operationally defined and measured; assessment instruments such as Vineland Adaptive Behavior Scale, AAIDD Adaptive Behavior Scale- School: Second Edition (ABS-S: 2) and Developmental Behavior Checklist (DBC) can be used to evaluate children abilities in different domains. Then, ABA intervention method is performed to alter target behaviors and finally, the rate of changing behavior can be revealed in the repeated measurement (81-85)

In Iran, home based lovaas approach was performed for treating autism, and the results showed that it was effective to improve social interaction, speech and language, play and behavior skills in autistic children (86). Furthermore, the effect of Applied Behavior Analysis (ABA) intervention method was demonstrated on autistic children who had acquired significant improvements in suitable behaviors (87). In another research, three therapeutic interventions (drug, education and combined therapy) were administered to autistic children. The results showed that while risperidone therapy positively affected stereotyped behavior and hyperactivity, education (according to Lovaas approach) improved social communication and language development of autistic children (88). The effectiveness of parent-child interaction therapy was investigated in four young children with high functioning autism, and the result showed a decrease in their behavioral problems (89). In another study, social stories as a social skills training was evaluated in autistic children, and the results indicated that this intervention was effective to decrease autistic behavior and improve social development in autistic children (90).

7. Mental health of ASDs mothers

Since it seems that parents of children with ASDs experience some stresses such as stigma, blame and insufficient social support in developing countries (91, 92), several studies have been conducted to investigate parental problems, especially in mothers, in Iran. A scientific research indicated a significant difference in parenting stress and coping strategies (emotion focused and problem-focused) variables between mothers with autistic children and mothers who had normal children ; also a significant correlation was observed between stress levels and emotion-focused coping strategies in mothers with autistic children (93). Another study investigated personality characteristics and attachment style in mothers with autistic children in comparison with mothers who had normal children. This study showed a significant difference in Neuroticism versus Emotional stability, not other characteristics. Also no significant difference was observed in the attachment style between the two groups. Based on the results, while mothers with autistic children could be in the Neurotic group, mothers with normal children were almost in the emotionally stable group (94). The correlation between personality characteristics and coping strategies was studied in parents who had children with ASDs; the study indicated no significant difference in coping strategies between fathers and mothers of children with ASDs. However, original thinking, sociability and vigor characteristics were significantly different between them (95). In another study, parental stress was compared in mothers of autistic children with mothers who had normal children, and the results indicated higher scores of parental stress for mothers of autistic children (96). The results of another investigation showed that 27.5% of the mothers with autistic children had mental disorders, and a significant correlation was observed between insufficient coping strategies and mental health (97).

Some interventions were performed to reduce mental problems in mothers with autistic children. A preliminary investigation showed that the symptoms of stress, depression, and anxiety of mothers with autistic children were relatively reduced by guided imagery via music (98). In another study, the group counseling was administered to a group of mothers with autistic children and the results indicated significant differences in the family performance and marital satisfaction scores in mothers who had received group counseling compared to control group (99).

8. Summary

The first preliminary study to investigate the frequency of ASDs in university students was conducted by Nejatisafa (2003); while the scores were significantly higher for men than women, the results showed the frequency of 120 out of 1000 adult participants (35).

In school children, the rate of 19 per 1000 for autistic disorder and 5 per 1000 for Asperger syndrome seem more than the reported ASDs prevalence in developed countries. In this clinical study, no significant correlation was observed between gender and age, diagnosis and severity of the symptoms in ASDs children. The research indicated the brain stem abnormality in severe autistic children which may result in intensifying the autism symptoms. Social interaction and stereotyped behaviors were investigated between autistic and MR children. The results showed higher mean scores of qualitative damage to social interaction and stereotyped behaviors in autistic children compared to MR children. We diagnosed ASDs children using qEEG in comparison with normal children. Considering that the relaxed eye-opened condition in alpha band was the best condition to discriminate between children with ASDs and normal group, the ASDs had significant lower spectrogram criteria values ($p<0.01$) at Fp1, Fp2, F3 and T5 electrodes and lower values ($p<0.05$) at T3, P3 and O1 electrodes. Spectrogram criteria had displayed more abnormalities in the left brain hemisphere and prefrontal lobe in children with ASDs. Magnitude Squared Coherence values at 171 pairs of EEG electrodes in the relaxed eye-opened condition illustrated more abnormalities in the connectivity of temporal lobes with other lobes in gamma frequency band in children with ASDs. It should be noted that one study pointed the gamma frequency band as the best discriminant in children with Asperger compared to the normal group. Asperger children had significant lower spectrogram criteria values ($p<0.01$) at Fp1 electrode, and lower values ($p<0.05$) at Fp2 and T6 electrodes. Coherence values at 171 pairs of EEG electrodes displayed the connectivity at (T4, P4), (T4, Cz), (T4, C4) electrode pairs and (T4, O1) had significant differences ($p<0.01$) in the two groups in the gamma band. The prefrontal and right temporal lobes had more abnormalities based on using spectrogram, and coherence values showed more abnormalities in the connectivity of right temporal lobe with the other lobes in the gamma frequency band in Asperger children.

In pharmacotherapy, typical antipsychotics have been replaced with atypicals that combine dopamine and serotonin receptor antagonist. The effects of pentoxifylline added to risperidone in comparison with placebo plus risperidone in the treatment of autistic disorder. The Aberrant Behavior Checklist Community Rating Scale indicated lower scores for irritability, lethargy, social withdrawal, stereotyped behavior, hyperactivity, noncompliance and inappropriate speech in autistic children who used pentoxifylline plus risperidone. Autistic children who received piracetam plus risperidone might have experienced synergistic effects of medications. Topiramate with risperidone demonstrated reduced scores for irritability, stereotypic behavior, hyperactivity and noncompliance in comparison with using placebo plus risperidone in autistic children. Combination of celecoxib with risperidone in comparison with risperidone plus placebo, caused significant differences between the two groups and the results showed reduced scores for irritability, lethargy and stereotyped behaviors in autistic children.

In Iran, home based lovaas approach was performed for the treatment of ASDs, and the results showed that it was effective in improving the social relationships, speech and language, play and behavior skills in PDD children. The effect of ABA intervention was demonstrated in autistic children who had acquired significant improvements in behaviors. The results of another investigation showed that 27.5% of the mothers with autistic children had mental disorders, and a significant correlation was observed between insufficient coping strategies and mental health.

It seems that Autism Spectrum Disorders are unknown in developing and developed countries and parents who have children with ASDs suffer from lack of social support. Although several studies have been conducted on ASDs in Iran, still they are not sufficient, especially in ASDs epidemiology and etiology. Because of the essential role of cultural factors in better understanding and improvement of ASDs, more comprehensive researches in prevalence, etiology, diagnosis and treatment of ASDs should be performed in many countries including Iran.

9. Acknowledgment

We thank our colleagues of child and adolescent Zafar clinic and the staffs of Roozbeh hospital and the personals of Psychiatry and Psychology Research Centre (PPRC) of Tehran University of Medical sciences for their kind cooperation.

10. References

[1] First MB, Frances A, Pincus HA. DSM-IV-TR: Handbook of differential diagnosis. United States of America: American Psychiatric Publishing; 2002.

[2] Parker S, Zuckerman B, Augustyn M. Developmental and behavioral pediatrics, 2 th ed. United States of America: Lippincott Williams & Wilkins; 2005.

[3] Howlin P. Autism and Asperger syndrome, 2 th ed. United States of America: Routledge; 2005.

[4] Mohammadi MR, Akhondzadeh S. Autism Spectrum Disorders: Etiology and Pharmacotherapy. Curr Drug ther 2007; 2: 97-103.

[5] Newschaffer CJ, Croen LA, Daniels J, Giarelli E, Grether JK, Levy SE, et al. The epidemiology of autism spectrum disorders. Annu Rev Public Health 2007; 28: 235-258.

[6] Gomez SL, Torres RMR, Ares EMT. Reviews on Autism. Rev Latinoam Psicol 2009; 41: 555-570.

[7] Grafodatskaya D, Chung B, Szatmari P, Weksberg R. Autism spectrum disorders and epigenetics. J Am Acad Child Adolesc Psychiatry 2010; 49: 794-809.

[8] Bowler DM. Autism spectrum disorders: psychological theory and research. England: John Wiley and Sons; 2007.

[9] Lord C, Rutter M, Le Couteur A. Autism Diagnostic Interview-Revised: a revised version of a diagnostic interview for caregivers of individuals with possible pervasive developmental disorders. J Autism Dev Disord 1994; 24: 659-685.

[10] Wing L, Leekam SR, Libby SJ, Gould J, Larcombe M. The Diagnostic Interview for Social and Communication Disorders: background, inter-rater reliability and clinical use. J Child Psychol Psychiatry 2002; 43: 307-325.

[11] Chlebowski C, Green JA, Barton ML, Fein D. Using the childhood autism rating scale to diagnose autism spectrum disorders. J Autism Dev Disord 2010; 40: 787-799.

[12] Skuse D, Warrington R, Bishop D, Chowdhury U, Lau J, Mandy W, et al. The developmental, dimensional and diagnostic interview (3di): a novel computerized assessment for autism spectrum disorders. J Am Acad Child Adolesc Psychiatry 2004; 43: 548-558.

[13] Matson JL, Wilkins J, Gonzalez ML, Rivet TT. Reliability of the Autism Spectrum Disorder-Diagnostic For Children (ASD-DC). Res Autism Spectr Disord 2008; 2: 533-545.
[14] Matson JL, Gonzalez ML, Rivet TT. Reliability of the Autism Spectrum Disorder-Behavior Problems for Children (ASD-BPC). Res Autism Spectr Disord 2008; 2: 696-706.
[15] Matson JL, LoVullo SV, Rivet TT, Boisjoli JA. Validity of the Autism Spectrum Disorder-Comorbid for Children (ASD-CC). Res Autism Spectr Disord 2009; 3: 345-357.
[16] Matson JL, Worley JA, Fodstad JC, Chung KM, Suh D, Jhin HK, et al. A multinational study examining the cross cultural differences in reported symptoms of autism spectrum disorders: Israel, South Korea, the United Kingdom, and the United States of America. Res Autism Spectr Disord 2011; 5: 1598-1604.
[17] Matson JL. Clinical Assessment and Intervention for Autism Spectrum Disorders. USA: Academic Press; 2008.
[18] Pfeiffer BA, Koenig K, Kinnealey M, Sheppard M, Henderson L. Effectiveness of sensory integration interventions in children with autism spectrum disorders: a pilot study. Am J Occup Ther 2011; 65: 76-85.
[19] McPheeters ML, Warren Z, Sathe N, Bruzek JL, Krishnaswami S, Jerome RN, et al. A systematic review of medical treatments for children with autism spectrum disorders. Pediatrics 2011; 127: e1312-1321.
[20] Coben R, Linden M, Myers TE. Neurofeedback for autistic spectrum disorder: a review of the literature. Appl Psychophysiol Biofeedback 2010; 35: 83-105.
[21] Corbett BA, Gunther JR, Comins D, Price J, Ryan N, Simon D, et al. Brief report: theatre as therapy for children with autism spectrum disorder. J Autism Dev Disord 2011; 41: 505-511.
[22] Bernier R, Mao A, Yen J. Psychopathology, families, and culture: autism. Child Adolesc Psychiatr Clin N Am 2010; 19: 855-867.
[23] Zachor D, Yang JW, Itzchak EB, Furniss F, Pegg E, Matson JL, et al. Cross-cultural differences in comorbid symptoms of children with autism spectrum disorders: An international examination between Israel, South Korea, the United Kingdom and the United States of America. Dev Neurorehabil 2011; 14: 215-220.
[24] Lee HJ. Cultural Factors Related to the Hidden Curriculum for Students With Autism and Related Disabilities. Intervention in school and clinic 2011; 46: 141-149.
[25] Zaroff CM, Uhm SY. Prevalence of autism spectrum disorders and influence of country of measurement and ethnicity. Soc Psychiatry Psychiatr Epidemiol 2011; published online.
[26] Baron-Cohen S, Scott FJ, Allison C, Williams J, Bolton P, Matthews FE, et al. Prevalence of autism-spectrum conditions: UK school-based population study. Br J Psychiatry 2009; 194: 500-509.
[27] Brugha TS, McManus S, Bankart J, Scott F, Purdon S, Smith J, et al. Epidemiology of autism spectrum disorders in adults in the community in England. Arch Gen Psychiatry 2011; 68: 459-465.
[28] Prevalence of autism spectrum disorders - Autism and Developmental Disabilities Monitoring Network, United States, 2006. MMWR Surveill Summ 2009; 58: 1-20.

[29] Fombonne E. Epidemiology of pervasive developmental disorders. Pediatr Res 2009; 65: 591-598.

[30] Ehlers S, Gillberg C. The epidemiology of Asperger syndrome. A total population study. J Child Psychol Psychiatry 1993; 34: 1327-1350.

[31] Kadesjo B, Gillberg C, Hagberg B. Brief report: autism and Asperger syndrome in seven-year-old children: a total population study. J Autism Dev Disord 1999; 29: 327-331.

[32] Williams JG, Higgins JP, Brayne CE. Systematic review of prevalence studies of autism spectrum disorders. Arch Dis Child 2006; 91: 8-15.

[33] Shamsi-pour M, Yonesian M, Mansouri A. Epidemiology of autism: recent challenges in prevalence of autism and its risk factors. Journal of health and knowledge 2010; 5: 133.

[34] Ghanizadeh A. A preliminary study on screening prevalence of pervasive developmental disorder in schoolchildren in Iran. J Autism Dev Disord 2008; 38: 759-763.

[35] Nejatisafa AA, Kazemi MR, Alaghebandrad J. Autistic features in adult population: evidence for continuity of autistic symptoms with normality. Advanced in cognitive science 2003; 5: 34-39.

[36] Khoushabi K, Pouretemad HR. Prevalence of pervasive developmental disorders according to gender in a sample of Iranian children referred to treatment and rehabilitation centers. Journal of Hamedan University of Medical Sciences 2006; 13: 58-60.

[37] Jannati M. Epidemiology of autism in exceptional students in Mashhd. MA thesis in psychology of exceptional children field. Islamic Azad University of Birjand; 2001.

[38] Nickl-Jockschat T, Michel TM. [Genetic and brain structure anomalies in autism spectrum disorders. Towards an understanding of the aetiopathogenesis?]. Nervenarzt 2011; 82: 618-627.

[39] Dodds L, Fell DB, Shea S, Armson BA, Allen AC, Bryson S. The role of prenatal, obstetric and neonatal factors in the development of autism. J Autism Dev Disord 2011; 41: 891-902.

[40] Voineagu I, Wang X, Johnston P, Lowe JK, Tian Y, Horvath S, et al. Transcriptomic analysis of autistic brain reveals convergent molecular pathology. Nature 2011; 474: 380-384.

[41] Griswold AJ, Ma D, Sacharow SJ, Robinson JL, Jaworski JM, Wright HH, et al. A de novo 1.5 Mb microdeletion on chromosome 14q23.2-23.3 in a patient with autism and spherocytosis. Autism Res 2011; 4: 221-227.

[42] Hughes JR. Update on autism: a review of 1300 reports published in 2008. Epilepsy Behav 2009; 16: 569-589.

[43] O'Roak BJ, State MW. Autism genetics: strategies, challenges, and opportunities. Autism Res 2008; 1: 4-17.

[44] Muhle R, Trentacoste SV, Rapin I. The genetics of autism. Pediatrics 2004; 113: e472-486.

[45] Mansouri M, Chalabianlou GR, Malekirad AA, Mosaded AA. The comparison of factors affecting the theory of mind development in autistic and normal children. Arak Medical University Journal 2011; 13: 115-125.

[46] Salmanian M. Visual memory of shapes and face in children with ASDs as compared to normal children. MS thesis in cognitive psychology. Institute for cognitive science studies; 2010.

[47] Ghanizadeh A, Mohammadi MR, Sadeghiyeh T, Alavi Shooshtari A, Akhondzadeh S. Symptoms of Children with Autism Spectrum Disorder, a Clinical Sample. Iran J Psychiatry 2009; 4: 165-169.

[48] Sasanfar R, Haddad SA, Tolouei A, Ghadami M, Yu D, Santangelo SL. Parental age increases the risk for autism in an Iranian population sample. Mol Autism 2010; 1:2.

[49] Abolfazli R, Mirbagheri SA, Zabihi AA, Abouzari M. Autism and Celiac Disease: Failure to Validate the Hypothesis of a Possible Link. Iranian Red Crescent Medical Journal 2009; 11: 442-444.

[50] Hamidi Nahrani M, Sedaei M, Fatahi J, Sarough Farahani S, Faghihzadeh S. Auditory brainstem responses in autistic children in comparison with normal children. Audiology 2008; 16: 16-22.

[51] Bahari Gharagoz A, Hassanpour A, Amiri SH. Social interactions and repetitive behavior of autistic and trainable mentally retarded children. Developmental Psychology 2010; 7: 39-47.

[52] Sheikhani A, Behnam H, Mohammadi MR, Noroozian M. Evaluation of Quantitative Electroencephalography in Children with Autistic Disorders in Various Conditions Based on Spectrogram. Iran J Psychiatry 2007; 3: 4-10

[53] Niedermeyer E, Lopes da Silva F. Electroencephalography: Basic principles, clinical applications, and related fields, 5th ed. Philadelphia: Lippincott Williams & Wilkins; 2005.

[54] Sheikhani A, Behnam H, Mohammadi MR, Noroozian M, Mohammadi M. Detection of Abnormalities for Diagnosing of Children with Autism Disorders Using of Quantitative Electroencephalography Analysis. J Med Syst 2010.

[55] Noroozian M, Sheikhani A, Behnam H, Mohammadi MR. Abnormalities of Quantitative Electroencephalography in Children with Asperger Disorder Using Spectrogram and Coherence Values. Iran J Psychiatry 2008; 3: 64-70

[56] Ahmadlou M, Adeli H, Adeli A. Fractality and a wavelet-chaos-neural network methodology for EEG-based diagnosis of autistic spectrum disorder. J Clin Neurophysiol 2010; 27: 328-333.

[57] Campbell M, Adams P, Perry R, Spencer EK, Overall JE. Tardive and withdrawal dyskinesia in autistic children: a prospective study. Psychopharmacol Bull 1988; 24: 251-255.

[58] Anderson LT, Campbell M, Adams P, Small AM, Perry R, Shell J. The effects of haloperidol on discrimination learning and behavioral symptoms in autistic children. J Autism Dev Disord 1989; 19: 227-239.

[59] Shattock P, Kennedy A, Rowell F, et al. Role of neuropeptides in autism and their relationships with classical neurotransmitters. Brain Dysfunct 1990; 3: 328 -345.

[60] Campbell M, Schopler E, Cueva, J, Hallin A. Treatment of autistic disorder. J Am Acad Child Adolesc Psychiatry 1996; 35: 134-143.

[61] Tsia LY. Psychopharmacology in autism. Psychosom Med 1999; 61: 651-665.

[62] McCracken JT, McGough J, Shah B, et al. Risperidone in children with autism and serious behavioral problems. N Engl J Med 2002; 347: 314 -321.

[63] Posey DJ, McDougle CJ. The pharmacotherapy of target symptoms associated with autistic disorder and other pervasive development disorders. Harv Rev Psychiatry 2000; 4: 45-63.

[64] Levy SE, Hyman SL. Novel treatments for autistic spectrum disorders. Ment Retard Dev Disabil Res Rev 2005; 11: 131-142

[65] Akhondzadeh S, Fallah J, Mohammadi MR, Imani R, Mohammadi M, Salehi B, et al. Double-blind placebo-controlled trial of pentoxifylline added to risperidone: effects on aberrant behavior in children with autism. Prog Neuropsychopharmacol Biol Psychiatry 2010; 34: 32-36.

[66] Akhondzadeh S, Tajdar H, Mohammadi MR, Mohammadi M, Nouroozinejad GH, Shabstari OL, et al. A double-blind placebo controlled trial of piracetam added to risperidone in patients with autistic disorder. Child Psychiatry Hum Dev 2008; 39: 237-245.

[67] Rezaei V, Mohammadi MR, Ghanizadeh A, Sahraian A, Tabrizi M, Rezazadeh SA, et al. Double-blind, placebo-controlled trial of risperidone plus topiramate in children with autistic disorder. Prog Neuropsychopharmacol Biol Psychiatry 2010; 34: 1269-1272.

[68] Akhondzadeh S, Erfani S, Mohammadi MR, Tehrani-Doost M, Amini H, Gudarzi SS, et al. Cyproheptadine in the treatment of autistic disorder: a double-blind placebo-controlled trial. J Clin Pharm Ther 2004; 29: 145-150.

[69] Mohammadi MR, Akhondzadeh S. A double-blind placebo controlled trial of celecoxib added to risperidone in children with autistic disorder. Under publishing.

[70] Ghanizadeh A. Targeting of glycine site on NMDA receptor as a possible new strategy for autism treatment. Neurochem Res 2011; 36: 922-923.

[71] Ghanizadeh A. Targeting neurotensin as a potential novel approach for the treatment of autism. J Neuroinflammation 2010; 7: 58.

[72] Zachor DA, Ben-Itzchak E, Rabinovich AL, Lahat E. Change in autism core symptoms with intervention. Res Autism Spectr Disord 2007; 1: 304-317.

[73] Reed P, Osborne LA, Corness M. The real-world effectiveness of early teaching interventions for children with autism spectrum disorder. Except Child 2007; 73: 417-433.

[74] Callahan K, Shukla-Mehta S, Magee S, Wie M. ABA versus TEACCH: the case for defining and validating comprehensive treatment models in autism. J Autism Dev Disord 2010; 40: 74-88.

[75] Granpeesheh D, Tarbox J, Dixon DR. Applied behavior analytic interventions for children with autism: a description and review of treatment research. Ann Clin Psychiatry 2009; 21: 162-173.

[76] Bolte S. [Psychobiosocial interventions for autism]. Nervenarzt 2011; 82: 590-596.

[77] Gould E, Dixon DR, Najdowski AC, Smith MN, Tarbox J. A review of assessments for determining the content of early intensive behavioral intervention programs for autism spectrum disorders. Res Autism Spectr Disord 2011; 5: 990-1002.

[78] Peters-Scheffer N, Didden R, Korzilius H, Sturmey P. A meta-analytic study on the effectiveness of comprehensive ABA-based early intervention programs for children with Autism Spectrum Disorders. Res Autism Spectr Disord 2011; 5: 60-69.

[79] Zachor DA, Ben Itzchak E. Treatment approach, autism severity and intervention outcomes in young children. Res Autism Spectr Disord 2010; 4: 425-432.

[80] Hume K, Boyd B, McBee M, Coman D, Gutierrez A, Shaw E, et al. Assessing implementation of comprehensive treatment models for young children with ASD: Reliability and validity of two measures. Res Autism Spectr Disord 2011; 5: 1430-1440.
[81] Matson JL. Applied Behavior Analysis for Children with Autism Spectrum Disorders. USA: Springer; 2009.
[82] Fisher WW, Piazza CC, Roane HS. Handbook of Applied Behavior Analysis. USA: The Guilford Press; 2011.
[83] Carter AS, Volkmar FR, Sparrow SS, Wang JJ, Lord C, Dawson G, et al. The Vineland Adaptive Behavior Scales: supplementary norms for individuals with autism. J Autism Dev Disord 1998; 28: 287-302.
[84] Perry A, Flanagan HE, Dunn Geier J, Freeman NL. Brief report: the Vineland Adaptive Behavior Scales in young children with autism spectrum disorders at different cognitive levels. J Autism Dev Disord 2009; 39: 1066-1078.
[85] Brereton AV, Tonge BJ, Mackinnon AJ, Einfeld SL. Screening young people for autism with the developmental behavior checklist. J Am Acad Child Adolesc Psychiatry 2002; 41: 1369-1375.
[86] Dalvand H, Dehghan L, Feizy A, Hosseini SA. The effect of home based Lovaas approach on social interaction, Speech and language, Play and behavior skills, and intensity of autism in young children with Autism. Modern Rehabilitation 2009; 3: 3.
[87] Golabi P, Alipour A, Zandi B. the effect of intervention by ABA method on children with autism. Research on exceptional children 2005; 5: 33-54.
[88] Arman S, Hakiman S, Golabi P. Three therapeutic methods for autistic children: a clinical trial. Journal of Isfahan Medical School 2005; 23: 44-48.
[89] Hatamzadeh A, Pouretemad H, Hassanabadi H. The effectiveness of parent-child interaction therapy for children with high functioning autism. World Conference on Psychology, Counselling and Guidance 2010; 5: 994-997.
[90] Bahmanzadegan Jahromi M, Yarmohammadian A, Mousavi H. Efficacy of social skills training in autistic behaviors and social development in children with autism disorder through social stories. New findings in psychology 2009; 3: 79-93.
[91] Chimeh N, Pouretemad HR, Khoramabadi R. Need assessment of mothers with autistic children. Journal of family research 2007; 3: 697-707.
[92] Ghanizadeh A, Alishahi MJ, Ashkani H. Helping families for caring children with autistic spectrum disorders. Arch Iran Med 2009; 12: 478-482.
[93] Khoushabi K, Farzad Fard SZ, Kakasoltani B, Pouretemad HR, Nikkhah HR. Coping strategies and stress in mothers with autistic children in comparison with mothers with normal children. Journal of family research 2010; 6: 87-97.
[94] Ghobari Bonab B, Estiri Z. A comparative study on personality characteristics and attachment style in mothers of children with and without autism. Research on exceptional children 2006; 6: 787-804.
[95] Rajabi Damavandi G, Poushineh K, Ghobari Bonab B. the relationship between personality characteristics and coping strategies in parents of children with ASDs. Research on exceptional children 2009; 9: 133-144.

[96] Khoramabadi R, Pouretemad HR, Tahmasian K, Chimeh N. A comparative study of parental stress in mothers of autistic and non autistic children. Journal of family research 2009; 5: 387-399.
[97] Poretemad HR, Khoushabi K, Afshari R, Moradi S. Coping strategies and mental health in autistic children mothers. Journal of family research 2006; 2: 285-292.
[98] Mohammadi A, Pouretemad HR, Khosravi G. An initial examination of the effect of guided imagery via music on reduction of stress, depression, and anxiety of mothers with autistic children. Journal of family research 2005; 1: 289-303.
[99] Arman S, Zareei N, Farshidnejad AA. Efficacy of group counseling on mothers with autistic children. Research in Behavioral Sciences 2004; 2: 48-52.

10

Autism Spectrum Disorders in Africa

Muideen O. Bakare[1] and Kerim M. Munir[2,3]
[1]*Child and Adolescent Unit, Federal Neuropsychiatric Hospital, Enugu*
[2]*Division of Developmental Medicine, Department of Medicine, Boston Children's Hospital,*
[3]*Department of Psychiatry, Harvard Medical School*
[1]*Nigeria*
[2,3]*USA*

1. Introduction

"………. Perhaps, in the future, there will be some African history to teach. But at present there is none, or very little: there is only the history of the Europeans in Africa. The rest is largely darkness………… And darkness is not a subject for history" – Hugh Redwald Trevor-Roper.

This chapter is necessitated so that similar comments to Trevor-Roper's on African history would be avoided as it relates to autism spectrum disorders in Africa, even though there are limited research works relating to autism spectrum disorders in Africa at present.

Since Leo Kanner first reported autism in his classical paper titled, "Autistic disturbances of affective contact" in 1943 (Kanner, 1943), knowledge and research about autism spectrum disorder have been on the increase in Europe and North America. However, the situation in Africa had remained largely obscured until about the last decade.

The pioneer works on autism spectrum disorders in Africa had been by Longe and Asuni (Longe & Asuni, 1972) and Lotter (Lotter, 1978; Lotter, 1980) about three decades after the first report of autism spectrum disorder by Kanner in 1943 (Kanner, 1943). Lotter discussed cross-cultural perspectives on childhood autism. Africa, because of its peculiar socio-cultural environment may have divergent conception on various aspects of autism spectrum disorder compared to that envisaged in the Western culture (Bakare et al, 2009a). In the same vein, cultural factors have recently been documented to influence characterization, diagnosis and treatment of autism spectrum disorder worldwide (Bernier et al, 2010).

It may be important to recall therefore that until about two and half decades ago, autism spectrum disorder was thought to be exclusively an illness peculiar to Western civilization. The existing evidence then suggested that autism occurs mostly in countries with high technological development, high level of industrialization and with salience of nuclear family system. However autism spectrum disorder was also believed to be relatively uncommon even in Western Europe and North America at that time. Nevertheless, the idea that autism may not exist in Africa was further supported by very infrequent report of cases on the continent and other parts of the world outside the West. These observations led Sanua to raise a debate and a pertinent question in 1984 in a paper entitled, "Is infantile autism a universal phenomenon? An open question" (Sanua, 1984).

While Sanua's question (Sanua, 1984) is yet to be satisfactorily answered because of lack of large scale epidemiological study of autism spectrum disorders in sub-Saharan Africa, evidence accruing through case reports before and after Sanua's question suggest that autism spectrum disorders indeed also occur in the African continent (Longe & Asuni, 1972; Lotter, 1978; Dhadphale et al, 1982; Bakare & Ikegwuonu, 2008). However, many aspects of autism spectrum disorders in Africa remain obscured. Some aspects of autism spectrum disorders in Africa over the period of year 2000 to 2009 were recently documented in a review by Bakare and Munir (2011).

2. Epidemiology of autism spectrum disorders in Africa and among Africans

Available literature revealed that the prevalence of autism spectrum disorders among Africans living in Africa differs from that among Africans living outside the continent and will be reviewed separately.

2.1 Epidemiology of autism spectrum disorders among Africans living in african continent

In an attempt to answer the question as to whether autism spectrum disorders occurred in Africa prior to Sanua's important inquiry of 1984, Lotter (1978) screened children with intellectual disabilities in nine major cities of six African countries, which included Ghana, Nigeria, Kenya, Zimbabwe, Zambia and South Africa. Lotter found 9 out of the 1,312 children with intellectual disabilities studied in these countries to meet the eligibility criteria to be classified as having autism, a rate which was 1 in 145 (Lotter, 1978). Because the screening was among children with intellectual disabilities , Lotter (1978) had expected to find a rate of about 1 in 20 based on the then epidemiological data in the West (Lotter, 1966). In addition to the finding on prevalence of autism spectrum disorders in the 1978 study on African continent, which Lotter admitted fell short of epidemiological survey, a number of other observations were made as follows: First, the combination of behaviors constituting criteria for autism occur in African children (Lotter, 1980). Second, there was a preponderance of boys among children who exhibited such behavior combination and such presentation tended to be more common among African children with moderate to severe intellectual disabilities (Lotter, 1980). Third, there was overrepresentation of children of parents of high socio-economic class among the children described as having features of autism (Lotter, 1980). Fourth, there were certain differences in frequency of specific behaviors between African children and children from Western Europe and North America, notable of which is stereotypic repertoire of behavior which was observed to be less common among African children compared to their counterparts in the West (Lotter, 1980). This is important because the stereotypic repertoire of behavior is an aspect of the main criteria for diagnosing autism spectrum disorders (Lotter, 1980).

A literature review to date shows no school or community based epidemiological studies of autism spectrum disorders in the African continent. The only available study that is closely related was focused on prevalence of autism spectrum disorder among children with developmental disorders in the Arab countries (Seif Eldin et al, 2008). This study (Seif Eldin et al, 2008), however included two Northern African countries, namely, Egypt and Tunisia, with predominantly Arabic populations. Prevalence of autism spectrum disorders among children with developmental disorders in Egypt and Tunisia were documented to be 33.6%

and 11.5% respectively (Seif Eldin et al, 2008). The prevalence figures are quite higher if compared against the earlier finding by Lotter who documented a prevalence of 9 in 1,312 (approximately 0.7%) among intellectually disabled children (Lotter, 1978).

In a clinic based population study in south-eastern Nigeria, prevalence of autism spectrum disorders had been noted to be 0.8% of the total population of children that attended the clinic over a one year period (Bakare et al, 2011a).

There is a need for both community and school-based studies on epidemiology of autism spectrum disorders in Africa. This is not only to know the present true prevalence in Africa to afford comparability with European and North American data, but to answer so many other questions on characteristics of African children with autism spectrum disorders as raised by Lotter in his paper on cross cultural perspectives on childhood autism (Lotter, 1980). Lotter (1980) observed, "These preliminary findings need to be corroborated and extended, in conjunction with better descriptions of normal early childhood development. Most of the children we saw in Africa were already over six years old, and little good information about early development could be obtained. We do not know therefore whether the age and pattern of onset of autism in Africa is similar to Western cases. .....Special difficulties arise also because the onset of autism coincides with a period of vulnerability to physical disease in the second year of life." Lotter (1980) further observed, "The African autistic children were all mentally retarded, with at best, very little speech. We do not know therefore whether the peculiar autistic patterns of speech use occur in Africa, or generally whether, and how, autism develops in African children of normal intelligence. All the children we saw were living in cities, most having been raised there. We know nothing therefore of the occurrence of autism in rural villages, in which most of the African populations still live." From Lotter's (1980) observations, there are therefore so many questions still awaiting answers on characteristics of African children with autism spectrum disorders.

2.2 Epidemiology of autism spectrum disorders among Africans outside african continent

Prevalence of autism spectrum disorders among Africans living in Europe had also been examined by three studies (Gillberg et al, 1995; Gillberg & Gillberg, 1996; Barnevick-Olsson et al, 2008). Gillberg et al (1995) observed a higher prevalence of autism spectrum disorders among children in Goteborg, Sweden born to mothers from Uganda compared to children of the indigenous Swedish mothers in the general population. They (Gillberg et al, 1995) documented a prevalence of 15% autism spectrum disorders among children of mothers from Uganda, which was noted to be two hundred times higher than in the general population of children in Goteborg, Sweden. This trend of higher prevalence of autism spectrum disorders among children of African immigrants in Europe was further confirmed by Gillberg and Gillberg (1996).

Like Gillberg et al (1995) and Gillberg & Gillberg (1996) studies, Barnevick-Olson et al (2008) study was conducted outside African continent and also in Sweden. Barnevick-Olsson et al (2008) documented significantly higher prevalence of autism spectrum disorders among children of Somali parents living in Sweden compared to non-Somali group. Children of Somali parents living in Sweden were found to have a prevalence of 0.7% autism spectrum disorders compared with approximately 0.2% in non-Somali group. Barnevick-Olsson et al (2008) concluded that their findings warrant further investigation into why children of

Somali parents living in Sweden tend to have higher prevalence of autism spectrum disorders, suggesting possible vitamin D etiological hypothesis among other factors might be responsible for this findings (Bakare et al, 2011b).
While Zaroff and Uhm (2011) recent review supported the evidence that there is variation in prevalence of autism spectrum disorders across cultures and regions, a standard community based epidemiological data for African sub-region is presently lacking.

3. Diagnosis of autism spectrum disorders in Africa

Diagnosis of autism spectrum disorders in Africa follows the criteria for diagnosing autism spectrum disorders specified in International Classification of Diseases, tenth edition (ICD - 10) (WHO, 1992) and Diagnostic and Statistical Manual of Mental Disorders, fourth edition, Text Revision (DSM - IV-TR) (APA, 2000). These criteria are based on impairments in areas of social interaction, communication and restricted repetitive and stereotyped patterns of behavior, interests and activities.
However, variations do exist as shown by literature originating from Africa on symptoms presentation and co-morbid conditions.

3.1 Symptoms presentation

Aside from the core symptoms of autism spectrum disorders in the areas of impairments in social interaction, communication and restricted, repetitive repertoire of behavior, one common presentation of symptoms found in over fifty percent of the cases reported in literature coming from Africa is lack of expressive language, i.e., predominantly non-verbal cases (Belhadj et al, 2006; Mankoski et al, 2006).
Belhadj et al (2006) reported 51.2% of non-verbal cases of autism spectrum disorders in their clinic. Mankoski et al (2006) observed 71.0% of non-verbal cases of autism spectrum disorder in the cohort of patients in their study. The trend of excess non-verbal cases of autism in African children as observed by Belhadj et al (2006) and Mankoski et al (2006) concurred with the trend of observation documented by Lotter (Lotter, 1980) . However, Mankoski et al, (2006) concluded that this observation might be as a result of local diagnostic practice. The inference of these findings is that based on population of children with autism spectrum disorders presenting to orthodox medical care and current diagnostic practice in Africa, the population of non-verbal cases diagnosed with autism spectrum disorders out-stripped those who are verbal.
The true picture of autism spectrum disorders in the general population of African children needs to be ascertained; whether there is an actual overrepresentation of non-verbal cases or that the population of children who were referred to orthodox medical care was likely to be skewed towards being non-verbal cases. Again, future epidemiological studies of characteristics of children with autism spectrum disorders in Africa might be the sources of answer to this unresolved question.

3.2 Co-morbid conditions associated with autism spectrum disorders in Africa

Of the co-morbid conditions diagnosed in association with autism spectrum disorders among African children and documented in the literature coming from Africa, intellectual disabilities are more common.

Belhadj et al (2006) found co-morbid intellectual disability in over 60% of cases in their clinic. Other noted co-morbid conditions in association with autism spectrum disorders among African children included epilepsy (Belhadj et al, 2006) and oculocutaneous albinism (Bakare & Ikegwuonu, 2008). Co-morbidity of epilepsy and intellectual disability in association with autism spectrum disorders found by the study from Tunisia is an interesting finding (Belhadj et al, 2006) as it corroborated the observation of Mankoski et al (2006) from Tanzania, that autism spectrum disorder in Africa is rarely diagnosed exclusively of intellectual disability. This observation is also in tandem with that of Lotter documented about three decades earlier (Lotter, 1980). Therefore, the relationship between autism spectrum disorder and intellectual disability among African children need to be further explored in well designed clinical and epidemiological studies.

The possibility also exist that more severe non-verbal cases of autism spectrum disorders with intellectual disability are likely to present to orthodox medical practice for help, largely because the symptoms may become intolerable to the parents. Many of the cases that are often less severe are likely to seek help from prayer houses, spiritualists and traditional healers (Bakare, 2006). This, possibly stemming from lay etiological explanation of autism spectrum disorders among Africans and African health care workers as documented by Bakare et al (2009a) in a study done in Nigeria.

Oculocutaneous albinism, though infrequently reported in association with autism spectrum disorder, had been observed to occur co-morbidly with autism spectrum disorder in Africa (Bakare & Ikegwuonu, 2008). The co-morbidity of autism spectrum disorders and oculocutaneous albinism had also been reported in some cases outside the African continent (Rogawski et al, 1978; DeLong, 2007). Bakare and Ikegwuonu (2008) suggested that further embryo-genetic studies into relationship between autism spectrum disorder and associated hypomelanotic skin disorders, including oculocutaneous albinism may provide useful clues to understanding etiology of autism spectrum disorders.

4. Etiology of autism spectrum disorders in Africa

Many etiological explanations have been proposed for autism spectrum disorders based on a number of studies coming from African continent. Discussion on these etiological explanations would be based on two major categories: etiological explanation based on opinions and etiological explanations based on scientific and clinical evidences.

4.1 Etiological explanation based on opinions

One study in Nigeria assessed the opinion of health care workers, specifically nurses, on their perceived etiology of autism spectrum disorders (Bakare et al, 2009a). A very significant proportion of 26.9% of the health care workers are of the opinion that etiology of autism spectrum disorders can be traced to supernatural causes. About fifty eight percent of these health care workers subscribed to natural causes as explanation for etiology of autism spectrum disorders, while 14.2% subscribed to preternatural causes, with rational explanations as yet unknown (Bakare et al, 2009a). The preternatural and supernatural etiological explanation for autism spectrum disorders as found in this study (Bakare et al, 2009a) is further substantiating the inseparable spiritual beliefs of Africans as it relates to etiological explanations for neuro-psychiatric disorders.

4.2 Etiological explanation based on scientific and clinical evidences

Several etiological hypotheses had been put forward for autism spectrum disorders and to date no definitive one is proven. Among the etiological hypotheses proposed by literature coming from Africa are post-encephalitic infections or sepsis preceding the onset of autism spectrum disorder symptoms, genetic factors, auto-immune factors, and vitamin D etiological hypothesis.

4.2.1 Post-encephalitic infections or sepsis preceding the onset of autism spectrum disorders

Mankoski et al (2006) in a case series documented cases of autism spectrum disorders following post-encephalitic infection/sepsis in a population of children from Tanzania. Because physical illnesses such as cerebral malaria and infectious diseases are common occurrence in African children under the age of five years, population of African children with symptoms of autism spectrum disorder setting-in following post-encephalitic infections may be substantially higher compared to that in high income developed countries where infectious diseases in children are not of public health significance. This brings to fore the observation of Lotter about three decades ago, that the age of onset of autism spectrum disorder may coincide with period of vulnerability to infectious diseases and other physical illnesses which may have greater likelihood for risk of infection and therefore neurological consequences among African children (Lotter, 1980). The specific roles played by post-encephalitic infection/sepsis on onset of autism spectrum disorders symptoms among African children need to be further examined.

4.2.2 Genetic factors

Genetic factors had been known worldwide to play a significant role in occurrence of autism spectrum disorders (Smalley, 1991; Muhle et al, 2004). Although the heritability of autism has been estimated to be as high as 90%, the genetic factors are heterogeneous, complex, and for the most part poorly understood. Epigenetic and environmental factors are also etiologically significant in autism (Muhle et al, 2004). The precise mechanisms of genetic inheritance of autism are presently being explored through methods of genome-wide screening, cytogenetic studies, and evaluation of candidate genes (Muhle et al, 2004). Evidence is accruing of similar genetic influences among African children as well (Arieff, 2010; Mostafa & Shehab, 2010). Although strong genetic association in etiology of autism spectrum disorders had been established, the specific model of inheritance is still unclear.

4.2.3 Auto-immune factors

Auto-immune factors have also been hypothesized as possible etiological explanations for autism spectrum disorders. The proposition of auto-immune factors as etiological explanation for autism spectrum disorders in Africa had largely been derived from studies coming from Egypt (Mostafa et al, 2008; Mostafa & Kitchener, 2009; Mostafa et al, 2010).

4.2.4 Vitamin D etiological hypothesis

Several studies had linked Vitamin D with autism and hypothesized that etiology of autism might be as a result of maternal and /or fetal Vitamin D deficiency (Grant & Soles, 2009;

Meguid et al, 2010). Most of these studies suggest that evidence for this hypothesis could be found in higher prevalence of autism spectrum disorders in higher latitudes, urban areas, and regions with intense air pollution and high precipitation where Vitamin D deficiency is likely to be common because of the reduced ultraviolet-B radiation essential for endogenous Vitamin D production (Grant & Soles, 2009, Bakare et al, 2011 b). Further observation that supports this etiological hypothesis of Vitamin D deficiency for autism spectrum disorder included the findings that autism may be more common in dark-skinned individuals living at higher latitudes compared to the light-skinned indigenous inhabitants (Gillberg et al, 1995; Barnevik-Olsson et al, 2008). The deduction is that at higher latitudes, dark-skinned individuals are less likely to maximize utilization of ultraviolet-B radiation in production of Vitamin D because of their skin color and therefore greater predisposition to risk of Vitamin D deficiency (Gillberg et al, 1995; Barnevik-Olsson et al, 2008). A number of these studies addressed Vitamin D etiological explanation for autism spectrum disorders in relation to Africans and African continent (Gillberg et al, 1995; Barnevik-Olsson et al, 2008; Meguid et al, 2010; Fernell et al, 2010).

5. Knowledge and awareness about autism spectrum disorders in Africa

The findings of many studies in Nigeria show a low level of knowledge and awareness about autism spectrum disorders in Africa, thereby compromising early recognition of the disorder and intervention to alleviate symptom severity (ANPPCAN, 2007; Bakare et al, 2008; Bakare et al, 2009b; Igwe et al, 2010; Igwe et al, 2011). African Network for the Prevention and Protection against Child Abuse and Neglect (ANPPCAN), Nigeria chapter, in a World Bank sponsored program carried out a survey to determine the level of knowledge and awareness of health care workers and the general public in Enugu, south-eastern Nigeria about autism spectrum disorders (ANPPCAN, 2007). The findings of the survey showed that there is very low level of knowledge and awareness about autism spectrum disorders among the general populace and a low to average level of knowledge and awareness among various categories of health care workers, with highest level of knowledge and awareness found among those health care workers working in psychiatric facilities (ANPPCAN, 2007). Using the template of findings and observations made during the ANPPCAN's study, a standard questionnaire for assessing knowledge of health care workers about autism spectrum disorders, aimed at early recognition was designed and validated (Bakare et al, 2008). Subsequent study done following ANPPCAN survey consistently was showing the same trend of low level of knowledge and awareness about autism spectrum disorders among the healthcare workers (Bakare et al, 2009b). It was further established that the ability of healthcare workers working in psychiatric facilities to recognize symptoms of autism spectrum disorder was better than their counterparts working in pediatric units/departments (Bakare et al, 2009b). Igwe et al (2010) examined level of knowledge about autism spectrum disorders among potential health care workers presently undergoing their training; they compared final year medical, nursing and psychology students of University of Nigeria in Enugu State, south-eastern Nigeria. Medical students were more likely to recognize symptoms of autism spectrum disorders, followed by nursing and then psychology students. Overall however, the level of knowledge of symptoms of autism spectrum disorder was low in the three groups of students (Igwe et al, 2010). In furtherance to this, Igwe et al (2011) examined knowledge of specialist pediatric and psychiatric nurses in Ebonyi State also in south-eastern Nigeria, establishing the same trend of low level of knowledge. They found association between improved knowledge and previous experience of participating in management of children with autism spectrum disorders and also noted that the ability of specialist psychiatric nurses in recognizing symptoms of autism spectrum disorders was slightly better than those of specialist pediatric nurses (Igwe et al, 2011).

The need to engage in education of health care workers and the general population in Africa on autism spectrum disorders cannot be ignored. This would enhance early recognition and interventions which had been observed to improve prognosis in individuals with autism spectrum disorders.

6. Summary

- It is established that symptoms of autism spectrum disorders occur among African children.
- To date, there have been no large scale epidemiological study on autism spectrum disorders in the African context. It is unclear whether the prevalence of autism spectrum disorders is different in rural and urban areas of Africa.
- The prevalence of autism spectrum disorders among children living in African continent is possibly lower than the prevalence among African children living in Europe and other high income developed countries. This disparity in prevalence need to be explained by future studies. The prevailing hypothesis of vitamin D etiological explanation for autism spectrum disorder is unlikely to explain the disparity in prevalence in its entirety.
- Period of onset of autism spectrum disorder symptoms among African children often coincides with period of vulnerability to physical illnesses and infectious diseases with neurological consequences, usually between the ages of two and five years. Etiology theory of post-encephalitic infection/sepsis preceding the onset of symptoms of autism spectrum disorder as observed in Tanzania study (Mankoski et al, 2006) may be reflecting this fact. This observation may also be confounded by the greater likelihood of exposure to infection/sepsis among African children in general. Given the high level of etiological and diagnostic heterogeneity implicit in autism spectrum disorders, these presentations may scientifically be highly informative.
- Based on presently available data, non-verbal cases of autism spectrum disorders outnumbered verbal cases in rate of presentation to orthodox medical care in Africa.
- Diagnoses of autism spectrum disorders in Africa are rarely made exclusively of intellectual disability. Therefore the relationship between autism spectrum disorders and intellectual disability need to be particularly explored in Africa.
- There are probable differences in clinical presentation of autism spectrum disorders among African children compared to that observed in Europe and North America. The symptoms of stereotypic repetitive repertoire of behaviors and activities which is one of the symptom domains for diagnosing autism spectrum disorder may be a less common occurrence in most African children with autism spectrum disorder.

- Etiology and pathogenesis of autism spectrum disorder in Africa and other parts of the world are still obscured, but complementary evidence point to both genetic ad epigenetic factors.
- Level of knowledge and awareness about autism spectrum disorder is low among the general population and health care workers in Africa. There is need for community education of the general population and continuous medical education for health care workers on issues relating to autism spectrum disorder. This would enhance early recognition and interventions and in turn improve prognosis.

7. Conclusions

Based on present state of knowledge and situation in Africa, more studies are needed to address the issue of epidemiology of autism spectrum disorder in Africa and characteristic presentation of autism spectrum disorders among African children. Genetic studies to unravel the etiology and pathogenesis of autism spectrum disorders are areas of research that also need to be focused on in Africa. Policy making attention to ease the burden of autism spectrum disorder and other childhood neuro-developmental disorders among affected African children and their care-givers is of import considering the observation of Mung'ala-Odera et al (2006) that burden of childhood neuro-developmental disorders is likely to increase in Africa as more children of age five years and below continue to survive because of anticipated improved health care system directed at infectious and communicable diseases.

8. Acknowledgement

This work was supported, in part, by the Fogarty International Center/NIH Mental Health & Developmental Disabilities (MH/DD) Program at the Children's Hospital Boston, Harvard Medical School (grant award no. D43 TW0005807, PI: K. Munir).

9. References

African Network for the Prevention and Protection against Child Abuse and Neglect (ANPPCAN), Nigeria Chapter (2007): Communique on a project to increase the level of awareness on autism and develop a mechanism for care and support of children with autism in Enugu State, South-Eastern Nigeria.

American Psychiatric Association (APA) (2000): Diagnostic and Statistical Manual of Mental Disorders; 4th Edition. Text Rev. Wahington, DC.

Arieff, Z, Kaur, M, Gameeldien, H, Merwe, L.V & Bajic, V.B (2010): 5-HTTLPR polymorphism: analysis in South African autistic individuals; Hum Biol; 82(3): 291 - 300.

Bakare, M.O (2006): Psychological disorders in Nigerian children and adolescents, and their peculiarities; In Embracing Identity while Nurturing Diversity; *[http://iacapap.ki.se/bulletins/Melbourne%20Supplement%202007.pdf]*

Bakare, M.O & Ikegwuonu, N.N (2008): Childhood autism in a 13 year old boy with oculo-cutaneous albinism: a case report; *J Med Case Reports*; 2: 56.

Bakare, M.O, Ebigbo, P.O, Agomoh, A.O & Menkiti, N.C (2008): Knowledge about childhood autism among health workers (KCAHW) questionnaire: description, reliability and internal consistency; *Clin Pract Epidemiol Ment Health;* 4: 17.

Bakare, M.O, Agomoh, A.O, Ebigbo, P.O, Eaton, J, Okonkwo, K.O, Onwukwe, J.U & Onyeama, G.M (2009a): Etiological explanation, treat-ability and preventability of childhood autism: a survey of Nigerian healthcare workers' opinion; *Ann Gen Psychiatry;* 8: 6.

Bakare, M.O, Ebigbo, P.O, Agomoh, A.O, Eaton, J, Onwukwe, J.U, Onyeama, G.M, Okonkwo, K.O, Igwe, M.N, Orovighwo, A.O & Aguocha, C.M (2009b): Knowledge about childhood autism and opinion among healthcare workers on availability of facilities and law caring for needs and rights of children with childhood autism and other developmental disorders in Nigeria; *BMC Pediatr* ; 9:12.

Bakare, M.O & Munir, K.M (2011): Epidemiology, diagnosis, etiology and knowledge about autism spectrum disorders (ASD) in Africa: perspectives from literatures cited in pubmed over the last decade (2000 -2009); *African Journal of Psychiatry* (In Press).

Bakare, M.O, Igwe, M.N, Odinka, P.C, & Iteke (2011a), O. Neuropsychiatric diagnosis and psychotropic medication prescription patterns in a mental hospital-based child and adolescent psychiatric service in Nigeria; *Journal of Health Care for the Poor and Underserved* (In Press).

Bakare, M.O, Munir, K.M, Kinney, D.K (2011b): Association of hypomelanotic skin disorders with autism: links to possible etiologic role of vitamin-D levels in autism?; *Hypothesis;* 9(1): e2.

Barnevick-Olsson, M, Gillberg, C, & Fernell, E (2008): Prevalence of autism in children born to Somali parents living in Sweden: a brief report; *Dev Med Child Neurol;* 50(8): 598 - 601.

Bejerot, S, & Humble, M (2008): Increased occurrence of autism among Somali children - does vitamin D deficiency play a role?; *Tidsskr Nor Laegeforen;* 128(17): 1986 - 1987.

Belhadj, A, Mrad, R, & Halayem, M.B (2006): A clinic and paraclinic study of Tunisian population of children with autism. About 63 cases; *Tunis Med;* 84(12): 763 - 767.

Bernier, R, Mao, A & Yen, J (2010): Psychopathology, Families and Culture: Autism; *Child Adolesc Psychiatr Clin N Am;* 19(4): 855 - 867.

DeLong, R (2007): GABA (A) receptor alpha 5 subunit as a candidate gene for autism and bipolar disorder: a proposed endophenotype with parent-of-origin and gain-of-function features, with or without oculocutaneous albinism; *Autism;* 11(2): 135 - 147.

Dhadphale, M, Lukwago, M.G, & Gajjar, M (1982): Infantile autism in Kenya; *Indian J Pediatr;* 49(396): 145 - 148.

Fernell, E, Barnevick-Olsson, M, Bagenholm, G, Gillberg, C, Gustafsson, S, & Saaf, M (2010): Serum levels of 25-hydroxyvitamin D in mothers of Swedish and of Somali origin who have children with and without autism; *Acta Paediatr;* 99(5): 743 - 747.

Gillberg, C, Schaumann, H, & Gillberg, I.C (1995): Autism in immigrants: children born in Sweden to mothers born in Uganda; *J Intellect Disabil Res;* 39(Pt 2): 141 - 144.

Gillberg, I.C & Gillberg, C (1996): Autism in immigrants: a population-based study from Swedish rural and urban areas; *J Intellect Disabil Res;* 40(Pt 1): 24 - 31.

Grant, W.B & Soles, C.M (2009): Epidemiologic evidence supporting the role of maternal vitamin D deficiency as a risk factor for the development of infantile autism; *Dermato endocrinol;* 1(4): 223 -228.

Igwe, M.N, Bakare, M.O, Agomoh, A.O, Onyeama, G.M, & Okonkwo, K.O (2010): Factors influencing knowledge about childhood autism among final year undergraduate medical, nursing and psychology students of University of Nigeria, Enugu State, Nigeria; *Ital J Pediatr;* 36: 44.

Igwe, M.N, Ahanotu, A.C, Bakare, M.O, Achor, J.U, & Igwe, C (2011): Assessment of knowledge about childhood autism among paediatric and psychiatric nurses in Ebonyi State, Nigeria; *Child Adoles Psychiatry Ment Health;* 5(1): 1.

Kanner, L (1943): Autistic disturbances of affective contact; *Nerv Child;* 2: 217.

Longe, C.I & Asuni, T (1972): Four cases of Infantile autism in Nigerian children; (Paper read at Third Pan African Psychiatric Conference, Khartoum. 1972).

Lotter, V (1966): Epidemiology of autistic conditions in young children: Prevalence; *Soc Psychiat;* 1: 124 - 147.

Lotter, V (1978): Childhood autism in Africa; *J Child Psychol Psychiatry;* 19(3): 231 - 244.

Lotter, V (1980): Cross cultural perspectives on childhood autism; *J Trop Pediatr;* 26(4): 131 - 133

Mankoski, R.E, Collins, M, Ndosi, N.K, Mgalla, E.H, Sarwatt, V.V, & Folstein, S.E (2006): Etiologies of autism in a case-series from Tanzania; *J Autism Dev Disord;* 36(8); 1039 - 1051.

Meguid, N.A, Hashish, A.F, Anwar, M, & Sidhom, G (2010): Reduced serum levels of 25-dihydroxy vitamin D in Egyptian children with autism; *J Altern Complement Med;* 16(6): 641 - 645.

Mostafa, G.A, El-Sayed, Z.A, El-Aziz, M.M, & El-Sayed, M.F (2008): Serum anti-myelin-associated glycoprotein antibodies in Egyptian autistic children; *J Child Neurol;* 23(12): 1413 - 1418.

Mostafa, G.A & Kitchener, N (2009): Serum anti-nuclear antibodies as a marker of autoimmunity in Egyptian autistic children; *Pediatr Neurol;* 40(2): 107 - 112.

Mostafa, G.A, El-Hadidi, E.S, Hewedi, D.H, & Abdou, M.M (2010): Oxidative stress in Egyptian children with autism: relation to autoimmunity; *J Neuroimmunol;* 219(1-2): 114 - 118.

Mostafa, G.A & Shehab, A.A (2010): The link of C4B null allele to autism and to a family history of autoimmunity in Egyptian autistic children; *J Neuroimmunol;* 223(1-2): 115 - 119.

Muhle, R, Trentacoste, S.V, & Rapin, I (2004): The genetics of autism; *Pediatrics;* 113(5): 472 - 486.

Mung'ala-Odera, V, Meehan, R, Njuguna, P, Mturi, N, Alcock, K.J, & Newton, C.R (2006): Prevalence and risk factors of neurological disability and impairment in children living in rural Kenya; *Int J Epidemiol;* 35(3): 683 - 688.

Rogawski, M.A, Funderburk, S.J, & Cederbaum, S.D (1978): Oculocutaneous albinism and mental disorder. A report of two autistic boys; *Hum Hered*; 28(2): 81 - 85.

Sanua, V.D (1984): Is infantile autism a universal phenomenon? An open question; *Int J Soc Psychiatry*; 30(3): 163 - 177.

Seif Eldin, A, Habib, D, Noufal, A, Farrag, S, Bazaid, K, Al-Sharbati, M, Badr, H, Moussa, S, Essali, A, & Gaddour, N (2008): Use of M-CHAT for a multinational screening of young children with autism in the Arab countries; *Int Rev Psychiatry*; 20(3): 281 - 289.

Smalley, S.L (1991): Genetic influences in autism; *Psychiatr Clin North Am*; 14(1): 125 - 139.

World Health Organization (WHO) (1992): *International Classification of Diseases, tenth edition (ICD - 10)*; WHO, Geneva. 1992.

Zaroff, C.M & Uhm, S.Y (2011): Prevalence of autism spectrum disorders and influence of country of measurement and ethnicity; *Soc Psychiatry Psychiatr Epidemiol*; Feb. 4 (Epub ahead of print).

Part 4

Sleep Disorders and Sexual Abuse in Autistic Children

11

Sleep Concerns and Disorders in Children with an Autistic Spectrum Disorder (ASD)

Oreste Battisti
Faculty of Medicine, University of Liège, Belgium

1. Introduction

The autistic spectrum disorder or ASD is frequently described or defined from several common characteristics during the periods of time concerning the wake time. More than many other situations, the investigations in ASD are difficult due to the particular personality encountered in this entity. This paper aims to present the interest of sleeping time study, owing to our experience and studies concerning sleep concerns in infants born prematurely, and in children suffering an ASD.

2. Definition of the autistic spectrum disorder or ASD and historical note

The ASD is included in the pervasive developmental disorders in the fourth edition text revision or DSM-IV-TR. That means that the original clinical description (Kanner's classic autism) has hardly changed with time, owing to the great variability of form and intensity in presentation. This clinical and biological entity contains a group of disorders (see Table I) with impairments in three major aspects: socialization, communication and behavior. It represents different clinical forms having however common social difficulties: a delay in language skills, an impaired social interaction, an impaired verbal or non-verbal communication, and repetitive, stereotyped or severely restricted activities and interests.

-	Classic autism or early infantile autism
-	Childhood autism (Kanner's autism)
-	Asperger syndrome or disorder
-	Atypical autism
-	Pervasive developmental disorder not otherwise specified
-	Childhood disintegrative disorder
-	Rett disorder

Table 1. The different forms of ASD

3. Diagnosis

It might happen, in most typical cases and with a short video recording, that the diagnosis is rapidly done. In most cases however, it will need time, after several observations and records of the CHAT or ADOS scales. One needs also to exclude the intervention of a mental retardation, an epilepsy, the effects of psychotropic drugs. The first signs may become prominent during infancy, and the diagnosis is merely done at three years, eventually sooner or later in life. In case of suspicion, it is highly recommended to address the infant to a specialized multidisciplinary team, after also an establishment of the IQ, a neuropsychological assessment, the assessment of hearing and vision .

4. Epidemiology, etiology, clinical description of ASD

The prevalence of ASD at 8 years of age has increased from 0.4 to about 2/1000 (range: 2-9 /1000. This observations is due to a combination of changes in case definition and an increased awareness together with more specialized developmental services. There is a male predominance with a male:female ratio of 4:1. One can also mention that ASD is present in siblings of an established ASD, in 2-8 percent. ASD is more frequently encountered in cases of monozygot twins and in case of prematurity. Associated following conditions are possibly found:

- Mental retardation;
- Seizures;
- Brain and cerebellum abnormalities (importance of MRI studies);
- Fetal alcohol syndrome;
- Phenylketonuria;
- Tuberous sclerosis;
- Chromosomal abdnormalities: Fragile X, Rett syndrome, Angelman syndrome, 15 q long arm duplication/triplication.

The causes or explanations of this entity are no yet elucidated, even if both genetics and environment seem to play a role in 10 to 25 % cases. It is likely that interactions between multiple genes (locus on chromosomes 15 and 16) are responsible, and that epigenetic factors and exposure to environmental modifiers contribute to the variable expression. Several biochemical abnormalities such as an impairment of intra cerebral folic acid, serotonine, catecholamines and the opiod systems have already been reported. Several studies concerning the outside and inside receptors to different neurotransmitters are in progress. Until now, the association with immunizations (mainly thimerosal as conservative) is not confirmed.

5. The building of a normal sleep architecture in infants

Before 6 months of age, in normal circumstances, the infant falls in sleep and goes directly in a REM or rapid eye movement phase and remains in it during about 55 minutes. REM phase is followed by a non REM phase which remains about 65 minutes. After 6 months of age, the infant falls in sleep and goes directly in a non REM phase, remains in it for about minutes 90-120 minutes, and it is followed by a REM phase for a period of about 45 minutes. A sleep cycle contains a REM and non REM phase. Sleeping night time contains 8 cycles until 12 months, 6 cycles from 12 to 24 months, and 5 cycles after this age. The repartition of all these cycle has an homogenous distribution through night before the 24 months of age, and more --distributed after midnight after this age. These facts are illustrated in the Figure 1.

It is known that this process is in correlation with the melatonin synthesis from tryptophan in the infant. We can summarize that physiology by the following points:

- Circadian rhythm is usually present between 3 to 6 months of age;

- The sun and the melatonin synthesis have an important role;
- The secretion (by the pineal gland) of melatonin becomes evident at 3 months of age, and it increases until 1 year of age, and thereafter remains stable until puberty;
- Its secretion and release shows an increasing level at around 7-8 pm, with a pic level at 2-3 am, an remains stable from 7 am until 7-8 pm;
- One can observe a significantly low level in case of epilepsy, ASD, diabetes, babies born before 32 weeks or with a birth weight below 1500 g and in babies born from addicted mothers.

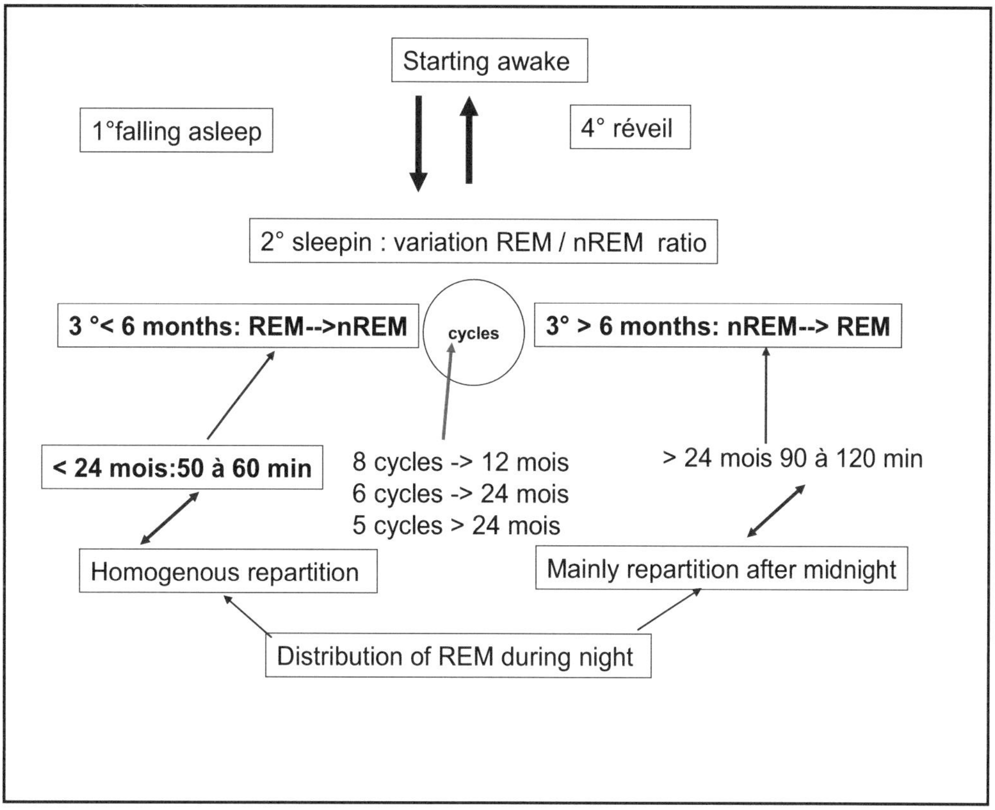

Fig. 1. The building of the normal sleep architecture in humans.

6. Sleep concerns in the autistic spectrum

In the ASD, the prevalence of sleep problems is between 44 and 83 % (in comparison of 30 % found in other population). It is not correlated to the IQ, although the degree of mental retardation tends to predict sleep impairment. Sleep disorders are hence more frequently encountered in children with an autistic spectrum.

The sleep disorders are not universal in autism, but they concerns about 55% of these beings. Good sleepers with ASD have fewer affective problems and satisfying social interactions.

Sleep disorders in ASD are listed in Table II.

- Insomnia.Here the parents report a prolonged time to fall asleep, a leter bedtime, a decreased sleep duration and continuity, an increased arousals, an early moorning wake time;
- Sleep disordered breathing;
- Bruxism;
- Arousal from sleep with confusion or wandering;
- Rhythmic movement disorder;
- Leg movements;
- Daytime sleepness

The most frequently encountered sleep disorder in ASD is insomnia;
One can understand that the expected building of normal sleep architecture (see above) is not easily encountered in ASD.
The sleep studies (polysomnography or better hypnology) in infants having sleep problems early in life are mainly indicated in situations concerned by the risk of cot death and the suspicion of epilepsy. Studies concerning behavioral difficulties in infants or children are not so few.

7. Observations in sleeping times of children having a ASD

In a group of 22 children with an ASD aged between 4 and 8 years, we find the following observations in a global polysomnography or hypnology (Table III): electrophysiology of brain, heart, muscles an retina, respiration, pulsed oxymetry, movements of whole body, sleep architecture, central and peripheral apneas.

- Obstructive sleep apnea due to enlarged tonsils;
- Obstructive sleep apnea due a tracheomalacia;
- Abnormal density of REM periods
- Abnormal distribution of REM periods;
- Monotony of source and trajectory of the electrophysiological vague.

In our experience of sleep analysis in children having a ASD diagnosis, the interesting observation is concerning the analysis of brain electrogenesis: in its emergence, its distribution and progression in the different cortical areas.
We found a combination of:

- A repetitive emergence of electrogenesis in the the left hemisphere (and more precisely around junction of frontal and temporal lobes) and
- A monotony and the spreading of that electrogenesis in the other cortical areas. (see Figure 2).

One possible hypothesis is that the observed abnormalities in wake time can be earlier observed in sleeping time. The loss of a normal variability in the usual neurological and behavioural moments in daily life could reflect a sort of (brain) internal self defensive attitude, an over and repetitive use of the same (being considered as safe and comfortable) circuitries among neurological pathways. This could lead to a sort of physical and emotional dependency, to a real fatigue of finally to much devoted cognitive and associated motor areas.
Together to these overuse and also underuse of brain areas, the concerned neurotransmitters are also overused or underused.

This could explain the following items in a strategy of self defense:

- the overfocusing areas of interest
- some periods of fatigue with suddenly an aggressive person against himself or an other person
- without the eventually need of adequacy on the moment of life
- without the need of waiting for or concerning the other
- without the need of integrating the task in the activities of a group
- without the approbation or interrogation (by listening to or looking at the other) in a task, or the use of a material.

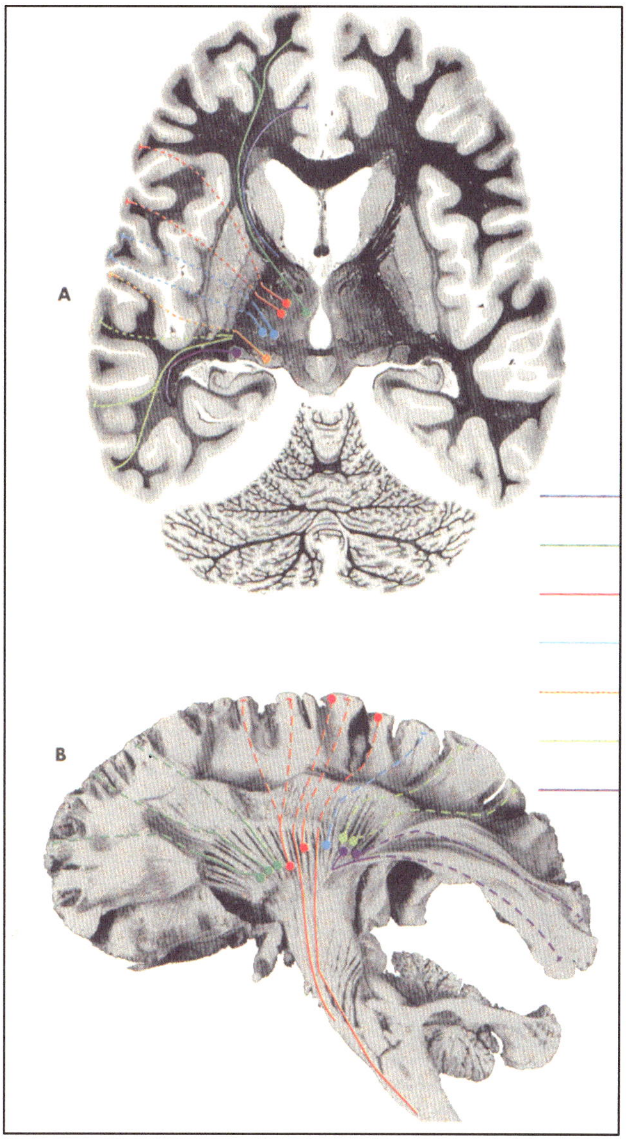

Fig. 2. Hypothetic fiber tracts repetitive activity in the autistic spectrum.

8. Integration of observation during sleeping and wake time for interventions and medications

As others, we find an association between sleep analysis and daytime functioning in ASD. Although it is difficult in this type of pathology, to determine whether poor sleep is the cause or result of a more problematic daytime functioning, or whether the severity is contributing to both poor sleep and more impaired daytime functioning, it seems plausible to imagine, as what can be seen in patients not having an ASD, that a better sleep time will contribute to a better daytime functioning and vice versa, and the more that is maintained over time, the more the resistance to possible perturbing factors will be high or low.

Autism therapies are designed to treat symptoms (mood instability, sleep disorder, agressivity) or interrupt the abnormal equilibrium when this is found (disturbed balance of neurotransmitters, disturbed brain input of tryptophan or folinic acid, disturbed pineal secretion of melatonin, disturbed endorphin secretion against neuropathic pain.

9. Behavioral and educational interventions

The therapies have the following nominations: the antecedent package, the behavioral package, the comprehensive behavioral treatment, the join attention intervention, the modeling, the naturalistic teaching strategies, the peer training package, the pivotal response treatment schedules, the schedules, the self-management, the story-based intervention package. Their goals are to improve the social functioning (decrease non functional or negative behaviors), to move the child toward independence (better communication, more adaptive skills, promote academic functioning and cognition).

These combined and adapted therapies to the given precise case should begin as soon as possible, with a minimum 25 hours/week schedule, 12 months per year

10. Medications

They should be associated to the behavioral, educational and environmental interventions.

Usually, the medications are given either to treat symptoms or to reestablish a normal brain input of mediators.

These are:

- psychotropic therapies targeting (as antagonists) dopaminergic and or serotoninergic receptors: haloperidol, risperidone, clomipramide.
- Anxiolytic when the patient is particularly anxious
- Mood stabilizers
- Vitamins (folinic acid, B6, B12)
- tryptophan
- Opiods antagonists (naltrexone)
- Sleep concerns medications.

It is interesting to remind here the neurobiology or chemistry of sleep.

Sleep and ASD have similar neurotransmitters intervening in the sleep-wake cycle: GABA, serotonin, histamine, melatonin. For all these 4 molecules, abnormalities are found in ASD

Any case is particular and request a fine analysis of daytime, sequence at bedtime, sleep time, but insomnia in ASD is particularly frequent.

After having discarded other causes (gastro-oesophageal reflux, severe atopic dermatitis, cow's proteins or other allergy, tracheomalacia, enlarged tonsils or adenoids), we can choose the best or most appropriate medication. In this point of view, melatonin, then a benzodiazepine, then an antihistamine drug given 1 hour before bedtime beside other therapies in daytime, could counteract the disturbed balance of neurotransmitter.

11. References

[1] Symons FJ, Byiers BJ, Raspa M, Bishop E, Bailey DB. Self-injurious behavior and fragile x syndrome: findings from the national fragile x survey. Am J Intellect Dev Disabil. 2010 Nov;115(6):473-81.

[2] Williams SR, Aldred MA, Der Kaloustian VM, Halal F, Gowans G, McLeod DR, Zondag S, Toriello HV, Magenis RE, Elsea SH. Haploinsufficiency of HDAC4 causes brachydactyly mental retardation syndrome, with brachydactyly type E, developmental delays, and behavioral problems. Am J Hum Genet. 2010 Aug 13;87(2):219-28. PubMed PMID: 20691407.

[3] Deonna T, Roulet-Perez E. Early-onset acquired epileptic aphasia (Landau-Kleffner syndrome, LKS) and regressive autistic disorders with epileptic EEG abnormalities: the continuing debate. Brain Dev. 2010 Oct;32(9):746-52. Epub 2010 Jul 15.

[4] Gillberg C. The ESSENCE in child psychiatry: Early Symptomatic Syndromes Eliciting Neurodevelopmental Clinical Examinations. Res Dev Disabil. 2010 Nov-Dec;31(6):1543-51. Epub 2010 Jul 14.

[5] Cortesi F, Giannotti F, Ivanenko A, Johnson K. Sleep in children with autistic spectrum disorder. Sleep Med. 2010 Aug;11(7):659-64. Epub 2010 Jul 4. Review.

[6] Wright B, Sims D, Smart S, Alwazeer A, Alderson-Day B, Allgar V, Whitton C, Tomlinson H, Bennett S, Jardine J, McCaffrey N, Leyland C, Jakeman C, Miles J. Melatonin Versus Placebo in Children with Autism Spectrum Conditions and Severe Sleep Problems Not Amenable to Behaviour Management Strategies: A Randomised Controlled Crossover Trial. J Autism Dev Disord. 2010 Jun 10. [Epub ahead of print]

[7] Stevens L, Tartaglia N, Hagerman R, Riley K. Clinical report: a male with Down syndrome, fragile X syndrome, and autism. J Dev Behav Pediatr. 2010 May;31(4):333-7.

[8] Miano S, Ferri R. Epidemiology and management of insomnia in children with autistic spectrum disorders. Paediatr Drugs. 2010 Apr 1;12(2):75-84.

[9] Carbone PS, Farley M, Davis T. Primary care for children with autism. Am Fam Physician. 2010 Feb 15;81(4):453-60.

[10] Coury D. Medical treatment of autism spectrum disorders. Curr Opin Neurol. 2010 Apr;23(2):131-6.

[11] Sung M, Fung DS, Cai Y, Ooi YP. Pharmacological management in children and adolescents with pervasive developmental disorder. Aust N Z J Psychiatry. 2010 May;44(5):410-28.

[12] Ekinci O, Arman AR, IÅŸik U, Bez Y, Berkem M. EEG abnormalities and epilepsy in autistic spectrum disorders: clinical and familial correlates. Epilepsy Behav. 2010 Feb;17(2):178-82. Epub 2009 Dec 29.

[13] Souders MC, Mason TB, Valladares O, Bucan M, Levy SE, Mandell DS, Weaver TE, Pinto-Martin J. Sleep behaviors and sleep quality in children with autism spectrum disorders. Sleep. 2009 Dec 1;32(12):1566-78.
[14] Wirojanan J, Jacquemont S, Diaz R, Bacalman S, Anders TF, Hagerman RJ, Goodlin-Jones BL. The efficacy of melatonin for sleep problems in children with autism, fragile X syndrome, or autism and fragile X syndrome. J Clin Sleep Med. 2009 Apr 15;5(2):145-50. Erratum in: J Clin Sleep Med. 2010 Aug 15;6(4):preceding 311. .
[15] Glickman G. Circadian rhythms and sleep in children with autism. Neurosci Biobehav Rev. 2010 Apr;34(5):755-68. Epub 2009 Dec 4. Review.
[16] Hughes JR. Update on autism: a review of 1300 reports published in 2008. Epilepsy Behav. 2009 Dec;16(4):569-89. Epub 2009 Nov 6. Review.
[17] Johnson KP, Giannotti F, Cortesi F. Sleep patterns in autism spectrum disorders. Child Adolesc Psychiatr Clin N Am. 2009 Oct;18(4):917-28. Review.
[18] Badoe EV. Classical Rett Syndrome in a Ghanaian child: a case report. West Afr J Med. 2009 Mar;28(2):134-6.
[19] Coury D, Jones NE, Klatka K, Winklosky B, Perrin JM. Healthcare for children with autism: the Autism Treatment Network. Curr Opin Pediatr. 2009 Dec;21(6):828-32. Review.
[20] Silva LM, Schalock M, Ayres R, Bunse C, Budden S. Qigong massage treatment for sensory and self-regulation problems in young children with autism: a randomized controlled trial. Am J Occup Ther. 2009 Jul-Aug;63(4):423-32.

12

Sexual Abuse in Autistic Children as a Risk Factor of Developing of Schizophrenia

Piotr W. Gorczyca[1], Agnieszka Kapinos-Gorczyca[1],
Katarzyna Ziora[2] and Joanna Oświęcimska[2]
[1]*Department of Psychiatry, Medical University of Silesia in Katowice*
[2]*Department of Paediatrics, Paediatric Endocrinology Unit,*
Medical University of Silesia in Katowice
Poland

1. Introduction

In this article the authors present the problem of sexual abuse in children with autism. The rates of sexually abuse for children with developmental disabilities are nearly two times greater than for typical children. Based on the prevalence of abuse and its association with various behaviors, clinicians should be observe the potential of abuse when these behaviors are changed. The results of the latest studies prove, however, that schizophrenia and other psychotic disorders can take place in patients diagnosed with autistic spectrum disorders (ASD). The sexual abuse of autistic children may be a risk factor of developing schizophrenia.

Some children with autism may be targeted for abuse by sexual offenders. Current estimates suggest that 1:3 girls and 1:10 boys will be sexually abused by the time they are 18 years old (Tang, Freyd, & Wang, 2007). The sexual offender is usually someone who is known and trusted by the child (Cavanagh Johnson, 1999, 2002). Offenders attempt to gain trust from potential victims. The rates of sexually abuse for children with developmental disabilities are nearly two times greater than for typical children and the effects of sexually abuse may be exacerbated by social isolation and alienation (Mansell, Sobsey and Moskal (1998). Some children with autism after sexual abuse may not have the skills to effectively communicate what happened to them. They are unable to understand the nuances of reciprocal conversation needed to disclose sexual abuse. The abused autistic children attempt to cope with these behaviors or to the development of new behaviors that were not previously present. Some studies suggests that autistic children who are nonverbal exhibit more behavioral difficulties than those who have verbal communication abilities (Dominick, Davis, Lanihart, Tager-Flusberg, & Folstein (2007). This may lead to frustration caused by the inability of others to understand what the child communicate. The fact that the child was sexually abused may be missed. Children who are sexually abused do not always display sexualized or concerning behaviors at all (Kendall-Tackett, Meyer Williams, & Finkelhor, 1993), so the presence or absence of sexualized behaviors cannot be a marker for whether or not a child has been sexually abused. Sexual abused children under age 7 have more hypersexual behavior, self-exposing, and victimizing sexual behaviors toward others (McClellan et al. 1996). In study of Mandell et al (2005) was reported that 18.5% of children with autism were physically 16.6% were sexually abused. Caregivers reported that 18.5% of children with autism had been physically abused and 16.6% had been sexually abused. Sexually abused children more likely had engaged in sexual acting out or abusive behavior, suicidal or other self-injurious behavior, had run away from home or had a psychiatric hospitalization. Based on the prevalence of abuse and its association with various behaviors, clinicians should be observe the potential of abuse when these behaviors are changed. Sullivan and Knutson (2000) found that the number of family stressors was associated with the risk of abuse, and Ammerman et al. (1994) found that lack of maternal social support was associated with it.

Westcott and Cross (1996) suggest that researchers examine more specific child, family, and social factors that may be associated with abuse. Mandell et al. (2005) also wrote about examine of autistic child`s community. Because of their social isolation and poor communication skills, children with autistic spectrum disorders may represent a group at particular risk of physical and sexual abuse (Howlin & Clements, 1995), although the only large-scale, community-based study published in this area found rates of abuse for children with autism similar to those in the general population (Sullivan & Knutson, 2000). For the most part, only case studies have characterized abuse among this group (Cook, Kieffer, Charak, & Leventhal, 1993; Perkins & Wolkind, 1991).

The majority of studies of the prevalence and correlates of abuse among children with disabilities were conducted using institutionalized samples, whereas most children with autism are served in the community (Jacobson & Mulick, 2000; Jarbrink & Knapp, 2001). Children with disabilities often have limited access to critical information pertaining to personal safety and sexual abuse prevention. Parents, caregivers, therapist and teachers of autistic children may experience high levels of stress. The social isolation of families with a child who was diagnosed with ASD can increase the risk of neglect or child abuse by the parent or the caregiver. We cannot ignore is a parent's/caregiver's lack of understanding of an autistic child's needs. Autism has been a mysterious condition for years. Parents and doctors have always been distressed when a young child who has previously seemed quite normal, begins to withdraw from social interactions and concern on the own world.

In the 1960s, Bruno Bettelheim made the notorious suggestion that autism is caused by emotionally distant parenting. The terms "refrigerator mothers" and "absent fathers" were coined. The idea was that even outwardly conscientious parents for some reason resented the very existence of their children, and the children, picking up on this, were so psychologically damaged, that they developed autism. The existence of these wrong theories has led to untold damage both to autistic children, their families and many others. These theories were later rejected, but the currency that they enjoyed for several years caused untold suffering to autistic child`s parents. Nowadays there is consensus that parental behavior plays no role whatsoever in causing autism. There are a number of incidents of horrific childhood abuse and neglect which nevertheless did not lead to autism developing. So modern scientists argue that certainly any parents who do not neglect and abuse their children cannot be blamed in any way for causing autism.

In comprehensive review of neurodevelopmental responses to trauma (sexual abuse), Perry and Pollard (1998) discuss how abuse can result in neuropsychiatric problems, including depressive disorders, ADHD, dissociative disorders, and developmental disorders. Infants and young children have immature central nervous system development, so distress may be unable to formulate a plan or to use words and withdrawal. In the middle of the 1980s the so-called "neurodevelopment" hypothesis of schizophrenia appeared (Murray and Lewis 1987, Weinberger 1987). In accordance with this theory the expression of certain genes or also of certain unspecified negative environmental factors, active in early development, lead to changes in the formation of the neuronal network, which are responsible for important psychic functions. These changes do not undergo expression until the period of adolescence, when they begin to appear in the disorganized thinking and productive symptoms. Even though the activity of the early negative factors do not appear in the early developmental stages through the appearance of psychotic symptoms, during this phase there exist many anatomical and neurophysiologic abnormalities, as well as defined characteristics and behaviors, by which people in whom schizophrenia will appear in the future can be distinguished from the general population (Rybakowski and Rajewski 2006).

In recent years some multiyear studies have been published that rate the frequency of psychotic disorders found in the same people in various developmental periods. In Kim-Cohen et al.(2003) the frequency of mental disorder found in subjects at the age of childhood is rated and their relationship with disorders found in them at the age of 26. In people in whom at the age of 26 schizophrenia and schizophrenic-like disorders appeared, anxiety disorders (2.5 times), depression (7.4 times), ADHD (4.5 times) as well as conduct disorder and/or oppositional defiant disorder had appeared more frequently up until the age of 15 than in other persons. These results show considerable sequential comorbidity in the case of schizophrenia, which may testify to a large generalization of developmental deficits connected with schizophrenia.

Childhood-onset schizophrenia appears to be clinically and neurobiologically continuous with the adult disorder (Nicolson and Rapoport 1995). From the 1970s childhood autism and schizophrenia have been regarded as unrelated and distinct disorders (Rutter 1972), although the creator of the concept of autism, Leo Kanner, tied this disorder with a very early likeness of schizophrenia. The results of the latest studies prove, however, that schizophrenia and other psychotic disorders can take place in patients diagnosed with autistic spectrum disorders (ASD). In Volkmar's and Cohen's study (1991) only one person (0,6%) among adolescents and adults diagnosed with autism presented symptoms of schizophrenia, whereas in Stahlberg's et al. (2004) 7,8% of adult patients diagnosed with ASD met the criteria for schizophrenia or other psychotic disorders.

Described also is the case of a family appearance of early childhood schizophrenia, childhood autism, and translocation (1;7) (p22;q21) (Yan et al 2000). Some scientists even maintain that autism may constitute a negative factor of risk in the later development of psychosis (Petty et al. 1984; Clarke et al.1989).

It seems that the multi-factored conditioning of childhood autism may result in the onset of schizophrenia at a slightly later age. Symptoms of autism are most likely to be nonspecific markers of severe early neurodevelopment, which confirms Sporn's et al. study (2004).

The next issue to interpret is sexual abuse of child. Sexually abused children more likely had engaged in sexual acting out or abusive behavior, suicidal or other self-injurious behavior, had run away from home, or had a psychiatric hospitalization. In adjusted multivariate models, the relationship between sexual abuse and sexual acting out, running away from home and suicidal attempts persisted. However it really seems very important to consider the potential of abuse when these behaviors appeared.

More studies about child sexual abuse concern after diagnosing autism, but less is before this illness. This fact can be a risk factor for developing autism and schizophrenia as well. The appearance of symptoms of schizophrenia in a person diagnosed with childhood autism, overlapping on the earlier likeness of the illness, fundamentally changes its hitherto course.

2. References

Tang, S. S. S., Freyd, J. J., & Wang, M. (2007). What do we know about gender in the disclosure of child sexual abuse? *Journal of Psychological Trauma, 6*, 1-26.

Cavanagh Johnson, T. (2002). Some considerations about sexual abuse and children with sexual behavior problems. *Journal of Trauma and Dissociation, 3*, 83-105.

Cavanagh Johnson, T. (1999). *Understanding your child's sexual behavior: What's natural and healthy.* Oakland, CA: New Harbinger Publications, Inc.

Mansell, S., Sobsey, D., & Moskal, R. (1998). Clinical findings among sexually abused children with and without developmental disabilities. Mental Retardation, 36,12-22

Dominick, K. C., Davis, N. O., Lainhart, J., Tager-Flusberg, H., & Folstein, S. (2007). Atypical behaviors in children with autism and children with a history of language impairment. *Research in Developmental Disabilities, 28*, 145-162.

Kendall-Tackett, K. A., Meyer Williams, L., & Finkelhor, D. (1993). Impact of sexual abuse on children: A review and synthesis of recent empirical studies. *Psychological Bulletin, 113*, 164-180.

Sullivan, P., & Knutson, J. (2000). Maltreatment and disabilities: A population-based epidemiological study. Child Abuse & Neglect, 24(10), 1257.1273.

Ammerman, R., Hersen, M., Van Hesselt, V., Lubetsky, M., & Sieck, W. (1994). Maltreatment in psychiatricaly hospitalized children and adolescents with developmental disabilities: Prevalence and correlates. Journal of the American Academy of Child & Adolescent Psychiatry, 33(4), 567.576.

Westcott, H., & Cross, M. (1996). This far and no further: Towards ending abuse of disabled children. Birmingham: Venture Press.

McClellan R., McCurry C., Ronnel M. et al. (1996). Age of onset of sexual abuse: relationship to sexually inappropriate behaviors. J Am Acad Child Adolesc Psychiatry 35: 1375-83.

Mandell DS, Walrath CM, Manteuffel B, Sgro G, Pinto-Martin JA (2005). The prevalence and correlates of abuse among children with autism served in comprehensive community-based mental health settings. *Child Abuse Negl.* Dec; 29(12):1359-72.

Howlin, P.,&Clements, J. (1995). Is it possible to assess the impact of abuse on children with pervasive developmental disorders? Journal of Autism and Developmental Disorders, 25(4), 337.354.

Cook, E., Kieffer, J., Charak, D., & Leventhal, B. (1993). Autistic disorder and post-traumatic stress disorder. Journal of the American Academy of Child & Adolescent Psychiatry, 32(6), 1292.1294.

Jacobson, J., & Mulick, J. (2000). System and cost research issues in treatments for people with autistic disorders. Journal of Autism & Developmental Disorders, 30(6), 585.593.

Bettelheim B. (1950), Love is not enough: the treatment of emotionally disturbed children. Free Press Glencoe, Il

Clarke DJ, LittleJohns CS, Corbett JA, Joseph S (1989) Pervasive developmental disorders and psychoses in adult life. *Br J Psychiatry* 155:692-699.

Kim-Cohen J, Caspi A, Moffitt TE, Harrington H, Milne BJ, Poulton R (2003), Prior juvenile diagnoses ion adults with mental disorder: developmental follow-back of a prospective- longitudinal cohort. *Arch Gen Psychiatry* 60: 709-717.

Murray RM, Lewis SW (1987), Is schizophrenia a neurodevelopmental disorder? *Brit. Med. J* 295: 681-682.

Nicolson R, Rapoport JL (1999), Childhood-onset schizophrenia: Rare but worth studying. *Biol Psychiatry* 46:1418-1428.

Perry BD, Pollard R (1998), Homeostasis, stress, trauma and adaptation-a neurodevelopmental view of childhood trauma. *Child Adolesc Psychiatr Clin N Am* 7:33-51.

Petty LK, Ornitz Em, Michelman JD, Zimmerman EG (1984), Autistic children who become schizophrenic. *Arch Gen Psychiatry* 41:129-135.

Rutter M (1972), Childhood schizophrenia reconsidered. *J Autism Child Schizophr* 2:315-337.

Rybakowski F, Rajewski A (2006), Czy we wszystkich zaburzeniach psychicznych obowiązuje model rozwojowy? *Psychiatr Pol* 2:191-203.

Sporn AL, Paddington AM, Gogtay N, Ordonem AE, Gornick M. Clasen L, Greenstein D, Tossell JW., Gochman P, Lenane M, Sharp WS, Straub RE, Rapoport JL (2004), Pervasive developmental disorder and childhood-onset schizophrenia: comorbid disorder or a phenotypic variant of a very early onset illness? *Biol Psychiatry* 55(10):989-994.

Stahlberg O, Soderstrom H, Rastam M, Gillberg C (2004), Bipolar disorder, schizophrenia, and other psychotic disorders in adults with childhood onset AD/HD and/or autism spectrum disorders. *J Neural Transm* 111(7): 891-902.

Volkmar FR, Cohen DJ (1991), Comorbid association of autism and schizophrenia. *Am J Psychiatry* 148(12):1705-1707.

Weinberger DR (1987), Implications of normal brain development for the pathogenesis of schizophrenia. *Arch Gen Psychiatry* 44: 660-669.

Yan WL, Guan XY, Green ED, Nicolson R, Yap TK, Zhang J, Jacobson LK, Krasnewich DM, Kumra S, Lenane MC, Gochman P, Damschroder-Williams PJ, Esterling LE, Long RT, Martin BM, Sidransky E, Rapoport JL, Ginns EI (2000), Childhood-onset schizophrenia /autistic disorder and t(1;7) reciprocal translocation: midentification of a BAC contig spanning the translocation breakpoint at 7q21. *Am J Med Genet* 96(6):749-753.

Part 5

Creativity, Psychiatry and Occupational Histories

13

Creativity Psychosis Autism and the Social Brain

Michael Fitzgerald
University of Dublin
Ireland

1. Introduction

From an evolutionary perspective the link between creativity and mental disorder is of critical importance to the progress of humanity (Fitzgerald, 1999; 2000; 2004; 2008; 2010). In relation to autism there is an overlap between a subgroup of persons with autism and creativity of genius proportions. A larger group show evidence of savant or special skills at a lower level of creativity.

In relation to psychosis persons have shown great creativity before their psychotic episode and John Nash the Nobel Prize winner has described this very well at a psychiatric congress and on television.

Nevertheless in relation to psychosis the greatest degree of creativity is shown in the relatives of persons with psychosis who have minor genetic loadings for psychosis and don't have a formal diagnosis of psychosis. This paper will also examine the relationship between psychosis and autism (Crespi and Badcock, 2008).

Paradoxically in relation to the social brain, this type of brain is not well adapted to creativity of genius proportions in the areas of mathematics, the sciences and engineering. It is the extreme male brain (Baron-Cohen, 1997), which is high in the capacity to systematise and low in empathy which is the most successful in this type of creativity.

The greatest example here is Isaac Newton (Fitzgerald, 1999) whose autism is widely accepted by psychiatrists and psychologists. It is interesting that later in life Newton had a psychotic episode, an example of comorbidity which is very common with autism.

Human kind from the start of recorded time has been fascinated with creativity. Over the centuries our understanding of genius has varied from one associated with place or person to one of inherent ability (Atkinson, 1993). In Greco-Roman times creativity was explained on the one hand by "devine fire", by "God's touch", by the idea that creativity was a product of "melancholy humour and of course the Muses" (Porter, 1998)

2. Genius and madness

This link between genius and psychiatric disorder has been made for thousands of years. Indeed, there has been almost equal interest in the relationship between genius and madness, and between genius and creativity. Arguably, much of this has stemmed from literary movements. It is with Romanticism, writes Porter (1998) that the 'indissoluble link between madness and artistic genius comes into its own as an autobiographical experience'.

Perhaps the man who first forged a theoretical link between genius and madness was the Italian psychiatrist and criminologist, Cesare Lombroso (1836-1909). He was rather fanatical on the subject and wrote numerous books that were translated and circulated widely. In *The Man of Genius*, which was first published in 1890, he declared that he had 'discovered genius', and with it the 'various characteristics of degeneration' that formed the basis of practically all forms of congenital mental abnormality (Murray 1989). In his work, he also provided descriptions of the perceived physical and social characteristics of geniuses. Geniuses were, he stated, 'short, emaciated, sterile, microcephalic, stupid, and ugly....lacking in tact, in moderation, in the sense of practical life, in the virtues useful in social "affairs" (Costwalk & Zegans 1993). Indeed, he was wrong in the physical characteristics but correct in terms of the social characteristics.
Steptoe (1988) stated that Plato emphasised the role of inspiration from the gods. Here he argued that poetic composition occurs in a "frenzy of divine madness". Broad (1977) noted that Seneca stated that "no great genius has ever existed without some touch of madness".
The poet John Dryden (Simonton, 1994) pointed out that "Great Wits are sure to Madness near ally'd - And thin Partitions do their Bounds divide".
Howe (1999) pointed out that for Immanuel Kant, genius was an "incommunicable gift that cannot be taught or handed on, but is mysteriously imparted to certain artists by nature, and dies with the person". This is true but of course part of the mystery is now resolved in the sense that genetic factors play a very significant role and particularly so in creativity of genius proportions. Gardner (1997) points out that "some traits that do not run in families may still be genetically transmitted according to a principle called emergenesis by which traits are passed on by a package of genes, but only if the entire package is transmitted".
Martindale (1996) points out that "for identical twins Waller 1993 found an intra class correlation of almost 0.60 from creative personality scales". It was very low for fraternal twins again because you need so many traits to come together. Martindale (1996) estimates that creativity is about as heritable as traits such as "eye colour or height". The genetics of High Functioning Autism put heritability at about 93%. This suggests that in terms of creativity of genius proportions particularly related to autism that the levels of heritability in relation to creativity are particularly high.

3. Mechanisms of creativity

Creative people with High Functioning Autism are obsessed with fundamental, bedrock discoveries. They can hyperfocus and become disconnected from the environment for long periods. Isaac Newton could focus for a number of days without interruption on a problem. This was part of his secret of success (Fitzgerald, 2004). These features are particularly seen in persons with High Functioning Autism and high mathematical ability (Fitzgerald and James, 2007). Dehaene (1997) points out that for mathematicians their "disproportionate and relentless passion for numbers and mathematics", is often sustained by their "inability to entertain normal relations with other fellow human beings". An example here is Ramanujan, a mathematician of genius (Fitzgerald, 2004).
There is absolutely no doubt that what Hans Asperger (1944) described as an "unconventional, unorthodox, strangely pure and original, akin to the intelligence of true creativity". Autistic intelligence is unconventional and unorthodox. It is persons with this thinking style who produce true creativity of genius proportions. These persons are often seen as being eccentric or having strange personalities.

4. Autistic savants

It is important to distinguish true creativity from autistic savantism. Autistic savantism relates to "a person with low intelligence who possesses an unusually high skill in some mental task like mental arithmetic, remembering dates or numbers for the performing other rote tasks at a remarkably high level" (Grossman, 1977).

The best explanation of savant talent has been put forward by O'Connor and Hermelin (1987). They point out that

a specific gift for art, music....tends to be self-contained, as are Fodor's modules, but it also includes its own aspects of central processing. We could thus regard savant ability as 'quasi-modular', ie being circumscribed by, but not restricted to, sensory perceptual processing.

Focussing on their savant activities, a personal with autism/Asperger's syndrome can then avoid a confusing, chaotic socio-emotional world.

Hermelin (2001) notes that some psychologists investigating 'creativity' have suggested that 'field independence' and 'diverse thinking' (ie forming unusual and unexpected associations) show the working of an original mind. This is what the individuals described in this book demonstrate. Hermelin asks whether such a tendency of 'field independence' in autistic perception and thought could help to account for the fact that most savants are autistic. I believe the answer is yes.

O'Connor and Hermelin (1987) feel that savants' ability is 'relatively independent of general mental development. It seems that the artists may have a richer and more acceptable store of visual images or forms, a picture lexicon'.

Sir Michael Rutter, in the foreword to Hermelin (2001), points out that 'the underlying feature is that the savants use the strategy of taking a mental path from single units to a subsequent higher order extraction of overarching patterns and structures'.

Treffert (2009) points out that the savant syndrome "is rare but one in ten autistic persons show some savant skills"; "the special skills are always accompanied by prodigious memory"; "savant skills do not fade or disappear; rather a pattern of replication to improvisation to creation is often seen". Savant skills are commoner in males as indeed is autism. In terms of true creativity an IQ of at least 120 is necessary. After that it is the personality characteristics of autism.

I have coined the term 'Asperger Savantism' to describe true creativity in persons with Asperger's Syndrome and IQ 120+

Mottron et al. (2009) emphasises "enhanced perception in autistic cognitive abilities" in savant syndrome. They note the "enhanced low-level operations; locally orientated processing as a default setting; greater activation of perceptual areas during a range of visuospatial, language, working memory or reasoning tasks; autonomy towards higher processes; and superior involvement in intelligence" in persons with autism. This enhances their savant abilities.

Synder (2009) points out that "savant's privileged access to lower level, less-processed information, before it is packaged into holistic concepts and meaningful labels. A strategy of building from the parts to the whole could form the basis for so-called autistic genius". Certainly persons with autism retain this ability to see the world through the eyes of the child, to see the world in detailed less holistic fashion.

What is it about autism from neurocognitive points of view that makes such great creativity possible? One aspect of this is the weak central coherence theory. (Frith, 1989). This means that these persons are poor at seeing the overall picture but have tremendous ability to see small details. This ability to focus on small details is partly responsible for their great creativity. They are not distracted by normal views of the world. Baron-Cohen (2003) emphasised the male brain theory of autism. This emphasised the superior abilities in systematising. Systematising refers to the ability to accumulate facts about the physical world in a systematic way (Lyons and Fitzgerald, 2005). This systematisation ability is of great value in science, engineering, etc. In short then Lyons and Fitzgerald (2005) point out the importance of specific cognitive style; persons being more object centred than people centred; very accurate at perceiving details; strong narrow interest; excellent memory and strong focus of attention.

5. Autism

The modern descriptions of autism were initially by Hans Asperger in 1938 then by Leo Kanner in 1943 and once again by Hans Asperger in 1944. Sadly Leo Kanner never referenced Hans Asperger even though they both came from the city, spoke the same language, and for a long time interacted with the same group of professionals. Leo Kanner saw his first case of Autism in 1938 (Kanner, 1943) the same time as Asperger's publication.

Hans Asperger (1944) in his paper Autistic Psychopathy in Childhood, is a very clear description of autism. This was later called Asperger's Syndrome by Lorna Wing (1981).

Hans Asperger (1944) recognised the possibility of "academic achievements". He wrote that in the vast majority of cases work performance can be excellent, and with this comes social integration. Able autistic individuals can rise to eminent positions and perform with such achievements. It is as if they had compensatory abilities to counterbalance their social deficiencies. Their unswerving determination and penetrating intellectual powers, part of their spontaneous and original mental activity, their narrowness and single-mindedness, as manifested in their special interests, can be immensely valuable and can lead to outstanding achievements in their chosen area. We can see in the autistic person, far more clearly than with any normal child, predestination for a particular profession from earliest youth. A particular line of work often grows naturally out of their special abilities. Hans Asperger was correct about this.

Autistic disorder (APA, 2000) is defined as a qualitative impairment in social interaction characterised by two of the following items (a) problems with the use of non-verbal behaviour, poor eye contact, failure to develop peer relations, lack of spontaneous seeking to share enjoyment and interests, and lack of social and emotional reciprocity. To make the diagnosis one also needs one item from the category of qualitative impairments in communication such as (1) delay in the development of spoken language, (2) problems with initiating or sustaining speech in those with language, (3) stereotyped and repetitive use of language, and (4) lack of spontaneous make believe play. Finally it is necessary to have one item from restricted repetitive and stereotyped patterns of behaviour either (1) preoccupation with some narrow interest, (2) preservation of sameness, (3) stereotyped and repetitive motor mannerisms, (4) persistent preoccupation with parts of objects. Finally there has to be an onset before three years of age.

Autism and Asperger's syndrome have never been successfully separated from neuropsychological point of view. There is a plan in DSM-V to have an overall diagnostic category called Autism Spectrum Disorder. High Functioning Autism and Asperger's syndrome are terms which have often been used for many years interchangeably.

Rausch and Johnson (2008) point out that Hippler and Klicpera (2003) state that a study of "74 clinical case records of children with Autistic Psychopathy (Asperger's syndrome) diagnosed by Asperger....revealed (at follow up) that 68% of the sample did meet ICD-10 criteria for autism". Mayes et al. (2001) stated that in relation to their research on "DSM-IV diagnosis of autism or Asperger's disorder. All children met the DSM-IV criteria for autistic disorder and absence of early speech delay. They conclude that a DSM-IV diagnosis of Asperger's disorder is unlikely or impossible". Accordingly evidence therefore favours a diagnosis of Autism Spectrum Disorder to cover the broad spectrum of autism and Asperger's syndrome.

6. Autism or schizophrenia?

For a period of time in the 20th century Autism was considered mistakenly as part of schizophrenia. Later it was realised that Autism had an onset generally before three years and schizophrenia typically showed itself in adolescence. Autism and schizophrenia can and do occur together by chance. The relationship is complex as Konstantareas et al (2000, 26) point out that co-morbid disorders maybe "(a) different expressions of the same disorder, (b) involve one disorder leading to another disorder, (c) be chance factors, (d) present different stages of the same disorder, (e) be separate but related disorders due to linked genes or environmental risk factors" (Kraemer, 1996).

Of course, delusions are not rare in the general population. Fleming & Martin (2010), 21, point out that "25% of people have reported voice hearing experience and 5-21% have reported delusions in studies of people from the general population". It appears that stress and anxiety play a role in the development of delusions. Tager-Flusberg & Dominick (2011) note that research has shown that "25% of boys with Asperger's Syndrome reported hallucinations or delusions".

Saulnier at al (2011) point out that there is "less association between ASD and schizophrenia than is observed between schizoid and schizotypal personality disorders". (Hollander at al, 2011).

There are significant overlapping features between Autism Spectrum Disorder and schizophrenia and also some clear differences. One of the major differences is that Autism Spectrum Disorders have an onset before three and schizophrenia has an onset in adolescence. Rausch and Johnson (2008) point out that in terms of social interaction Autism Spectrum Disorders show "impaired social interaction" while schizophrenia shows "limited social contact". In terms of non-verbal social skills they point out that in the Autism Spectrum Disorders there are "impaired non-verbal social behaviours" and in schizophrenia "reduced body language". In terms of body language they point out that in the Autism Spectrum Disorders there are "impaired body posture, impaired gestures" while in schizophrenia there is "posturing; reduced body language". In terms of eye contact they point out that in Autism Spectrum Disorders there is "impaired eye to eye gaze" while in schizophrenia "the face appears immobile and unresponsive, with grimacing". In terms of relatedness and social motivation they point out that in Autism Spectrum Disorders there is "failure to develop peer relationships" while in schizophrenia there is "avolition, limited social contacts". In terms of sharing and emotional reciprocity they point out that in the Autism Spectrum Disorders there are "lack of sharing interests with others' lack of social and emotional reciprocity, while with schizophrenia there is "Alogia, brief, laconic, empty replies; little interest in participating in social activities". The language difficulties in Autism Spectrum Disorders and schizophrenia can easily be confused. I often noticed persons with Autism Spectrum Disorders have very restricted dialogue and give very brief answers to questions. Their answers lack any elaboration. The same can happen in schizophrenia. Rausch and Johnson (2008) point out that "autistic subjects show worse performance on the facial recognition test than do schizophrenic subjects". Emotional perception is much more severely involved in autism than in schizophrenia. Both Autism Spectrum Disorders and schizophrenia have difficulty understanding irony, humour, metaphor, and proverbs. "Theory of mind impairments in schizophrenia tend to be less severe than in autism". (Rausch and Johnson, 2008, Paranoid thinking and psychotic episodes with delusions are not rare in Autism Spectrum Disorders (Abell et al, 2005). Both Autism Spectrum Disorders and schizophrenia can show rocking behaviour and stereotyped behaviour. They can both show odd mannerisms. Nevertheless persons with Autism Spectrum Disorders are far more rigid, inflexible, dominant and controlling in comparison to schizophrenia. They can show similar impairment in living skills but in acute psychosis or schizophrenia, in the acute phase the impairment in living skills is greater in schizophrenia.

Crespi and Badock (2008) proposed that psychosis and autism are diametrical disorders of the social brain. Indeed it was believed for a long time that they were one and the same and they both were covered by the term child psychosis. Later it was realised that there were very significant differences. Crespi and Badcock (2008) point out that autism shows a general pattern "of constrained overgrowth, whereas schizophrenia involves undergrowth". They also point out that "these disorders exhibit diametrical patterns for traits related to social brain development, including aspects of gaze, agency, social cognition, local versus global processing, language and behaviour". I don't find it as clear cut as this.

Konstantareas et al, (2001), noted that in their sample of persons with Autistic Disorder (35%) displayed one or more positive symptoms of schizophrenia, that "Autistic Disorder showed 'more negative symptoms' than schizophrenia and there was overlap in consistency of intellectual response, lack of interest in imitation, and extremes in activity level.

Thought Disorder is more strongly associated with schizophrenia than Autism. Another reason for misdiagnosis of Autism as schizophrenia is the impression given of Thought Disorder by persons with Autism which is well put by Katz (1989), as reported by Konstantareas (2001) "Some of them make remarks that are out of context, carry on conversations with themselves....or laugh at imaginary persons in their environment". These features are very common in ASD. The out of context remarks reveal problems in theory of mind.

Kostantareas et al (2001) showed in their study that "more patients with Autism than schizophrenia were rated as displaying negative symptoms such as affect flattening, alogia and attentional difficulties". There is considerable overlap in symptoms in Asperger's Syndrome / HFA and schizophrenia.

A delusion is partly the best explanation a person can come up with in the context of gene/ environment interaction. Sensory deprivation and extreme stress can lead to paranoid phenomena. I have the experience of a patient with Autism where one room was reconstructed in the home and this sent the patient into paranoid psychosis.

Delusions are more severe in schizophrenia than Asperger's syndrome. All autistic and psychotic phenomena are on a continuum of severity and are on spectrums or dimensions. Most conditions in psychosis are on dimensions and there is a great deal of overlap between psychiatric conditions.

7. The brain

The brains of persons with autism are unusual in the sense that they have atypical cerebral asymmetry. They also have problems with minicolumns of the brain which is the smallest functioning units of the brain (Casanova, 2008), Casanova (2008) points out that "it does appear that minocolumnar pathology may provide an overarching explanation to many of the signs and symptoms observed in autism. Supernumeracy minicolumns provide for cortical expansions and consequently brain growth. Resutls indicated that minicolumns were smaller and their components cells more dispersed than normal". The brain with its increased local connectivity is more creative in certain areas and the poor long range connectivity is a feature that is probably underlying the language and poor social skills. A study by Casanova, Switala, Trippe and Fitzgerald (2007) confirmed these findings in relation to three distinguished scientists.

Happe and Frith (2009) note the "possibility that developmental periods of exceptional brain plasticity may be extended in ASD. Life-long learnings may be of special importance in autism". This could increase creativity.

Lyons & Fitzgerald (2005) put (forward) the theory that right hemisphere impairment leads to a dysfunctional Self development in autism/Asperger syndrome. An optimally functioning RH is required for early intersubjective processes between infant and caretaker. The RH is dominant in the first years of human life when the major brain development during critical periods takes place. Substantial behavioural evidence of infants who later developed autism is supporting the theory of disrupted intersubjective behaviour. These infants did not engage in early mother-infant dyadic experiences which are vital for the maturation of the right brain system. In the majority of cases the causes can be traced to abnormal brain development beginning very early in development, probably in the embryo period. These abnormalities are the basis for the difficulties in deriving maximal advantage from environmental stimulation for children with autism/AS. Therefore, impairments in neurobiology affecting the RH both cause and interact with defects in intersubjectivity and later developing self processes. Cognitive neuroscience studies have shown that the right hemisphere plays a special role in personal relatedness which is intimately linked to the development of the Self. There is evidence for the centrality of the right brain in socio-emotional functioning, cognitive self related processes as shown in face-recognition and autobiographical memory studies as well as its importance for the development of a physical sense of self and its dominance for the Social Self in general. Based on neuropsychological and neurobiological evidence in autism/AS including lateralization evidence we advanced the theory that abnormal brain development particularly in the Right hemisphere due to genetic and/or environmental influences compromises the affective psychosocial development in autism/AS resulting in a disruption of intersubjectivity and leading to an atypical development of the Self.

8. Genetics

Freitag et al (2010) points out that "molecular genetic studies in autism disorder have come a long way from the early linkage studies, which aimed at describing a few loci and subsequently finding one of a few genes of major effect relevant for all cases of autistic disorder. It has now become clear, that autistic disorders are heterogeneous disorders, caused by several rare - most likely - monogenetic disorders (as fragile X syndrome, mutations in TSCI-TSCII, LAMBI, CNTNAP2, PTEN, DHCR7, SHANK3, NLGN3-4,

RPL10)". Freitag et al (2010) concludes that "despite the high-heritability estimates for autistic disorder, no major gene has been observed to be relevant for the majority of autistic disorder diagnoses. In contrast, rare mutations of large effect and a few common variants of small effect in several different genes, which are also involved in different cellular pathways, seem to be caused for many cases of autistic disorder. From a statistical point of view therefore, large autistic disorder and controlled samples are necessary, to prove the causability of specific rare mutations (including CNVs) or variants of small effect as risk factors for autistic disorder". Freitag et al (2010) recommends that it is important "to perform a detailed cytogenetics analysis in every individual with autistic disorder and additional testing for Fragile X syndrome in individuals with autistic disorder and low intelligence - mental retardation in clinical and research settings".

Happe and Frith (2009) points out that there is research focussing on "rare single-gene disorders with a high prevalence of autism, with a recent suggestion that some molecular defects in autism may interfere with mechanisms of synaptic protein synthesis linked, theoretically, to both cognitive impairment and savant skills". This may be important for understanding the genetics of talent and creativity.

Badcock (2008) points out that genomic imprinting means that "even though a child inherits half of its DNA from each parent, we now know that certain genes are only expressed if they come from one parent rather than the other". Children of older fathers and mothers have more children with autism (Badcock, 2008). Badcock (2008) also emphasised the possibility of "faulty genomic imprinting in schizophrenia".

There are some chromosomal regions which show the overlap for both autism and schizophrenia. These include 3p.3q.Xp. From a statistical point of view autism and schizophrenia can occur together (Rausch & Johnson (2008).

9. The social brain

Baron-Cohen et al (2003) points out that "empathizing is a drive to identify another person's emotions and thoughts, and to respond to these with an appropriate emotion. Empathizing allows you to predict a person's behaviour and to care about how others feel. A large body of evidence suggests that, on average, females spontaneously empathise to a greater degree than do males". Baron-Cohen et al (2003) points out that females are superior in "decoding non-verbal communication, picking subtle nuances from tone of voice or facial expression, or judging a person's character". These are all characteristics of a very well functioning social brain. These are all very valuable human characteristics which women on average have stronger traits of. Baron-Cohen et al (2003) points out that "there is evidence for a male advantage in systematising....and (doing) maths, physics and engineering". Baron-Cohen (2002) points out that on average females are better at "sharing and turn-taking"; are more sensitive to facial expressions; put more value in relationships; use more cooperative reciprocal language; and talk more about emotions. These are all evidence of a good social brain. Males with autism are typical examples of impaired brain functioning or high systematisation. It would appear that the minicolumns problems that I have described earlier increase local connectivity and decrease long range connectivity and these underlie the problems with social brain which of course are underpinned by genetic differences and neural cell migration difficulties in the utero and with problems after birth with pruning of nerve cells. This leads to often a larger brain which helps systematising and mathematical creativity but which inhibits the development of the social brain and good language.

A well functioning social brain has an emotional understanding of themselves and other people. They can put themselves in other people's 'shoes'. They can recognise when other people are happy or sad or in pain from the tone of their voice and from reading their faces and particularly their eyes. They can judge other people's emotional intentions. They can express caring words to a person in distress in a meaningful empathetic way. They can 'read' emotional subtext in a novel. They can share other people's emotions and reciprocate emotions. They can understand deception and lies at an average expectable level. If children at about 18 months don't show joint attention and pretend play and don't bring and show various objects and toys to parents they may be at risk of autism (Baron-Cohen, 1992).

Persons with autism show Theory of Mind Deficits (Baron-Cohen, 1995). By theory of mind he meant problems reading other people's minds, their intentions, their state of mind, their level of happiness or distress, and using this to predict what other people might do socially. These abilities are critical to a well functioning "social brain or mind".

They often have a very narrow and simple view of the social world and people. They have great difficulties with complex emotions. They have a very one dimensional view of the world. They have a very concrete view of things and take things very literally. They often have problems understanding symbolism, fiction, irony, humour, metaphors, double meanings, deception, and proverbs. These are all critical to social conversation and social understanding and to a well functioning 'social brain'. Nevertheless they are able to understand certain kinds of humour eg slapstick or the humour that mathematicians use (Lyons and Fitzgerald, 2004). These theory of mind difficulties mean that persons with autism often misinterpret other people's intentions and this makes them very anxious, phobic, or paranoid. Indeed they can develop paranoid delusions which are less severe than delusions ok persons with schizophrenia (Abell et al, 2005).

Because of their empathy or theory of mind difficulties they get very easily into social conflicts, become extremely controlling and dominating, and find it very difficult to resolve conflict. Indeed they can get stuck in a paranoid position in relation to another person. They have poor negotiating skills, poor capacity to give and take, poor social reciprocity, and have to win and insist that the other person give in and submit. They need help with understanding other's minds, the nature of social relationships, social nuance, social know-how, help in reading other people's minds, and seeing things from other's point of view. A lot of this can be subsumed under pragmatic language problems and mind reading skills problems. Therapy aimed at improving mind reading, using pragmatic language therapy can help in reading non-verbal behaviour.

As children and adults they are often bullied because they come across as naive and immature because of their mind reading skills deficits. This often leads to them being bullied and taken advantage of. It is hardly surprising they become very anxious, paranoid or depressed.

A very small group of persons with autism who best fit Asperger's (1938 / 1944) Autistic Psychopathy engage in serious criminal activity eg computer hacking and indeed up to and including murder. This very small subset of persons with autism overlap with Primary Psychopathy (Fitzgerald, 2010). This group also shows callous and unemotional traits (Fitzgerald, 2003) in childhood and later. They can be fascinated by fire setting, killing animals, and in poisons. Some of their behaviour can be experimental. The aggression in persons with this condition was well described by Hans Asperger. Psychosis and Autism can be easily confused as described in this chapter. It is important not to ignore positive or creative aspects.

10. References

[1] Barron-Cohen S. (1997). Are children with autism superior at folk physics. In: H. Wellman and K. Inagaki (Eds.). Children's Theories. New Directions for Child Development: Jossey-Bass.

[2] Crespi B., Badcock C. (2008). Psychosis and autism as diametrical disorders of the social brain. Behaviour and Brain Sciences, 31, 241 - 320.

[3] Fitzgerald M. (1999). Did Isaac Newton have Asperger's Disorder? European Child and Adolescent Psychiatry Journal, 8, 244.

[4] Fitzgerald M. (2000). Einstein: Brain and behaviour. Journal of Autism and Developmental Disorders, 30, 620 - 621.

[5] Fitzgerald M. (2004). Autism and Creativity: Is there a link between autism in men and exceptional ability? Brunner Routledge: New York.

[6] Fitzgerald M. (2008). Autism: Asperger's syndrome – History and First Descriptions. In: J. Rausch, M. Johnson, M. Casanova. Asperger's Disorder. Informa Health Care: New York.

[7] Fitzgerald M. (2010). Young, Violent & Dangerous to Know: Autism and Criminality. Nova Science Publishers, New York.

[8] Abell F., Hare D.J (2005), An Experimental Investigation of The Phenomenology of Delusional Beliefs in People with Asperger's Syndrome. Autism, 9, 5, 515-531.

[9] Asperger H (1938), Das psychisch abnormal kind Wiener Klinische Wochenschrift, 51: 1314-1317.

[10] Asperger H. (1944/1991). Die "autistischen Psychopathen" i.m Kindesalter. Archieves fur Psychiatric and Nervenkrankheiten, 177, 76-136. Translated by Uta Frith (Ed). Autism and Asperger's syndrome. Cambridge: Cambridge University Press, 1991, 37-92.

[11] Baron-Cohen S. Allen J. Sillberge (1992), Can Autism Be Detected at 18 Months? British Journal of Psychiatry, 161, 839-843

[12] Badcock C. (2008), The Imprinted Brain. Jessica Kinsley. Publishers: London

[13] Baron-Cohen S (2002). The Extreme Male Brain Theory of Autism. Trends in Cognitive Sciences, 6, 6, 248-254

[14] Baron-Cohen S (2003), The Essential Difference. Men, Women and the Extreme Male Brain. London: The Penguin Press

[15] Baron-Cohen S., Richler J., Bisarya D., Gurunathan N., Wheelwright S (2003). The Systematizing Quotient an Investigation of Adults with Asperger's Syndrome or High Functioning Autism and Normal Sex Differences. Philosophical Transactions of The Royal Society of London. Biological Sciences, 358, 361-374

[16] Broad J.H. (1977). Schizotypy. Edited by Gordon Claridge. Oxford: Oxford University Press.

[17] Casanova M (2008). Neuropathological Findings in Asperger's Syndrome. In: Asperger's Disorder. Edited by J. Rausch, M. Johnson, M. Casanova. Informa Health Care: New York

[18] Casanova M., Switala A., Trippe J., Fitzgerald M (2007). Comparative Minicolumnar Morphometry of Three Distinguished Scientists. Autism: International Journal of Research and Practice, 11, 6, 557-569

[19] Crespi B.J., Badcock C (2008). Psychosis and Autism as Diametrical Disorders of the Social Brain. Behavioural and Brain Sciences, 31, 284-320

[20] Dehaene S (1997). The Number Sense: How the Mind Creates Mathematics. New York: Oxford University Press
[21] Dryden J. Absalom and Archtophel. In: D.K. Simonton, Greatness: Who makes History and Why? New York: Guildford Press, 1994
[22] Fitzgerald M (2004). Autism and Creativity: Is There a Link Bewteen Autism in Men and Exceptional Ability? Brunner Routledge: New York
[23] Fitzgerald M (2010). Autistic Disorders and Psychopathy. Faculty of teh Psychiatry of learning Disability Annual Meeting, Royal College of Psychiatrist, 7th-8th October 2010, Leeds
[24] Fitzgerald M. (2010), Young, Violent & Dangerous to Know. Nova Science Publishers, New York.
[25] Fitzgerald M., James I (2007), The Mind of the Mathematician. John Hopkins University Press.
[26] Fitzgerald M (2003), Callous & Unemotional Traits in Asperger's Syndrome. Journal of the American Academy of Child & Adolescent Psychiatry, 42, 9, 1011
[27] Fleming M, Martin C (2010). Low Grade Psychotic Symptoms in a Non-Clinical Population. British Journal of Wellbeing, 1, 8, 21-23
[28] Fitzgerald M (1988), Antecedents to Asperger's Syndrome. International Journal of Research and Practice: Autism. 2, 4, 427-429
[29] Freitag C., Stall W., Klauck S., Duketis E., Waltes R. (2010). Genetics of Autistic Disorders: Review and Clinical Implications. European Child & Adolescent Psychatry, 19, 169-178
[30] Frith U (1989). Autism: Explaining the Enigma. Blackwell: Oxford
[31] Gardner H (1997). Extraordinary Minds: Portraits of Exceptional Individuals and an Examination of Our Extraordinariness. New York: Basic Books
[32] Grossman H (1977). Manual on Terminology and Classification in Mental Retardation. Washington DC: American Association on Mental Deficiency.
[33] Happe F., Frith U. (2009). Beautiful Otherness of the Autistic Mind. Philosophical Transactions of the Royal Society of London. Biological Sciences, 364, 1345-1350
[34] Hermelin B. (2001). Bright Splinters of the Mind. London: Jessica Kingsley Publishers, Kingsley
[35] Hippler K., Klicpera C. (2003). A Retrospective Analysis of the Clinical Case Records of 'Autistic Psychopaths' Diagnosed by Hans Asperger and His Team at the University Children's Hospital, Vienna. Philosophical Transactions of the Royal Society of London. Series B: Biological Sciences, 358, 291-301
[36] Howe M. (1999). Genius Explained. Cambridge: Cambridge University Press
[37] Kanner L (1943). Autistic Disturbances of Affective Contact. Nervous Child, 2, 217-250
[38] Konstantareas M, Hewitt T (2001). Autistic Disorder and Schizophrenia: Diagnostic Overlaps. Journal of Autism Developmental Disorders 31, 1, 19-28
[39] Kraemer H (1996). Bio-Statistical Recommendations. Journal of Autism Developmental Disorders 26, 150-154
[40] Lyons V., Fitzgerald M (2004). Humour in Autism and Asperger's Syndrome. Journal of Autism and Developmental Disorders, 34, 5, 521-531
[41] Lyons V., Fitzgerald M (2005). Asperger's Syndrome, Gift or Curse? Nova Scientific: New York

[42] Martindale C (1996). Genetics. In: M. Runco, s. Pritzker. Volume 1: Encyclopaedia of Creativity. Academic Press: London

[43] Mayes S., Calhoun S., Crites D (2001). Does DSM-IV Asperger's Disorder Exist? Journal of Abnormal Child Psychology, 29, 3, 63

[44] Mottron L., Dawson M., Soulieres I (2009). Enhanced Perception in Savant Syndrome: Patterns, Structure and Creativity. Philosophical Transactions of the Royal Society of London. Biological Sciences, 364, 1385-1391

[45] Murray P. (1989). Genius: The History of an Idea. Oxford: Basic Blackwell

[46] Ostwald P. Zegans L (1993). The Pleasures & Pleasures of Genius. Madison WI: International University Press.

[47] O'Connor N. Hermelin B (1987). Visual & Graphic Abilities of the Idiot Savant Artist Psychological Medicine 17, 79-90

[48] Porter R (1998). In: A. Steptoe (Ed). Forward: Genius and the Mind. Studies of Creativity and Temperament. Oxford: Oxford University Press

[49] Rausch J., Johnson M (2008). Diagnosis of Asperger's Disorder. In: J. Rausch, M. Johnson, M. Casanova (2008). Asperger's Disorder. Informa Health Care: New York

[50] Synder A (2009). Explaining and Inducing Savant Skills. Privilieged Access to Lower Level, Less-Processed Information. Philosophical Transactions of the Royal Society of London. Biological Sciences, 364, 1399-1405

[51] Steptoe A (1988). Genius and the Mind: Studies of Creativity and Temperament. Oxford: Oxford University Press

[52] H. Tager-Flusberg, K. Dominick (2011). Co-Morbid Disorder, Chapter 18 In E. Hollander, A. Kolevzon, J. Coyle (2011). Textbook of Autism Spectrum Disorders. American Psychiatric Publishing: Washington DC

[53] Treffert D (2009). The Savant Syndrome: An Extraordinary Condition. A Synopsis: Past, Present, Future. Philosophical Transactions of the Royal Society of London. Biological Sciences, 364, 1351-1357

[54] Waller N., Bouchard T., Lydden D., Tellegen A., Blacker D (1993). Why Creativity Does Not Run in Families. A Study of Twins Reared Apart, Psychological Enquiry, 4, 235-237

[55] Wing L (1981). Asperger's Syndrome – A Clinical Account. Psychological Medicine, Vol 11, 115-129

14

Psychiatric and Occupational Histories in Families of Children with Autism

G. Robert DeLong, Marie MacDonald and Vidya Krishnamurthy
Division of Pediatric Neurology and Division of Genetics and Metabolism, Department of Pediatrics, Duke University Medical Center
USA

1. Introduction

We have consistently found a high incidence of familial major affective disorder, especially bipolar disorder, among relatives of children with idiopathic autism compared to published incidences in the general population. [DeLong and Dwyer 1988] Psychiatric family histories of children with idiopathic autism revealed a dramatically higher incidence of affective disorder than the families of children with symptomatic neurological autism. These findings led us to advance the idea that an important segment of idiopathic autism is etiologically related to familial affective disorder.[DeLong 2004]]

Several subsequent controlled studies found a higher than expected incidence of familial psychiatric disorder, especially major affective disorder, in families of autistic probands, but these findings were minimized or ignored in large part. Larsson et al. [2005] in a careful epidemiological study in Denmark, identified two significant risk factors for autistic spectrum disorder: birth injury and familial affective disorder and psychosis, the second bearing the greater risk.

We have continued to find, in our clinics, a very strong association among idiopathic autism, major affective disorder, and another feature: special intellectual abilities or unusually high achievement, often in mathematical, scientific or computational areas. We have published our clinical observations showing a strong correlation among these three features: idiopathic autism, bipolar disorder and special intellectual abilities in family members in a retrospective open study.[DeLong et al, 2002] We have also pointed out the clinical analogies between idiopathic autism and major affective disorder, as well as the emerging similarities in neurochemistry, pharmacology, neuroimaging, and putative genetic linkages. [DeLong 2004]

The present study was undertaken to compare the family histories of autistic children with a suitable control population, with respect both to psychiatric history and special abilities. We considered that children with genetic or chromosomal disorders which confront their families with an equivalent burden regarding genetic and developmental significance would be a suitable control group. For this, we collaborated with members of the Duke Division of Genetics and Metabolism, who routinely see children with comparable developmental disorders in terms of severity and stress involved to the child's family, and who are accustomed to taking careful and complete family histories. Moreover, the importance of the family history is at least as apparent to the families of children with genetic/metabolic disorders as to families of children with autism - if not more so - so that their maximal cooperation is likely. We planned to determine the incidence of the same psychiatric disorders in both groups of families, utilizing a controlled prospective blinded study. The prior hypothesis was that relatives of children with idiopathic autism would have a higher incidence of familial psychiatric disorder, especially major affective disorder (bipolar disorder and major depression) than the relatives of children in the comparison group, in whom the incidence was expected to approximate the rates in the population at large. A second objective of the study was to determine and compare the occupational and academic achievements of the parents in the two groups, with the hypothesis that achievement reflecting special intellectual abilities would be higher in the autistic group.

2. Methods

The study was conducted jointly by the Duke University Division of Genetics and Metabolism and the Division of Pediatric Neurology. The control group consisted of families of children with major developmental disorders having diagnoses of defined genetic metabolic disorders, major chromosomal disorders, or neurofibromatosis. (Previous control studies of autism of this kind have uniformly utilized Down's syndrome children, which is subject to the possibility that Down's syndrome families may have a different incidence of psychiatric disorder from that of the general population. Including as controls children with varied diagnoses guarded against distortion by any unrecognized factor in family histories of children of any one diagnostic group.)

For the controls, successive families of children having one of the accepted diagnoses, seen in the clinic of the Division of Genetics and Metabolism, were invited to participate in the study. Participation consisted of taking a detailed and complete family history by the senior genetics fellow (VK), with emphasis on a structured psychiatric history and "special abilities and achievements" history, in the course of a comprehensive clinic visit with the family or during a telephone interview. The Family History Method (in which one or more family members, commonly the mother of the proband, is the informant) was used; this method has been shown to be accurate for major psychiatric illness, tending if anything to underestimate true incidence. Family history taking was structured to ensure uniform coverage of all pertinent relatives and all significant disorders [see Table 1.] and included questioning about first, second, and third order relatives of the probands. The study including the family history protocol was approved by the Duke Institutional Review Board. Thirty-four families participated in this phase of the study.

For the autistic probands, a similar complete family history was taken by a senior clinician (GRD), using the same structured outline, during the course of a comprehensive clinic visit. The study group of families of autistic children consisted of thirty-four successive families seen in the Duke Autism Clinic in whom complete family history was obtainable. All probands were diagnosed as having idiopathic autistic spectrum disorder (using DSM-IV criteria) after appropriate neurological, language and developmental assessments, including ADOS; none had detectable dysmorphic, neurological, genetic or chromosomal abnormalities. History taking utilized the same structured outline and the Family History Method, with mother or another family member - such as father or a grandparent -- as the informant. For some analyses, a larger (78) successive group of families of autistic probands was utilized.

In both the study and control groups, psychiatric diagnoses were made using DSM-IV criteria. Diagnoses were accepted if the history indicated they were made by a psychiatrist

or other physician, if the disorder caused significant chronic or recurrent disability, if appropriate psychotropic medication was used, or if hospitalization occurred. Suicide without other evidence was not taken to indicate a psychiatric diagnosis.
In addition to psychiatric diagnoses, parents' occupations and educational history were recorded. Data were recorded for all individuals in each family by diagnosis. Thus we could calculate the percentage of family members diagnosed with each specific diagnosis for each group (Genetic/Metabolic and Autistic). Data analysis utilized the chi square method to determine whether the incidence of specific disorders differed significantly between the study and comparison groups. (For analyses of the percentage of families who had one or more individuals with major affective disorder, a larger group of successive autism families (78) was utilized.)

1.	**Do you know of any nervous or mental disorder in the family?**
a.	Do you know of any other disorder of development among family members?
b.	Is there any family history of depression, alcoholism (or other substance [drug] abuse)? or extreme anxiety disorder?
c.	Is there any history of mental disorder? Bipolar disorder? Post-partum depression? IF SO: Any psychiatric hospitalization? Diagnosis by a psychiatrist? Use of lithium? Or other psychiatric medications? Duration of disability, if any? Schizophrenia?
d.	Is there anybody with social reclusiveness? With obsessive-compulsive disorder?
2.	**Are there any family members with unusual or special abilities, intelligence or talents? Any one with unusually high achievement?**
a.	Anyone with unusual scholarly or mathematical talents?
b.	Anyone with unusual artistic, musical, or mechanical abilities?
c.	Anyone with unusual memory abilities? E.g. photographic memory
d.	Anyone with strongly focused, narrow, intense interests in something?
3.	**Now go through the family pedigree individual by individual as indicated; e.g.:**
	Mother and mother's family:
a.	Have you been well? Any nervous or mental problems?
b.	Do you have brothers and sisters? Have they all been well? (Any nervous or mental problems?) Do they have children? Are those children well?
c.	How about your parents? Are they well? (Do they have any nervous or mental problems?) Do they have brothers and sisters? Any nervous or mental disorders among them that you know?
d.	Anyone with special abilities or achievement in your family?
	Father and father's family: (depending on respondent; here the form of questions assumes it is mother. If father, can use same language as above.)
a.	Is your husband (or: the child's father) well? Does he have any history of nervous or mental problems? If so, elaborate:
b.	Does father have any brothers or sisters? If so, how many? Are they well? Do they have any children? Are those children well?
c.	Are father's parents well? (Any nervous or mental disorders?) Do they have brothers and sisters? How many? Are they well? (etc.)
d.	On father's side, are there any individuals with unusual talents, abilities or achievement? What is father's employment or profession? What was (is) grandfather's employment or profession?

(Respondent: parent or principal caregiver (in practice, usually mother or both parents)

Table 1. Outline of Family History Questioning

3. Data storage and analysis

Data was transferred from the clinician taking the history directly to the data technician of the Autism Program and stored anonymously. Data compilation was done by a technician blind to the families' names or identifiers (which were discarded before this stage) and naïve as to the purpose of the study, including that she was and remained unaware of the initial hypotheses. Data were analyzed utilizing the following:

a. Presence or absence of bipolar disorder, major depression, schizophrenia; plus suicide, attempted suicide; psychiatric hospitalization; use of psychotropic medications.
b. Presence or absence of special abilities, unusual achievement or talents
c. Re each of the above, the incidence of each: i.e. no. having a specific diagnosis/total no. included in pedigree
d. The family history data from the group of autistic probands were compared with that from the group of control families, looking at:

1. The number of families (and percentage of families) having members with bipolar disorder and other specific psychiatric diagnoses.
2. The aggregate burden of major psychiatric disease in each group (i.e. the proportion of individuals in the aggregated families of each group having a history of major psychiatric disorders).
3. The same foregoing analysis was applied to special abilities and achievements.

Diagnosis of special ability or achievement is not systematized. We so classify anyone having doctoral-level education and/or work in scientific or mathematical fields, or a professional career in the arts (usually music), or masters level education and/or work in computer science, finance, engineering or related highly technical field. In addition, we so consider anyone with demonstrable photographic memory or similar prodigy of memory. These criteria are somewhat arbitrary, but derive from our clinical experience and if anything probably underestimate the true incidence.

4. Results

Incidence of familial psychiatric disorder by group

	Metabolic (n = 761)	Autistic (n = 566)	Chi square
Depression	4.86%	12.36%	$X^2 = 24.7, p<0.001$
Suicide	1.31%	1.41%	ns
Bipolar disorder	1.83%	3.71%	$X^2 = 4.3, p<0.05$
Psychiatric hosp.	0.26%	4.24%	$X^2 = 28, p<0.001$
Psychotropic meds	3.02%	5.65%	$X^2 = 5.6, p<0.025$
Schizophrenia	0.53%	1.06%	ns
Attempted suicide	0.26%	0.53%	ns

Table 2. Percentage incidence of psychiatric diagnoses in relatives by group

	Metabolic (n=34)	Autistic (n=78)
Families with bipolar/depression	20	61
Families without " "	14	17

$X^2 = 4.47, p<0.05$

Table 3. Families with individuals having major affective disorder by group

Autism group	
Fathers	Mothers
1. Architect	1. Architect
2. PhD computers	2. Psychologist
3. Engineer, civil	3. RN, Nurse
4. PhD law	4. MPH, public health
5. PhD, professor EE	5. *
6. PhD, professor language	6. *
7. PhD, professor, English	7. *
8. Lawyer	8. *
9. MA, CPA	9. BS, BA
10. Special forces, Army	10. MA, education
11. MD, physician	11. MD, physician
12. MA, banker	12. Architect
13. PhD, professor political sci	13. MS
14. BA, dietitian	14. RN, nurse
15. MS, electrical engineering	15. BS
16. Law librarian	16. *
17. BS, computer engineering	17. *
18. MA, English	18. MA, education
19. MS, computer engineering	19. MS, computer engineer
20. BS, science teacher	20. BS
21. BS	21. DDS, dentist
22. Graphic designer	22. Psychologist
23. Sales manager, 1 year college	23. GED
24. BS, civil engineer	24. *
25. Fireman	25. Dental assistant
26. BS, CEO	26. BS
27. Welder	27. Hairdresser
28. *	28. *
29. PhD, statistician	29. *
30. Computer work, music scholar	30. *
31. "high IQ", no career	31. Counsellor
32. PhD, professor education	32. RN
34. BA, CEO	33. BA, marketing director
35. MD, physician	34. *

Metabolic/genetic Group	
Fathers	Mothers
1. BS, golf course superintendent	1. Pharmacist
2. Marble worker	2. Waitress
3. Factory worker	3. *
4. PhD candidate	4. BA
5. *	5. GED
6. Forklift operator	6. Paramedic
7. Welder	7. Cashier
8. Mechanic	8. High school graduate
9. Roofing worker	9. *
10. *	10. *
11. BS, engineer/manager	11. BA
12. Insurance, project manager	12. Security
13. *	13. *
14. *	14. *
15. *	15. *
16. *	16. *
17. *	17. PhD, pharmacy
18. Cafeteria worker	18. "Slow learner"
19. BS, computer programmer	19. High school graduate
20. *	20. GED
21. Truck driver	21. *
22. Did not graduate high school	22. College, 2 years
23. BS, prison system	23. Dental assistant
24. Optician	24. *
25. *	25. *
26. PhD, music	26. Artist
27. Store manager	27. *
28. High school graduate, printing worker	28. BS
29. BS, mortgage industry	29. BA
30.AA (associate degree)	30.AA, veterinary tech
31. High school graduate, air force	31. College
32. *	32. *
33. Construction work	33. *
34. *	34. *
35. College student: literature and history	35. *

* no data

Table 4. Academic/Occupational Achievements of Parents

5. Discussion

This study confirms once again that the incidence of familial psychiatric disorder, especially major affective disorder, is increased in the families of children with idiopathic autistic spectrum disorder. More strikingly it demonstrates a pronounced increase in the incidence of special intellectual or academic gifts in family members, especially fathers, of children with idiopathic autism. In these respects it corroborates our earlier open studies showing strong correlation among idiopathic autism, familial major affective disorders, and special intellectual ability.[DeLong et al. 2002]

The current study is subject to critique. The family histories were taken by different individuals (VK for the genetic/metabolic families, GRD for the autism families); however, the same objective criteria were utilized by all investigators It may be that the family histories were taken more seriously by the autism families, many of whom were aware of the postulated link between autism and familial affective disorder. However, the families of the genetic/metabolic group were aware that their child had a genetic disorder and thus were presumably motivated to consider family history seriously. As it turned out, the incidences of major affective disorders in the control families approximated published population incidences, thus tending to give greater confidence in the results. In the autism families in the current study, 3.7% of first-, second- and third-degree relatives were reported to have bipolar disorder; this compares to 4.2% in our first study [DeLong and Dwyer, 1988] which included first- and second-degree relatives.

The larger number of relatives in the genetic/metabolic group as compared to the autism group (761 versus 566), for an equivalent number of families is unexplained. It is unlikely to be caused by less intense questioning of the autism families; if anything, we would suspect the opposite. It may be suggested that the higher incidence of familial psychiatric disorder may have the effect of decreasing fertility, or that higher educational status may yield the same result.

The data about academic achievement and occupations of parents, especially fathers, require scrutiny. Although a difference between the two groups was not surprising, the magnitude of the difference was astounding. Several possible contributing factors must be considered: 1) Referral bias: Our Autism Clinic is situated in an area of dense academic and research concentration (Research Triangle Park); but the Genetics clinic is in the same institution. Both clinics draw patients from the same geographic area, and both accept both private and staff patients indiscriminately. Though we have no definite information about this, outside providers may refer children to our Autism Clinic whom they consider to be favorable candidates for pharmacotherapy, which could result in an increased concentration of a certain subgroup of autistic children. Likewise, more educated families may be more insistent on further referral or more vigorous treatment efforts. While these factors may apply to some extent, they seem unlikely to account for all the difference between groups, and seemingly cannot account for the particular, rather narrow, strand of talent represented - primarily engineering, computation, or academic work at professional level. In the Genetic/Metabolic control group, these features are sparsely represented (4 of 24 (17%) compared to 26 of 33 (79%) in the Autism group). 2) Lower than normal ability in the comparison group: Fathers in the comparison group may have lower than expected academic talent or occupational achievement, possibly by virtue of the same genetic disorder expressed in their offspring. We have no data pertinent to this, and in any event, this would not account for the strikingly high achievements and talents identified in the Autism group. 3) Missing data: data are unavailable for eleven fathers of the control group versus one for the autism group. Even assuming all of those missing fell into the talented category - an unreasonable assumption to be sure - only 15 of 35 (43%) in the control group would be so characterized (versus 79% in the Autism group). 4) Investigator bias in selecting cases: The authors are not aware of such bias. Sequential cases were enrolled. Indeed, such "cherry-picking" of certain cases would have to be massive to account for the great differences found.

Overrepresentation of academic and computational ability in fathers of autistic children has been found and remarked repeatedly. We found a strong correlation among fluoxetine-responsive autism, bipolar disorder, and special intellectual abilities in an earlier study. [DeLong et al. 2002] Various authors have supported [Dor-Shav and Horowitz 1984; Wheelwright and Baron-Cohen 2001] a link between autism and special abilities. Others have not found a correlation of autism with socioeconomic status [Tsai et al 1982, Larsson et al. 2005]; we suggest this may be because special intellectual abilities and socioeconomic status are not correlated in any simple way; or perhaps more importantly, the correlation of special abilities in family members with autism only applies to a subgroup of autistic children, and is diluted if one looks at the entire population of individuals considered as autistic.

Cognitive hyperfunction - greater than normal function in certain areas - is an intrinsic part of autism, as manifested in the autistic child (savant features, increased visuo-spatial abilities)[Caron et al 2004] and in the parents and other relatives (unusual intellectual abilities). Any comprehensive theory of autism must account for this hyperfunction. [see for example Nurmi et al 2003] That is why the finding of increased learning and memory ability in mice with GABRA5 gene knockout is so intriguing.[Collinson et al 2004] GABRA5 has been linked with autism; it has been linked with bipolar disorder; and it has been shown that knocking it out produces increased learning and memory [see DeLong 2007]. We have speculated that the special abilities seen in fathers of autistic children may be due to decreased expression of GABRA5, while the autism itself may result from some further distortion of the expression of the same gene, or that plus other neighboring genes, by imprinting.

6. Summary

This investigation was undertaken to clarify the psychiatric and cognitive characteristics of members of the families of autistic children. We were especially interested in the fathers, because of our experience and that of others suggesting that fathers of autistic children may have unusual intelligence or other cognitive gifts, and/or may have an increased incidence of major affective disorders. A control group was chosen from children referred to genetics clinic with various genetic developmental diagnoses thought to entail an effect on family anxiety and need to investigate family history comparable to that imposed by autism. Detailed family history questioning was carried out according to a structured interview (outlined herein).

Results indicated a significant .increase in incidence of psychiatric disorders in family members in the autism families, especially depression, bipolar disorder, and psychiatric hospitalization. Most striking, however, were the remarkably high academic and occupational attainments of the fathers of the autistic children. 79% of these fathers had high academic or occupational achievement compared to 17% of the fathers from the control group. These results reinforce extensive evidence of an association of high cognitive ability with autism, and must be explained in any comprehensive hypothesis of autism.

7. Acknowledgments

We are grateful to the families for their cooperation, and to the John A. Jones Family Trust for their continuing support.

8. References

Caron MJ, Mottron L, Rainville C, Chouinard S. (2004) Do high functioning persons with autism present superior spatial abilities? Neuropsychologia 42:467-481.

Collinson N, Kuenzi FM, Jarolimek W, Maubach KA, Cothliff R, Sur C, Smith A, Otu FM, Howell O, Atack JR, McKernan RM, Seabrook GR, Dawson GR, Whiting PJ, Rosahl TW. (2002) Enhanced learning and memory and altered GABAergic synaptic transmission in mice lacking the alpha 5 subunit of the GABAA receptor. J Neurosci. 22:5572-5580.

DeLong GR, Dwyer J. Correlation of family history with specific autistic subgroups: Asperger syndrome and bipolar mood disease. J Autism Devel Disorders 1988;18:593-600.

DeLong R and Nohria C (1994) Psychiatric family history and neurological disease in autistic spectrum disorders. *Dev.Med.Child Neurol.* 36 (5):441-448

DeLong GR, Ritch CR, Burch S.(2002) Fluoxetine response in children with autistic spectrum disorders: correlation with familial major affective disorder and intellectual achievement Dev Med Child Neurol.44:652-9.

DeLong R (2004) Autism and familial major mood disorder: are they related? *J Neuropsychiatry Clin.Neurosci.* 16 (2):199-213

DeLong GR. GABA(A) receptor alpha5 subunit as a candidate gene for autism and bipolar disorder: A proposed endophenotype with parent-of-origin and gain-of-function features with or without oculocutaneous albinism. Autism 2007;11:135-147.

Dor-Shav NK, Horowitz Z. (1984) Intelligence and personality variables of parents of autistic children. Journal of Genetic Psychology 144(1st half):39-50.

Larsson HJ, Eaton WW, Madsen KM, Vestergaard M, Olesen AV, Agerbo E, Schendel D, Thorsen P, Mortensen PB. (2005) Risk factors for autism: perinatal factors, parental psychiatric history, and socioeconomic status. Am J Epidemiol. 161(10):916-25

Nurmi EL, Dowd M, Tadevosyan-Leyfer O, Haines JL, Folstein SE, Sutcliffe JS.(2003) Exploratory subsetting of autism families based on savant skills improves evidence for genetic linkage to 15q11-13. J Am Acad Child Adolesc Psychiatry 42: 856-63

Tsai L, Stewart MA, Faust M, Shook S. Social class distribution of fathers of children enrolled in the Iowa Autism Program. J Autism Dev Disord 12: 211-221.

Wheelwright S, Baron-Cohen S. The link between autism and skills such as engineering, maths, physics and computing: a reply to Jarrold and Routh. (2001) Autism. 5:223-7.

Part 6

Moral Judgment and Criminal Law

15

Moral Judgment in Autism

Hirotoshi Hiraishi
Cognition & Learning section, Primate Research Institute, Kyoto University, Japan

1. Introduction

Haidt (2001) defined morality as an evaluation (good or bad) of the actions or character of a person and is made with respect to a set of virtues held to be obligatory by a culture or subculture. This definition remarks its nature shortly but it does not express all aspects of morality. So what is morality? What is the role of morality in our human society? Is morality nature or nurture? There are many questions about morality. Therefore, it is needed to review the history of moral study first and list related theories.

In the first period, morality is dealt as a philosophical problem. Plato was the first person to think ethics philosophically in the 4th century B.C.. In the next period, Socrates turned the philosophical/theoretical questions to the practical human questions. After that, Aristotle discussed morality in his book "Nicomachean Ethics". As same as Socrates, Aristotle thought ethics as practical matters. In the Aristotle's work, his main insistence was that good behavior is moderate behavior, not extreme behavior, and good life would be given by the appropriate/moderate judgment in each situation. His theory affected tons of later philosophers. In the third period, morality was treated as social philosophy. In 1759, Adam Smith wrote "The Theory of Moral Sentiments" from the view point of social philosophy. In his work, he discussed that the impartial spectator's view makes human act as unobjectionable and judge the propriety of other's behaviors. In the fourth period, morality is dealt from the view of development. In the 20th century, Piaget (1932) proposed his moral developmental theory that morality has been acquired through a childhood and Kohlberg (1969) improved Piaget's theory. The contexts of their theories would be explained later. After that, Eisenberg (1979) shed the light on the positive aspect like pro-social values of moral development although prohibition is needed when a child learns morality in their theories. Moreover, Turiel (1980, 1983) proposed a new moral developmental theory that morality and social convention are different and they have different developmental processes. These almost theories are focused on moral development but Gilligan (1982) focused on the moral differences between genders that males are justice-based moral evaluations and females are care-based ones. As same as Gilligan (1982), Eisenberg (1989) gave an equivalent value to justice-based and care-based moralities and used the next six levels; self-centered reasoning, needs-oriented reasoning, stereotyped and/or approval-oriented reasoning, empathetic reasoning, partly internalized principles, and strongly internalized principles. Like these, many moral theories has been proposed.

One of the most remarkable moral theories was proposed by Piaget (1932). Piaget was a developmental psychologist and proposed the genetic epistemology in intelligence that comes from the mixture of the cognitive development as the ontogeny and the history of science and technology as the phylogeny. This embryological parallelism assisted to raise a problem whether morality is innate or not. Therefore, it is needed to think moral development from the phylogenic view. Almost of our human behaviors are evolved from ancient animal's ones. This means that the key of moral acquisition is in the duplicated things between humans and other animals. Those are fitness and society. Fitness is very important for creatures to live and not only humans but also other animals have societies that are specific to each species. These two things have a very close relationship. For example, some animals are gregarious for avoiding predator animals and others are solely. Of course, human ancestors are thought to gather in crowds for avoiding predators. This gathering effect reduces the risk of individuals hunted and as the result it increases the fitness of the escaped individuals. Moreover, the behavior of one of a group members affects to the other members (i) positively, (ii) none (neutrally) or (iii) negatively in a group. These differences are divided from the view point of the affected individual's fitness. Cosmides and Tooby (1992) speculated that human have evolved to be able to detect a cheater easily. This theory is that animals act as increasing their inclusive fitness and when the cheaters decrease other's inclusive fitness, the others feel the negative effect from the cheaters' act. Therefore human evolve as stopping cheating acts. Therefore, we can think of this cheater detection system as a kind of or the origin of morality. Pardales (2002) described that moral judgment plays an important role in our attempts to lead our lives meaningful. In other words, the reason why moral judgment is important for human life is to avoid risks from the surroundings and to enhance fitness. From these, morality plays an important role in keeping each society. However, there is a strange example. That is incest. Incest that is sexual intercourse between close relatives would be usually avoided in animals, because it decreases the fitness genetically in the following generations. In human, although incest is "legally" prohibited in almost our human societies now, the ruling class drawn on incest for keeping their wealth and the derived influence in their class until medieval age.

When thinking about animals, there is no morality like human. Why do not animals have morality like us? Tse (2006) said that humans still have associative learning in common with other animals but humans have one-shot learning of associations among arbitrary categories of things and events. This suggests that because one-shot associative learning is needed to moral acquisition, it is hard for animals to get morality. Moreover, categorical learning that needs try and error is difficult to animals, even primates without human.

From Tse (2006), there is a possibility that moral judgment can be seen as a kind of well-trained moral knowledge tasks. There is a ward "moral intuition" that means moral assessments, judgments, or responses to someone's behavior in actual or hypothetical scenarios, where these responses typically occur quickly or automatically and carry with them a strong feeling of authority or appropriateness but where one need not be (and often is not) aware of any conscious reasoning process that leads to this assessment. Intuition, in this sense, is meant to contrast with moral judgments that are reached on the basis of some extended process of deliberate or explicit reasoning. A recent fMRI study showed that Japanese chess ("Shogi") experts activate the precuneus area of parietal lobe that is related to episodic memory and visualizing images rather than amateurs when they choose the next

step with longtime and the experts activate the caudate nucleus that is related to goal-directed behavior rather than the amateurs did not activate when players choose the next step as quick as they can (Wan et al., 2011). This means that repetitive training/learning changes brain activities and forms specific neural networks that belong to each by each and we can use those different neural networks for each situation flexibly. From their study, it can be thought that morality is not innate. In other words, the neural base is just the base and appropriate moral judgment needs this moral neural bases and moral knowledge. Moreover, appropriate moral judgment is learnt through our daily lives with try and error.
Emotion that is the most basic human function that comes from earlier species and is related to limbic system plays an important role for moral judgment. The examples of moral emotion are guilt, shame, embarrassment and pride (Haidt, 2003). Although babies do not have these emotions, from the view point of moral development, it is thought that the first step of morality begins from like and dislike during babyhood. For a baby, the only way to express his/her will is crying and smiling. This is very nascent and basic behavior to tell his/her demands. Then this faddiness is discharge of emotion. Like this, we human have emotion since we are babies. This means that the limbic system is the key part of morality in brain.

1.1 Moral development in typical developed people

As written above, Piaget (1932) proposed the moral developmental theory. The main claim of their theories is that human learn morality from prohibition from others and conventional rule is their keyword. Piaget's theory is composed of 4 stages; one is the period of sensory-motor intelligence (0-2 yrs old), one is the period of operational period (2-7 yrs old), one is the concrete operational period (7-12 yrs old) and the other one is the period of formal operations (12 yrs old and onwards). This Piaget's theory focused on the development of intelligence and morality is acquired according to the development of intelligence. Kohlberg (1969) improved the Piaget's moral development theory from the view point of developmental stage of morality with children's reaction to moral dilemmas and reconstructed into 3 levels that each level contains 2 stages; one is the pre-conventional level (obedience and punishment orientation stage and self-interest orientation stage), one is the conventional level (interpersonal accord and conformity stage and authority and social-order maintaining orientation stage) and the other one is the post-conventional level (social contract orientation stage and universal ethical principles stage). The Kohlberg's theory is constructed on the thought that the development of morality is related with the development of cognitive ability and role-taking ability.
Recently, neuroimaging studies revealed the relationship between morality and other cognitive abilities (especially "Theory of Mind", emotion and reasoning) (See review; Casebeer, 2003). "Theory of Mind" is a new theory and it has been focused in these decades. "Theory of Mind" is an ability to attribute independent mental states to self and others in order to explain and predict behavior, has been suggested to arise from a dedicated, domain-specific, and possibly modular cognitive mechanism (Premack, D. and Woodruff, G., 1978; Leslie, A., 1987). Keeping our social lives appropriately needs smooth communications between each other and read the situations around us. Reading the situation correctly is important, because we survive through negative situations. This reading situation behavior needs "Theory of Mind" and Hayashi (2009, 2010) reported "Theory of Mind" in children, especially from the view point of omission and commission.

He suggested that "Theory of Mind" is related to child development and morality. As same as Hayashi (2009, 2010), Wimmer et al. (1985) reported young children's conception of lying. They studied young children's conception of lying from the view point of development and moral intuition. These findings showed (a) that young children's moral intuition about lying is quite advanced as compared to their definition of "to lie" and (b) that children's realist definition of "to lie" carries a strong negative moral connotation that overrides their usual subjectivist moral intuitions.

These studies showed developmental changes of child in many cognitive abilities and morality. However, because the development of morality would be affected by many social and cognitive environments, further studies are needed to reveal the overall picture of the morality.

1.2 Brain activity during moral judgment in typical developed people

In this decade, the number of neuroimaging studies about moral judgment has been increased and moral dilemma studies gave new evidences. Those studies showed many activated brain areas; prefrontal cortex and orbito-frontal cortex (Broadmann area 10), superior temporal sulcus and amgdala (Greene and Haidt, 2002) and these brain areas suggest that morality is related to emotion, "Theory of Mind" and reasoning, too (Casebeer, 2003).

Greene and Haidt (2002) reviewed brain activities related to moral judgment. They guessed that reasoning, emotion and "theory of mind" is the components of moral judgment from the comparison of previous moral judgment neuroimaging studies and other studies. However, the participants of these neuroimaging studies are typical developed adults and the brain activities are already fixed. Therefore, it is not well known how the developmental change of morality.

However, the stimuli used in these moral judgment neuroimaging studies were mainly negative things. Moll et al. (2002) also reported the brain activities of typical developed participants during moral dilemma tasks. In their study, the negative moral emotion of participants was elicited and this helped them to judge the morality of it. At the same time, they insisted that participants compare some parallel imaginary outcomes and choice the one which they judge it one of the most appropriate. As same as Greene et al. (2002), Moll et al. (2002) reported that orbito-frontal cortex has dedicated sub-regions specialized in processing specific forms of social behaviors.

There is another view that moral judgment is a kind of reward related decision-making. From this view point, the brain areas activated by moral judgment may overlap the brain areas activated by decision-making or reward. There are many reward and decision-making related neuroimaging studies. These studies showed that

Hiraishi et al. (2007) researched brain activity during moral judgment that compared typical developed children and autistic children. In the study, typical developed children showed orbito-frontal cortex activity rather than autistic children. Moreover, my unpublished behavioral data showed that judging-bad is faster than judging-good and that judging-bad does not activated orbito-frontal cortex rather than judging-good. These results suggested that judging-good and judging-bad might use different neural circuit. Moreover, this fast judging-bad time rather than judging-good one can reinforce the view point of fitness. The situation that a person judges as bad is to be avoided.

Harenski et al. (2008) examined based on the Gilligan's theory (1982) showed that moral sensitivity is different between genders in neural mechanisms. Their evidence is that females activated posterior and anterior cingulated and anterior insula and males activated superior temporal sulcus rather than each other gender during moral judgment.
Harenski et al. (2010) gave evidence that the ventro-medial prefrontal cortex may contribute more to moral deliberation than moral intuition, whereas the temporo-parietal junction may contribute more to moral intuition than to moral deliberation. My unpublished data showed that judging-good (moral deliberation) needs longer time than judging-bad (moral intuition) and judging-good activated orbito-frontal cortex more but judging-bad deactivated there.
However, there are few studies that clarify the changes of moral development and its related brain activities from child to adult.

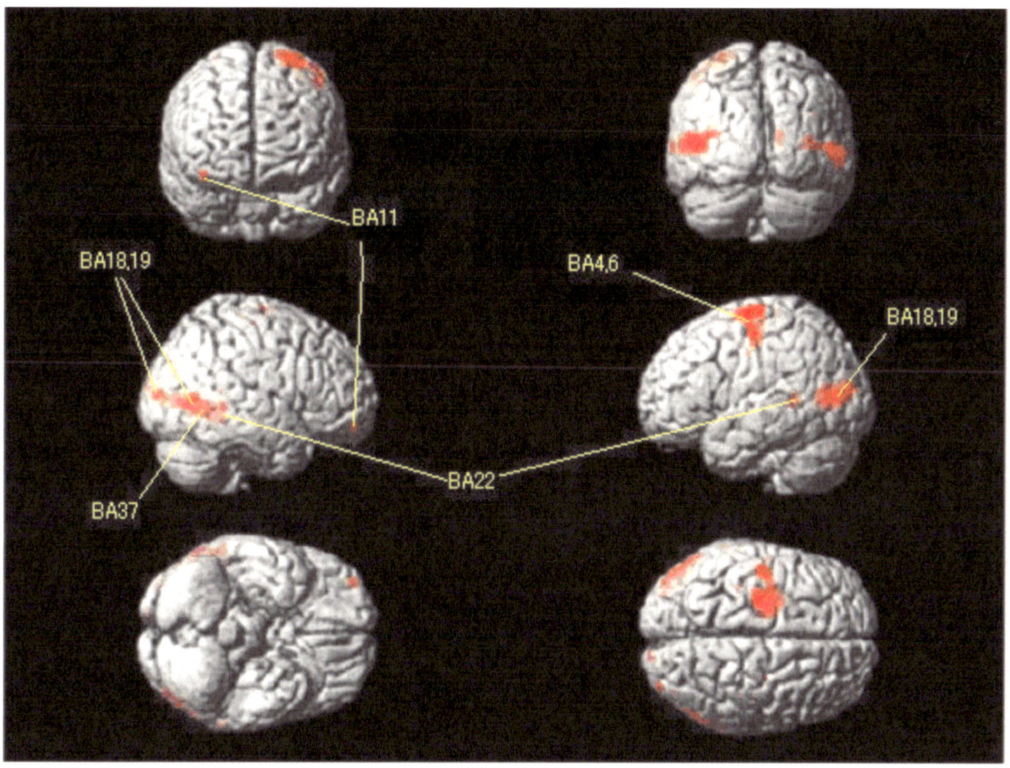

Fig. 1. An example of brain activity induced by moral judgment in a typical developed child (13yrs old). Those are left BA 4, 6, 18, 19, 22 and right BA 11, 18, 19, 22, 37.

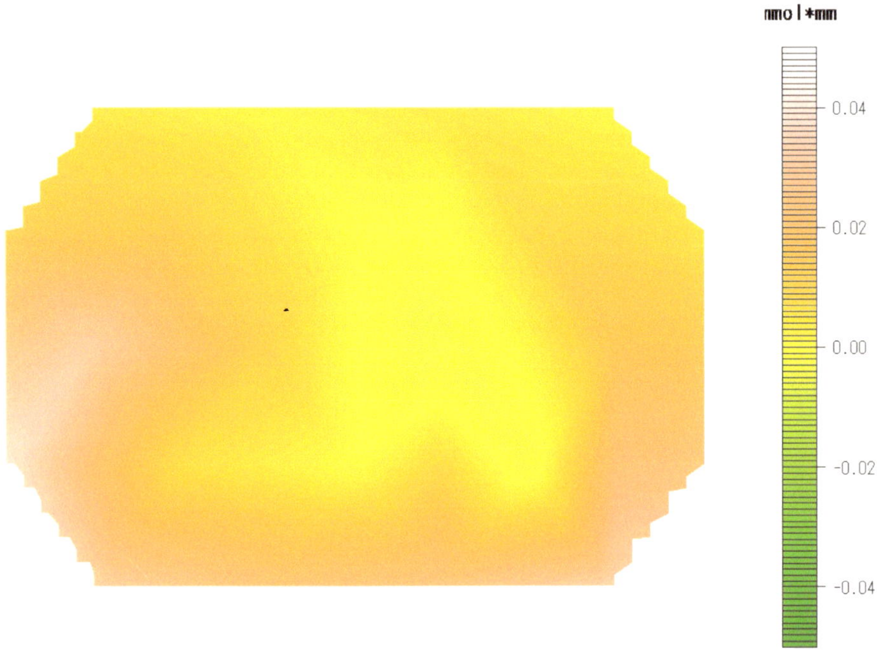

Fig. 2. Brain activity induced by moral judgment as good. The left side is the right hemisphere and the right side is the left one. The top is superior and the bottom is inferior.

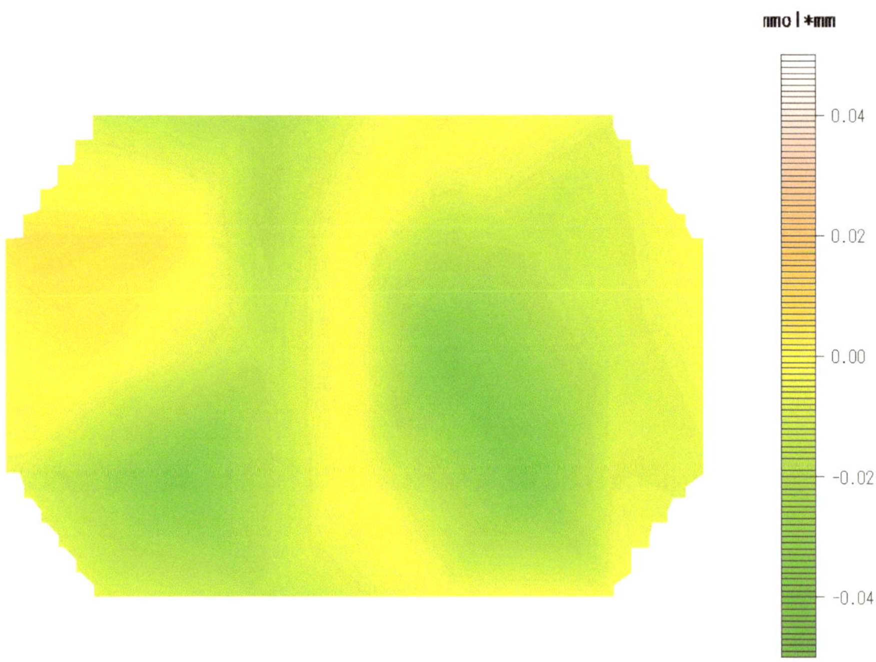

Fig. 3. Brain activity induced by moral judgment as bad. The left side is the right hemisphere and the right side is the left one. The top is superior and the bottom is inferior.

1.3 Autistic moral judgment and its development

Autism is diagnosed by behavioral features (qualitative impairment in social interaction, qualitative impairments in communication, and restricted repetitive and stereotyped patterns of behavior, interests and activities) and the cause comes from abnormalities of the central nerve system (APA, 2000). In Japan, one of the major complaints of autistic children is sometimes shoplifting. After that, they are diagnosed as autism. Almost autistic people have some deficits in their cognitive aspect and these deficits affects negatively to their social lives. Moreover, it is well known that autistic people are difficult to learn unwritten rules like morality. The number of autistic moral judgment study is very few and those studies investigated moral judgment from the view point of "Theory of Mind".

Autism is one of pervasive developmental disorders characterized by qualitative abnormalities in reciprocal and social interactions and in patters of communication, and by restricted and stereotyped repetitive repertoire of interests and activities and they have abnormality in their central nervous system (World Health Organization, 1992). Like this, autism is diagnosed by behavioral features. However, almost of them have many disorders in the cognitive aspect. Sometimes, these features give negative effects to their social lives. Baron-Cohen et al. (1985) adopted "Theory of Mind" to autistic people and pointed out that they lack "Theory of Mind". For example, they are difficult to read a situation. This may related to their deficits of "Theory of Mind".

There is one study about moral understanding in children with autism (Grant et al., 2005). Their study focused on "theory of mind" mainly and reasoning and executive functions. Their result is that children with autism have deficits in complex reasoning and executive functions. Not only autistic children but also typical developed children do not make it clear the relationship between acquirement of morality and its related social abilities.

1.4 Brain activity during moral judgment in autistic people

There is only one neuroimaging study about autistic moral judgment (Hiraishi et al., 2007). They reported that the orbito-frontal cortex was not activated in autistic children (Fig. 1.) although the brain area was activated in typical developed children (Fig. 2.) when they judged the morality of a behavior of the protagonist in a picture (Table 1). Because previous neuroimaging studies of moral judgment in typical developed persons showed that orbito-frontal cortex is one of the most moral related brain areas (Haidt and Greene, 2002; Casebeer, 2003), this is one of the most important evidence that autistic children deficits kinds of moral activities. However, Hiraishi et al. (2007) reported that the judgments of morality in autistic children are appropriate. This means that autistic children acquired moral knowledge properly but they did not use them properly in their daily lives. These are sound like a contradiction. Moreover, there are some suggestions that autism is sometimes lack their prefrontal cortex activities including orbital area. These suggested that further studies are needed to the lack of the prefrontal cortex activities during moral judgment in autism and moral knowledge.

Because the behavioral data suggested that autistic children can judge morality correctly as same as typical developed children did, the difference of the OFC activation Autistic children judge morality appropriately in their study. This means that other neural circuit activity in autism might compensate orbito-frontal cortex activity in typical developed people during moral judgment. However, because the stimuli in this study contain both good and bad situations, the brain activities induced by judging-good and judging-bad are not divided into each judgment. Therefore, further study is needed to make it clear whether judging-good and judging-bad are processed in different neural networks and it is adopted the relationship between judging-good and judging-bad and those neural networks in autistic people as same as typical developed people.

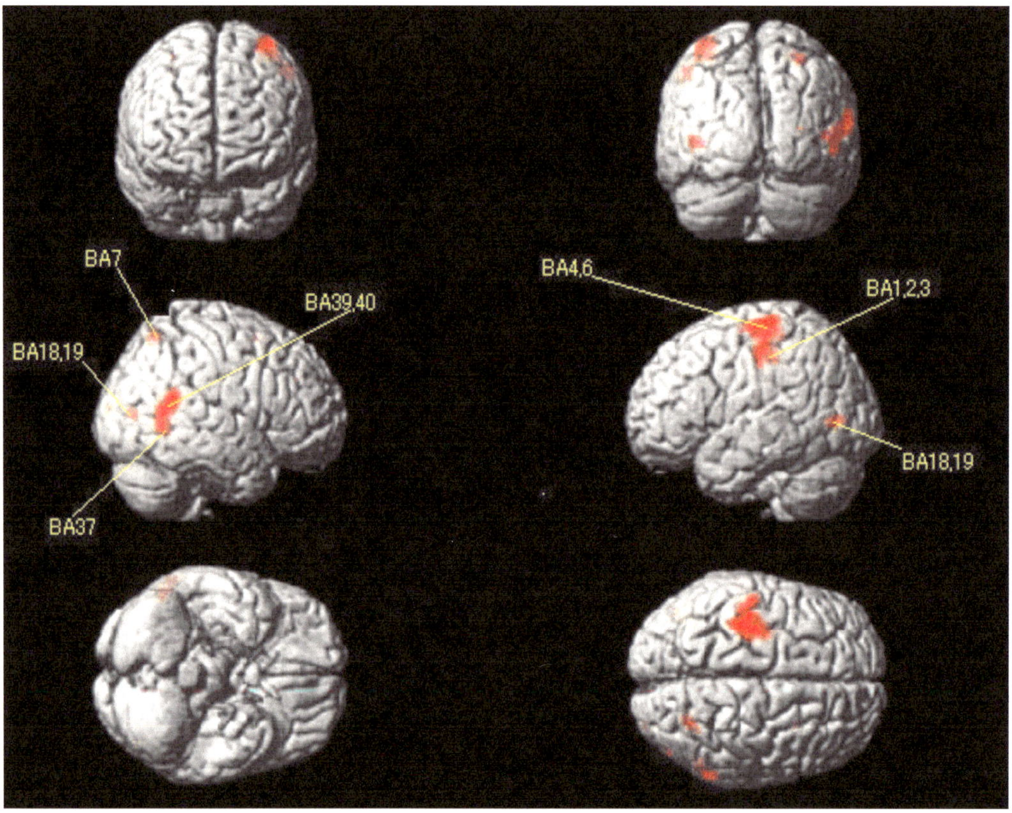

Fig. 4. An example of brain activation induced by moral judgment in a child with Asperger's syndrome. Those are left BA1, 2, 3, 4, 6, 19 and right BA 7, 18, 19, 37, 39, 40. This is the color version of the figure in Hiraishi et al. (2007).

participant	hemisphere	brain activated area (BA)													
TD1	left				4		6			18	19	22			
	right								11	18	19	22	37		
TD2	left				4					18	19				
	right								11	18	19				
AD1	left	1	2	3	4		6				19				
	right							7		18	19		37	39	40
AD2	left	1	2	3	4	5	6	7	11	18	19				
	right								11	18	19				

Table 1. Activated brain area (BA:Broadman area) by moral judgment

2. Future study

Although the number of moral study has been increased day by day, the information is not enough to understand the essence of morality. Almost previous moral judgment study used a common method that compares negative situation and negative situation and their participants are typical developed adults. Moreover, in these studies, participants were asked which situation is worse. Of course, judging a negative situation is important for enhancing a person's fitness because it will give avoidance from that situation. However, judging a good situation may not be in the same line. Avoiding a good situation will not give more fitness than nothing.

Not only almost previous studies used negative moral situations as stimuli, but also participants were asked to judge the morality compared with negative situations. However, there are many situations that moral judgment is needed not only a negative situation but also a positive situation.

The developmental process of morality is mainly known from the behavioral studies. It is needed to investigate (1) the comparison of positive situation and another positive situation, (2) positive moral judgment, (3) developmental changes, (4) the relationship between other brain activities between ToM and emotion reasoning and (5) the brain activities of them. These results would suggest us better way that the autistic children acquire morality easily.

Although there are relationships between morality and other cognitive abilities that are needed to live appropriate social lives (e.g. "Theory of Mind"), it is not still unknown the developmental association between them.

There is a possibility that morality is composed of two different brain networks that one is related to negative moral judgment and another one is related to positive one (Young et al., 2011).

There is only one study that reported moral understanding in children with autism (Grant et al., 2005). They discussed that moral reasoning is related to "Theory of Mind" and deficits in complex reasoning and executive functions. However, there is no study to make it clear the role of emotion in moral judgment. In autistic people, moral judgment and moral understanding is different thing. There is a possibility that autistic children have moral knowledge but they do not judge appropriate morality in the real situation (Hiraishi et al., 2007). O'Neill and Petrinovich (1998) showed cross-cultural study of moral intuitions. In their case, Taiwanese students those are representatives of the Eastern culture and U.S.A. students those are representatives of the Western culture were compared and they showed similar reactions to moral dilemma tasks. Their study showed not only fundamental but also derivative moral attitudes are not so different between cultures and suggested that the cultural effect is low in morality. As the examples of their study, here I show the episode of the emperor Gaozu of Han and the Ten Commandments in the Bible. The Emperor Gaozu of Han remade the law from details to fundamentals; "Punish offenders who murders, hurts and thieves". The Ten Commandments is a list of religious and moral imperatives in the Bible. Both of them punish a person who attacks to others and threats others' wealth and family, and latter one admonishes to make good social relationships between neighbors. Like these, morality is affected by religion and culture. Therefore, cross-cultural moral study would be needed.

Moreover, social skill training (SST) is recently used to get the skills for communicating with others smoothly. The targets of SST are not only typical developed persons and children but also persons and children with developmental disorder. However, there are still few studies that clarify the relationship between behavioral changes that induced by SST and the related brain activity changes. The gathering of these reports would make a new way to assist autistic people to live comfortable in our human society that is mainly composed of typical developed people.

3. Acknowledgment

At first, I appreciate the offer by InTech and the support of Ms Lorkovic. This is a very good opportunity for me to review my research. Next, I want to thank Dr. Hashimoto who gave me this interesting research topic. At last, I am deeply grateful to my parents and my family.

4. References

American Psychiatric Association. (2000). Text Revision of the Diagnostic and Statistical Manual of mental disorders fourth edition.

Baron-Cohen, S., Leslie, A., Frith, U., 1985. Does the autistic child have a'theory of mind'? Cognition 21, 37–46.

Casebeer, WD. (2003). Moral cognition and its neural constituents. Nature Reviews Neuroscience 4, 840-847.

Cosmides, L. and Tooby, J. (1992). Cognitive adaptations for social exchange. In J. Barkow, L. Cosmides and J. Tooby (Eds.), *The adapted mind* (pp. 163-228). New York: Oxford University Press.

Eisenberg-Berg, N. (1979). Development of children's prosocial moral judgment. Developmental Psychology, 15, 128–137.

Eisenberg, N. (1989). The development of prosocial values. In N. Eisenberg, J. Reykowski, & E. Staub (Eds.). Social and moral values: Individual and social perspectives. Hillsdale, NJ: Erlbaum.Gilligan, C. (1982). In a different voice. Harvard University Press.

Grant, CM., Boucher, J., Riggs, KJ., and Grayson, A. (2005). Moral understanding in children with autism. Autism, 9(3), 317-331.

Greene, JD and Haidt, J. (2002). How (and where) does moral judgment work? TRENDS in Cognitive Sciences, 6(12), 517-523.

Greene, J.D., Sommerville, R.B., Nystrom, L.E., Darley, J.M., & Cohen, J.D. (2001). An fMRI investigation of emotional engagement in moral Judgment. Science, Vol. 293, Sept. 14, 2001, 2105-2108.

Haidt, J. (2001). The Emotional Dog and Its Rational Tail: A Social Intuitionalist Approach to Moral Judgment. Psychological Review, 108(4), 814-34.

Hayashi, H. (2009). Is there a developmental difference in recognizing harm through action and inaction (commission and omission) based on first-order mental states? Psychologia, 52, 209-218.

Hayashi, H. (2010). Young children's moral judgments of commission and omission related to the understanding of knowledge or ignorance. Infant and Child Development, 19, 187-203.

Hiraishi et al (2007). A Preliminary fMRI Study of Moral Judgment Task in High Functioning Autistic Children. No To Hattatsu. 39 (5); 360-5. (Article in Japanese).

Joyce, R. (2006). *The Evolution of Morality*. Massachusetts, U.S.A.: MIT Press.

Kohlberg, L. (1969). Stage and sequence: The cognitive -developmental approach to socialization. In D. Goslin (Ed.). *Handbook of socialization theory and research.* Chicago: Rand McNally.

Leslie, A., (1987). Pretence and representation: The origins of 'theory of mind'. Psychol. Rev. 94, 412–426.

O'Neill, P. and Petrinovich, L. (1998). A Preliminary Cross-Curtural Study of Moral Intuitions. Evolution and Human Behavior. 19(8)349-367.

Pardales, M. J. (2002) So, how did you arrive at that decision? Connecting moral imagination and moral judgement, Journal of Moral Education, 31(4), 429–436.

Petrinovich, L and O'Neill, P. (1996). Influence of wording and framing effects on moral intuitions. Ethology and Sciobiology. 17(3)145-71.

Piaget, J. (1932). *The moral judgment of the child.* New York: Free Press.

Premack, D., Woodruff, G., (1978). Does the chimpanzee have a 'theory of mind'? Behav. Brain Sci. 4, 515–526.

Smith, A. (1759). "The Theory of Moral Sentiments"

Tse, P. (2006). How the evolution of symbolic cognition transformed human morality. In:Sinnott-Armstrong, W. (Ed.), Moral Psychology, Volume 1: The Evolution of Morality. MIT Press.

Turiel, E. (1980). The development of social-conventional and moral concepts. *Moral development and socialization*. Allyn and Bacon, INC.

Turiel, E. (1983). The development of social knowledge: Morality and convention. *Cambridge, England: Cambridge University Press.*

Young, L et al. (2011). Neural evidence for "intuitive prosecution": The use of mental state information for negative moral verdicts. Soc Neurosc.

Wimmer, H. Gruber, S., and Perner, J. (1985). Young Children's Conception of Lying: Moral Intuition and the Denotation and Connotation of "to Lie". Developmental psychology. 21(6) 993-5.

16

Autism Spectrum Disorders and the Criminal Law

Ian Freckelton
Senior Counsel, Melbourne, Australia; Professor, Law Faculty, Department of Forensic Medicine and School of Psychology and Psychiatry, Monash University, Australia

1. Introduction

While criminal offending by persons with Autism Spectrum Disorders is rare (*see R v George*, 2004: at [44]; see also Bishop, 2008), the symptoms of such disorders have the potential to be relevant to almost every aspect of the criminal justice process from interviews with suspects by the police, to accused persons' fitness to stand trial, a variety of defences to which accused persons may be entitled, especially self-defence, mental impairment/insanity, provocation and diminished responsibility, and to the sentencing process. For over 20 years there have been suspicions (see eg Tantam, 1988) that persons with such disorders may not just be alienated from the general community, but have been over-represented in the criminal justice population. "In 2004 the National Autistic Society in the United Kingdom (2004: 4) stated: "There is (sic) no data on the proportion of people with autism in the prison population. The NAS is aware of reports from families of distressing encounters with the police where an individual's condition has not been recognised, or where their needs are not properly understood in prison.Without an informed and flexible approach to management custodial sentences can be highly punitive and completely unproductive for a person with autism, and it is important that their increased vulnerability to abuse is recognised.""

Recent court decisions in the United Kingdom, Australia, New Zealand and Canada are notable for their exploration of ways in which such disorders, especially Asperger's disorder, have the potential to exclude or mitigate criminal responsibility and culpability.

This chapter explores issues arising in the criminal law for persons with the Autism Spectrum Disorder that most often arises in criminal law proceedings: Asperger's disorder, often described as high functioning autism. It does so by analysing recent court decisions in a number of countries and reflecting upon the extent to which expert evidence is enabling courts to evaluate effectively the ramifications of the disorder within the context of determining criminal responsibility and culpability.

1.1 Autism spectrum disorders and criminal offending

The link between Autism Spectrum Disorders and conduct with the potential to engage the criminal justice system dates back to the early research in the area during the 1940s. Dr Asperger described one of the children whom he assessed in his landmark study, Fritz V, as quickly becoming "aggressive" and "attacking other children", while he observed Harrow L to attack other children, to gnash his teeth, to hit out blindly and to show "social unconcern in sexual play with other boys", allegedly going as far as attempted homosexual acts (Asperger, 1994; see though Miller and Ozonoff, 1997). Dr Asperger identified as features that his subjects had in common impairments in social maturity and social reasoning, as well as in communication and control of emotions. Amongst other reasons, this led him to propose for their pathology the term "childhood autistic personality disorder" (Autistische Psychopaten im Kindesalter) (see also Chawarska, Klin and Volkmer, 2006; Carly, 2008; O'Reilly and Smith, 2008; Patrick, 2008, Freckelton, 2011).

An issue that goes to the heart of Autism Spectrum Disorders and to their relevance to criminal conduct is the propensity of those with them to act in a socially unacceptable and/or criminal manner (see Langstrom et al, 2009; Warren, 2006). More research in this regard is needed with most analyses being based on small and potentially unrepresentative samples. As noted above, Dr Asperger himself identified within his seminal study a variety of forms of antisocial behaviour. Wing (1981) noted that four of the 34 cases to which she referred in her research had a history of bizarre antisocial acts. Mawson, Grounds and Tantam (1985) four years later explored the link between violence and Asperger's in a case study. Simblett and Wilson (1993) in 1993 described three persons diagnosed with Asperger's as having "severe temper tantrums" and two with violent behaviour (see too Everall and Lecouteur, 1990). Barry-Walsh and Mullen (2004) accepted that "Given the low prevalence of Asperger's Syndrome, it is not clear how commonly violent and potentially criminal behavior occurs" but contended that "Consistently a direct relationship between the offending and the clinical features of the syndrome has been identified. This is usually placed in the context of deficits in social relatedness or rigidity in thought and behavior." Freckelton and List (2009) commenced a process of analyzing court decisions in which Asperger's had figured, arguing for the need for better forensic understanding of the disorder.

Relatively little attention has been given as yet to the forensic repercussions of Autism Spectrum Disorders (see though Murrie et al, 2002; Silva, Ferrari and Leong, 2003; Barry-Walsh and Mullen, 2004; ; Haskins and Silva, 2006; Langstrom et al, 2009; Freckelton and List, 2009, Freckelton, 2011). An important aspect of the link between them and violence may be the fact that around 65 per cent of adolescents diagnosed with Asperger's disorder, for instance, also have a mood disorder, generally an anxiety disorder, but also a higher than normal incidence of depression and bipolar disorder (see Ghaziuddin, Tsai and Ghaziuddin, 1991; Gillot, Furniss and Walter, 2001; Duggal, 2003; Volkmar, State and Klin, 2009; for a forensic example see *Chandler v The Queen*, 2010).

Interaction with the criminal justice system for those with such disorders is not only as offenders. Klin, Volkmar and Sparrow (2000: p6) have observed that those with Asperger's syndrome are the "perfect victims" for criminal or tortious bullying behaviour in a variety of contexts (see eg *R v EH*; 2008 *R v JO*, 2008). They are also less likely than their peers to report such victimisation "as they have impaired Theory of Mind abilities; that is, they have difficulty determining the thoughts and intentions of others in comparison to their peers" (Atwood, 2007: 109). A consequence of this is that they may be particularly vulnerable in custodial environments, although, ironically, they are likely to adapt well to penitential routines (Paterson, 2005). They can become unusually anxious and depressive in either the work or residential contexts if they experience change; they tend to be somewhat inflexible and to be poor adaptors to new situations. Their propensity to situation-generated distress raises the potential for those with Autism Spectrum Disorders to respond to stimuli in what appear to be excessive or anomalous ways.

The limitations of complainants with Autism Spectrum Disorders can also lead to the contention on behalf of defendants that such witnesses are unreliable in their evidence (see Paterson, 2008). On occasions, this will be a legitimate concern but, often, those with the disorder will be guileless, accurate, albeit unadorned, historians in their accounts. In short, they may be punctiliously reliable in their narratives, although the impression that they create in what they say may be otherwise..

However, the greater prominence of those with Autism Spectrum Disorders in the criminal justice system is as defendants. In this regard it could be argued that the deficits that are intrinsic to such disorders are particularly pertinent to capacity to be interviewed and function effectively within the trial process, their ability to foresee the possibility or probability of the effects of their behaviour, as well as their capacity to cope with stressors in traumatic situations and interpret others' behaviour (see *R v Mueller,* 2005: [92]; see too *McC v Regina*, 2007).

In Australia forensic attention came to be given to Asperger's after the forensic psychiatrist, Dr Sale, concluded that Martin Bryant, the murderer of 37 people at Port Arthur in Tasmania in 1996, had Asperger's (Mullen, 1996). Since that time in both Australia and other countries increasing attempts have been made to argue on behalf of accused persons with Asperger's disorder that they either lack criminal responsibility or that their criminal culpability is of a lesser level than that of "normal" defendants. It is apparent from many of the courts' decisions over the past decade that judicial officers at first instance and on appeal have had very limited familiarity with Autism Spectrum Disorders and have required expert assistance from psychiatrists and clinical psychologists with expertise in the area not just to disabuse them of the potential for drawing wrong inferences but to enable them to factor symptoms informedly into their instructions to juries and into their own decision-making.

More to the point, however, is the fundamental relationship between the deficits associated with Autism Spectrum Disorders and functional vulnerabilities in relation to criminal behaviour. Anecdotally, there are at least preliminary data to support a portrait of autistic offending, characterised by criminal activities that tend to be engaged in: physical violence, sexual assault, stalking, arson, and computer and internet offences (Freckelton, 2011).

In evaluating whether such a portrait is accurate, it is important to have regard to the social deficits inherent in Autism Spectrum Disorders, and the consequential limitations of socialisation associated with those deficits. For example, in relation to sexual assault, there is evidence that sexually assaultative behaviour occurs in the context of the inability of a person with an autistic disorder to interpret the victim's negative response to sexual overtures. The offender experiences normal sexual impulses, as well as a desire to interact socially with the object of such impulses. The offender attempts to engage the target of his (occasionally her) affection by physical touching or direct sexual contact, but is unable to interpret the other person's facial expression, tearfulness, or verbal response as being threatened or repelled by such a direct, possibly sudden, advance. In that context, the object of affection feels intimidated and frightened, even terrified, by what to the initiator is a benign, even affectionate, overture. The initiator is puzzled, even distressed, by the realisation that "something is seriously wrong", struggling to interpret the meaning of verbal or non-verbal cues or running away. He understands that he has committed a social offence, but is unable to construct a coherent whole from the signals he has received (Freckelton and List, 2009).

Similarly, in relation to physical violence, the clinical picture is not of a reservoir of simmering rage, or of an acute persecutory oversensitivity to imagined slights. It is, rather, more likely to occur in face of what is experienced as a sudden, distressing invasion of personal space (Freckelton and List, 2009). The reaction by the person with an autism spectrum disorder can be instant and intense, reflecting a primitive fight or flight response to threat. It is not connected with dislike, or with emotionally experienced interpersonal rage; it is, rather, an impulsive response arising from highly attuned personal radar to what is experienced as a repugnant, intolerable intrusion. In that context, what is to the perpetrator a reflexive self-protective stance is, to the object, an experience of physical, even violent, assault. The person with an autism spectrum disorder may well be perplexed by the intensity of the reaction by the other person, although distressed that he or she had caused such an unexpected, confusing, and severe response.

In the context of the arsonist with an Autism Spectrum Disorder, there is often an obsessive preoccupation with flames, cinders, colours and heat, rather than an intention to damage property or put lives at risk. There is a gulf between the focus of the perpetrator and the distress and anger of the property owner. Similarly, for the person with an Autism Spectrum Disorder who engages in stalking whether in person or by the internet, the intention is often to learn more about the person or to communicate with them than to cause distress or to harass.

For those with an Autism Spectrum Disorder computer access to the internet creates a world of intellectual stimulation with few emotional demands. It also affords a forum for working through obsessions and interests that has few boundaries. However, boundaries in terms of precluded access to some sites and the risk for cyberstalking impose limitations that can create legal difficulties.

In each of these cases, there tends to be no malice involved and little by way of mischievous or destructive impulse. In each, the person with an Autism Spectrum Disorder tends to be acting reflexively, but without the capacity to synthesise, interpret, and appropriately respond to such signals. Often there is impairment of inhibitions which would in others moderate such conduct.

In making clinical or forensic findings about such behaviour, it is necessary to draw a fundamental distinction between the social deficits of a person with an Autism Spectrum Disorder and those associated with psychopathy.

In psychopathy, there is a genuine lack of empathic attachment to others, who are viewed instrumentally rather than as equivalent humans with whom it is possible to develop a genuine relationship. The psychopath is motivated by self-interest or unexamined impulse, unmitigated by the governance of intrinsic morality or the concern for the consequences to victims of criminal acts (Freckelton and List, 2009). The person with an Autism Spectrum Disorder, by contrast, seeks relationships (sometimes inappropriately) and can maintain a precise, if narrowly eccentric, moral framework, even though the behaviour and framework may be misconstrued by reference to ordinary community and legal standards.

As illustrations of the potential significance of Autism Spectrum Disorders for both the determination of criminal responsibility and for the sentencing process, the following sections of this paper analyse important decisions in the United Kingdom, New Zealand, Australia, and Canada in which Asperger's disorder has figured prominently.

2. The United Kingdom

a. The Sultan decision

In *Sultan v The Queen* (2008) a man with Asperger's disorder appealed to the United Kingdom Court of Appeal against findings of guilt by a jury on counts of rape and indecent assault of his wife.

The Trial. Mr Sultan had been diagnosed prior to his conduct the subject of the charges with a morbid jealousy disorder and his wife, from whom he was alienated, had taken an intervention order against him. It was common ground that sexual interaction took place on the evening in question. Mr Sultan's wife maintained that it had been wholly non-consensual. Mr Sultan contended that it had been consensual and initiated by his wife. Certain of Mr Sultan's conduct at the trial, including overtly reading a book during his wife's evidence was odd and would have been difficult for the jury to interpret informedly. Put another way, there was a risk that they would misinterpret it and draw adverse inferences from it.

The New Evidence. Subsequent to the trial and the sentence of four years imprisonment imposed upon Mr Sultan, he was diagnosed with Asperger's disorder. On appeal he sought to adduce evidence of this diagnosis as further evidence on the basis that "a sufferer, such as the appellant, is liable to misunderstand in real time the signs and even straightforward indications of those with whom he comes into contact" (*Sultan,* 2008: at [10]) and that, had the diagnosis been known at the time of the trial, the issue of intention would have been contested.

The Appeal. The Court of Appeal accepted (*Sultan,* 2008: at [19]) that:

> Asperger's Syndrome is a developmental disorder which begins to manifest itself sometime in the early childhood of the patient. Its precise cause is unknown but genetic factors and peri-natal trauma are thought to be possible contributory causes. Because it is a developmental disorder its presence is constant: unlike psychotic illness it does not come and go. It is a disorder which has only become understood in recent years. Its essential features are severe and sustained impairment in social interaction and restricted, repetitive patterns of behaviour, interests and activities. It causes clinically significant impairment in social, occupational and other important areas of functioning. In contrast to autistic disorder, there are no clinically significant delays or deviance in language acquisition, although more subtle aspects of social communication may be affected.

It observed a significant discrepancy between Mr Sultan's verbal IQ (117) and performance IQ (87), which was said to be consistent with Asperger's, and heard evidence from a psychologist that Mr Sultan's "speech had an odd prosody with an almost telegraphic quality; his language was formal and tangential, displaying an apparent inability to understand the needs of the listener; his discourse was repetitive and returned to preoccupations which superficially resembled delusions; he struggled with non-literal uses of language, having difficulty in understanding metaphors, irony, sarcasm or humour." (*Sultan,* 2008: at [20]) An assessing psychologist observed (*Sultan,* 2008: at [21]):

> The period of inpatient assessment has demonstrated the extent to which problems in executive function and understanding others' beliefs can disable someone who is otherwise intellectually very able. Thus his rigid belief in his illegal detention has resulted in long periods of time when Mr Sultan has refused to interact with members of the multidisciplinary team. He has refused to read letters sent to him by his legal team, maintaining that he is already a free man and that these letters have no interest or

> value to him (despite patient explanation that they related to the ongoing appeal process)...maintaining instead that our only function was to 'appraise the trauma suffered by an innocent man in prison'...

The Court of Appeal accepted that the new evidence could have affected the trial in one or more of three ways (*Sultan*, 2008: at [34]): "First, it would have enabled a defence for the first time to be based on the requirements of mens rea. Secondly, it would have enabled the jury to view the defendant before them not solely on the basis of whether what he said happened was at all credible, but more importantly on the basis of whether he was honest about what he believed to have been the situation, even if the facts were otherwise as [his wife] said them to be. Thirdly, it might have gone some way to explain to the jury why the appellant was behaving so oddly at trial, such as reading a book during [his wife's] evidence." Accordingly, the court quashed the convictions and ordered a new trial. For accused persons with Asperger's this is a most important decision.

b. The McKinnon saga

The saga of Gary McKinnon is illustrative of a number of issues in relation to the Autism Spectrum Disorders and the criminal law. McKinnon is a British subject who, between 2001 and 2002, gained unauthorised access to computers belonging to the United States Army, Navy, Department of Defense and the National Aeronautic and Space Administration. In the course of his access he installed a suite of hacking tools and deleted a range of data which caused large numbers of computers variously to shut down, to become inoperable, and to become vulnerable to other intruders. It was alleged that his conduct caused risk to the United States defence system. In addition, he copied files onto his own computer system. It was alleged against him that his conduct was intentional and calculated to influence and affect the United States government by intimidation and coercion, damage being caused to computers "by impairing their integrity, availability and operation of programmes, systems, information and data on the computers, rendering them unreliable. The cost of repair totalled over $US700,000." (*McKinnon*, 2007: [6]).

The computer compromises were traced to computers in Mr McKinnon's house and forensic analysis identified him as the perpetrator. He was interviewed under a request for legal assistance and admitted responsibility for the conduct. He stated that he had copied files onto his computer from American computers and had deleted log files on the American computers so as to conceal his activities. He stated that his targets were high level United States Army, Navy and Airforce computers and that his ultimate goal was to gain access to the United States military classified information network. He admitted leaving a message on one computer that read:

> US foreign policy is akin to Government-sponsored terrorism these days. ... It was not a mistake that there was a huge security stand down on September 11 last year ... I am SOLO. I will continue to disrupt at the highest levels (McKinnon, 2007: [8]).

In 2006 an application was successfully made before the Bow Street Magistrates' Court to extradite Mr McKinnon to the United States to stand trial for a range of criminal offences. He lodged an appeal to the High Court (*McKinnon v USA*, 2007) on many legal grounds. It was unsuccessful, as was a further appeal to the House of Lords (*McKinnon v The United States of America*, 2008). In 2009 he took an action for judicial review (*McKinnon v Secretary of State for the Home Department*, 2009) on the basis that within weeks of the House of Lords decision Mr McKinnon, for the first time, was diagnosed with Asperger's syndrome. Accordingly, representations were made to the Secretary of State that she should not proceed with the extradition on the basis that she held a residual discretion to decline the application because Mr McKinnon's health condition would make his extradition to the United States oppressive. She did not accede to the submissions and the High Court found by application of principles of statutory construction that she had not made an error. However, it was also contended on Mr McKinnon's behalf that the Secretary did not do justice to the submission on his behalf that if convicted he faced a real risk of imprisonment in a "super-max prison" in Colorado where he would be subject to conditions that would infringe his entitlements under the *Human Rights Act 1998* (UK).

Expert evidence was given by a psychologist, Dr Berney, that "It would be consistent with this diagnosis that Mr McKinnon does not appreciate the relative priorities of societal rules and so has difficulty in judging what is serious offence and what is minor and balancing this against the perceived rightness of his cause. The nature of Asperger syndrome is to hinder the development of the close, confiding relationship that would allow him to test his perception of his activities and behaviour against the way that they might be seen by others. Although he does discuss the possibility of conspiracy, he is less able to accommodate conflicting opinions and to modify his views so leaving him with a rather black-and-white perception of his world." (*McKinnon v Secretary of State for Home Affairs*, 2009: [15])

He asserted too that Asperger's syndrome left Mr McKinnon vulnerable to the "stress of social complexity" and "if he finds himself in circumstances where he is unable to withdraw from complex environments into something more autism-friendly, he is likely to develop a pathological anxiety state and, given the presence of the developmental disorder he will be prone to develop an acute, psychotic disorder" (*McKinnon v Secretary of State for the Home Department*, 2009: [12]) Dr Berney suggested that other prisoners were unlikely to have sympathy for Mr McKinnon's difficulties and that transplanting him into the culture of a United States prison would be particularly difficult for him. Professor Baron-Cohen, a psychologist, expressed the view that there was "a high risk of serious deterioration of Mr McKinnon's mental health if he were to be incarcerated in the USA pre-trial or post conviction. It is also important to bear in mind that if separated from his parents and partner and put into the traumatic environment of prison, there is a risk that he would attempt to take his own life." (*McKinnon v Secretary of State for the Home Department*, 2009: [12]) He subsequently reported that:

> [Mr McKinnon's] difficulties in relation to possible detention in prison may relate to his social awareness and empathy difficulties but in my mind they relate more to his current depression and anxiety. The latter centres on his fears of being raped by other prisoners of being physically assaulted by prison guards and he has talked about preferring suicide as an option rather than being put in such a threatening environment. It is not about the environment (I have no idea if his fears are based on any real risks of this) but about his perception of what prison would be like. My previous report identified that he is suffering from an anxiety disorder (panic attacks) over and above his AS. If Gary were subject to long-term detention in solitary confinement it is my view that it will likely to exacerbate his depression and increase the risk of suicide. I would also add that in my view Mr McKinnon does not have the social skills to cope with prison. He is unlikely to be able to negotiate his way through a social group of other prisoners in such a way as to be accepted. Nor is he likely to be able to make

relationships, and may offend others through expressing his opinions in a very blunt and direct undiplomatic fashion. But as stated under point 2 above, I don't think it is his social skills that are the main risk factor for his mental health. Rather, his mental health is already very poor from having suffered from anxiety and depression over many years at not knowing what is going to happen to him. Dislocation from the support of his family and girlfriend may be other key risk factors that might exacerbate his already poor mental health. I would anticipate that the particular features of a prison environment that would be traumatic for Mr McKinnon as a person with AS is that he would suffer from the following:

1. Aggression from other prisoners
2. Aggression from prison guards
3. Being expected to share a cell with someone
4. Loud noise and other forms of sensory overload which he would find aversive
5. Having to live in a large group of people when the natural state of people with AS is to withdraw.

I also anticipate that if Mr McKinnon was presented with any sensory sensitivities then that would exacerbate the impact of prison conditions on him such as harsh lighting, loud noises etc. I have a real concern that he would not survive a term of imprisonment. I am stating this as strong assertion because to put a vulnerable adult who has a disability into a situation of imprisonment when that adult has [stated] that suicide would be preferable, to avoid the suffering that he fears he will experience in a prison, is a decision that should carry with it some responsibility for any consequences. The courts for example, should not be able to claim that they were unaware of the risks prison might pose to Mr McKinnon if he suffers a complete psychiatric breakdown or commits suicide. The courts should have it on their record that if they order him to be detained, it is in the full knowledge that this outcome is a serious and dangerous possibility. My impression is that even being put on a plane to stand trial in the US, even if he were not imprisoned, might be too traumatic for him to manage. Inevitably it would involve some detention whilst awaiting a court hearing in the USA, which may push his already high anxiety to intolerable levels. (*McKinnon v Secretary of State for Home Affairs*, 2009: [23])

However, the submissions fell on unsympathetic ears both before the Secretary of State and the High Court. In October 2008 the Treasury Solicitor on behalf of the Secretary of State acknowledged that Dr Berney and Dr Baron-Cohen had identified the stressful and destabilising effects of extradition, and the likely consequences on Mr McKinnon's mental health. However, he observed that they had provided no explanation as to why it was said that proceedings in the United States would be of such a different order of magnitude in terms of their effect as to be likely to lead to a significant deterioration in his mental health. The information in relation to Mr McKinnon's Asperger's syndrome might lead a United States court to grant him bail. However, if he failed in a bail application, the Secretary commented that "he is to be extradited to a country with a highly developed awareness of psychiatric illness and which has procedures for ensuring that those in custody receive appropriate care." Therefore, although extradition to the United States would cause him "certain stress and may exacerbate any illness from which he currently suffers", The Secretary of State did not accept that his condition could not be appropriately treated.

Lawyers acting on behalf of Mr McKinnon then urged the DPP to prosecute Mr McKinnon in England. When the DPP declined, they challenged this decision, as well as that of the

Secretary of State. The Court declined to entertain the application insofar as it pertained to the potential for Mr McKinnon to be detained in a supermax prison. It held that the decision about whether to prosecute was that of the DPP and could not in these circumstances be challenged.

In considering the expert evidence in relation to Mr McKinnon's Asperger's syndrome it observed that it was important to place it in perspective:

> ...despite having had AS in childhood his condition has, so far, not necessitated any type of treatment or medical intervention. He is aged 42. He faced arrest and interview by the police, arrest on an extradition warrant, an extradition hearing, the order for his extradition, and litigation in the High Court and House of Lords, all no doubt deeply stressful events without this leading to any acute events requiring intervention. Although the symptoms of his undiagnosed AS would have been manifested throughout the proceedings, there was no suggestion (until very recently) that the act of ordering, or effecting, extradition would give rise to any type of acute event (as has been the case in some of the cases dealing with severe depression). Neither the symptoms of his disorder, some of which were apparent to his close family and loved ones, nor his depression (which, according to his mother, was diagnosed "some time ago") have, until very recently, led to the Claimant being treated or to being the subject of investigation or of medical reports, let alone to an application under section 91 of the 2003 Extradition Act.
>
> The difficulties encountered by the Claimant "not being able to cope with sharing a cell or fitting in with a group and being traumatised by the loud noise" apply to "many adults" with AS, yet they too may face the possibility of prison. According to the National Autistic Society, 1 in 100 children has ASD, and over 300,000 adults in the UK have ASD (which includes more serious disabilities than AS). The availability of appropriate expertise is patchy in this country, and it is not to be supposed that a prison sentence served by the Claimant in this country would not present him with difficulties. The availability of appropriate expertise here is described as "patchy", and the same is probably true of the USA; and in both countries, it is likely that services in prison are not as well resourced as those in the community. (*McKinnon v Secretary of State for Home Affairs*, 2009: [78]-[79])

The Court was satisfied that any United States sentencing court would properly take into account Mr McKinnon's condition in terms of the nature and extent of any sentence of imprisonment imposed, as well as where it should be served. In addition, it was satisfied that if the United States authorities were not prepared to agree to his repatriation, that was a matter which the sentencing court would take into account. It noted that United States prisons were serviced by both psychologists and psychiatrists and took into account evidence that a treatment plan may well be prepared "geared primarily to assisting with adaptation to the correctional environment specifically relating to institution rules, disruptive or potentially disruptive behaviour, and functioning within the prison culture, particularly communication issues within the prison setting. It may well be determined that Mr McKinnon will need to learn a completely different set of communication strategies for the prison setting compared with the normal social setting." (*McKinnon v Secretary of State for Home Affairs*, 2009: [79])

The Court treated the assurances of various United States witnesses about how Mr McKinnon would be looked after in the United States penitential system "as having substantial value.

Certainly, the Secretary of State was and is entitled to do so. Of course, these assurances do not amount to cast-iron guarantees of appropriate care during the Claimant's sentence. But they are the considered assurances of a friendly state, indeed of a state with which this country has close relations. (*McKinnon v Secretary of State for Home Affairs*, 2009: [79])

The Court stated that:

> it had no doubt that he will find extradition to, and trial and sentence and detention in the USA, very difficult indeed. His mental health will suffer. There are risks of worse, including suicide. But if I compare his condition with those considered in the authorities to which I have referred above, even taking full account of the (in my view undesirable) possibility of his being prosecuted in this country, his case does not approach Article 3 severity. ." (*McKinnon v Secretary of State for Home Affairs*, 2009: [89])

It determined that it had not been established that the Secretary of State's decision letter contained any error of law. The McKinnon series of decisions highlight complexities about the impact that imprisonment may be regarded as having for those with Autism Spectrum Disorders, depending on both its harshness and the extent of available psychiatric care (see Freckelton 2011a).

3. New Zealand

a. Glover v Police

New Zealand's major decision on the significance of Asperger's disorder for the criminal law is the High Court's decision in *Glover v Police* (2009). Mr Glover had damaged Mr Bauer's property on two separate occasions in July and November 2008. He described himself as a "road safety activist". He was of the view that a footpath was needed to run past the front of Mr Glover's property. However, to his considerable consternation the Council had licensed Mr Bauer to use a garden area at the front of Mr Bauer's property as part of his front garden.

In purported assertion of his and others' rights to the use of the area in front of Mr Bauer's house, Mr Glover interfered with and caused damage to Mr Bauer's garden area. At his summary trial Mr Glover argued that he had acted with lawful justification, excuse or a "claim of right" to do what he had done. However, his defence was not accepted and he was convicted and ordered to pay $NZ30 reparation and to undertake 40 hours' community work. He appealed against the sentence.

The issue before the court at first instance and then on appeal was the relevance of the fact that Mr Glover suffered from Asperger's disorder. It was argued that both the gravity of his offending and the direct and indirect consequences of a conviction needed to be considered in light of the nature of the disorder and its effects on his behavior. Professor Attwood had originally diagnosed his condition and contended that a conviction would lead to an increase in Mr Glover's alienation, frustration and despair.

The sentencing judge had regarded Mr Glover's offending at the more serious end of the scale, having regard to the fact that the conduct was repeated, the victim was 86 years of age, the distress caused to the victim and the degree of premeditation on the part of Mr Glover. He declined to place much weight on Mr Glover's Asperger's disorder. He took into account Mr Glover's three previous convictions and a previous discharge without conviction, as well as the fact that Mr Glover had exhibited no remorse, indicating that he would continue his conduct, regardless of the orders of the court.

On appeal Clifford J was provided with a report from a forensic psychiatrist, Dr Justin Barry-Walsh. He accepted that the syndrome was relevant for the assessment both of the gravity of his offending and of the consequences for him of conviction. Justice Clifford concluded that Mr Bauer's rigidity of thought and inflexibility contributed to Mr Glover's offending. He proceeded from this proposition to the finding that Mr Glover's offending "must be regarded as significantly less than that of a healthy and rationally thinking person." (*Glover v Police,* 2009: [21]; see too possibly R *v Burkett,* 2006) He found Mr Glover's strong interest in road safety to be a manifestation of his "syndrome" and concluded that Mr Glover was not motivated by criminal intent or malice (see also *R v Walker,* 2008) but by his ideological position on road safety matters.

Justice Clifford also found that Mr Glover's Asperger's went "a considerable way to explain his failure to express remorse or to offer to make amends, which appear to be a result of his rigidity of mind and egocentric perspective."

All told, he found that the property damage was "in effect minor and easily remedied" and that his offending was of relatively minor gravity. Dr Barry-Walsh expressed the view that:

> He is vulnerable to depression and more sensitive to apparently minor grievances and setbacks than other people. His response to such setbacks may be disproportionate and severe. It is likely Mr Glover would have difficulty in accepting a conviction was reasonable and further in accepting the reasonableness of any sentence. Further, he lacks the capacity to adopt a pragmatic, flexible approach to the circumstance and therefore I think it unlikely he would put aside his strong sense of entitlement and injustice. Consequently I believe it likely that the impact of a sentence upon Mr Glover would be greater than it would be towards other people. It is possible he would experience an increase in frustration and despair as speculated by Prof Attwood; it is also plausible that he would not be able to accept the conviction or sentence and would continue to consider he had been wronged and to ruminate upon such findings. It is possible that he would become depressed. (*Glover v Police,* 2009: [27])

Justice Clifford also heard from Mr Glover's parents who emphasised the significance for their son of his efforts in relation to road safety and concluded that "A conviction against him for these activities would therefore be regarded by him as a matter of considerable significance." (*Glover v Police,* 2009: [28]) He noted that Dr Barry-Walsh's views about depression were conditional, in the sense that he was expressing no more than the potential for depressive consequences to flow from a conviction for Mr Glover. He stated that he had been informed that the incidents had occasioned the opportunity for Mt Glover to consider carefully his behaviour and to ensure that his road safety initiatives in the future would be carried out within a lawful framework - "notwithstanding his subjective views as to the appropriateness of that framework." (*Glover v Police,* 2009: [30]) Accordingly, he determined that given the centrality to Mr Glover's life of those interests, it was appropriate to place considerable reliance on the significance of Asperger's disorder in assessing the consequences to him of the imposition of a conviction. He held that convictions would have an effect "out of all proportion to the gravity of his offending" and discharged him without conviction, thereby quashing the order for community work. The case exemplifies scenarios in which obsessive anti-social behaviour, which is also technically criminal, may be generated for a person with an Autism Spectrum Disorder by virtue of their disorder.In such a situation, only a moderate emphasis on punishment by a sentencer is clinically legitimate.

b. R v Walker

In a 2008 case before the New Zealand High Court at first instance (*R v Walker*, 2008) the accused's Asperger's disorder once more was central to the sentence imposed upon him. Owen Walker pleaded guilty to a series of computer fraud offences committed when he was aged between 16 and 18 years of age. Mr Owen developed and used software that enabled him to remotely control infected computers which collectively formed a robot network, known as a "bot net". He installed his bot code on tens of thousands of computers. The code automatically disabled antivirus software. The court was informed that Mr Walker's code was considered by international cyber crime investigators to be amongst the most advanced bot programming encountered. While his software had the potential to be used to conduct fraudulent financial transactions, there was no evidence that it had been employed for that purpose.

Mr Walker had no previous convictions and had a good background and reputation. He had been tentatively diagnosed as having a mild form of Asperger's syndrome as a child, although latterly his symptoms had decreased in conjunction with his being encouraged to socialize more. He described his offending as having been motivated principally by curiosity – "to see what he could do." He showed signs of remorse and was prepared to pay reparation. A psychologist, Mr Laven, classified him as being of low to medium risk of reoffending.

Justice Potter accepted that Mr Walker had a "diminished understanding in relation to the nature of his offending" (*R v Walker*, 2008: [17]), partly because of having Asperger's disorder. He concluded that Mr Walker's conduct was carried out simply to demonstrate to himself that he could inflict the kind of harm that resulted – "he was unaware of the nature of the harm that his activities could cause and was immature to the extent that he was unable, or failed, to set proper boundaries for himself in relation to his undoubted ability and expertise in the use of computers." (*R v Walker*, 2008, at [25]). He also took into account that Mr Walker had received offers of employment from large corporations active outside New Zealand and also that the New Zealand Police were interested in employing him. Justice Potter formed the view that Mr Walker had a "potentially outstanding future" (*R v Walker*, 2008: [37]) and discharged him without conviction. The decision is an example of pragmatic sentencing of a person with an Autism Spectrum Disorder factoring into a sentence the potential for a person's skills (and obsessions) to be constructively directed.

4. Australia

a. The Parish decision

In *Parish v DPP* (2007) a person with Asperger's disorder appealed against a decision of a magistrate to find him guilty of two common assaults upon a woman whom he met on a train.

Proceedings before the Magistrate. At first instance, a Magistrate accepted the complainant's evidence, which was to the following effect. She said that on 6 January 2006 at about 5.00pm she took a train from the city to Box Hill after spending time in the city with her boyfriend. Prior to entering the train, she noticed Mr Parish looking at her. On entering a relatively empty carriage, Mr Parish sat diagonally opposite her. Very soon after the train started its journey, Mr Parish pushed his calf against hers. She tried to move her leg away from his. He also changed positions and sat directly in front of her, with his hands over his knees. He then placed his hands on top of her knees. At this stage she was looking out the window, trying to ignore him. He then rubbed his hands on top of her knees. She did not speak to him or attempt to change seats.

When she got to Box Hill Station, she waited back and allowed Mr Parish to alight first. She then stood beside the train to make sure that Mr Parish was away from her. She then proceeded to take the escalator but felt a hand on top of her hand. She turned around and noticed that it was Mr Parish. He was standing on the step below her and, as the escalator was going up, he rubbed her lower back and her upper buttocks. She gave evidence that she was scared and was unable to move through the people surrounding her on the escalators. Again she said nothing to him.

After alighting from the escalator, she went to look for her sister and broke down in tears when telling her what had happened. On the recommendation of family members, she made a complaint to the police. Mr Parish was identified from CCTV photographs.

On being interviewed, Mr Parish denied any recollection of the events and said he had no memory of the alleged incident with the complainant. However, he did admit, in his record of interview, that he had rubbed his leg against girls on trains before. He said:

> I put my leg close to her and see if she doesn't mind. And if she kind of does then I won't do it anymore. She didn't seem I suppose at the time she didn't seem she probably didn't seem to mind. (*Parish*, at [10])

He was asked whether it had occurred to him that perhaps the complainant might have been frightened and not known what to do? He answered: "Err no at the time it didn't" (*Parish*; at [11]). He was further asked: "Why did you rub her leg with yours?" His answer was: "It was kind of ... I'm not as you say a very confident person, I'm more of a touchy feely sort of person and that was kind of my way of trying to get to know her a little bit" (*Parish* at [11]). He was then asked if such behaviour excited him and he responded: "It wasn't, it wasn't sexual. It wasn't for excitement or sexual. It was more a way of me trying to get to know her, to see if something would come out of it; a relationship or something" (*Parish*: at [11]).

The following exchange took place:

> Question: "How many women have you tried to meet by rubbing their legs?". Answer: "I don't know. Maybe four". Question: "Have you ever had any success?". Answer: "Err, once". Question: "Yeah? What, that turned into a relationship, did it?". Answer: "Not exactly, but ...". Question: "Did you see this woman to be scared, quite frightened as to a person she doesn't know by this sort of thing happening to her on the train?". Answer: "Yes, I can see that". Question: "Especially on the escalator as well, the same person gets off and rubs her on the bottom. Can you see she may be frightened and may be feeling a bit violated?". Answer: "Yeah". (Parish: at [12])

Mr Parish was charged with a counts of indecent assault and 2 counts of indecent assault.

Mr Parish's defence arose out of his having been recently diagnosed with Asperger's disorder. Evidence was given by Dr Nicole Reinhardt, who had been treating Mr Parish, about the nature of the disorder, including that "a person born with Asberger's (sic) is born without the brain capacity to understand, interpret and act in the social world - they have to be taught in a concrete way the rules of social behaviour." Further, she said, people affected by the disorder are unable to pick up non-verbal cues - a subtle cue probably would not even register. Dr Reinhardt expressed the view that Mr Parish would have been unlikely to have been aware that the complainant was not consenting to his actions.

During her evidence-in-chief, Dr Reinhardt said as follows (*Parish*: at [16]):

> Question: "Can you say what level of sexual understanding or development from your dealing with Mr Parish in the light of his condition, what level of understanding, appreciation, development he had in that area?".
>
> Answer: "At the time that I assessed Phillip and subsequent appointments I have had with Phillip, overseeing his treatment, Phillip had no understanding of how ... he has no understanding of how to make same sex friends, just in a friendship way. For example, he doesn't know how long it is you have to speak to somebody before they might be your friend. Or is that they have to offer their phone number to establish that they might be your friend. In terms of meeting a potential partner of the opposite sex, Phillip has no idea how that would happen or how he would come to have a sexual encounter with a person of the opposite sex. He had this idea that perhaps ... he's not good, he knows he's not good at expressing himself verbally. Pragmatics, part of the disorder, he was aware he's not good with words, so had an idea that perhaps the way that you do it is you might use your hands ... and that might be a way of ... and if somebody doesn't object, that might mean that they want to be your girlfriend. He didn't know, when he had discussions about this, that you would interact with that person verbally, and that all the sophisticated steps that are involved in meeting a potential partner. He had no idea, so again, an early primary school aged concept."

Under cross-examination, Dr Reinhardt was asked a question in relation to the fact that the complainant moved away from Mr Parish and there was a break before she had gone up the escalator. Dr Reinhardt said (*Parish*: at [17])

> The interpretation of that behaviour for a person with Asberger's disorder ... might be: M'hm, she might be interested, she might have enjoyed sitting next to me, em, I'll follow her and see if I can get any more data to enter into my information about that social interaction ... em ... again unless there was this pronounced verbal and non-verbal communication that this isn't OK in concert ... would he have understood that this wasn't OK for that person. Remembering at the same time that a person with Asberger's disorder cannot interpret and understand other subtle cues that we would have. So, for example, tense body posture that the person, the victim, would have been no doubt showing ... where her eyes were looking ... all of that would have just been ... it wouldn't have even gone into Phillip's thinking, ... (indistinct) (long pause). I might just add, I'm giving you clinical anecdotes and observations, but em there are hard empirical data to show that people with Asberger's disorder cannot pick up cues."

The magistrate found Mr Parish not guilty of the first charge of indecent assault as the prosecution had not established a sexual connotation to the assault or that Mr Parish's intent was sexual. He also found in relation to the further charge of indecent assault that the prosecution had not proved beyond reasonable doubt that Mr Parish did not believe that the victim was consenting or might have been consenting to his overtures. However, he found the common assault to be in a different category and, while consent can be a defence to common assault, such as sporting contact or perhaps restraint of liberty, the case did not fall into these areas and the charges were made out.

The Appeal. On behalf of Mr Parish it was argued on appeal on a question of law that in the circumstances of the case the prosecution had failed to negative a consent element in the charges of assault. Justice Robson accepted on the basis of authorities that in the case of common assault a distinction should be drawn between contact of such a nature that if done to another person consent is no answer and those cases where the prosecution bears the burden of negativing consent (*Parish*: at [117]). He found that he was dealing with the latter category and that "where assault is being used to include battery, the definition of the offence is the actual intended use of unlawful force to another person without his consent or any other lawful excuse." He concluded that the prosecution, therefore, bore the onus of establishing that Mr Parish intended to use force on the complainant without her consent - this was necessary to establish the necessary intentional element to the criminal conduct. He found that Mr Parish had raised the issue of consent but, even if he were wrong in that, the prosecution still bore the onus of establishing that Mr Parish was aware that the complainant was not consenting or might not be as it bore the onus of establishing that the complainant did not consent. The result of this was that Robson J found that the magistrate had made an error of law in finding the common assault charges made out. He allowed the appeal and quashed the finding of guilt in relation to the escalator assault but proceeded to hear further submissions about the train assault in respect of which the magistrate made no finding related to Mr Parish's awareness. He stressed that his decision was confined to the circumstances of Mr Parish's disability - "his being a sufferer of Asberger's (sic) Syndrome and the unfortunate impact that it has on Mr Parish's ability to deal with other people. I would expect that in the case of a person who was not suffering from Asberger's Syndrome or having a similar disability, that the prosecution would be able to easily establish the necessary awareness on the part of any person who did what Mr Parish did" (*Parish*: at [126]).

The decisions both at first instance and on appeal, therefore, constitute important examples of how the symptomatology of Asperger's can impact upon the capacity of a defendant to form the necessary intent for criminal offences to be established.

b. The HPW decision

In *DPP v HPW* (2011) the Victorian Court of Appeal heard an appeal brought by the prosecution contending that the sentencing judge at first instance had wrongly found a causal connection between HPW's Asperger's disorder and his sexual offending, had erred in imposing a manifestly inadequate sentence and had inadequately cumulated the penalties he imposed for a significant number of sex offences. HPW was found guilty at first instance of eight charges, three of which were representative of many instances of offending, committed against his biological daughter during a time when she was aged 11 and 12. They involved multiple instances of oral, digital and anal penetration as well as instances of masturbation and of encouraging the family dog to lick his daughter's vagina.

When interviewed by the police, HPW admitted sodomising his daughter and explained that it was "just as an experiment". He said by way of explanation that "it was just sexual gratification for myself" and commented that he was "probably a psycho". HPW was aged 47 at the time of sentencing and without prior convictions. He had served a lengthy period of time in the army until he was discharged in 2007 for not handing back some hand grenades. He had two children from a marriage that lasted over a decade, after which he formed a relationship that involved bestiality and anal sex with another woman. A psychologist who examined him concluded that the offending with his daughter concluded when "he realized what he was doing".

HPW's Asperger's Disorder went undiagnosed until after the criminal charges were laid. A psychologist who assessed him concluded (*HPW*, at [37]) that he had "significant deficits in social interaction; restricted behaviour, interests and activities; clinically significant impairment in social or other important areas of functioning; no apparent language impairment; and no apparent cognitive impairment. He is somewhat atypical on his awareness of his deficiencies in empathy and friendship skills."

Dr Kennedy, a psychologist whose report was tendered at the plea hearing, stated (HPW, at [47]):

> In this case, victim empathy should be commented on for specific reasons, particularly in relation to [HPW]'s cognitive distortion associated with the offences. In this matter, he has reported that while carrying out the sexual offences he considered that [his daughter] *was experiencing the sexual abuse in a matter-of-fact way* as if the activities were normal, and nothing more than her daily activities.
>
> Discussion of this issue occurred at some length. I should note that [HPW] did not appear to be attempting to minimise this behaviour in this [sic], but *was attempting to explain how he saw [his daughter's] response to the sexual abuse*. He thought at the time for her, it was "something to do ... as if it was an activity such as playing cards or watching TV" that *had no impact on her at an emotional level*. When asked about his understanding of the effects of the sexual abuse on [his daughter], he reported in a very distinct way that the impact has been "huge ... I think I've ruined her ... she'll never be able to see me in the same light ... it will be very difficult for her with partners in the future".

He added (*HPW*, at [50]) that:

> [There is a] focus on deficient empathy, which is clearly relevant in this case, interpersonal naivety which appears to be the case in this matter, sexual frustration which is clearly relevant in this case, and immediate confession, which from my understanding, is also present. Additionally, there are sexual preoccupations, which do appear relevant in this case.

Dr Kennedy expressed the view that at the time of his offending HPW was unaware of the distress he was causing to his daughter but contended that since that time he had acquired genuine empathy and remorse. He observed that there had been no grooming process, as is often seen in sex cases.

The Court found that the evidence of the expert gave no support for the foundation of the plea made on HPW's behalf, and which was (wrongly) accepted by the sentencing judge that HPW misread his daughter's behaviour as providing encouragement to him by hints or signals, to engage in the sexual offending (cp *Hopper v The Queen*, 2003, at [40], [54], [68]). Tate JA (*HPW*, at [53]) found that the psychologist's opinion:

> suggested that the sexual offending occurred in a context in which (1) the respondent had sexual preoccupations with his daughter, fantasising about her in a manner reflective of his previous unusual sexual relationship with an earlier partner of whom his daughter reminded him; (2) he was sexually frustrated with his current partner; (3) his level of alcohol abuse led to disinhibition; and (4) his deficient empathy meant that he believed that his sexual offending was having no emotional impact on his daughter. Dr Kennedy's

opinion did not provide a proper evidentiary base supporting the finding of the sentencing judge that the respondent 'may have misinterpreted [his] daughter's cues'.

She found that the plea by counsel misrepresented the expert report. To the extent that Dr Kennedy had commented "it is highly likely that [HPW's] behaviour is best explained by the presence of an Autism Spectrum Disorder", Tate JA found that it could not support the proposition that there was a causal connection between his conduct and his misreading of his daughter's behavioural cues. This led Tate JA (with Neave and Mandie JJA agreeing) to find a sentencing error. They also found that HPW's Asperger's disorder should not have led to a significant moderation in the sentence imposed upon him, and that his sentence was not sufficiently cumulated to reflect the "debased and humiliating nature of the offending, the core breach of trust, or the effect of the offending upon [HPW's] daughter" (at [82]).

While the Court did not generally find that HPW's Asperger's reduced his moral culpability for the purposes of sentencing, it did accept that it was appropriate to view his disorder as a mitigating factor to the extent that it was likely to make his service of a sentence in prison more burdensome. It ordered his sentence to be increased from seven and a half years' imprisonment with a non-parole period of five years and six months to nine years and six months' imprisonment with a non-parole period of sex years and six months. The appellate decision makes the important point that the fact alone that a person has an Autism Spectrum Disorder does not necessarily exculpate or even mitigate an accused person's conduct.

5. Canada

5.1 The R v Kagan decision

In *R v Kagan* (2007) McDougall J of the Supreme Court of Nova Scotia in a judge-alone trial heard a charge that Mr Kagan committed an aggravated assault contrary to s268 of Canada's Criminal Code. It was incumbent on the prosecution under Canadian law to prove that a reasonable person, in the circumstances, would inevitably realise that the force Mr Kagan applied would put the complainant (Mr Kinney) at risk of suffering some kind of bodily harm. Mr Kagan accepted that he had used "bear spray" – a form of repellant containing certain active ingredients called capsaicin and dihydrocapsaicin, often referred to as pepper spray - on Mr Kinney. He also conceded using a pocket knife to stab Mr Kinney in an area of his back which caused him to suffer significant and potentially life-threatening injuries, including a punctured lung. Mr Kagan maintained that he had acted in self-defence. Under Canadian law, to determine whether Mr Kagan acted in lawful self-defence the following three issues had to be considered:

1. Was Mr Kagan unlawfully assaulted by Mr. Kinney?
2. Did Mr Kagan use force against Mr Kinney because he reasonably feared that Mr. Kinney would kill or seriously injure him?
3. Did Mr Kagan use force against Mr Kinney because he reasonably believed that he could not otherwise save himself from being killed or seriously injured by Mr Kinney?

The issue was not what an outsider would have reasonably perceived but what the accused reasonably perceived, given his situation and his experience. Expert evidence was adduced for Mr Kagan to explain that he suffered from Asperger's disorder and the effects that the disorder might have exercised upon his perceptions in the circumstances of conflict with Mr Kinney.

Dr Glancy, a psychiatrist, gave evidence (*Kagan*: at [28]-[30]) that:

> Persons suffering from Asperger's quite often have difficulty developing peer relationships. This is noticeable at any early age. They are usually slow in reaching developmental milestones. They seldom develop long-lasting peer relationships. They appear strange or odd to others. They fail to maintain eye-to-eye contact in conversation with others. They have difficulty feeling and expressing emotions and understanding the emotions of others. They can be quite blunt which can be perceived as rude by those they interact with. They tend to suffer from mild paranoia and have a lower tolerance of change which can lead to frustration. They develop anxiety when things are not the way they fervently wish them to be.
>
> Asperger's patients are typically loners. They can be awkward or clumsy when they are young but they can develop quite good motor skills as they get older.
>
> Since they do not normally develop long-lasting or warm relationships with others, they are usually distrustful of others.Asperger's sufferers like structure and routine in their lives. In stressful situations they can develop a heightened level of anxiety.
>
> Defence counsel put to Dr Glancy a bare hypothetical scenario which included the events that took place on the day that Mr Kagan sprayed Mr Kinney with bear spray and then stabbed him. In Dr Glancy's opinion the hypothetical person with Asperger's would have felt a rising level of paranoia and anxiety. He would have felt increasingly persecuted as tensions escalated between him and the other hypothetical figure. He would have felt trapped. As the perceived intimidation continued, he would have become fearful for his life. The escalation of the tension would have made him feel that an attack was becoming more imminent. The hypothetical assailant would have felt that the bear spray would only provide temporary protection from attack and thus he would feel it necessary to use the knife to protect his own life.

In cross-examination by Crown counsel, the issue of moving from the hypothetical to the specific scenario arose. Dr Glancy expressed the opinion that Mr Kagan's mental condition would not have prevented him from knowing that what he did was wrong. He felt that Mr Kagan was capable of making rational choices but if he was paranoid then he would have been extremely sensitised to the feeling of being trapped. Dr Glancy likened the situation to that of a battered woman and her distorted perceptions of threat. However, he said that his views were dependent upon evidence that Mr Kinney was a violent man and that living with him was a negative experience for Mr Kagan. The evidence as to this was dubious.

Justice McDougall commented (*Kagan*: at [34]) that "These insights into the mind of a person suffering from Asperger's and specifically the mind of Mr Kagan at the time of the incident are helpful in assessing the evidence provided by the accused." (cp *R v Tarr*, 2009L at [34]) He noted that Dr Glancy had warned of the risks of drawing adverse inferences from the obsessiveness and pedantry of Mr Kagan. Ultimately, however, McDougall J concluded that he was an unreliable witness and preferred the account of Mr Kinney. He stated that he made his evaluations mindful of the Asperger's syndrome of Mr Kagan:

> In the case of Paul Kagan's testimony his demeanor on the witness stand and the answers he provided to questions put to him by both defence and Crown counsel has to be evaluated taking into consideration Dr Glancy's diagnosis. Dr Glancy described Mr Kagan as being pedantic. Indeed, he exhibited this characteristic by repeating most every question that was put to him by counsel before attempting to answer it. On occasion he would ask the question to be repeated over and over again before offering a

> response. On other occasions he would seek clarification of a question to the point where he appeared to be searching for the reason or purpose for the question. In many instances this left the Court with the impression that Mr Kagan was attempting to provide an answer that he thought would be better for the Court to hear. This, in my opinion, has affected his credibility. This, and the numerous inconsistencies in his testimony between this trial and the first trial have left me in doubt as to the truthfulness of some of the answers he has given. (*Kagan*: at [37])

Justice McDougall found that a variety of Mr Kinney's habits irritated Mr Kagan and prompted confrontations between the two men, initiated by Mr Kagan. However, he concluded that it would not have been reasonable for Mr Kagan to fear that Mr Kinney was about to either kill him or cause him grievous bodily harm. He also found that it was not reasonable for Mr Kagan to have used the force that he did against Mr Kinney on the assertion that he could not otherwise save himself from apprehended death or grievous bodily harm. There is no indication, therefore, that McDougall J accepted that Mr Kagan's perceptions may have been distorted at the relevant time by his Asperger's symptomatology. His reasons for this are not articulated, leaving the potential that the expert evidence did not effectively educate the court about the potentially relevant effects of the disorder upon the accused man's perceptions and anxieties.

However, at the sentencing hearing, McDougall J imposed a non-custodial sentence to be served in the community, having heard evidence not only about Mr Kagan having Asperger's but about the "steps taken by the offender to follow the recommended counselling and other treatment devised to help him better understand and to deal with the symptoms of Asperger's Syndrome" (*Kagan*: at [22]) and his successful attendance at university in the period between the offending and the date of imposition of sentence. Although he rejected the defence of self-defence based upon Asperger's, he explicitly accepted that "The condition ... does affect the way the offender interprets the words and actions of those he might encounter. His condition must be considered in arriving at an appropriate sentence in this particular case." (*Kagan*: at [37])

Like the decision of the Victorian Court of Appeal in *DPP v HPW* (2011), the decision of McDougall J constitutes an important reminder that the mere presence of Asperger's disorder in a defendant will not automatically exculpate them or even, necessarily, reduce their moral culpability for criminal conduct.

6. Forensic issues

By virtue of Autism Spectrum Disorders being a pervasive developmental disorder, it is apparent that they have the potential to impact upon almost every aspect of criminal responsibility and also to raise the likelihood of certain kinds of offending. As already indicated, reported cases in which the defendant has Asperger's have tended particularly to include offences of physical violence, sexual violence, fire-setting, stalking and computer offences. In respect of each of these impoverished empathy, poor sensitivity, low responsivity and obsessionality have the potential to lay the groundwork for the commission of the offending. In turn, this has ramifications for both the criminal responsibility and culpability of the conduct.

Those with Autism Spectrum Offences are likely to be found fit to be interviewed by police more often than they should be (see eg *R v Maxwell*, 2007: at [43]). The difficulty is that while such persons may be intellectually capable of understanding questions and giving articulate answers, they may be more compliant and deferential than other interviewees (see North, Rissell and Gudjonsson, 2005), and may also be particularly fearful of figures in authority who place them under what they experience as pressure by their authoritarian manner and their questioning style. A difficult issue in evaluating the voluntariness of a police interview that has taken place with a person with an Autism Spectrum Disorder is to assess their capacity to make an independent and free decision as to whether or not to participate in such an interview. Expert evidence on the issue from a mental health professional with knowledge of the disorder is necessary (see Freckelton and Selby, 2009). Another forensic issue is the need for provision of counter-intuitive guidance to decision-makers (judges, juries and magistrates) about the risks of drawing over-ready (and inaccurate) inferences from the unusual manner of interviewees with Autism Spectrum Disorders. This consideration applies both to interview and trial behaviour by those with Autism Spectrum Disorders.

Finally, the language of persons with Autism Spectrum Disorders can be eccentric, tangential, formal and easily capable of misinterpretation. The following is an example of questioning in court to a person with Asperger's disorder who had assaulted someone invading their space, as in the following hypothetical dialogue:

Q: So when he wouldn't leave, you decided to attack him?

A: I wanted to be left alone.

In this example, an inference of intention could easily be made, when no such intention actually existed (see Freckelton and List, 2009).

Those with Autism Spectrum Disorders are generally likely to be accounted fit to stand trial as in most jurisdictions the threshold for fitness is quite low(see Freckelton and Selby, 2009). Those with the disorder will often be able to understand the nature of a trial, the various participants in it, will be able to follow the evidence, albeit with some limitations, and will be able to give instructions to their legal representatives. It is only in cases of considerable complexity or where (usually because of particular stress) their paranoia is close to pathological levels that their ability to participate in the criminal justice system will become legally problematic. Where it is their distress levels that are highly elevated and impacting upon their capacity to participate in the proceedings, medication may be able to play a constructive role. Importantly, given the lifetime nature of the disorder, and the limited extent to which it is responsive to clinical intervention, a decision of unfitness to stand trial may not be attractive to those providing legal advice to defendants with Autism Spectrum Disorders (as in the case of persons with intellectual disability or personality disorders) because of the draconian consequences that follow from such a decision. This is especially so when the charges preferred are not serious.

The most controversial forensic issue in relation to Autism Spectrum Disorders is the capacity of those with such disorders to be able to appreciate the nature and quality of their conduct or that it is wrong - the orthodox tests for insanity and mental impairment. In this regard, the disorders share some features with the developmental deficit that enables children over the age of criminal responsibility in some circumstances to plead as a defence that, although they committed the criminal act, nonetheless they were not criminally responsible on the basis that they were *doli incapax* (see R v M, 1977; *R v Whitty*, 1993; *C v DPP*, 1995; Blazey-Ayoub, 2003) - they did not know that what they did was wrong.

Those with Autism Spectrum Disorders tend to be preoccupied with constituent elements of behaviour (their own and others') and sub-tasks, with limited capacity to foresee the consequences of their behaviour and also its likely impact upon their victims. They are more likely than others to be obsessed by a perceived grievance (see eg *Glover v The Police*, 2009) or by a characteristic of the victim or something associated with the victim. This tends to deny or at least reduce for them the inhibiting mechanisms that militate against other members of the community engaging in socially unacceptable behaviour. They can be capable of thoughtful deliberation before acting, but under conditions of stress or, if feeling overwhelmed or confused, can behave impulsively and erratically (see Attwood, 2007: p234). Barry-Walsh and Mullen (2004: at p104) have appropriately raised this question: "if social conventions and connectedness are opaque to them how can they authentically appreciate that their actions are morally wrong (as opposed to a concrete understanding that certain behavior may provoke a predictable and unpleasant response from others?" However, as with the issue of fitness to stand trial, there are good strategic reasons why those representing defendants with Autism Spectrum Disorders may be loathe to raise a defence of insanity/mental impairment because of the grim consequences in terms of custodial detention that follow from such a determination.

It is possible that Autism Spectrum Disorders may constitute an "abnormality of mind" for the purposes of a partial defence of diminished responsibility to murder (see *R v Reynolds*, 2004), where such a defence exists. The main issue will be the extent to which the symptomatology affected the defendant's thinking at the relevant time.

It has been argued on occasions that because of having an Autism Spectrum Disorder a defendant was prone to misinterpret the behaviour of another as threatening (see eg *R v Mrzljak*, 2004: at [88]). This has the potential, for instance, to enable a defence of self-defence or provocation (where it exists) if latitude is given to take account of the peculiar characteristics of a person with the disorder. However, it remains incumbent upon the defendant in such matters to establish the preconditions for the defence (see eg *Kagan*, 2007). Alternatively, it has been argued that because of such a disorder defendants failed to appreciate cues and communications which would have alerted others that their behaviour was distressing or not resulting in consent (see eg *Parish*, 2007; *Sultan*, 2008; *Hopper*, 2003). This has the potential to constitute a full defence if the prosecution cannot adequately prove the intentional element of the offending. The existence of an Autism Spectrum Disorder in an accused can go to the issue of either the basic intention to commit the relevant act at all (eg, due to motor clumsiness or diminished appreciation of exactly what the person was doing) or to the specific intention to cause any required results (due to a lack of thought about consequences).

Another relationship between Asperger's disorder and criminal offending can be the development of obsessions and fixations. Example in this regard are to be found especially in computer offending such as that engaged in by McKinnon in the United Kingdom and Mr Walker in New Zealand, Barry Walsh and Mullen (2004) described:

- an arson offender with Asperger's who had an unusual facility for mathematics and became absorbed in the flickering of different forms of flames;
- a stalker who became fixated on professionals who had been involved in his care;
- an arson offender with a fascination for moving objects, Second World War aircraft and then a radio station - when he could no longer hear the radio station clearly he set fire to the organisation that interrupted his access to his favoured station, displaying no regret for his behavior;
- an arsonist with a preoccupation with electronics who assaulted his father when confronted with his fire-setting behaviour; and

- a child sex offender with repetitive and obsessive behaviours.

On a significant number of occasions the submission has been put at the sentencing stage of criminal proceedings that offenders with Asperger's disorder have reduced levels of culpability for their offending (see eg *R v Petroulias, 2008; R v Walker*, 2008: at [17]; *DPP v HPW*, 2011). This has potential repercussions for the imposition of a sentence that has as its objectives punishment, specific deterrence (deterrence of the individual concerned) and general deterrence (deterrence of others in the community). It is also pertinent to the ongoing need of the community to be protected from the person to be sentenced. However, the relevance of Asperger's depends upon the circumstances of offending and whether there is a causal nexus between the disorder and the conduct of the offender. There are occasions where such a nexus will not be established and the only impact of the disorder for the purposes of sentence will be its effect upon the burdensome nature of imprisonment as many persons with the disorder will struggle with the dynamics of jail (see eg *DPP v HPW*, 2011, see also Freckelton, 2011).

It is important for courts to be informedly assisted by suitable expert evidence by psychiatrists and psychologists in cases where the person charged (or found guilty) has an Autism Spectrum Disorder so as to appreciate better what can be the subtle repercussions of the disorder for the conduct in which the person has engaged. The consequences of Autism Spectrum Disorders for persons' states of mind in different situations and also for the effect that imprisonment may have upon them lie outside the realm of competence of many mental health practitioners meaning that suitable referral and commissioning of forensic opinions is fundamentally important if courts are to be adequately guided and assisted.

As Debbaudt (2002: 16) observed: "Recognition and response is the key for law enforcement professionals to understand the needs of the rising autistic population. Most importantly, law enforcers need to recognise the signs of autism in order to provide for the welfare and safety of all citizens and to avoid needless litigation".

7. Cases

C v DPP [1995] 2 All ER 43
Chandler v The Queen [2010] VSCA 338
DPP v HPW [2011] VSCA 88
Glover v Police [2009] HC 1150
Hopper v The Queen [2003] WASCA 153
McKinnon v USA [2007] EWHC 762 (Admin)
McC v Regina [2007] NSWCCA 25
McKinnon v The United States of America [2008] UKHL 59
McKinnon v Secretary of State for the Home Department [2009] EWHC 170 (Admin)
McKinnon v Secretary of State for Home Affairs [2009] EWHC 2021 (Admin)
Parish v DPP [2007] VSC 494
R v Burkett [2006] NZHC 800
R v EH [2008] QCA 67;
R v George [2004] NSWCCA 247; (2004) 149 A Crim R 38
R v JO [2008] QCA 260.
R v Kagan (2007) 261 NSR (2d) 285; (2008) 261 NSR (2d) 168.
R v M (1977) 16 SASR 589

R v Maxwell (2007) 314 NBR (2d) 191
R v Mrzljak [2004] QCA 420.
R v Mueller [2005] NSWCCA 47
R v Petroulias (No 36) [2008] NSWSC 626
R v Reynolds [2004] EWCA Crim 1834
R v Tarr, 2009 NSPC 2
R v Walker [2008] NZHC 1114
R v Whitty (1993) 66 A Crim R 462*Sultan v The Queen* [2008] EWCA Crim 6
United States v Lange [2006] USCA7 220; 445 F 3d 983.

8. References

Asperger H; tr. and annot. Frith U (1991) [1944]. Autistic Psychopathy' in Childhood. In Frith U. *Autism and Asperger Syndrome.* Cambridge University Press. pp.37–92. ISBN 0-521-38608-X.

Attwood T. 2007. *The Complete Guide to Asperger's Syndrome.* London. Jessica Kingsley Publishers. ISBN 978 1 84642 559 2

An Examination of the Links between Autistic Spectrum Disorders and Offending Behaviour in Young People". Internet Journal of Criminology: 1-32 http://www.internetjournalofcriminology.com/Bishop%20-%20Autistic%20Spectrum%20Disorders%20and%20Offending%20Behaviour%20in%20Young%20People.pdf, viewed 12 May 2011.

Barry-Walsh, J. .and Mullen, P. 2004. Forensic Aspects of Asperger's Syndrome" *Journal of Forensic Psychiatry and Psychology* 15(1): 96-107.

Chawarska, K. Klin, A. and Volkmer, F.R. 2008. *Autism Spectrum Disorders in Infants and Toddlers.* New York. Guilford Press. ISBN 1593856490, 9781593856496.

Carly, M.J. 2008. *Asperger's from the Inside Out.* New York. Perigee.

Crofts T. 2003. Doli Incapax: Why Children Deserve Its Protection" *Murdoch Electronic Journal of Law.* 10(3) http://www.murdoch.edu.au/elaw/issues/v10n3/crofts103_text.html, viewed 21 March 2011.

Debbaudt, D. (2002). *Autism, Advocates and Law Enforcement Professionals.* London: JKP

Duggal, H.S. 2003. Bipolar Disorder with Asperger's Disorder. *American Journal of Psychiatry* 160: 184-185.

Enayati, J. Grann, M. Lubbe, S and Fazel, S. (2008). Psychiatric Morbidity in Arsonists Referred for Forensic Psychiatric Assessment in Sweden. *Journal of Forensic Psychiatry and Psychology* 19(2): 139-147

Everall I. and Lecouteur A. 1990. Fire Setting in an Adolescent Boy with Asperger's Syndrome (1990) *British Journal of Psychiatry* 157: 284-287.

Freckelton I (2011), "Asperger's Disorder and the Criminal Law". *Journal of Law and Medicine*, 18: 677-694.

Freckelton I (2011a) Cruel and Unusual Punishment of Prisoners with Mental Illnesses: From Oates to Plata. *Psychiatry, Psychology and Law.* 18(3): 329-340

Freckelton I. and List D., 2009. Asperger's Disorder, Criminal Responsibility and Criminal Culpability. *Psychiatry, Psychology and Law.* 16(1): 16-40.

Freckelton, I. and Selby, H. 2009. Ex*pert Evidence: Law, Practice, Procedure and Advocacy.* 4th edn. Sydney. Thomson.

Ghaziuddin M., Tsai L. and Ghaziuddin N. 1991. "Brief Report: Violence and Asperger's Syndrome, a Critique" (1991) *Journal of Autism and Developmental Disorders* 21: 349-354.

Gillot A., Furniss F. and Walter A. 2001. Anxiety in High-functioning Children with Autism. *Autism.* 5: 277

Haskins B.G. and Silva J.A., 2006. Asperger's Disorder and Criminal Behavior: Forensic Psychiatric Considerations. *Journal of the American Academy of Psychiatry and Law* 34: 374-384: http://www.jaapl.org/cgi/reprint/34/3/374.pdf, viewed 17 March 2011.

Klin A., Volkmar F.R. and Sparrow S.S., 2000. Asperger Syndrome. New York. Guilford Press. ISBN 1572305347, 9781572305342.

Langstrom N., Grann, M., Ruchkin V., Sjostedt, G. And Fazel, S. 2009. Risk Factors for Violent Offending in Autism Spectrum Disorder: A National Study of Hospitalized Individuals. *Journal of Interpersonal Violence.* 24(8): 1358-1370.

Mawson D., Grounds A. and Tantam D. 1985. Violence and Asperger's Syndrome: A Case Study. *British Journal of Psychiatry* 147: 566- 569.

Miller J.N. and Ozonoff S. 1997 Did Asperger's Cases Have Asperger's Disorder? *Journal of Child Psychology and Psychiatry* 38: 247-252.

Mullen P.E. 1996. Forensic Report: http://kildall.apana.org.au/autism/articles/bryant.html, viewed 17 March 2011.

Murrie, D.C., Warren J., Kristiansson M. and Dietz PE. 2002. Asperger's Syndrome in Forensic Settings. *International Journal of Forensic Mental Health.* 1(1): 59-70.

National Autistic Society (2004). A Place in Society (National Autistic Society: London).

North A., Russell A. and Gudjonsson G., An Investigation of Potential Vulnerability During Police Interrogation of Adults with Autism Spectrum Disorder: A Focus on Interrogative Suggestibility and Compliance. Paper presented at the 1st International Symposium on Autism Spectrum Disorders in a Forensic Context, Copenhagen, Demark, September 2005.

Paterson P. 2008. How Well Do Young Offenders with Asperger's Syndrome Cope in Custody?"*British Journal of Learning Disabilities.* 36(1): 54-58.

Patrick N.J. 2008. *Social Skills for Teenagers and Adults with Asperger Syndrome.* New York. Jessica Kingsley.

Schwartz-Watts, D. 2005. Asperger's Disorder and Murder. *Journal of the American Academy of Psychiatry and Law* 33(3): 390-393.

Silva J.A., Ferrari M.M. and Leong G.B. 2003. Asperger's Disorder and the Origins of the Unabomber" *American Journal of Forensic Psychiatry* 24: 5-8.

Simblett G and Wilson D. 1993. Asperger's Syndrome: Three Cases and a Discussion. *Journal of Intellectual Disability Research* 37: 85-94.

Tantam D, "Lifelong Eccentricity and ocial isolation. I. Psychiatric, social, and forensic aspects". Br J Psychiatry. 153: 777-782.

Volkmar F.R., State M. and Klin A. 2009, Autism and Autism Spectrum Disorders: Diagnostic Issues for the Coming Decade. J Child Psychol Psychiatry.;50(1-2):108-15.

Warren A., 2006. Asperger's Syndrome and Autistic Spectrum Disorders in the Courts. Paper presented at the National Judicial College of Australia Conference, Science, Experts and the Courts: http://njca.anu.edu.au/Professional%20Development/programs%20by%20year/2006/Science%20and%20courts/Anthony%20Warren.pdf, viewed 7 April 2011.

Wing L. 1981. Asperger's Syndrome: A Clinical Account. *Psychological Medicine* 11: 115-129.

Part 7

Diagnosis of Autism Spectrum Disorders and a Financial Side

17

The Financial Side of Autism: Private and Public Costs

Deanna L. Sharpe and Dana L. Baker
University of Missouri
Washington State University
United States

1. Introduction

First identified by Leo Kanner in the early 1940s, autism is a biologically based developmental disorder that impairs an individual's ability to communicate, build relationships, and relate appropriately to the environment (Kanner, 1943). Diagnosis is usually made in early childhood after a multi-disciplinary assessment of behavior, developmental level, and communication ability. Boys are four times as likely as girls to be affected (Fombonne, 2003a, 2005).

Initially, autism was considered a rare disorder. An early epidemiological study conducted in England in the 1960s documented a 0.05% prevalence rate (4.5 per 10,000) (Lotter, 1966). Prior to the 1980s, recorded incidence of autism disorder in the United States was also low, affecting about 1 in every 2,000 children (Fombonne, 2009; Rutter, 2005). In the 1990s, the American Psychiatric Association broadened diagnostic criteria and included Asperger's syndrome and Pervasive Developmental Disorder - Not Otherwise Specified (PDD-NOS) with Autism Disorder under Autism Spectral Disorder (ASD)(Centers for Disease Control, 2009). In this article, the terms autism and ASD are used interchangeably.

Autism is now known to affect children world-wide, regardless of race, ethnicity, or socio-economic status (Naqvi, 2009). Documented prevalence rates vary. In the United States, the current ASD prevalence rate is 1 in every 110 births (1 in 70 boys) (Centers for Disease Control, 2009), representing an average increase of 57% over 2002, 600% over the last two decades (Dawson, 2010; Wang & Leslie, 2010). Prevalence rates in Western Europe, Canada, and Australia are similar to those in the United States (Grossman & Barrozo, 2007; Naqvi, 2009), whereas rates in Japan and China are somewhat higher (Naqvi, 2009; Wong & Hui, 2008). Prevalence rates in Western Europe and Canada are similar to those the United States. In recent years, the number of cases in Latin America, Asia, the Middle East, and Africa has increased as well (Grossman & Barrozo, 2007).

No consensus regarding cause exists (Fombonne, 2003b). Reasons for the surge in incidence of autism are ardently debated. Autism has no known genetic or biological markers. Diagnosis relies on observation of behavior and professionals may differ in application of diagnostic criteria. Some have argued that the recent surge in numbers simply reflects increased awareness of symptoms and better diagnostic tools (Cohen & Spenciner, 1996;

Gernsbacher, et al., 2005). Others counter that while improved understanding of autism may account for some of the increase; it fails as a satisfactory explanation of all of the growth in diagnosed cases (Yazbak, 2003).

Autism can be an expensive disorder. Diagnosis and therapeutic intervention can be a lengthy and labor intensive process. Families can spend more than $50,000 per year on autism-related therapies such as applied behavioral analysis (ABA) (National Conference of State Legislatures [NCSL], 2010). Treatment may involve use of costly foods or dietary supplements. Prescription of psychotropic medications can lead to frequent use of the medical system. Health care costs for individuals with ASD can be as much as 45% higher than otherwise comparable individuals without ASD (Croen, et al., 2006). Further, individuals with ASD are likely to have other types of disabling medical conditions, increasing use of inpatient and outpatient care services (Mandell, et al., 2006).

ASD-related costs are not limited to the cost of therapeutic or medical intervention. As with other forms of childhood disability, parents of a child with autism often face greater outlays of time and money than they would for a neurologically typical child for things such as specialized childcare and educational materials. Caregiving demands can force parents to reduce work hours or leave the labor market (Gould, 2004)

ASD is now considered a significant and growing public health concern due to the rapid increase in prevalence and high cost of therapeutic interventions and care (Newschaffer & Curran, 2003; Grossman and Barrozo, 2007). Greater understanding of the costs associated with ASD is needed to guide service planning, allocation of private and public sector resources to those affected by autism, and evaluation of market systems and public policies that affect access to and cost of autism-related services.

This article reviews what is currently known about the type, amount, and distribution of autism-related financial costs relative to family and society. Estimates of the broad social costs of autism are compared. Components of the financial burden on family members are examined. Current avenues to sharing some of this financial burden with the public and private sector are reviewed. The article concludes with recommendations for future research.

2. Total cost of autism: Estimates and issues

Autism is complex. Considerable heterogeneity exists among those affected by it. A wide spectrum of health care, education, and social service agencies provide diagnostic services, therapeutic interventions, and medical care related to autism, each with their own recordkeeping standards and data considered relevant. Sharing of information or data across agencies is limited. In addition, most of the costs borne by families of children with autism occur outside the market and are difficult to quantify. These facts make it challenging to obtain a comprehensive measure of autism-related expenditures. To date, no single representative data base captures all of the costs and expenditures related to autism spectrum disorders. Consequently, to inform public policy decisions, researchers have used available data and estimates in efforts to quantify ASD-related expenditures.

Given the challenges in data collection, the prominent role of medical care in the lives of children with ASD, and the availability of medical data, much attention has been given to measurement or estimation of medical costs and expenditures. Researchers have assessed use and cost of health care for children with ASD (e.g. Croen et al, 2006; Liptak, et al., 2006), and have developed broader measures that account for the indirect as well as the direct costs associated with ASD (e.g. Ganz, 2006, 2007). Researchers have used survey data (e.g. Järbrink & Knapp, 2001), institutional or government health care usage and cost data (e.g. Shimabukuro et al., 2008; Wang & Leslie, 2010) or constructed synthetic expenditure estimates using published cost and use data and prevalence rates (e.g. Ganz, 2006, 2007). Incidence of autism is worldwide. Research on the costs associated with ASD has been conducted in the United States (e.g. Croen, et al. 2006), the United Kingdom (Järbrink & Knapp, 2001), Sweden (Järbrink, 2007), and, recently, China (Xiong et al. 2011) and Egypt (Mendoza, 2010). More remains to be learned about autism-related costs in developing countries, however.

Key findings of recent studies of autism-related costs conducted in the United States and abroad are summarized in Table 1. To facilitate comparison, all monetary values in the table have been converted to 2011 United States dollars. A brief review of each study follows.

Croen, et al. (2006) used data from the Kaiser Permaente Medical Program in Northern California, a large group health care plan, to compare health care utilization and expenditures of children aged 2 to 18 with and without ASD. On every measure considered the health care cost for children with ASD was higher. Children with ASD had higher average total clinic, pediatric and psychiatric outpatient visits. A larger percent of children with ASD had inpatient and outpatient hospitalizations (3% vs. 1% for inpatient and 5% vs. 2% for outpatient). Children with ASD were about twice as likely to use gastrointestinal medications and 9 times more likely to use psychotherapeutic medications. Average cost for children with ASD were twice as high as other children for hospitalization, clinic visits, and prescription medications. Age and gender adjusted total cost per member was on average almost 3 times higher for children with ASD. Among children that had psychiatric conditions, total average annual costs were 45% higher for children who also had ASD.

Liptak, et al. (2006) also examined the health care use and expenditures of children with ASD. Instead of using data from one specific health care provider however, researchers examined cross sectional data from 3 national surveys: the Medical Expenditure Panel Survey, the National Ambulatory Medical Care Survey, and the National Hospital Ambulatory Care Survey. Similar to Croen, et al. (2006), Liptak et al. (2006) found that, as compared with other children, children with ASD had more outpatient visits, physician visits, and prescription medication. Also, physician visits for children with ASD lasted an average of about 15 minutes longer than those of children without ASD. Annual medical expenses for children with ASD were over 7 times higher.

Mandell, et al. (2006) used Medicaid data from Allegheny County, Pennsylvania from 1994 to 1999 to compare medical expenses of minor aged children with and without an autism diagnosis. Total expenditures equaled the sum of reimbursed charges per person per year for ambulatory care, emergency care, hospitalization, psychiatric hospitalization and psychiatric outpatient care. Average expenditures were calculated using data on only those with that expense. Average annual Medicaid spending for children with ASD was 3.5 times that of children with mental retardation and nine times that of other children, largely due to dissimilar inpatient and outpatient psychiatric expenditures.

Leslie and Martin (2007) conducted a comprehensive assessment of health care spending on children with ASD age 17 and under using a large, national database containing claims information from the private health plans of large employers. This estimate was compared with that of children that had a mental disorder using inflation-adjusted annual figures 2000 though 2004. Health care spending equaled the sum of actual amounts paid by the patient (e.g. deductible or co-pay), the patient's insurance plan and any other insurance for inpatient, outpatient, and pharmaceuticals.

Authorship	Data Source	Sample	Expenditures Developed Country per person per year estimates
Croen et al. 2006	Kaiser Permanente Northern CA 2003-2004	3,053 children with autism diagnosis	Total Medical: $3,190 Inpatient: $1,650 Meds: $847 Other: $660
Liptak et al. 2006	National sample from MEPS 1997-2000	31 children with autism diagnosis	Total Medical $8,140 Inpatient: $968 Meds: $1,287 Other: $5,830
Mandell et al. 2006	Allegheny County, PA Medicaid data 1994-1999	334 children with autism diagnosis	Total Medical $13,200 Inpatient: $9,130 Other: $4,070
Leslie and Martin 2007	Large US self-insured employers	256,646 children with mental disorder diagnosis 2000-2005	Total Medical $6,995
Wang and Leslie 2010	Medicaid data for 42 states; fee-for-service	2,184,677 children with mental disorder diagnosis; 49,921 with autism, 19,621 with other ASD	Autism: $27,400 Other ASD: $24,410 Total health care cost per 10,000 for children with ASD $2,024,326
			Developed Country: lifetime estimates
Järbrink and Knapp 2001	Center of Economics data & survey of 250 parents	228 children with autism or high functioning autism	Autism $2,293,250 High Functioning Autism $859,000
Ganz 2006	Synthetic estimate		$3,783780
Knapp, et al., 2007	Synthetic estimate		Low Functioning: $8.1 million High Functioning: $4.9 million
Xiong, et al., 2011	Clients in 3 Beijing rehab. institutions	227 children; 61 with ASD	$2,984
Mendoza 2010	Probability sample Greater Cairo Region	174 persons with ASD	Direct financial costs for surveyed households ranged between $37,560- $55,080

Table 1. Summary of cost and expenditure studies for individuals with ASD; all monetary amounts converted to 2011 US$. Table adapted from Bouder, et al. (2009).

Treated prevalence of ASD was low relative to other mental disorders reported in the database. But, over the 5 years of the study, ASD prevalence increased 101.1%, which was a substantially higher rate than all other mental disorders except bipolar disorder at 106%.

Expenditure among ASD patients was relatively high, however. Between 2000 and 2004, mean ASD expenditures increased 26.1% per patient. Computing total health care expenditures per 10,000 covered lives, the researchers found expenditures for ASD patients increased markedly over the 5 years, from $47,378 per 10,000 (2000$) to $114,710 per 10,000 (2004$), a 142.1% increase. They note, however, that in the context of the data utilized in the study, ASD related expenditures were smaller than those associated with more common mental health conditions. As a comparison, hyperactivity had the highest cost burden with an average of $406,238 during the same time frame.

Wang and Leslie (2010) examined trends in health care expenditures associated with ASD using Medicaid from 42 states. Their focus was children aged 17 or younger who were continuously enrolled from 2000 to 2003 in fee-for-service Medicaid with a mental disorder diagnosis. Treated prevalence of ASDs in the data increased almost 29% over the four years observed, the largest increase among the mental disorder diagnostic groups. Average total health care expenditures per treated child were $27,400 (2011 US$) for autism; $24,410 (2011 US$) for any other ASD. Total health care expenditures for ASDs per 10,000 covered lives increased 32.8% between 2000 and 2003.

A few studies have attempted to estimate lifetime costs. Järbrink and Knapp (2001) used autism prevalence rates and cost data from several prior national research studies and reports to estimate costs associated with service use, lost productivity of those with autism, and family time cost and expenses in Britain. They considered two scenarios. The average lifetime cost for someone with autism and an additional learning disability was £2.94 million ($4.77 million 2011 US$). For someone with high functioning autism, lifetime cost was estimated to be £785,000 ($1,274,840 2011 US$). For both groups, living support was the highest expense at 87% of total cost for those with autism and an additional learning disability and 40% of total cost for those with high functioning autism. They note that their estimates were highly sensitive to prevalence rates. Drawing on then current research, they used a prevalence rate of 5 per 10,000 (Fombonne, 1998).

Rather than survey parents regarding the specific costs that they bear, Ganz (2006, 2007) relied on published cost and usage data from various sources to estimate total costs associated with having a child with autism. Ganz classified costs as direct and indirect. Direct costs included the value of goods and services consumed as well as medical and nonmedical costs. Indirect cost focused on value of employment-related productivity lost by individuals with autism and their families as a result of autism-related time demands. Since these costs were not observed in the market, an opportunity cost approach was used to estimate their value. This approach is based in economic theory of opportunity cost. It identifies the value of other services that could have been obtained had resources not been consumed by or for individuals with autism.

Knapp, Romeo, and Beecham (2007) calculated aggregated cost of ASD for the United Kingdom. Data on prevalence, level of functioning, place of residence, and cost per individual were drawn from national surveys, published research, own prior studies and expert opinion. Individual level costs were multiplied by estimated prevalence rates, stratified by age (0 - 3, 4-11, 12-17, adult), level of functioning (high or low), and residence (foster/residential care or private family household).

Average annual costs per child ranged between £16,185 and £62,536 ($26,220 and $101,308, 2011 US$) for children with low functioning ASD, depending on age and residential placement. For children with high functioning ASD, the range was £1,214 to £21,090 ($1,967 to $13,076 2011 US$). It was assumed all high functioning children would reside at home with family. Average annual cost per adult ranged between £14,124 and £75,840 ($22,880 and $122,861 2011 US$) for low functioning adults and between £13,076 and £67,514 ($21,183 and $109,373 2011 US$) for high functioning adults. These adult estimates do not include value of lost employment for the person with ASD at either level of functioning or the value of welfare benefits for low functioning adults. Considering lost employment would add, on average, an amount equivalent to $34,154 to average annual cost per adult. Considering welfare benefits would add approximately $1,500 to $10,860 (US$), depending on residential status.

Aggregate annual national cost for all children with ASD was £2.7 billion ($4.3 billion 2011 US$) with about 63% of that cost attributed to children with low functioning ASD. Aggregate annual national cost for all adults with ASD was £25 billion ($40.5 2011 US$), with about 66% of that cost attributed to adults with low functioning ASD. Knapp et al. (2007) estimated lifetime costs for someone with low functioning ASD at £4.7 million ($7.6 2011 US$) and at £2.9 million ($4.6 2011 US$) for high functioning ASD.

Incidence of autism is world-wide. Two recent studies examined costs associated with ASD in developing countries. As in the United States, prevalence rates of ASD in China have grown dramatically. Prior to 1980, average prevalence of ASD in China was close to 2 per 10,000, whereas after 1980 it has been 14.8 per 10,000. Median prevalence of ASD among children aged 2 to 6 from 2000 on is 10.3 per 10,000 (Sun & Allison, 2010).

Xiong et al. (2011) used data from 227 parent interviews to calculate difference in family income, living expenses, and economic assistance between families with and without a child with autism. Living expenses included spending on education, health care, as well as such things as clothing, "caring cost," and "amusement cost." Result of this calculation was deemed to be the annual financial burden of raising a child with autism. Researchers found cost was highest for families with a child with autism, followed by families with a child with a physical disability and mental disability. Bivariate regression analysis indicated that autism was a significant predictor of family spending on education, medical, caring, and clothing, but not for amusement or educational toys.

Mendoza (2010) conducted the first known study of autism-related costs in Egypt using survey data gathered from a probability sample of 165 households in the Greater Cairo Region. In contrast to the United States and European countries, Mendoza found few families used ASD interventions or institutionalized autism-related services, citing lack of knowledge about ASD and effective interventions, limited state or community resources, limited financial resources, and pessimism regarding the family member with autism as reasons why. Most individuals with ASD (91.2%) relied on immediate family for care; family members expected to continue to provide that care for the lifetime of the disabled member. The widespread use of home based care resulted in direct financial cost estimates that were considerably lower than similar estimates obtained in developed countries. The majority of costs were for non-medical items such as special education, skills training, or camps rather than for medical services, prescription medication, or behavioral therapy.

Examining results across these expenditure studies, several conclusions may be drawn. Provision of services to those with ASD requires a large investment of family and social resources. Consequently, meeting the needs of those with ASD generates significant opportunity costs for all sectors of society. Care costs for those with ASD are several times higher than that of other individuals, both with and without disability. For those with ASD, medical costs in general and pharmacology costs in particular appear to be a large share of expenditures. Both annual and lifetime cost estimates can vary greatly, depending on such things as the age of the individual, residential situation (family vs. institutional), and degree of function. Costs associated with ASD in developed countries with established social service, education, and medical sectors are considerably higher than costs in developing counties that lack such services. Worldwide, families bear a significant portion of the financial burden of ASD. In developing countries, virtually all of the care costs fall to family. The portions of the caregiving burden that family cannot sustain will inevitably spillover to society in one form or another.

An obvious and major weakness of all cost estimates is that they are highly sensitive to the assumptions made regarding any component part. Counts and costs are documented for such things as physician visits, but value of non-market costs such as reduction in parent employment is difficult to capture and monetize. Government and community resources can differ greatly by state, let alone by country, reducing ability to make meaningful comparisons. In absence of any other methods, the estimates are useful. But, clearly, a superior method would be development and use of comprehensive, longitudinal data collections on the characteristics and expenditures of those with ASD across the lifespan.

3. Family cost burden

Autism spectrum disorder places an enormous burden on families. Some costs such as out-of-pocket expenditures for diagnosis and treatment can be quantified. Other costs such as the value of lost leisure and employment time, and lost income can be estimated. Still other costs such as increased stress, disruption of family life, or reduced time with other family members can only be recognized. Relatively few studies have attempted to measure the cost of the informal care provided by family members. Each of these studies has used a different methodology and examined the question from a somewhat different perspective.

Endeavoring to improve methods for gathering data on family informal care, Järbrink, et al. (2003) conducted a pilot study with 15 families in the United Kingdom that had one or more children with autism between ages 4 and 10. Families were asked to keep a diary of autism-related time and money expenditures for 14 days. Questionnaires were also administered. The authors used parent records and questionnaire responses to determine the average cost of informal care, select out-of-pocket expenses, service use, and income losses. They also compared the type and amount of data gathered by each method and evaluated the strength and weakness of each approach.

Children in the study varied in severity of the disorder and presence of other disorders. Of the seventeen children in the study, eleven had an autism diagnosis, three were diagnosed with atypical autism, two had Asperger syndrome and one had semantic pragmatic disorder. Several of the children had some type of co-morbidity. Seven children had some degree of mental retardation. Two had chronic bowel syndrome, one had epilepsy and another had gluten intolerance.

Parents reported spending nearly 60 hours per week caring for their child due to autism spectral disorder. They estimated that if their child was not on the autism spectrum, they would have spent an average of 40 hours per week in other activities with about half of those hours (22 hours) allocated to paid work. Interestingly, several reported that if there were there no need to care for their child, their amount of unpaid work would actually decrease because paid work would replace current volunteer activities. Parents estimated they lost 11 hours of leisure per week due to care for their child.

Järbrink et al. (2003) found that average total out-of-pocket expenditures per child for goods and services other than education, early intervention therapy, health services and medications were about 52% higher in the diary survey than the questionnaire. They concluded use of long recall periods in expenditure studies would likely underestimate out-of-pocket spending noting that smaller outlays were apparently forgotten when completing the six month retrospective in the questionnaire.

Service use expenses were divided among education (mean weekly cost £223.82 or $363.48 2011 US$), early intervention therapy (mean weekly cost £144.38 or $234.47 2011 US$) and health and social services (£20.12 or $32.67 2011 US$). All of the children were either in a special school setting (e.g. boarding school or private school) or had special support in a mainstream school. Ten of the children received early intervention therapy where parents paid about a third of the cost. Health and social service cost focused on in-patient hospital care, social services respite care and clinical psychologist appointments.

Although all parents reported that their child's condition had a negative effect on career or income, only eleven could give a numerical estimate of that loss. Average weekly loss reported by parents was £231 ($375 2011 US$) with a median of £250 ($406 2011 US$). Most estimates were in the range of £200 to £450 ($325 to $731 2011 US$) per week.

Combining cost estimates for education, early intervention therapy, health and social services, voluntary support, medication, other costs paid by parent (e.g. for damages, certain food or clothing, toys), and income losses, Järbrink, et al. (2003) determined that the total societal cost for a child with autism in the study was £689 ($1,119 2011 US$) if the only time cost considered was reported income lost. However, if a human capital approach were used to place a value on time spent in informal care, weekly cost would increase to £855 ($1,388 2011 US$)

Using data gathered in the Family Experiences with Autism survey, Sharpe and Baker (2007) assessed responses from 333 parents of minor age children with autism to investigate factors associated with experiencing financial problems. Parents were asked about use various types of interventions including Applied Behavioral Analysis, speech and language, sensory integration, diet modification, special education, music therapy, riding therapy, and medical intervention. Parents also reported on unreimbursed out-of-pocket expenses for medical doctor or therapy, prescription and nonprescription drugs, and education expenses. Two unique contributions of their study were use of multivariate analysis to identify significant contributors to experiencing financial problems while holding demographics and economic resources constant and use of qualitative methods to identify themes in parent report of experiences.

Comparing the characteristics of those who did and who did not report having financial problems in the past 12 months due to autism, the researchers found that, among those reporting financial problems, a significantly higher proportion had autism limit family activities and had unreimbursed out-of-pocket expenses for doctor or therapy services, prescription and non-prescription drugs, and medical interventions. A significantly lower proportion in this group had used speech and language therapy or special education. No significant difference was found between the two groups for child age, use of Applied Behavioral Analysis (ABA), sensory integration, diet modification, music or riding therapy, income levels, receipt of public services, and rural residence, suggesting similar experience across all families in the sample for these items.

Two results stood out in the multivariate analysis of factors affecting likelihood of financial problems. First, utilizing medical interventions and having unreimbursed out-of-pocket expenditures for medical doctor or therapy or for education expenses were significant factors in increasing the likelihood of financial problems (by 121%, 264%, and 289%, respectively). Second, consistent with previous research and as would be expected, those with annual income under $40,000 were more likely to have financial problems than those with annual incomes of $60,000 or more. These results suggest that, while all families with a child with autism may struggle to meet the demands of the disorder, for low income families the demands can quickly outstrip family resources. For that reason, special attention needs to be given to low income families in the design and delivery of programs and public policy.

The researchers also used qualitative research methods to identify common themes in parent report of reasons for financial difficulty. Most were caught between rising expenses and reduced income. One of most salient sources of financial pressures according to the parents was the high cost of therapy, especially Applied Behavioral Analysis, as well as special foods or supplements. Medical expenses of other family members could increase as well. As one parent reported, "other family members need[ed] counseling and medication to cope with the stress of living with an autistic child." (Sharpe & Baker, 2007, p. 259)

Another common source of financial struggle was lost income due to reducing work time to manage care of the child. This situation exacted an emotion cost as well. Many of the parents expressed anguish or anger at having to leave the labor market or desperation and fear when considering how to meet financial demands with the income loss. An important insight given by the parents was that care management extended well beyond meeting the child's physical needs. Parents reported struggles with insurance providers to obtain or continue coverage for health related services; protracted battles with school administrators to obtain specific education services or starting to home school their children in an attempt to meet their educational needs. Scheduling and transportation to various therapies and medical appointments also took a toll on parent time. Other sources of financial pressure included replacing items broken, damaged, or destroyed by the child and retraction of public program support due to a misunderstanding of program rules.

A poignant aspect of parent report was the extent to which parents mortgaged their own future to obtain therapy and services for their children with autism. Parents cashed out their retirement investments, sold stock, drained the equity in their home, and borrowed money to the point that bankruptcy seemed inevitable. One desperate family reported "My husband and I often do not eat lunch or dinner because we have no money left to buy food for ourselves ...We are hard pressed to make a choice between heat for our family and food" (Sharpe & Baker, 2007, p. 259).

3.1 Family financial planning issues

Planning the financial future of a family with a child on the autism spectrum is a complex process. There are many important considerations not shared by families with neurotypical children. Family ability to engage in financial planning varies greatly. As noted, funding autism treatment can devastate the financial resources of some families and leave little hope for rebuilding the spent wealth. Seeking ways to help a child with autism, families have taken out a home equity loan, charged credit cards to the limit, or declared bankruptcy after exhausting their financial resources. Although a parent's desire to secure help at any cost is understandable, these actions have long term financial consequences for family and potentially society as well. In absence of reform of methods to fund autism treatment, families in this situation will continue to struggle to maintain income and may have to seek help from relatives and public assistance programs just to cover basic expenses.

The unique characteristics of children with ASD leads to wide variation in future care needs. High functioning children may require expensive intense therapy while young, but then incur minimal to no additional autism-related expenses in adolescence or adulthood. Children in this group may be able to support themselves as adults. In this situation, family financial plans could focus on funding post-secondary education and training.

Financial plans for a child that is mid-range to low functioning are quite different. Parents must arrange for care to continue after their death. Attention must be paid to lifestyle, legal, financial, and government benefit issues. Decisions must be made regarding where the disabled person will live, behavior management, education and employment activities, as well as social and religious activities.

Wills and trusts can be used to distribute parental assets to benefit the disabled child. Careful planning is needed to ensure the disabled individual receives what he/she is entitled to receive and assets transferred from financial gifts, bequests, or other sources do not jeopardize other potentially important sources of income or health care support such as Supplemental Security Income or Medicaid. Arrangements need to be made to provide professional money management, oversight of use, maintenance of government or other benefits, and protection of assets. Guardians, conservators, and trustees need to be named. Power of attorney to act on behalf of the disabled person may need to be executed along with end of life health directives. Plans should be reviewed annually and changes made as necessary.

4. Cost sharing: Public and private sector

Central to public policy discussion of autism is deliberation regarding who should share the cost of treatments, to what extent, and by what mechanisms. Much attention has been focused on access to and funding for applied behavioral analysis (ABA). ABA uses discrete trial training help individuals with ASD learn life, social and communication skills. ABA is an early intervention therapy that appears to be most effective when applied in the preschool years. Since it is delivered one-on-one with a trained therapist, it is very expensive. But, because its efficacy has been supported in the scientific literature, it is highly sought after by families with a child with autism as a therapeutic intervention.

Families in the United States have sought respite from the high costs of ASD in the federal Individuals with Disabilities Education Act (IDEA), state Medicaid waivers, and state health insurance mandates. Although each of these items offer some help for families with a child with autism, program structure and funding limits often curtail the type and amount of help actually received from these programs.

4.1 IDEA

The Individuals with Disabilities Education Act (IDEA) is a federal law passed in 1990 that addresses education needs of children with disabilities from birth to either age 18 or 21, depending on the disability. The intent of IDEA was to guarantee a free and appropriate education for every child with a disability, including ASD. Under IDEA, schools have typically offered speech and language therapy. Although speech and language therapy is important for most children with ASD, recently, attention has focused on provision of Early Intensive Behavioral Intervention (EIBI), usually in the form of Applied Behavioral Analysis (ABA). Given the high expense of ABA, parents have requested that school districts provide, fund, or reimburse them for ABA therapy for their child under the "free and appropriate" provision of IDEA. When refused, some parents have taken schools to court. Generally, when schools have correctly processed a student's Individual Education Plan, have hired qualified staff, used research-supported practices in educational programs, and collected meaningful data to monitor student progress and program effectiveness, courts have ruled in the schools favor (Yell & Drasgow, 2000).

As a practical matter, however, in times of cutbacks in education funding, school districts cannot afford the high cost of ABA therapy for each child with an autism diagnosis. Even if they could, they could not hire necessary personnel. Public schools are short more than 12,000 special education teachers, and the shortage is expected to rise as teachers retire or leave teaching. Consequently, in practice, "appropriate education" does not mean ideal, nor is it necessarily what parents believe is best for their child (Tarkan, 2002).

4.2 Medicaid waivers

Medicaid is a means-tested program designed to help persons that have low income and resources access health care. The program is funded by the federal and state governments. Although Congress and the federal Centers for Medicare and Medicaid Services have established the general rules for program operation, each state administers its own Medicaid program. Consequently, eligibility criteria can differ somewhat from state to state.

Medicaid waivers allow states to provide home and community based services to individuals that do not meet all eligibility criteria but, without the services provided by the waiver, would require long term institutional care. Total cost to Medicaid to provide services under the waiver cannot exceed what Medicaid would have paid for service in an appropriate institutional setting.

In 2007, Colorado, Indiana, Maryland and Wisconsin were the only states with Medicaid waivers focused specifically on children with autism. Since that time, Indiana, Kansas, Maryland, Massachusetts, Missouri, Montana, Nebraska, North Dakota, and Pennsylvania have received Medicaid waivers for autism. Most of these autism waivers focus on provision of service to children, although Pennsylvania has a waiver specifically for adult autism (Centers for Medicare and Medicaid Services [CMS], 2011). In a majority of the remaining states, autism is included in the state's definition of developmental disability and covered under a Medicaid developmental disability waiver. A few states, however, explicitly exclude autism from the state developmental disability definition unless the person also has mental retardation (Spigel, 2007).

Unfortunately, in practice, relatively few individuals with autism can obtain services under a waiver. Since persons must otherwise require long-term institutional care to be eligible, those at the high functioning end of the autism spectrum could not qualify. To control costs, states can cap waiver enrollment leading to long waiting lists. In states that focus on providing early intervention behavior therapy under the waiver, children on a long waiting list might no longer be eligible for services once an opening occurred (Spigel, 2007).

Future Medicaid funding is another concern. Medicaid represents about one-fifth of total state spending (National Association of State Budget Officers, 2010), making it one of the largest components of state budgets. The severe national recession in the late 2000s squeezed states between substantial declines in revenue and increased demand for public services, including Medicaid. According to the National Association of State Budget Officers, fiscal years 2009 and 2010 were two of the most difficult years for state budgets since the Great Depression. Attempting to meet budget shortfalls, 41 states made mid-year budget cuts during fiscal 2009; 39 states did so in 2010 (National Association of State Budget Officers, 2010). Across all states, Medicaid and education (K-12 and higher education) bore the brunt of these budget cuts. Given a slow economic recovery, tight state budgets are expected to continue into 2012 and beyond, thus restricting resources available to fund services for families that have a child with autism.

4.3 State health insurance mandates

The health insurance industry has generally excluded or strictly limited coverage for autism-related diagnosis and treatment, arguing that therapies such as ABA are an education intervention that should be funded by the public schools instead of health insurance. In recent years, diligent lobbying efforts from autism advocacy groups and families with a child with autism have resulted in passage of insurance mandates for autism in many states. In fact, a majority of the laws providing coverage for autism has been passed in the last three years (National Conference of State Legislatures [NCSL], 2010).

A health insurance mandate is a requirement that state law places on health plans or insurance providers in that state. Mandates typically force health plans or insurance providers to extend coverage to a broader population than they otherwise would. Some states only require that certain types of coverage be offered. Individuals and employers can accept or reject the coverage, giving the purchaser some control over policy content and cost. Other states disallow choice and require the mandate to be a part of all policies sold in the state (American Speech-Language Hearing Associates [ASHA] 2011)

Living in a state with an autism health insurance mandate does not guarantee adequate coverage of autism-related treatment or medication, however. Individuals along with small and medium sized employers purchase health insurance in the market. Large employers have the resources to self-insure. Self-insured plans are governed by the Federal Employee Retirement Income Security Act (ERISA) and are exempt from state law. Currently, 55 % of enrollees in a private sector plan are in a self-insured plan (Fernandez, 2010).

As of March 2011, all states except Alaska, Delaware, South Dakota, and Wyoming had passed a state insurance mandate related to autism diagnosis and treatment. Eighteen states have a mental health parity law that may include autism spectrum disorder as a covered mental illness: Alabama, Arkansas, California, District of Columbia, Georgia, Hawaii, Michigan, Minnesota, Mississippi, Nebraska, North Carolina, North Dakota, Ohio, Rhode Island, Utah, Virginia, Washington and West Virginia. Mental health parity laws mean that financial payments (e.g. co-pays or deductibles) or treatment limits (e.g. number of visits) for mental health services cannot be more restrictive than limits for medical/surgical benefits (ASHA, 2011).

Maryland, New York, Oklahoma, and Tennessee have limited autism mandates. In general, these mandates focus on medical conditions. Insurers cannot deny otherwise available coverage simply because treatment is used to diagnose or treat autism spectrum disorder. Coverage for treatment related to autistic disorder is restricted and only available for a child under age 18 or 19, depending on the state (ASHA 2011).

Almost half of the states have broad autism mandates that delineate coverage for assessment, diagnosis and treatment of autism spectrum disorders. These states are Arizona, Colorado, Connecticut, Florida, Illinois, Indiana, Iowa, Kansas, Kentucky, Louisiana, Maine, Massachusetts, Missouri, Montana, Nevada, New Hampshire, New Jersey, New Mexico, Oregon, Pennsylvania, South Carolina, Texas, Vermont, and Wisconsin. In five of these states - Kansas, Massachusetts, Missouri, Nevada, and Vermont - the mandates became effective January 1, 2011 (ASHA, 2011).

Consistent with the documented importance of early intervention (Chasson, et al., 2007; Jacobson, et al. 1998), the mandates in these states target provision of services to young children. In South Carolina, for example, an individual must be diagnosed with an autism spectrum disorder at age eight or younger to be covered. Texas sets the age of diagnosis at age nine. Coverage is typically limited to those aged under age 18, although Illinois and Pennsylvania extend coverage to age 21.

With a few exceptions, state mandates cap benefits at $36,000 per year. Kansas reduces the cap for children age 7 to 18 from $36,000 to $27,000 per year. Kentucky made a distinction between large and individual / small group health benefit plans. Benefits in large group health plans were capped at $50,000 per year for children age 1 through their 7th birthday and $1,000 per month for children age 7 through 21. In individual and small group health benefit plans, the cap was set at $1,000 per month per covered individual. South Carolina capped behavioral therapy coverage at $50,000 per year. Two states set lifetime dollar limits on coverage. In Louisiana, that limit is $144,000. In New Mexico, it is $200,000 (ASHA, 2011).

4.3.1 Effect of mandates

Since state Autism Mandates are still relatively new, it will take time to see their full effect. In the short run, though, it is clear that mandates increase premiums. Whether the increase is problematic is debated. Critics argue that premium increases create loss. Some portion of individual policy holders will drop coverage because they can no longer afford to pay the premiums. The cost of paying claims would then be spread over a smaller pool of policy holders. If individuals leave the insurance market, a majority of remaining policy holders would be employers. It is argued that higher premiums would pass to workers in the form of lower net wages or loss of employment. Results of empirical studies of these expected effects have been inconclusive, however. (Boulder, et al., 2009; Collins et al., 2005, Hopkins & Zweifel, 2005, Klerman & Goldman, 1994, Sommers, 2005, Wolaver et al., 2003).

Actuaries with The Council on Affordable Health Insurance estimate an autism mandate will increase the cost of health insurance by about 1 percent, but caution that increasing prevalence rates coupled with coverage of more services could drive premiums up 1 to 3 percent (Bunce, 2009). But, autism is only one of many mandates that state legislatures imposed on insurance providers in recent years. Between 2004 and 2010, the number of insurance mandates for all types of issues across the states rose 18% from 1,823 to 2,156.

Taking the broad spectrum of mandates into consideration, actuarial estimates of aggregate premium increase runs between 10 to 50 percent (Bunce, 2010). Currently, Rhode Island has the largest number of mandates at 69, whereas Idaho has the least at 13 (Bunce & Wieske, 2010). The total cost of meeting all mandates rather than the marginal cost to meet an autism mandate needs to be considered.

Advocates of autism mandates concede that premiums increase, but they take a human capital investment perspective and argue that monies spent in early intervention will be repaid later in the form of reduced expenditures to care for those with ASD. There is research supporting that perspective. Jacobson et al, (1998) conducted a relatively early cost/benefit evaluation of providing early intensive behavioral intervention (EIBI) for children with ADS aged 2 to 5, using representative cost data from Pennsylvania. Their model assumed EIBI could have three potential outcomes. Some children would be able to engage in regular classroom instruction without support once the intervention ended. Other children would still require special education. Some children would need intensive special education. Given the range in treatment effectiveness and expected outcome, they estimated that cost savings in constant dollars would range from $187,000 to $203,000 ($263,670 to $286,230 in 2011$) per child for ages 3 to 22 years and from $656,000 to $1,082,000 ($924,960 to $1,525,620 in 2011$) per child for ages 3 to 55 years. Given initial costs of $33,000 to $50,000 ($46,530 to $70,500 in 2011$) per year for EIBI, they argue that although EIBI would have a modest effect on cost-benefit balance in the short run, cost in the long run would be greatly outweighed by potential savings.

In a similar vein, Chasson et al. (2007) compared costs associated with 18 years of special education to cost to implement 3 years of Discrete Trial Training as an early intervention in Texas. They estimate that by implementing 3 years of early intervention, the state of Texas would save $208,500 ($223,095 2011$) per child across 18 years of education. Given a conservative estimate of 10,000 Texas children with ASD, they estimate overall savings of EIBI would be $2.9 billion ($3.1 billion 2011$).

5. Health care reform

In 2008, President Obama made a campaign pledge to support a federal mandate requiring coverage for autism treatments. On March 23, 2010 he signed the Patient Protection and Affordable Care Act (PPACA). Seven days later, PPACA was amended by the Health Care and Education Reconciliation Act of 2010.

PPACA introduces significant change in the health care market in the United States. The law places new requirements on individuals, employers, and health plans regarding possession and coverage of health insurance. The law also restructures the private health insurance market, sets minimum standards for health coverage and provides financial help to certain individuals and small employers to secure health insurance (Fernandez, 2010).

State exchanges will be used to offer a variety of health care plans. Each plan must offer a package of "essential benefits" as outlined in the Affordable Care Act. Of interest to the autism community is inclusion of mental health and substance abuse disorder services, including behavioral health treatment as well as preventive and wellness services and chronic disease management in the so-called "essential benefit list".

The autism community sees the new law as a win as it will reduce or eliminate opportunity for health insurance companies to impose pre-existing condition exclusions, excessively long waiting periods before coverage begins, or rescissions of coverage.

Further, ability of insurers to set annual or lifetime caps on coverage will be limited (Autism Speaks, 2011b).

Still, these changes may not go far enough. Not all health plans will be bound by the new law. The only plans required in 2014 to cover essential benefits will include plans offered by state-based exchanges where individuals and businesses purchase coverage, and plans offered in the individual and small group market outside the exchange. Existing coverage, plans offered in large group market outside of the exchanges, and self-insured plans will not be required to supply the essential benefit package to the insured. Thus, in many ways, the new law does not move far beyond the state mandates already in place.

Those state mandates were due, in large part, to the lobbying efforts of Autism Speaks, a large autism advocacy organization. Reviewing provisions of the new law as they related to the autism community, Autism Speaks, still saw room for improvement, reaffirming a commitment to state and federal lobbying efforts to "make effective health care coverage a reality for the autism community and to bring about an end to discrimination of individuals with autism by the insurance industry." The group does not see health care reform ending the problem of high medical costs for a child with autism, though the law may lessen the severity of those costs. Consequently, they will continue efforts to "make autism insurance reform a reality for all Americans living with autism "(Autism Speaks, 2011b).

6. Future considerations

It is clear that, in the future, attention must turn to study of ASD-related issues in a global context. Epidemiological studies conducted since 2000 confirm ASD is found worldwide. For example, according to these studies, the estimated incidence of ASD in children is 4.3 to 5.5 per 10,000 in Australia (Williams et al., 2005), 4.5 per 10,000 in North America (Barbaresi, et al., 2005), 5.9 per 10,000 for Chinese children in Hong Kong (Wong & Hui, 2008), 8.3 per 10,000 in the United Kingdom (Powell, et al., 2000), 8.6 per 10,000 among the Danish (Lauritsen, et al., 2004), 18 per 10,000 in Saudi Arabia (Yazbak, 2004) and 27.2 per 10,000 in Japan (Honda, et al. 2005).

Recently, in the first comprehensive study of autism prevalence in a total population sample, an international research team estimated the prevalence rate of ASDs in South Korea at 1 in 38 children (Autism Speaks, 2011c). Taken together, these figures indicate that a significant portion of the world's population faces the challenges of ASD and will continue to do so in the years to come.

Despite growth in epidemiological studies such as these, the specific percentage of persons with ASD that could benefit or have benefited from education, medical, and social services in developed or developing countries is not known. There are several reasons for this lack of knowledge. It is challenging to establish diagnostic criteria that are consistent across countries. Diagnostic criteria are behavioral rather than biologic. Cultures can differ in behavioral social norms such as eye contact or expected timing of speech development, making it difficult to identify autism-related behavior (Daley & Sigman, 2002; Naqvi, 2009). Culture can also influence views of behavior, perceived need for treatment and the type of treatment offered. For example, in a study of incidence and treatment of ASD in China, Clark and Zhou (2005) report that only in the last ten years has autism been broadly recognized among Chinese service providers. Few Chinese professionals are trained in the diagnosis and effective treatment of ASD. The small number of treatment programs that exist are only found private schools and hospitals in large cities. Traditional Chinese medicine sees autism as a "Yin" disorder displayed in social isolation, lack of communication, and apathy. Herbal medicines, acupuncture, and relaxation are common treatments. Only rarely do children on the autism spectrum receive sensory integration training or applied behavioral analysis. No formal education programs exist for children with autism in China.

Another issue that limits accurate count of those with ASD is that knowledge of behavioral indicators may be limited, especially in developing countries (Naqvi, 2009). Even when individuals with ASD have been identified, access to services is a function of public and private resource levels and these levels vary widely across family, as well as across country and culture. An additional factor is that, although there is general agreement among professionals that early therapeutic intervention helps children improve communication and relationship skills, it is also recognized that not all children respond to therapy and, among those that do, gains are not equal (Canadian Institutes of Health, 2007). Currently, even in developed countries with a long history of providing ASD-related services, no mechanism exists to coordinate service delivery or track level and outcome of service use. These limitations will need to be addressed and overcome before the efficiency and effectiveness of ASD service delivery in the global community can be improved.

Much remains to be learned regarding public and private costs of diagnosis and treatment as well as cost of lifetime care for those on the autism spectrum in the global community. Of necessity, much of the data in this chapter has come from the United States and other developed countries, as that is where the vast majority of research on autism related costs has been conducted. But, the costs associated with treatment and care of someone with autism have no cultural bounds.

Initial research on autism diagnosis and service delivery in developing countries suggests that diagnosis can be a cumbersome and frustrating process, access to effective therapeutic services is often limited to nonexistent, and the greater part of the burden of care rests on family members (see, for example, Al-Salehi, et al., 2009; Daley, 2002; Mendoza, 2010; Tuman, et al., 2008). More research is needed within countries to determine the most effective and efficient means to improve diagnosis and service delivery in the context of a given country, culture, and governmental structure. In addition, research is needed across cultures to better understand the types of ASD-related needs and costs that transcend culture as well as to compare care models in an effort to build a set of best practices.

Development of effective means of information sharing across culture is critical in the quest to improve efficiency and reduce costs in programs, education, medical, and social services. To build a foundation for research, screening along with diagnostic instruments and processes need to be standardized across countries and cultures, while attending to cultural relevance and sensitivity when translating the instruments used. To strengthen the science underlying treatment recommendations, treatment modalities need to be vetted both across cultures and across various populations within cultures. Fortunately, advances in computer technology, Internet access, and electronic data storage and management systems make sharing of information much easier and cheaper now as compared with times past.

To help achieve these ends, Autism Speaks, an autism advocacy group in the United States, has recently launched two coordinated efforts. In 2002, Autism Speaks began development of the Autism Epidemiology Network in collaboration with the United States Centers for Disease Control and Prevention. The long run goals of this effort are to develop a network that facilitates exchange of information and research collaboration on epidemiological activities across countries, to draw on successful international collaboration models that have been applied to other health conditions as a way to identify best practices, and to foster use of epidemiology as a tool for understanding the causes of autism through making comparisons across diverse genetic, environmental, social and cultural situations.

In 2008 Autism Speaks formed an international collaboration with North, South, and Central America for autism-related research and service training. The international collaboration has a four-fold purpose. First, it is to increase public and professional awareness of autism spectrum disorders outside the United States. A similar campaign in the United States has been instrumental in building support for passage of state and federal legislation focused on improving research and services. Second, it is to develop and validate screening and diagnostic tools that can be used across cultures. Tools such as these enhance cross cultural comparisons and can improve the ability of researchers to identify possible causes of ASD. Third, it is expected that collaborative research will be facilitated through the sharing of epidemiologic ideas and practice. To date, close to 80 researchers representing over 30 different countries have engaged in collaborate research under this initiative. Finally, the collaboration strives to build service capacity by providing professional development, technical assistance, content development, and education for service providers (Autism Speaks, 2011a).

Expanding the collaborative efforts that Autism Speaks has made to facilitate research development to include additional countries will be an important step in improving diagnosis and treatment of ASD worldwide. In addition, methods of information exchange developed in the research, diagnostic, and service provider training communities could serve as model for efficiently and effectively connecting families with a child with autism with service providers, including medical personnel and educators, as well as community, insurance, and social service agencies.

7. Conclusion

Research on expenditures related to ASD underscores the fact that the disorder imposes high costs on immediate family as well as society. Families of those with ASD shoulder a large part of the burden of ASD-related costs, especially in developing countries where few public or community resources exist. Not only are there direct costs such as dollars out-of-pocket for therapy and medical care not covered by insurance, there are also the indirect and intangible but no less real costs of lost opportunity, reduced productivity, attention largely focused on the child with ASD to the exclusion of other family members, increased stress, and a forever changed family structure.

Persons with ASD benefit from education, medical, and social services. But, the question of how to allocate payment of these services between the public and private sector is ardently debated. Neither sector has unlimited resources. Research is an important means of finding effective ways to lessen the burden of ASDs. Certainly, more needs to be learned regarding the cause of autism and reasons for the diversity in the presentation and progression of the disorder. Given limits to both private and public resources, scientific study designed to identify which interventions and therapies are most effective in helping a child with autism learn, develop, and become productive are necessary. Reasons why certain therapies work with some children and not others need further investigation. Although ABA is currently considered the behavioral intervention with the greatest support from the scientific community, there is still much debate about its efficacy. More studies of different therapeutic interventions that follow strict standards of scientific inquiry are needed. Longitudinal studies would be particularly useful in judging the long term benefits of various types of interventions for ASD. Ways to improve efficiency and reduce cost in program delivery also need to be evaluated.

Recent increase in the number of Medicaid autism waivers and state autism mandates in health insurance as well as the coming implementation of health care reform offer researchers a rich source of natural experiments in determining the effects of change in public policy on the welfare of persons with ASD. Research in ASD-related cost could benefit from taking a systems perspective and investigating how the various sectors that serve those with ASD might collaborate both to enhance service delivery and reduce costs. For example, a child whose digestive problems are eased by medication will likely be a better learner. A child who learns through behavior therapy how to express and resolve frustrations may be able to reduce behavior modifying medications. Other types of synergies may exist as well.

In the public policy arena, cost/benefit analysis of programs and policies designed to help families with a child with autism is needed to inform resource allocation. Programs and agencies exist that can help families that have a child with autism, but there is little coordination of effort among these. Further, current programs and policies for those with ASD can fall short of meeting the pressing needs of families. Resources available to families can be location specific. Differences in state administered Medicaid programs and state insurance waivers can create some dramatic inequities between residents of different states. Recently, media highlighted the situation of two families. One family lived a state without an autism insurance waiver and paid $1,000 per week for behavior therapy. The other family lived in a state where an autism insurance waiver required health insurers to cover costly behavior therapy. They paid $3,000 per year for the same type of therapy (FoxNews, 2008). Ways to reduce such inequities need to be sought.

Looking to the future, today's young child with ASD will become tomorrow's adult. At least some portion of high functioning individuals with ASD could be employed, but they will likely need help mastering the technical and communication skills needed to obtain and retain employment. Family support for individuals currently receiving home care must inevitably decline either through drain on family financial resources or the aging and death of parents who have been the main caretakers. Options for these individuals need to be considered now.

Rising numbers of individuals with ASD and the high cost of their care make it important to continue to press for advances that will provide genuine help for these individuals and their families. Coordinated efforts from a variety of sectors including medical, educational, research, community, insurance, public policy is needed. Much remains to be learned about how best to invest today in the development of children with ASD to create a better future for them, their families, and society.

8. References

Al-Salehi, S. H., Al-Hifthy, E. H., & Ghaziuddin, M. (2009). Autism in Saudi Arabia: Presentation, clinical correlates, and comorbidity. *Transcultural Psychiatry*, 46, 340-347.

American Speech-Language-Hearing Association (2011). State Insurance mandates for autism spectrum disorder. March 7, 2011, Available from

http://www.asha.org/advocacy/state/state-insurance-mandates-autism/
Autism Speaks (2011a). Global Autism Public Health initiative. May 11, 2011, Available http://www.autismspeaks.org/science/research/initiatives/gaph.php
Autism Speaks (2011b). Health care reform: What does it mean for the autism community? March 24, 2011, Available from http://www.autismvotes.org/site/apps/nlnet/content2.aspx?c=frKNI3PCImE&b=3930723&ct=8129903
Autism Speaks (2011c) New study reveals autism prevalence in South Korea estimated to be 2.6% or 1 in 38 children. May 20, 2011, Available from http://autismspeaks.org/press/south_korea_autism_prevalence_study.php
Barbaresi WJ, Katusic SK, Colligan RC, Weaver AL, & Jacobsen SJ. (2005). The incidence of autism in Olmsted County, Minnesota, 1976-1997: results from a population-based study. *Archives of Pediatric and Adolescent Medicine*,159, 37-44.
Boulder, J. N., Spielman, S., & Mandell, D. S. (2009). Brief report: Quantifying the impact of autism coverage on private insurance programs. *Journal of Autism Developmental Disorders*, 39, 953-957.
Bunce, V. C. (2009). The growing trend toward mandating autism coverage. *The Council on Affordable Health Insurance's Issues & Answers*, 152, March.
Bunce, V. C. (2010). Trends in state mandated benefits, 2010. *The Council on Affordable Health Insurance's Policy Trends*, October.
Bunce, V. C., & Wieske, J. P. (2010). Health insurance mandates in the states 2010. Council for Affordable Health Insurance. March 24, 2011, Available from http://www.cahi.org
Canadian Institutes of Health (2007). Report on the national autism research symposium. May 10, 2001, Available from http://www.cihr-irsc.gc.ca/e/36237.html
Centers for Disease Control (2009). Prevalence of autism spectrum disorders - autism and developmental disabilities monitoring network, United States, 2006. March 4, 2011, Available from http://www.cdc.gov/mmwr/preview /mmwrhtml/ss5810a1.htm
Centers for Medicare and Medicaid Services (2011) Medicaid waivers and demonstrations list. March 23, 2011, Available from https://www.cms.gov/ MedicaidStWaivProgDemoPGI /MWDL/list.asp
Chasson, G. S., Harris, G. E., & Neely, W. J. (2007) Cost comparison of early intensive behavioral intervention and special education for children with autism. *Journal of Child and Family Studies*, 16, 401-413.
Clark, E., & Zhou, Z. (2005). Autism in China: From acupuncture to Applied Behavior Analysis. Psychology in the Schools, 42(3), 285-295.
Cohen, L., & Spenciner, L. (1996). Assessment of social-emotional development in young children. In M. J. Breen & C. R. Fiedles (Eds.), *Behavioral approach to assessment of youth with emotional/behavioral disorders: A handbook for school-based practioners* (pp. 503-580). Austin, TX: PRO-ED.
Collins, S., Davis K, & Ho, A. (2005). A shared responsibility: US employers and the provision of health insurance to employees. Inquiry 2005, 42(1), 6-15.
Croen, L., Najjar, D., Ra, T., Lotspeich, L., & Bernal, P. (2006). A comparison of health care utilization and costs of children with and without autism spectrum disorders in a large group-model health plan. *Pediatrics*, 118(4), e1203-e1211.

Daley, T. C. (2002). The need for cross-cultural research on the pervasive developmental disorders. *Transcultural Psychiatry*, 39(4), 531-550.

Daley, T. C., & Sigman, M. D. (2002). Diagnostic conceptualization of autism among Indian psychiatrists, psychologists, and Pediatricians. *Journal of Autism and Developmental Disorders*, 32(1), 13-23.

Dawson, G. (2010). The changing face of autism requires rethinking policy needs. Social Policy Report, 24(2), pp. 22-23.

Fernandez, B. (2010). Self-insured health insurance coverage. Congressional Research Service.

Fombonne, E. (1998). Epidemiological surveys of autism, in F. R. Bolkmar (Ed.) *Autism and Pervasive Developmental Disorders*, pp. 32-63. Cambridge, MA: Cambridge University Press.

Fombonne, E. (2003a). Epidemiological surveys of autism and other pervasive developmental disorders: An update. *Journal of Autism and Developmental Disorders*, 33(4), 365-382.

Fombonne, E. (2003b). Modern views of autism. *The Canadian Journal of Psychiatry*, 48(8), 503-505.

Fombonne, E. (2005) Epidemiological surveys of pervasive developmental disorders. In F. Volkmar, R. Paul, A Klin, D Cohen (Eds.) *Handbook of Autism and Pervasive Developmental Disorders*. pp. 42-69 Hoboken, NJ: Wiley.

Fombonne, E. (2009). Epidemiology of pervasive developmental disorders. *Pediatric Research*, 65, 591-598.

Fox News (2008, October 20) Parents want states to mandate insurance coverage for autism treatments http://www.foxnews.com/printer_friendly_story /0,3566,440823,00.htmlHillman, R. E., Kanafani, N., Takahashi, T. N., & Miles, J. H. (2000). Prevalence of autism in Missouri: Changing trends and the effect of a comprehensive state autism project. *Missouri Medicine*, *97*(5), 159-163.

Ganz, M. L. (2006). The costs of autism, In S. O. Moldin & Rubenstein, J. L. R. (Eds.). *Understanding Autism: From Basic Neuroscience to Treatment* pp. 475-502. Boca Raton, FL: Taylor and Francis Group.

Ganz, M. L. (2007). The lifetime distribution of the incremental societal costs of autism. *Archives of Pediatric and Adolescent Medicine*, 161, 343-349.

Gernsbacher, M. A., Dawson, M., & Goldsmith, H. H. (2005). Three reasons not to believe in an autism epidemic. Current Directions in Psychological Science, 14(2), 55-58.

Gould, E. (2004). Decomposing the effects of children's health on mother's labor supply: Is it time or money? *Health Economics*, 13(6), 525-541.

Grossman, L., & Barrozo, P. (2007). The next global human rights issue: Why the plight of individuals with autism spectrum disorder requires a global call to action. *Autism Advocate*, 4, 8-12.

Honda H, Shimizu Y, Imai M, & Nitto Y. (2005). Cumulative incidence of childhood autism: a total population study of better accuracy and precision. *Developmental Medicine and Child Neurology*, 47,10-18.

Hopkins, S, & Zweifel P. (2005). The Australian health policy changes of 1999 and 2000: A evaluation. *Applied Health Economics and Health Policy*, 4(4) 229-238.

Jacobson, J. W., Mulick, J. A., & Green, G. (1998). Cost-benefit estimates for early intensive behavioral intervention for young children with autism-general model and single state case. Behavioral Interventions, 13,201-226.

Järbrink, K., & Knapp, M. (2001). The economic impact of autism in Britain. *Autism*, 5(1), 7-22.

Järbrink, K., Fombonne, E., & Knapp, M. (2003). Measuring the parental, service and cost impacts of children with autistic spectrum disorder: a pilot study. Journal of Autism and Developmental Disorders, 3(4), 395-402.

Järbrink, K. (2007). The economic consequences of autistic spectrum disorder among children in a Swedish municipality. *Autism*, 11(5), 453-463.

Kanner, L. (1943). Autistic disturbances of affective contact. *The Nervous Child*, 2, 217–250.

Klerman J. & Goldman D (1994). Job loss due to health insurance mandates. *Journal of the American Medical Association*, 272(7), 552-556.

Knapp, M., Romeo, R., & Beecham, J. (2007). The economic consequences of autism in the UK. Foundation for People with Learning Disabilities. London.

Lauritsen MB, Pedersen CB, & Mortensen PB. (2004). The incidence and prevalence of pervasive developmental disorders: a Danish population-based study. *Psychological Medicine*,34, 1339-1346.

Leslie, D. L., & Martin, A. (2007). Health care expenditures associated with autism spectrum disorders. *Archives of Pediatric and Adolescent Medicine*, 161(4), 350-355.

Liptak, G, Stuart,T., & Auinger, P. (2006). Health care utilization and expenditures for children with autism: Data from US national samples. *Journal of Autism and Developmental Disorders*, 36, 871-879.

Lotter, V. (1966). Epidemiology of autistic conditions in young children, I: Prevalence. *Social Psychiatry*, 1, 124-137.

Mandell, D., Cao, J., Ittenbach, R., & Pinto-Martin, J. (2006). Medicaid expenditures for children with autistic spectrum disorders: 1994 to 1999. *Journal of Autism and Developmental Disorders*, 36(4), 475-485.

Mendoza, R. L. (2010). The economics of autism in Egypt. *American Journal of Economics and Business Administration*, 2(1), 12-19.

Naqvi, N. (2009). Prevalence and services outside of Europe and North America. May 20, 2010. Available http://www.hunter.cuny.edu/school-of-education/special-programs-and-centers/regional-autism-center/repository/files/NNaquviprevalenceoutsideUS.pdf/view

National Association of State Budget Officers (2010). *The Fiscal survey of states: Fall 2010*. Washington, DC: National Association of State Budget Officers.

National Conference of State Legislatures (2010) Insurance coverage for autism. March 22, 2010. Available from http://www.ncsl.org/?tabid=18246

Newschaffer, C., & Curran, L. (2003). Autism: An emerging public health problem. *Public Health Reports*, 118(5), 393-399.

Powell, J. E., Edwards, A., Edwards, M., Pandit, B.S., Sungum-Paliwal, S.R., & Whitehouse W. (2000). Changes in the incidence of childhood autism and other autistic spectrum disorders in preschool children from two areas of the West Midlands, UK. *Developmental Medicine and Child Neurology*, 42(9),624-628.

Rutter, M. (2005). Incidence of autism spectrum disorders: Changes over time and their meaning. Acta Paediatrica, 94, 2-15.

Sanua, V.D. (1984). Is infantile autism a universal phenomenon? An open question. International Journal, *Social Psychiatry*, 30 (3), 163-177.

Sharpe, D. L. , & Baker, D. L. (2007). Financial issues associated with having a child with autism. *Journal of Family and Economic Issues*, 28, 247-264.

Shimabukuro, T. T., Grosse, S. D., & Rice, C. (2008). Medical expenditures for children with an autism spectrum disorder in a privately insured population. *Journal of Autism and Developmental Disorders*, 38, 546-552.

Sommers B (2005). Who really pays for health insurance? The incidence of employer-provided health insurance with sticky nominal wages. International Journal of Health Care Finance and Economics 5(1) 89-118

Spigel, S. (2007). Medicaid autism waivers and state agencies serving people with autism. OLR Research Report 2007-R-0319. Retrieved March 20, 2011 from http://www.cga.ct.gov/2007-rpt/2007-R-0319.htm.

Sun, X., & Allison, C. (2010). A review of the prevalence of autism spectrum disorder in Asia. *Research in Autism Spectrum Disorders*, 4, 156-167.

Tarkan, L. (2002). Autism therapy is called effective, but rare. New York Times. Retrieved May 25, 2005 from http://www.spedalliance.com/autism.htm

Tuman, J. P., Roth-Johnson, D., Baker, D. L., & Vecchio, J. (2008). Autism and special education policy in Mexico. *Global Health Governance*, 2(1), 1-22)

Wang, L., & Leslie, D. L. (2010). Health care expenditure for children with autism spectrum disorders in Medicaid. *Journal of the American Academy of Child & Adolescent Psychiatry*, 49(11), 1165-1171.

Williams K, Glasson, E.J., Wray, J., Tuck, M., Helmer, M., Bower, C. I., & Mellis, C. M. (2005) Incidence of autism spectrum disorders in children in two Australian states. *Medical Journal of Austrailia*, 182 (3), 108-111.

Willingham, V. (2008), Parents press for autism insurance coverage. CNN.com/Health. March 22, 2011. Retreived 3/22/11 from http://edition.cnn.com/2008/HEALTH/conditions/10/17/autism.insurance/index.html.

Wolaver A, McBride T & Wolfe B (2003), Mandating insurance offers for low-wage workers: An evaluation of labor market effects. *Journal of Health Politics Policy and Law* 28(5), 883-926.

Wong, V. C. N. & Hui, S. L. H. (2008). Epidemiological study of autism spectrum disorder in China. *Journal of Child Neurology*, 23(1),67-72.

Yazbak, F. E. (2003). Autism in the United States: A perspective. *Journal of American Physicians and Surgeons*, 8(4), 103-107.

Yazbak, F. E. (2004). Autism seems to be increasing worldwide, if not in London. British Medical Journalo, 328, (7433), 226-227.

Yell, M. L., & Drasgow, E. (2000). Litigating a free appropriate education: the Lovaas hearings and cases. *Journal of Special Education*, 33, 205-214.

Xiong, N., Yang, L., Yu, Y., Hou, J., Li, J., LI., Y, & Liu, H (2011). Investigation of raising burden of children with autism, physical disability and mental disability in China. *Research in Developmental Disabilities*, 32, 306-311.

Part 8

Basic Science and Autism Spectrum Disorders

18

Early Behavioural Alterations in Mouse Models of Autism Spectrum Disorders: A Step Forward Towards the Discovery of New Therapeutic Approaches

Bianca De Filippis, Emilia Romano and Giovanni Laviola
Sect. Behavioural Neuroscience, Dept. Cell Biology & Neuroscience, Istituto Superiore di Sanità, Roma, Italy

1. Introduction

Historically, research in non-human beings, primarily rodents, has played a fundamental role in understanding neural dysfunctions underlying pathological conditions and how they can be treated. To date, several animal models have been proposed to recapitulate autism spectrum disorders (ASD).

We can never fully recapitulate human neuropsychiatric symptomatology in non-human beings; some symptoms, such as low self-esteem and suicidal ideation, are impossible to model in mice. Moreover, brain anatomy between humans and mice is considerably different (i.e. the cerebral cortex is highly elaborated in humans). However, the brains of vertebrates have a common structural organization in which the cerebral cortex is intimately interconnected with subcortical structures that are well conserved across mammals (Tecott, 2003). Furthermore, many fundamental physiological and behavioural responses have been evolutionarily conserved between species. The study of these responses in lower species can therefore provide a better understanding of the neural circuits and the genetic factors subserving them and, through inference, of human behaviour and disease.

One of the criteria that are commonly used to validate an animal model (McKinney, 1984) is based on a conceptual analogy of the proposed model to the causes of the human disease (*construct validity*). Mutant mice with a targeted mutation in a gene implicated in a given neuropsychiatric disorder, neuroanatomical lesions, prenatal drug exposures, and environmental toxins offer examples of putative causes of human diseases that can be replicated in animal models.

The etiopathogenesis of autism however has not been clearly elucidated so far and diagnosis of ASD is mainly based on presentation of three core symptoms: profound alterations in social interaction, communication deficits and stereotyped behaviours (i.e. repetitive behaviours and restricted interests). Different approaches have therefore been adopted to model these pathologies in rodents. Table 1 provides a schematic view of currently available mouse models of ASD-like symptomatology.

1.1 Lesions models

One approach is to generate defects in brain regions that are analogous to neurochemical or anatomical abnormalities seen in autism. This includes models obtained after neonatal lesions of brain areas abnormal in autistic patients, such as the cerebellum, the amygdala (Wolterink et al., 2001) or the medial prefrontal cortex (Bobee et al., 2000). Indeed, those models suggest that lesions in specific brain regions leads to the development of specific or general behavioural abnormalities that are comparable to those observed in autism. Importantly, the age at which the lesion is made has a significant impact on the phenotypic outcome (Auvray et al., 1989; Daenen et al., 2002; Wolterink et al., 2001), thus highlighting the need for a better understanding of the role played by abnormal development in ASD pathophysiology.
Although such models actually reproduce altered behaviours related to ASD-like traits, the lesions employed destroy entire brain regions and do not reproduce the underlying genetic or developmental pathways of autistic spectrum disorders. These models are thus quite useful, but bear little *construct validity*.

1.2 Enviromental models

The search for environmental causes of autism arose from the observation that autism prevalence has considerably increased over the last 20 years and monozygotic (MZ) twins do not show complete concordance for autism. In fact, environmental challenges during prenatal and early postnatal periods are known to modify brain development and result in behavioural abnormalities and cognitive deficits that appear later in life (Landrigan, 2010).
Among the environmental factors that may have an etiological role in autism, in utero exposures to teratogens, including valproic acid, a commonly used antiepileptic drug, thalidomide, a sedative drug, and misoprostol, an abortifactant, have been proposed to increase incidence of autism (Dufour-Rainfray et al., 2010). Mouse models have therefore been produced by means of prenatal or neonatal environmental challenges, including early exposure to valproic acid, inflammatory agents and anticonvulsant exposure of the fetus. Immunological abnormalities have also been suspected to be involved in autism [reviewed in (Krause et al., 2002) and (Torres, 2003)] and several groups have described behavioural deficits in rodents as a consequence of immunological challenges or anomalies (Patterson, 2002; Shi et al., 2003; Vojdani et al., 2003). Those include, among others, exposure during gestation to Trichinella spiralis (Rau, 1983), neonatal exposure to Borna virus (Hornig et al., 1999; Pletnikov et al., 1999); reviewed in (Pletnikov et al., 2003) and prenatal exposure to maternal antibodies (Singer et al., 2009).
In all of these cases, the environmental nature of the perturbations potentially reproduces the conditions experienced by developing human subjects. Additionally, compared to lesions of selected brain areas, the action of these chemical and infectious agents is usually reported to provoke global effects on the brain, thus more closely resembling ASD pathophysiology.

1.3 Genetic mouse models

In the last decades, gene targeting procedures have been developed for the introduction into pre-determinated sites in the genome of planned mutations (null mutations as well as more subtle changes which alter, but do not eliminate gene function). Although genetic modifications can be engineered in the rat and even in higher mammals, the mouse is uniquely amenable to these techniques (Chaible et al., 2010). The development and application of novel molecular technologies has therefore led to an explosion in the use of mice in neuropsychiatric research as in other biomedical disciplines, with the creation of mouse models with genetic aberrations characteristic of human clinical disorders (Tecott, 2003).

Mouse models	*Behavioural alterations (compared to wt mice)*	*References*
	Mice bearing genetic mutations	
BTBR T+tf/J	Social approach ↓ Reciprocal social interactions ↓ Juvenile play ↓ Repetitive behaviours ↑ Unusual repertoire of UVS	(McFarlane et al., 2008; Scattoni et al., 2008; Silverman et al., 2010)
NL-3 KO	Motor activity ↑ Social novelty preference ↓ PPI ↔ UVS ↓ Seizure susceptibility ↔ Sucrose preference ↔	(Radyushkin et al., 2009; Tabuchi et al., 2007)
En2 KO	Juvenile play ↓ Learning and memory ↓ Social behaviour ↓ Motor coordination ↓	(Cheh et al., 2006; Kuemerle et al., 2007)
Gabrb3 KO	Social behaviour ↓ Explorative behaviour ↓ Attention ↓ Seizure susceptibility ↑	(Chandra et al., 2008)
CAPS2 KO	Social interaction ↓ Hyperactivity Abnormal sleep-wake rhythm Anxiety in unfamiliar environments ↑	(Sadakata & Furuichi, 2010)
glut3 +/-	UVS ↓ SHIRPA ↔ Social behaviour ↓ Learning and memory ↓ Cognitive flexibility ↓ Abnormal motor stereotypies	(Zhao et al., 2010)
GAP43 +/-	Anxiety-like behaviour ↓ Social approach ↓ Sociability ↓	(Zaccaria et al., 2010)
Mthfr +/-	Recognition memory ↓ Hyperactivity	(Levav-Rabkin et al., 2011)
V1aR KO	Anxiety-like behaviours ↓ Social recognition ↓	(Bielsky et al., 2004)
Dvl1-deficient	Abnormal social interaction Abnormal sensorimotor gating	(Lijam et al., 1997)
	Gene-environment interaction	
Orpm -/-	UVS ↓ Maternal potentiation ↓ Attachment behaviour ↓	(Moles et al., 2004)

Mouse models	*Behavioural alterations (compared to wt mice)*	*References*
patDp/+	UVS ↓ Anxiety-like behaviours ↑ Generalized fear Spatial learning ↔ Sociability ↓	(Nakatani et al., 2009)
NL-4 KO	UVS ↓ Social Interaction ↓ Social Memory ↓	(Jamain et al., 2008)
MALTT	Hyperactivity Social behaviour ↓ Hyperactive circling stereotypy	(Hamilton et al., 2011)
Exposure (E11) in utero to VPA	Sociability ↓	(Roullet et al., 2010)
Exposure (E14-E17) to B(a)P in $Cpr^{lox/lox}$ mice	Response to novelty ↓	(Sheng et al., 2010)
Exposure (P14) to VPA in GSTM1-/- mice	Play behaviour ↓	(Yochum et al., 2010)
Neonatal exposure to GVG in Mthfr+/- mice	Body weight ↔ Recognition memory ↓ Anxiety-related behaviour ↔ Activity ↑	(Levav-Rabkin et al., 2011)
Reelin $^{rl/+}$	Reversal learning ↓ Social behaviour ↔ Coordination ↔ Anxiety-related behaviour ↓ Motor impulsivity ↑	(Laviola et al., 2009; Macri et al., 2010; Ognibene et al., 2007a)
Neonatal thimerosal in SJL Mice	Motor coordination ↔ Social interaction ↔ Social recognition ↔ Anxiety-like behaviour ↔ Sensory gating ↔	(Berman et al., 2008)
	Brain lesions	
5,7-DHT (P0)	Exploratory behaviours ↓ Sensory motor reflex↔	(Hohmann et al., 2007)

Table 1. Selection of mouse models of ASD.

Abbreviations: KO: knockout; *UVS:* ultrasonic vocalizations; *PPI:* prepulse inhibition; *SHIRPA*: protocol for comprehensive phenotype assessment; *BTBR:* inbred mouse strain; *NL-3*: neuroligin-3, *En2*:engrailed genes, *Gabrb3:* gene, which encodes the β3 subunit of the GABAA receptor; *CAPS2*: Ca2+-dependent activator protein for secretion 2; *glut3:* Neuronal glucose transporter isoform 3; *GAP43:* growth-associated protein-43; *Mthfr*: methylenetetrahydrofolate reductase gene;*V1aR:* Vasopressin V1a Receptor; *Dvl1:* Dishevelled, *Orpm:* μ-opioid receptors; *patD*: paternal duplication of mouse chromosome 7 corresponding to the region of human chromosome 15; *NL-4:* neuroligin-4; *MALTT:* multiple autistic-like transgenic traits; *nervous: nervous gene mutation;* *VPA:* valproic acid; *B(a)P:* benzo(a)pyrene; *Cpr:* Cytochrome p450 reductase; *GSTM1:* glutathione-S-transferaseM1; Thimerosal (sodium ethylmercury thiosalicylate) is an antimicrobial preservative used in numerous vaccines; *GVG: vigabatrin; Rl:* reelin gene; *5,7-DHT:* 5,7-dihydroxytryptamine. ↔: unaltered; ↓: reduced; ↑: increased.

Thanks to these advances in the field of genetics and the discovery of relevant loci for autism susceptibility identified by association or linkage studies in human populations (Lintas & Persico, 2009), several mouse models that reflect genetic alterations associated with autism have been developed in recent years. Those mouse models provide useful tools to address the genetic hypothesis of autism and investigate genetic factors which are thought to contribute to the expression of ASD.

Known genetic causes of nonsyndromic ASD include gene copy number variations (i.e., submicroscopic deletions and duplications) (Weiss et al., 2008) or single gain- or loss-of-function mutations in identified genes (Lintas & Persico, 2009; Serajee et al., 2006). A great deal of interest has been recently devoted to the potential involvement of mutations in synaptic genes encoding for Neuroligin-3 (NL-3), Neuroligin-4 (NL-4), and Neurexin-1 (NX-1), which are cell adhesion proteins at nerve cell synapses, and SHANK3, which is a synaptic scaffold protein in autism susceptibility. Based on the rare-occurring mutations identified in the ASD population, mouse models carrying mutations in these genes have recently been generated (Berkel et al., 2010; Jamain et al., 2003; Kim et al., 2008; Laumonnier et al., 2004; Moessner et al., 2007). In line with findings from neuroimaging and genetic studies that indicate abnormalities in both structural and functional brain connectivity in autism, those mouse models recapitulate autism symptomatology, thus indicating that aberrant signaling between nerve cells may cause the ASD phenotype in the affected patients. Interestingly, NLGN3 expression was found to be reduced in several brain regions of mice exposed in utero to valproic acid, such as the hippocampus (Kolozsi et al., 2009), thus increasing the relevance of this gene for ASD.

Mutant animals displaying targeted gene mutation for neurotransmitters and developmental genes that may regulate social behaviours constitute another example of transgenic models of ASD. These include oxytocin knockout mice, which display deficits in social recognition and social memory (Bielsky & Young, 2004; Young, 2001), and vasopressin receptor subtype 1b knockout mice, which display reduced social motivation and aggression (Lim et al., 2005; Young, 2002). Indeed, the *construct validity* of those models is quite low. However, given that deviant social development is one of the core symptoms of autism and related disorders, they incorporate a conceptual analogy to the symptoms of the human disease, thus bearing high *face validity* (McKinney, 1984). In fact, children with classic autism are unable to "read" other people, ignoring them and often strenuously avoiding eye contact.

Most of the current mouse models of ASD have used reverse genetics, going from an a priori target (i.e. a specific genetic alteration) to phenotype. A different classical method for identifying unknown and potentially unpredicted genetic contributions to phenotypes is the forward genetics approach, first identifying a relevant phenotype and then elucidating the genetic underpinnings.

Relevant phenotypes include behavioural symptoms, neuroanatomical pathology, neurophysiological responses, and neurochemical abnormalities. Given the prominent role of behavioural symptoms in the diagnosis of ASD, particular attention in ASD research has been so far devoted to one of the disease components or endophenotypes that can be modeled in animals: behavioural abnormalities. A number of studies have described deficits in social, communication, and/or stereotypic domains in mouse models of ASD (see Table 1). However, only a few of these models have reported deficits in all

ASD-related behavioural domains. Among them, the most extensively studied is the BTBR inbred strain.

Initially, BTBR mice attracted a great deal of attention as a potential model for social deficiencies in general, and more specifically for the social and stereotypical changes that are characteristic of ASD. As a matter of fact, low levels of social behaviour (Bolivar et al., 2007; McFarlane et al., 2008; Moy et al., 2007) and poor social learning in the transmission-of-food-preference assay (McFarlane et al., 2008) have been reported in this strain. Core symptoms of ASD also include repetitive behaviours, a broad class of behaviours linked by repetition, rigidity, and invariance. Moreover, some children with autism never develop meaningful speech and fail to develop reciprocal communication either by speech, gestures, or facial expressions. For those who do, speech differs from that in normal children as stereotypic speech that may involve echolalia, pronoun reversal, and unusual inflections and intonations may be displayed. Although stereotyped behaviours have been less investigated than social behaviours in BTBR mice, high levels of repetitive self-grooming have been consistently observed (McFarlane et al., 2008; Yang et al., 2009; Yang et al., 2007a; Yang et al., 2007b). An unusual pattern of ultrasonic vocalizations has also been evidenced in BTBR mice. This behavioural abnormality is thought to represent a behavioural homolog to communication deficits (Scattoni et al., 2008; Scattoni et al., 2011). As a matter of fact, although mice do not use language, they do display social communication mechanisms. In particular, rodents communicate predominantly in the ultrasonic range of sound frequencies (Nyby et al., 1978). Ultrasonic vocalizations are emitted by mice under different social conditions throughout their life span. Pups separated from the nest emit vocalizations, and parents use them to locate the pup and retrieve it to the nest (D'Amato et al., 2005; Scattoni et al., 2009; Scattoni et al., 2008) (see below). Calls have also been reported in juveniles during social play and in adults during reproductive encounters and/or social investigation (Holy & Guo, 2005; Nyby et al., 1983; Panksepp et al., 2007; Sales, 1972). Interestingly, abnormal ultrasonic vocalizations emission was found at all the ages tested in BTBR mice (Scattoni et al., 2008; Scattoni et al., 2011). Early in development, BTBR pups showed an unusual pattern of vocalizations and a more frequent, loud harmonics than controls, thus resembling the atypical vocalizations seen in some autistic infants. As adults, BTBR mice when tested in three different social contexts displayed lower levels of both vocalizations and social investigation, thus confirming previous findings in pups of social communication deficits. Recently, however, a complete absence of the corpus callusum has been reported in this strain, which has not been clearly associated with ASD neuroanatomical changes. (Wahlsten et al., 2003).

Spontaneous mouse mutants have furthered our understanding of biological systems for more than one hundred years. One of the molecules that are under examination as a risk factor, playing a role in autism and schizophrenia, is Reelin (RELN). Reelin is a glycoprotein of the extracellular matrix that plays a key role in migration and positioning of neurons, thus bearing a fundamental neurodevelopmental role in the laminar and columnar organization of the cortex (Andersen et al., 2002; Costa et al., 2001; Costa et al., 2002; Keller & Persico, 2003). As a consequence, normal cortical development and mature function depend on appropriate levels of reelin protein, its receptors, and its cytoplasmic adapter, disabled-1 (Dab1) (Deguchi et al., 2003). Support for reelin's involvement in autism include finding of decreased RELN mRNA, decreased reelin protein, decreased mRNA for Dab1 (Fatemi et al., 2002a; Fatemi et al., 2005). Reduced plasma levels of reelin have been also reported in patients with autism (Fatemi et al., 2002a).

The deletion of a wide portion of the gene coding for reelin, which is highly conserved between the mouse (symbol *Reln*) and the human (symbol *RELN*) (Fatemi et al., 2002b), arose spontaneously in mice, showing autosomic recessive transmission. The homozygous reeler mouse completely lacks the protein, presenting an impaired phenotype characterized by striking neurological signs (dystonia, ataxia, tremor) and severe alterations in the architecture of laminar structures like the cerebral cortex, the cerebellum and the hippocampus (Caviness & Rakic, 1978; Goffinet, 1990; Goffinet et al., 1984). When levels of Reelin are reduced by 50% as in heterozygous mice compared to wild-type, lamination defects in the SNC and the classical reeler phenotype are not evident. The HZ phenotype, however, shows subtle neuro-anatomical and behavioural abnormalities (Laviola et al., 2006; Liu et al., 2001; Ognibene et al., 2007a; Ognibene et al., 2007b; Salinger et al., 2003; Tueting et al., 1999), thus suggesting a higher validity of the heterozygous mutation to model ASD.

Interestingly, mice haploinsufficient for the reelin gene have reduced numbers of cerebellar Purkinje cells, which is the most frequent neuropathologic finding in autism, and progressive loss of Purkinje cells of the cerebellum in the first weeks of life has been highlighted in heterozygous reeler mice (Marrone et al., 2006). Given the role played by reelin in the development of the central nervous system, this model has been extensively studied during the early phases of development (see below).

1.4 Monogenic syndromes associated with autistic-like behaviour

Among the genetic mutant lines which are expected to model ASD, some are based on the introduction in mouse genome of monogenic aberrations underlying syndromes associated with autistic-like behaviours. These include, among others, loss of methyl-CpG-binding protein-2 (Mecp2), a gene responsible for Rett syndrome.

Rett syndrome (RTT), classified together with autism into the DSM-IV in the group of the pervasive developmental disorders, affects primarily girls with a prevalence of 1 on 10.000 births. ASD core symptoms are associated with severe cognitive and physical impairments in RTT patients. Mutations in the MeCP2 gene, a transcriptional regulator binding to methylated CpGs (Dragich et al., 2000; Jorgensen & Bird, 2002), have been recognized as clear etiological factors in about 90% of classical RTT cases. This advance in RTT research allowed the generation, by means of strategies employing gene targeting, of several lines of mice carrying endogenous MeCP2 mutations (De Filippis et al., 2010b; Ricceri et al., 2008).

Although the causes of this syndrome have been clarified, the mechanisms leading to the severe, progressive and specific neuronal dysfunctions when these genes are mutated are currently unknown. RTT mouse models are therefore expected to be enormously beneficial for determining the functional outcome and the effects on organic and cellular functions of gene mutations and can have translational value in offering preclinical surrogate markers to evaluate treatment efficacy (Crawley, 2007). Indeed, although the behavioural characterization of some of these mutant mice, is at the moment far from complete, indications are available suggesting that their high *construct validity* [i.e. the extent to which a model reproduces the etiology and pathophysiology of a disorder (McKinney, 1984)] is accompanied by a high *face validity* [i.e. the degree to which a model resembles the symptoms of a disorder (McKinney, 1984)], as MeCP2 mutant mice have been reported to recapitulate many RTT symptoms (De Filippis et al., 2010a; De Filippis et al., 2010b; Ricceri et al., 2008).

2. Behavioural phenotyping

Given that the eziopathogenesis of ASD is still unclear, the primary diagnostic indicators are abnormal behaviours, rather than biochemical, neuroanatomical or other physiological indices. In this line, behavioural phenotyping plays a crucial role in the validation of mouse models of autism spectrum disorders and, accordingly, a number of behavioural assays have been developed that capture and model aspects of ASD-like core symptoms (Crawley, 2007).

Determining whether a proposed mouse model for autism recapitulates one or more of the core clinical symptoms can in fact provide valuable insight as to the functional impact of altered genes or environment. Moreover, since behaviour is the ultimate output of brain, behavioural phenotyping of mouse models of autism provides functional information hardly detectable using molecular, cellular or histological evaluations. Such functional information is not only helpful to identify the role of specific genes in neuropathologies, but it also provides a framework for understanding the role of genes in behaviour, identifying key stages of human brain development, and, eventually, targets for potential therapeutic interventions. To unravel the effects of genetic manipulations, deviations from the normal range of strain-specific behaviours and the age-dependent onset of normal response patterns can be investigated.

Another behavioural phenotyping strategy can be based upon the study of selected brain regions and of those neurochemical systems specifically targeted by genetic alterations: to assess their functional integrity, behavioural tasks known to be controlled by those circuits could represent a powerful tool and a very sensitive assay. Furthermore, the analysis of deviations in response to challenge with psychoactive drugs (direct receptor agonists or antagonists, acting on specific neurotransmitter systems) can complement this strategy. The use of drug challenge may indeed unmask neurobehavioural alterations not detectable under baseline testing conditions and provide crucial information on neurobiological impairments that can be subsequently confirmed in vitro (Bignami, 1996).

Table 1 summarizes our current knowledge on the behavioural phenotypes of the available mouse models of autism. Several reviews have already addressed this issue. However, no one is available dealing with the study of the early phases of development in mouse models of ASD.

2.1 Behavioural phenotyping of the early phases of development: The earlier the better

Typical clinical presentation strongly suggests that brain development is aberrant during early postnatal life in individuals with autism. Although the primary developmental disruptions have not been identified, redundancy of neurodevelopmental processes has been demonstrated in patients' brains. Early interventions may however be valuable even if they do not address autism's etiology; in line with the observation that neurodevelopment is regulated by multiple environmental factors, some studies suggest the efficacy of early behavioural treatments in contrasting ASD symptomatology, likely as a consequence of increased brain plasticity (Dawson & Zanolli, 2003; Kasari et al., 2006; Kashinath et al., 2006). Targeting the regulation of early neurodevelopmental processes and increasing neural plasticity may thus represent suitable pharmacologic interventions for young children with autism. Given the strict interplay between genes and environment during the development of a healthy individual, the possibility of an early intervention can result particularly important for autistic patients to reduce most of the carry-over consequences of a deviant developmental trajectory. However, in spite of the clear value placed on early behavioural interventions for autism and suggestions to develop developmentally focused pharmacologic treatments (Rubenstein & Merzenich, 2003; Whitaker-Azmitia, 2001), few studies have addressed this issue in ASD research.

In models of human neurodevelopmental disorders, developmental analyses are expected to provide a behavioural phenotype on which potential therapeutic strategies could be tested starting from the early phases of development, when recovery could be more likely. Time of onset of selected somatic changes and the time of first appearance of various reflexes and behavioural patterns show a remarkable regularity, providing an effective tool to assess possible neurobehavioural/developmental alterations (Bignami, 1996). Particularly in models of neurodevelopmental disorders, it seems therefore critical to conduct behavioural phenotyping during the developmental period (Branchi & Ricceri, 2002; De Filippis et al., 2010a). As well as defining an Alzheimer animal model via its behavioural characterization only in the pre-weaning phase could be at least considered hazardous, it is similarly limiting and inappropriate to describe adult, but not infant or adolescent behaviour in animal models of neurological disorders such as autism with an early onset and developmental pathology. Moreover, in transgenic and knockout mice, developmental analysis can shed light on gene effects not accessible when studying adulthood alone. Behavioural testing during ontogeny can help our understanding of how a genetic manipulation affects central nervous system function in ontogeny and it can represent an appropriate strategy to identify possible compensatory and/or unexpected effects (Branchi & Ricceri, 2002). Since the development of different neural systems is differentially timed, the ontogenetic analysis of associated behavioural phenotypes can, for instance, represents a powerful strategy to investigate the effects of genetic manipulations on different brain functions before the occurrence of possible compensatory events.

Within the field of developmental psychobiology, the neurobehavioural profile of developing rodents has been extensively characterized (Hofer & Shair, 1991; Spear, 1990). A number of tests and experimental protocols are now available that take into account the practical constraints imposed by the peculiar physiological and behavioural responses of an immature subject. Although many of the behavioural tests were originally developed for rats, they have been successfully adapted to mouse competencies and now allow the performance of robust measurements of several aspects of the neonatal mouse behavioural repertoire (Bignami, 1996; Cuomo et al., 1996). Keeping in mind Pat Bateson's cardinal view of neurobehavioural development in mammals, as a process akin to the metamorphosis of a caterpillar into a butterfly, we can investigate appropriate behavioural endpoints for each selected maturational step, and use standardized methodological procedures to assess sensory-motor, emotional and cognitive domains in developing mice. However, this knowledge is rarely exploited by neurobiologists working with transgenic and knock-out mice (Branchi & Ricceri, 2002). To date such studies are primarily focused on adult phenotyping and neglect the crucial information provided by the study of ontogeny. Table 2 provides an overview of the behavioural analyses so far carried out on neonatal pups in mouse models of ASD. To better address the importance of behavioural phenotyping the early phases of development in these models, a focus will be made on two mouse models carrying genetic mutations related to ASD: the heterozygous reeler mice and the Mecp2-308 model for Rett syndrome. Which kind of tests can be applied to rodent pups and how our knowledge can benefit from a refined behavioural analysis of the early phases of development will be illustrated.

Mouse models	*Behavioural domains*			*References*
	UVS	**Motor reflex and coordination**	**Cognition and emotion**	
patDp/+	P5-14 ↑ Peak delayed	Not tested	Not tested	(Nakatani et al., 2009)
En2 KO	Not tested	Surface-righting↔ Negative geotaxis ↔ Mid-air righting ↓ Grip strength ↓	Not tested	(Cheh et al., 2006; Kuemerle et al., 2007)
MALTT	P3-7 ↔ P8-14 ↑	Not tested	Not tested	(Hamilton et al., 2011)
BTBR T+tf/J	P1-12 ↑	P2-14 Somatic growth and somatosensory reflexes: Advanced maturation	P9 Homing ↑	(Scattoni et al., 2008)
Orpm-/-	P4-8-12 ↓	Not tested	Not tested	(Moles et al., 2004)
nervous $^{nr/nr}$	Not tested	P1-12 Coordination ↓ Exploration ↓	P1-12 T-maze↓ P13–17 Morris maze ↓	(Lalonde & Strazielle, 2003)
Reln $^{rl\text{-}orl}$	Not tested	P1-12 Coordination ↓ Exploration ↓	P1-11 T-maze↓ P13–17 Morris maze ↓	(Lalonde et al., 2004)
Heterozygous Reeler	P7-11 ↓	P7-11 Coordination↔	P9 Nest-seeking↓	(Laviola et al., 2009; Macri et al., 2010; Ognibene et al., 2007b)
Neonatal exposure to vigabatrin (GVG) in Mthfr+/- mice	Not tested	Coordination ↔ Strength ↔ Righting reflex ↔	Not tested	(Levav-Rabkin et al., 2011)
Neonatal thimerosal in SJL Mice	Not tested	P8-10 Negative geotaxis ↔ Righting reflex ↔ Proto-ambulatory locomotion ↔	Not tested	(Berman et al., 2008)
Prenatal (E11) VPA	Not tested	P12-16 Eye opening: delayed	P9 Nest-seeking ↓	(Kolozsi et al., 2009)
Exposure (E11) to VPA	Not tested	P12-16: Eye opening: delayed	P9-11 Latency nest-seeking↑	(Roullet et al., 2010)

Table 2. Early behavioural alterations in mouse models of autism.

Abbreviations: KO: knockout; *UVS:* ultrasonic vocalizations; *patDp:* paternal duplication of mouse chromosome 7 corresponding to the region of human chromosome 15; *En2:* Engrailed genes; *MALTT:* multiple autistic-like transgenic traits; *nervous:* nervous gene mutation; *BTBR:* inbred mouse strain, *Orpm:* μ-opioid receptors; *Reln* $^{rl\text{-}orl}$: mice with the Orleans mutation; *GVG: vigabatrin; Thimerosal* (sodium ethylmercury thiosalicylate): antimicrobial preservative used in vaccines; *Mthfr+/-*, methylenetetrahydrofolate reductase gene; *VPA:* valproic acid. ↔: unaltered; ↓: reduced; ↑: increased.

2.1.1 Early behavioural alterations in the heterozygous reeler mouse as a model of ASD

Reelin plays a prominent neurodevelopmental role. Brain levels of this glycoprotein are in fact very high during late fetal life and gradually decline during late childhood to achieve a plateau during adolescence (Forster et al., 2006).

As previously mentioned, in rodents, ultrasonic vocalizations are emitted by pups when separated from the mother. Provided that these pup vocalizations elicit maternal orientation/approach and retrieval (Cohen-Salmon et al., 1985; Noirot, 1972; Smotherman et al., 1974) and reduce attacks or rough manipulation by the dam (Noirot & Richards, 1966), they are now widely recognized as precocious and reliable indexes of pups communicative/social behaviour, and are thought to constitute a marker on emotional/affective condition early in development (Farrell & Alberts, 2002a; Farrell & Alberts, 2002b; Santucci et al., 1994). Moreover, ultrasound vocalizations can be quantitatively analysed, can be elicited by measurable stimuli, and can be recorded with limited handling of the pup. On postnatal day (pnd) 7, null mutant reeler mice emitted fewer calls than wt controls, and heterozygous subjects emitted ultrasound vocalizations at an intermediate level (Laviola et al., 2006). These results confirm the relevance of these mice as behaviourally interesting model of early communication deficits in ASD.

We also detected effects of reelin gene dosage on behavioural and neuro-physical maturation during the first week of postnatal life: compared to wild-type littermates, null mice showed developmental retardation of the righting reflex (pnd 3) and a decelerated maturation of grasping reflex (around pnd 11) (Laviola et al., 2006). Neonatal grasping reflex and levels of general locomotion in infancy failed to show any difference between heterozygotes and wild-type subjects, thus suggesting that 50% of reelin level availability is sufficient to avoid major alterations in motor development (Macri et al., 2010).

The homing test paradigm allows a measurement of neonatal social recognition and early motivation towards a relevant social stimulus, i.e. the nest odor, as early as pnd 9. At this developmental stage, pups are able to coordinate body movements and move toward the nest. However, as their eyes are still closed, they recognize the nest by olfactory stimuli. Heterozygozous mice were found to be impaired in this test and these effects were apparently independent of general locomotion (Alleva et al., 1985; Laviola et al., 2006), thus suggesting an association with the reciprocal interaction deficits observed in autistic patients early in infancy (Rutgers et al., 2004).

As a whole, these results are particularly intriguing as some subtle alterations in early phases of development have been described in children later diagnosed for autism (Teitelbaum et al., 2004). Autism spectrum disorders are complex and multifactorial psychiatric diseases (Agid et al., 1999) and recent studies have emphasized the importance of gene–environment interaction in the etiology of these disorders (Tsuang, 2000). Indeed, while genetic vulnerability can be predictive of later-onset disorders, it is unlike that monogenic alterations can fully reproduce the underlying causes of ASD. Environmental factors can clearly exacerbate, or sometimes, mitigate the biological consequences of genetic alterations (Jobe & Harrow, 2005). More studies are therefore needed which address the interaction between genetic vulnerability and secondary external agents for the development of a given disease (Gottesman & Hanson, 2005).

In this framework, we hypothesized that lower expression of reelin could represent a factor of vulnerability for development of ASD-like symptomatology and that environmental

factors could either improve or worsen the behavioural outcome. To address this issue, we evaluated in a series of different studies, the effects of gene-enviroment interaction on the early behavioural phenotype of the mouse model. Three experimental manipulations were used as environmental challenges during the ontogenetic window: prenatal exposure to an organophosphate pesticide, maternal separation and estradiol treatment during early postnatal life (Laviola et al., 2006; Macri et al., 2010; Ognibene et al., 2007b).
For the latter, in line with the 'extreme-male brain theory' (Knickmeyer & Baron-Cohen, 2006) which suggests that elevated fetal testosterone levels may favor the onset of ASD symptoms, estradiol treatment on pnd 5 significantly affected the performance of heterozygous reeler mice in the homing test (Macri et al., 2010). Unexpectedly, the other two environmental challenges normalized the early behavioural phenotype of null mice (Laviola et al., 2006; Laviola et al., 2009; Laviola et al., 1990; Ognibene et al., 2007a; Ognibene et al., 2007b): both prenatal exposure to an aceticholinesterase agent (Chlorpirifos) and repeated maternal separation seemed to restore wt-like levels of ultrasound vocalization emission in homozygous reeler mice. Moreover, in contrast with our predictions, reelin deficiency seemed to play a protective role against maternal separation in the homing-test, where a reduced motivation towards the nest was found in separated mice. However, no effects of the treatment were found in mutant mice.
These results suggest that gene-related early behavioural alterations can be modulated by environmental factors, thus supporting the need for further studies during ontogenesis in mouse models of ASD. As a matter of fact, this kind of studies clearly represents a first step toward a better understanding of the underlying causes of ASD-like symptoms and, hopefully, toward the discovery of therapeutic interventions targeted at the early phases of life.

2.1.2 Early alterations in mouse models of Rett syndrome

One essential feature of RTT is an apparently normal prenatal and perinatal development until about 6-18 months of age, followed by a regression period, characterized by both a profound loss of acquired developmental skills in the areas of social contact, communication and hand use and a deceleration of head growth, usually leading to microcephaly. At the end of this period, which is extremely variable in duration, lasting few years in some individuals, development reaches a plateau associated with a wide variety of RTT peculiar symptoms (for a detailed review of symptoms see: (Hagberg, 2002; Mount et al., 2001).
In line with clinical observations, a peculiar progression of symptoms has been evidenced in all the RTT mouse models described so far (Ricceri et al., 2008). As a matter of fact, all of them experience an early developmental phase where no obvious deficits (i.e. visible by gross examinations) can be detected and after the onset of symptoms, undergo an escalating worsening until their premature death.
Increasing evidences from clinical studies, however, support the presence of early defects (i.e. during that developmental phase previously regarded as asymptomatic) (Charman et al., 2002; Kerr et al., 1987). Studies of family home videos, recorded before the disorder was clearly manifested (Charman et al., 2002; Kerr et al., 1987), would confirm that girls with RTT, during the first months of life, are not completely asymptomatic as it was thought. Motor deficits during the first 6 months of life (e.g. abnormal general movements and finger movements) (Einspieler et al., 2005) as well as alterations in communicative behaviours during the first 2 years of life (e.g. limited gestural communication) (Tams-Little & Holdgrafer, 1996) have been reported. Moreover, developmental delays and pre-regression abnormalities correlate in RTT girls with the severity of symptoms shown later on during development (Kerr & Prescott, 2005).

The analysis of the behavioural phenotype in RTT mouse pups confirmed the presence of subtle alterations during the so called "pre-symptomatic phase" (De Filippis et al., 2010a; De Filippis et al., 2010b). In particular, by means of a scale adapted to very young rodents, a delay in the acquisition of single reflexes and motor skills in both sexes was evidence in Mecp2-null mice (Fox, 1965; Ricceri et al., 2008) from postnatal day (PND) 4 to 21 (Picker et al., 2006; Santos et al., 2007). Interestingly, on PND 5 mutant males were also characterised by an abnormal emission of ultrasonic vocalizations and a different pattern of calls throughout the first postnatal week compared to WT controls. Females also showed an increase in ultrasonic vocalizations during the whole first week with a peak on PND 7.
Shortly after the creation of Mecp2-null mice, a mouse which expresses a truncated form of Mecp2 gene (Mecp2-308) has been generated (Shahbazian et al., 2002). In line with clinical observations that report a milder phenotype in RTT patients carrying C-terminal deletions of Mecp2 (about 10 % of RTT cases) (Chahrour & Zoghbi, 2007), this RTT mouse model shows both a later onset of symptoms [6 weeks of age (Shahbazian et al., 2002)] as well as a longer life expectation than the null mutants (De Filippis et al., 2010a; De Filippis et al., 2010b; Ricceri et al., 2008). In Mecp2-308 mutant male mice, a picture of increased arousal and hyperactivity and reduced motor coordination was evidenced during the first postnatal days. In contrast with null mutant mice, impaired emotional communicative behaviour in this mouse model involved a significant decrease in ultrasound vocalizations emission.
This discrepancy suggests that the behavioural phenotype of models carrying different mutations in the Mecp2 gene do not necessarily overlaps, thus supporting previous reports (Belichenko et al., 2008; Ricceri et al., 2008). Indeed, BDNF levels, a gene-target of Mecp2 (Chang et al., 2006), are decreased in Mecp2-null mice (Schaevitz et al., 2010), while appear not altered in Mecp2-308 mice (Ricceri et al., 2011), suggesting that the truncated form of Mecp2 could retain some of its functions, thus contributing to the milder neurobehavioural phenotype of Mecp2-308 mice. As clinical studies support the presence of differences in the clinical manifestation of the syndrome in RTT patients carrying different mutations in the Mecp2 gene, our results strongly support the need for further studies aimed at elucidating the genotype-phenotype correlation in RTT. Indeed, thanks to the development of international databases, many step forwards have been made in the study of genotype-phenotype correlations in clinical research. The availability of RTT mouse models carrying different mutations in the Mecp2 gene now offers the unique opportunity to preclinical research to uncover the neurobiological correlates of such clinical observations.
In the brain of RTT mouse models, morphological and functional alterations have also been reported to be evident early in development, thus preceding the appearance of gross behavioural changes. These include, among others, overall reduction in brain size (Saywell et al., 2006; Stearns et al., 2007) and imbalance between inhibitory and excitatory synaptic transmission in the ventrolateral medulla (Medrihan et al., 2007). Moreover, a longitudinal study (from birth to postnatal day 42) investigating the concentrations of major neurotransmitters in the brain of MeCP2-null mice, reported smaller concentrations of biogenic amine in the brain of mutant mice when compared with WT. Interestingly, this difference became larger with increasing age. Modifications in BDNF expression, early neuronal morphology and cortical synaptic plasticity were also confirmed in pre-symptomatic mice (Belichenko et al., 2008; Chang et al., 2006; Dani et al., 2005).
Taken together, these results suggest that some subtle alterations are already evident in both RTT patients (quite before the pre-regression period) and mouse models. A better

investigation and characterization of the pre-symptomatic phase in RTT mouse models could therefore be extremely worthwhile for a better understanding of the neurobiological correlates of these behavioural alterations and for the development of new therapeutic approaches targeted at early intervention in RTT.

3. Conclusion

As demonstrated by the large number of models that have been generated so far, several efforts have been made in ASD research. Increasing the validity of mouse models, by identifying new potential models and investigating further the existing ones, is however mandatory in order to fully recapitulate ASD neuropathological signs and symptomatology. A prominent role is expected to be played by behavioural techniques in this process. As a matter of fact, behavioural phenotyping represents a valuable tool to be exploited for both the identification and the validation of models. Moreover, as already discussed, once behavioural alterations have been detected, they represent markers to evaluate the efficacy of potential therapeutic approaches.

As diagnosis of ASD is mainly based on detection of core symptoms, the fundamental role of behavioural phenotyping has been widely acknowledged in ASD research. It is however worth mentioning that refined analyses of the behavioural phenotype in mouse models should not neglect the early phases of development. Such analyses are in fact expected to advance our knowledge on the developmental disruptions that take place in the brains of patients, thus considerably increasing the probability to find a cure that can be administered early in development. Such an approach would be extremely beneficial for patients as it would allow passing over the consequences of aberrant developmental trajectories.

In conclusion, good mouse models and refined behavioural analyses should be definitely regarded as fundamental prerequisites for advancing our knowledge in ASD research, and many efforts are expected from this field in this direction.

4. Acknowledgments

Preparation of this book chapter was supported by Foundation Jerome Lejeune (France) and E-Rare EuroRett grants (to G.L. as P.I); the "ADHD-sythe" young investigator program ("under 40" call) and as Italian partner of the EU project "NeuroGenMRI" (ERAnet "PrioMedChild"), Italian Ministry of Health (to Walter Adriani as P.I.); Italia-USA project 11US/11, Italian Ministry of Health (to Enrico Alleva as P.I.)

5. Summary

Research in animal models, primarily rodents, has played a fundamental role in elucidating behavioural and neurological dysfunctions as well as the contribution of specific gene alterations and gene-environment interactions to the phenotype of some forms of neurodevelopmental pathologies. As the etiopathogenesis of autism has not been clearly elucidated so far and diagnosis is mainly based on presentation of three core behavioural symptoms (profound alterations in social interaction, communication deficits and stereotyped behaviours), different approaches have been adopted to model these pathologies in rodents. This chapter provides an overview of currently available mouse models of autism spectrum disorders (ASD)-like symptomatology.

The need for refined analyses of the behavioural phenotype in mouse models of ASD, which should not neglect the early phases of development, is also emphasized. Since behaviour is the ultimate output of brain function, behavioural phenotyping of these models provides integrated and reliable information hardly detectable using molecular, cellular or histological evaluations. Such functional information is also helpful to identify the role of specific genes -- and potential innovative molecular targets for therapy -- in neuropathologies and their interaction with the environment. As diagnosis of ASD is mainly based on detection of core behavioural symptoms, the fundamental role of behavioural phenotyping has been widely acknowledged in ASD research. However, only few studies have investigated the early phases of development in mouse models of ASD.

A number of tests and experimental protocols are now available that take into account the practical constraints imposed by the peculiar physiological and behavioural responses of an immature subject. Developmental analyses in fact provide a framework for understanding key stages of human brain development and unraveling deviations from the normal range as well as the age-dependent onset of normal response patterns.

Several reviews have already addressed our current knowledge on the behavioural phenotypes of the available mouse models of autism. However, very little literature is available dealing with the study of the early phases of development in mouse models of ASD. The present paper therefore provides an overview of the behavioural analyses so far carried out on neonatal pups in mouse models of ASD, particularly focusing on the heterozygous reelin mouse (haploinsufficient for the gene Reelin) and mouse models of Rett syndrome.

Such analyses are expected to advance our knowledge on the developmental disruptions that take place in the brains of patients, thus considerably increasing the potential for prevention or the identification of therapeutic approaches that can be administered early in development. Given the strict interplay between genes and environment during the development of a healthy individual, the possibility of an early intervention can result particularly important for autistic patients to reduce most of the carry-over consequences of a deviant developmental trajectory.

6. References

Agid, O., Shapira, B., Zislin, J., Ritsner, M., Hanin, B., et al. (1999). Environment and vulnerability to major psychiatric illness: a case control study of early parental loss in major depression, bipolar disorder and schizophrenia. *Mol Psychiatry*, Vol. 4 (2), Mar, pp. (163-172)

Alleva, E., Laviola, G., Tirelli, E. & Bignami, G. (1985). Short-, medium-, and long-term effects of prenatal oxazepam on neurobehavioural development of mice. *Psychopharmacology (Berl)*, Vol. 87 (4), pp. (434-441)

Andersen, T.E., Finsen, B., Goffinet, A.M., Issinger, O.G. & Boldyreff, B. (2002). A reeler mutant mouse with a new, spontaneous mutation in the reelin gene. *Brain Res Mol Brain Res*, Vol. 105 (1-2), Sep 30, pp. (153-156)

Auvray, N., Caston, J., Reber, A. & Stelz, T. (1989). Role of the cerebellum in the ontogenesis of the equilibrium behavior in the young rat: a behavioral study. *Brain Res*, Vol. 505 (2), Dec 29, pp. (291-301)

Belichenko, N.P., Belichenko, P.V., Li, H.H., Mobley, W.C. & Francke, U. (2008). Comparative study of brain morphology in Mecp2 mutant mouse models of Rett syndrome. *J Comp Neurol*, Vol. 508 (1), May 1, pp. (184-195)

Berkel, S., Marshall, C.R., Weiss, B., Howe, J., Roeth, R., et al. (2010). Mutations in the SHANK2 synaptic scaffolding gene in autism spectrum disorder and mental retardation. *Nat Genet*, Vol. 42 (6), Jun, pp. (489-491)

Berman, R.F., Pessah, I.N., Mouton, P.R., Mav, D. & Harry, J. (2008). Low-level neonatal thimerosal exposure: further evaluation of altered neurotoxic potential in SJL mice. *Toxicol Sci*, Vol. 101 (2), Feb, pp. (294-309)

Bielsky, I.F., Hu, S.B., Szegda, K.L., Westphal, H. & Young, L.J. (2004). Profound impairment in social recognition and reduction in anxiety-like behavior in vasopressin V1a receptor knockout mice. *Neuropsychopharmacology*, Vol. 29 (3), Mar, pp. (483-493)

Bielsky, I.F. & Young, L.J. (2004). Oxytocin, vasopressin, and social recognition in mammals. *Peptides*, Vol. 25 (9), Sep, pp. (1565-1574)

Bignami, G. (1996). Economical test methods for developmental neurobehavioral toxicity. *Environ Health Perspect*, Vol. 104 Suppl 2, Apr, pp. (285-298)

Bobee, S., Mariette, E., Tremblay-Leveau, H. & Caston, J. (2000). Effects of early midline cerebellar lesion on cognitive and emotional functions in the rat. *Behav Brain Res*, Vol. 112 (1-2), Jul, pp. (107-117)

Bolivar, V.J., Walters, S.R. & Phoenix, J.L. (2007). Assessing autism-like behavior in mice: variations in social interactions among inbred strains. *Behav Brain Res*, Vol. 176 (1), Jan 10, pp. (21-26)

Branchi, I. & Ricceri, L. (2002). Transgenic and knock-out mouse pups: the growing need for behavioral analysis. *Genes Brain Behav*, Vol. 1 (3), Aug, pp. (135-141)

Caviness, V.S., Jr. & Rakic, P. (1978). Mechanisms of cortical development: a view from mutations in mice. *Annu Rev Neurosci*, Vol. 1, pp. (297-326)

Chahrour, M. & Zoghbi, H.Y. (2007). The story of Rett syndrome: from clinic to neurobiology. *Neuron*, Vol. 56 (3), Nov 8, pp. (422-437)

Chaible, L.M., Corat, M.A., Abdelhay, E. & Dagli, M.L. Genetically modified animals for use in research and biotechnology. *Genet Mol Res*, Vol. 9 (3), pp. (1469-1482)

Chandra, S., Tjarks, W., Lorey, D.R., 2nd & Barth, R.F. (2008). Quantitative subcellular imaging of boron compounds in individual mitotic and interphase human glioblastoma cells with imaging secondary ion mass spectrometry (SIMS). *J Microsc*, Vol. 229 (Pt 1), Jan, pp. (92-103)

Chang, Q., Khare, G., Dani, V., Nelson, S. & Jaenisch, R. (2006). The disease progression of Mecp2 mutant mice is affected by the level of BDNF expression. *Neuron*, Vol. 49 (3), Feb 2, pp. (341-348)

Charman, T., Cass, H., Owen, L., Wigram, T., Slonims, V., et al. (2002). Regression in individuals with Rett syndrome. *Brain Dev*, Vol. 24 (5), Aug, pp. (281-283)

Cheh, M.A., Millonig, J.H., Roselli, L.M., Ming, X., Jacobsen, E., et al. (2006). En2 knockout mice display neurobehavioral and neurochemical alterations relevant to autism spectrum disorder. *Brain Res*, Vol. 1116 (1), Oct 20, pp. (166-176)

Cohen-Salmon, C., Carlier, M., Roubertoux, P., Jouhaneau, J., Semal, C., et al. (1985). Differences in patterns of pup care in mice. V--Pup ultrasonic emissions and pup care behavior. *Physiol Behav*, Vol. 35 (2), Aug, pp. (167-174)

Costa, E., Davis, J., Grayson, D.R., Guidotti, A., Pappas, G.D., et al. (2001). Dendritic spine hypoplasticity and downregulation of reelin and GABAergic tone in schizophrenia vulnerability. *Neurobiol Dis*, Vol. 8 (5), Oct, pp. (723-742)

Costa, E., Davis, J., Pesold, C., Tueting, P. & Guidotti, A. (2002). The heterozygote reeler mouse as a model for the development of a new generation of antipsychotics. *Curr Opin Pharmacol*, Vol. 2 (1), Feb, pp. (56-62)

Crawley, J.N. (2007). Mouse behavioral assays relevant to the symptoms of autism. *Brain Pathol*, Vol. 17 (4), Oct, pp. (448-459)

Cuomo, V., De Salvia, M.A., Petruzzi, S. & Alleva, E. (1996). Appropriate end points for the characterization of behavioral changes in developmental toxicology. *Environ Health Perspect*, Vol. 104 Suppl 2, Apr, pp. (307-315)

D'Amato, F.R., Scalera, E., Sarli, C. & Moles, A. (2005). Pups call, mothers rush: does maternal responsiveness affect the amount of ultrasonic vocalizations in mouse pups? *Behav Genet*, Vol. 35 (1), Jan, pp. (103-112)

Daenen, E.W., Wolterink, G., Gerrits, M.A. & Van Ree, J.M. (2002). The effects of neonatal lesions in the amygdala or ventral hippocampus on social behaviour later in life. *Behav Brain Res*, Vol. 136 (2), Nov 15, pp. (571-582)

Dani, V.S., Chang, Q., Maffei, A., Turrigiano, G.G., Jaenisch, R., et al. (2005). Reduced cortical activity due to a shift in the balance between excitation and inhibition in a mouse model of Rett syndrome. *Proc Natl Acad Sci U S A*, Vol. 102 (35), Aug 30, pp. (12560-12565)

Dawson, G. & Zanolli, K. (2003). Early intervention and brain plasticity in autism. *Novartis Found Symp*, Vol. 251, pp. (266-274; discussion 274-280, 281-297)

De Filippis, B., Ricceri, L. & Laviola, G. (2010a). Early postnatal behavioral changes in the Mecp2-308 truncation mouse model of Rett syndrome. *Genes Brain Behav*, Vol. 9 (2), Mar 1, pp. (213-223)

De Filippis, B., Ricceri, L. & Laviola, G. (2010b). Investigating Rett syndrome through genetic mouse models: pre-symptomatic, clearly symptomatic phases and innovative therapeutic approaches. In: *Transgenic and Mutant Tools to Model Brain Disorders*. A. V. Kalueff & C. L. Bergner, pp. (151-178), Humana Press Inc, 1601-183X (Electronic)

1601-183X (Linking), Totowa

Deguchi, K., Inoue, K., Avila, W.E., Lopez-Terrada, D., Antalffy, B.A., et al. (2003). Reelin and disabled-1 expression in developing and mature human cortical neurons. *J Neuropathol Exp Neurol*, Vol. 62 (6), Jun, pp. (676-684)

Dragich, J., Houwink-Manville, I. & Schanen, C. (2000). Rett syndrome: a surprising result of mutation in MECP2. *Hum Mol Genet*, Vol. 9 (16), Oct, pp. (2365-2375)

Dufour-Rainfray, D., Vourc'h, P., Tourlet, S., Guilloteau, D., Chalon, S., et al. (2010). Fetal exposure to teratogens: Evidence of genes involved in autism. *Neurosci Biobehav Rev*, Vol. 35 (5), Apr, pp. (1254-1265)

Einspieler, C., Kerr, A.M. & Prechtl, H.F. (2005). Is the early development of girls with Rett disorder really normal? *Pediatr Res*, Vol. 57 (5 Pt 1), May, pp. (696-700)

Farrell, W.J. & Alberts, J.R. (2002a). Maternal responsiveness to infant Norway rat (Rattus norvegicus) ultrasonic vocalizations during the maternal behavior cycle and after steroid and experiential induction regimens. *J Comp Psychol*, Vol. 116 (3), Sep, pp. (286-296)

Farrell, W.J. & Alberts, J.R. (2002b). Stimulus control of maternal responsiveness to Norway rat (Rattus norvegicus) pup ultrasonic vocalizations. *J Comp Psychol*, Vol. 116 (3), Sep, pp. (297-307)

Fatemi, S.H., Halt, A.R., Realmuto, G., Earle, J., Kist, D.A., et al. (2002a). Purkinje cell size is reduced in cerebellum of patients with autism. *Cell Mol Neurobiol*, Vol. 22 (2), Apr, pp. (171-175)

Fatemi, S.H., Snow, A.V., Stary, J.M., Araghi-Niknam, M., Reutiman, T.J., et al. (2005). Reelin signaling is impaired in autism. *Biol Psychiatry*, Vol. 57 (7), Apr 1, pp. (777-787)

Fatemi, S.H., Stary, J.M. & Egan, E.A. (2002b). Reduced blood levels of reelin as a vulnerability factor in pathophysiology of autistic disorder. *Cell Mol Neurobiol*, Vol. 22 (2), Apr, pp. (139-152)

Forster, E., Jossin, Y., Zhao, S., Chai, X., Frotscher, M., et al. (2006). Recent progress in understanding the role of Reelin in radial neuronal migration, with specific emphasis on the dentate gyrus. *Eur J Neurosci*, Vol. 23 (4), Feb, pp. (901-909)

Fox, W.M. (1965). Reflex-ontogeny and behavioral development of the mouse. *Anim Behav*, Vol. 13, pp. (234-240)

Goffinet, A.M. (1990). Cerebellar phenotype of two alleles of the 'reeler' mutation on similar backgrounds. *Brain Res*, Vol. 519 (1-2), Jun 11, pp. (355-357)

Goffinet, A.M., So, K.F., Yamamoto, M., Edwards, M. & Caviness, V.S., Jr. (1984). Architectonic and hodological organization of the cerebellum in reeler mutant mice. *Brain Res*, Vol. 318 (2), Nov, pp. (263-276)

Gottesman, II & Hanson, D.R. (2005). Human development: biological and genetic processes. *Annu Rev Psychol*, Vol. 56, pp. (263-286)

Hagberg, B. (2002). Clinical manifestations and stages of Rett syndrome. *Ment Retard Dev Disabil Res Rev*, Vol. 8 (2), pp. (61-65)

Hamilton, S.M., Spencer, C.M., Harrison, W.R., Yuva-Paylor, L.A., Graham, D.F., et al. (2011). Multiple autism-like behaviors in a novel transgenic mouse model. *Behav Brain Res*, Vol. 218 (1), Mar 17, pp. (29-41)

Hofer, M.A. & Shair, H.N. (1991). Independence of ultrasonic vocalization and thermogenic responses in infant rats. *Behav Neurosci*, Vol. 105 (1), Feb, pp. (41-48)

Hohmann, C.F., Walker, E.M., Boylan, C.B. & Blue, M.E. (2007). Neonatal serotonin depletion alters behavioral responses to spatial change and novelty. *Brain Res*, Vol. 1139, Mar 30, pp. (163-177)

Holy, T.E. & Guo, Z. (2005). Ultrasonic songs of male mice. *PLoS Biol*, Vol. 3 (12), Dec, pp. (e386)

Hornig, M., Weissenbock, H., Horscroft, N. & Lipkin, W.I. (1999). An infection-based model of neurodevelopmental damage. *Proc Natl Acad Sci U S A*, Vol. 96 (21), Oct 12, pp. (12102-12107)

Jamain, S., Quach, H., Betancur, C., Rastam, M., Colineaux, C., et al. (2003). Mutations of the X-linked genes encoding neuroligins NLGN3 and NLGN4 are associated with autism. *Nat Genet*, Vol. 34 (1), May, pp. (27-29)

Jamain, S., Radyushkin, K., Hammerschmidt, K., Granon, S., Boretius, S., et al. (2008). Reduced social interaction and ultrasonic communication in a mouse model of monogenic heritable autism. *Proc Natl Acad Sci U S A*, Vol. 105 (5), Feb 5, pp. (1710-1715)

Jobe, T.H. & Harrow, M. (2005). Long-term outcome of patients with schizophrenia: a review. *Can J Psychiatry*, Vol. 50 (14), Dec, pp. (892-900)

Jorgensen, H.F. & Bird, A. (2002). MeCP2 and other methyl-CpG binding proteins. *Ment Retard Dev Disabil Res Rev*, Vol. 8 (2), pp. (87-93)

Kasari, C., Freeman, S. & Paparella, T. (2006). Joint attention and symbolic play in young children with autism: a randomized controlled intervention study. *J Child Psychol Psychiatry*, Vol. 47 (6), Jun, pp. (611-620)

Kashinath, S., Woods, J. & Goldstein, H. (2006). Enhancing generalized teaching strategy use in daily routines by parents of children with autism. *J Speech Lang Hear Res*, Vol. 49 (3), Jun, pp. (466-485)

Keller, F. & Persico, A.M. (2003). The neurobiological context of autism. *Mol Neurobiol*, Vol. 28 (1), Aug, pp. (1-22)

Kerr, A.M., Montague, J. & Stephenson, J.B. (1987). The hands, and the mind, pre- and post-regression, in Rett syndrome. *Brain Dev*, Vol. 9 (5), pp. (487-490)

Kerr, A.M. & Prescott, R.J. (2005). Predictive value of the early clinical signs in Rett disorder. *Brain Dev*, Vol. 27 Suppl 1, Nov, pp. (S20-S24)

Kim, H.G., Kishikawa, S., Higgins, A.W., Seong, I.S., Donovan, D.J., et al. (2008). Disruption of neurexin 1 associated with autism spectrum disorder. *Am J Hum Genet*, Vol. 82 (1), Jan, pp. (199-207)

Knickmeyer, R.C. & Baron-Cohen, S. (2006). Fetal testosterone and sex differences in typical social development and in autism. *J Child Neurol*, Vol. 21 (10), Oct, pp. (825-845)

Kolozsi, E., Mackenzie, R.N., Roullet, F.I., deCatanzaro, D. & Foster, J.A. (2009). Prenatal exposure to valproic acid leads to reduced expression of synaptic adhesion molecule neuroligin 3 in mice. *Neuroscience*, Vol. 163 (4), Nov 10, pp. (1201-1210)

Krause, S., Langrock, M. & Weiss, M. (2002). Influence of seasonal variations in training loads on selected amino acids and parameters of the psychoimmunological network in a swimming team. *Int J Sports Med*, Vol. 23 (5), Jul, pp. (380-387)

Kuemerle, B., Gulden, F., Cherosky, N., Williams, E. & Herrup, K. (2007). The mouse Engrailed genes: a window into autism. *Behav Brain Res*, Vol. 176 (1), Jan 10, pp. (121-132)

Lalonde, R., Hayzoun, K., Derer, M., Mariani, J. & Strazielle, C. (2004). Neurobehavioral evaluation of Reln-rl-orl mutant mice and correlations with cytochrome oxidase activity. *Neurosci Res*, Vol. 49 (3), Jul, pp. (297-305)

Lalonde, R. & Strazielle, C. (2003). Motor coordination, exploration, and spatial learning in a natural mouse mutation (nervous) with Purkinje cell degeneration. *Behav Genet*, Vol. 33 (1), Jan, pp. (59-66)

Landrigan, P.J. (2010). What causes autism? Exploring the environmental contribution. *Curr Opin Pediatr*, Vol. 22 (2), Apr, pp. (219-225)

Laumonnier, F., Bonnet-Brilhault, F., Gomot, M., Blanc, R., David, A., et al. (2004). X-linked mental retardation and autism are associated with a mutation in the NLGN4 gene, a member of the neuroligin family. *Am J Hum Genet*, Vol. 74 (3), Mar, pp. (552-557)

Laviola, G., Adriani, W., Gaudino, C., Marino, R. & Keller, F. (2006). Paradoxical effects of prenatal acetylcholinesterase blockade on neuro-behavioral development and drug-induced stereotypies in reeler mutant mice. *Psychopharmacology (Berl)*, Vol. 187 (3), Aug, pp. (331-344)

Laviola, G., Ognibene, E., Romano, E., Adriani, W. & Keller, F. (2009). Gene-environment interaction during early development in the heterozygous reeler mouse: clues for modelling of major neurobehavioral syndromes. *Neurosci Biobehav Rev*, Vol. 33 (4), Apr, pp. (560-572)

Laviola, G., Sedowofia, K., Innes, J., Clayton, R. & Manning, A. (1990). Genetic differences in maternal behaviour patterns in mice administered phenobarbital during pregnancy. *Psychopharmacology (Berl)*, Vol. 102 (3), pp. (383-390)

Levav-Rabkin, T., Blumkin, E., Galron, D. & Golan, H.M. Sex-dependent behavioral effects of Mthfr deficiency and neonatal GABA potentiation in mice. *Behav Brain Res*, Vol. 216 (2), Jan 20, pp. (505-513)

Levav-Rabkin, T., Blumkin, E., Galron, D. & Golan, H.M. (2011). Sex-dependent behavioral effects of Mthfr deficiency and neonatal GABA potentiation in mice. *Behav Brain Res*, Vol. 216 (2), Jan 20, pp. (505-513)

Lijam, N., Paylor, R., McDonald, M.P., Crawley, J.N., Deng, C.X., et al. (1997). Social interaction and sensorimotor gating abnormalities in mice lacking Dvl1. *Cell*, Vol. 90 (5), Sep 5, pp. (895-905)

Lim, M.M., Bielsky, I.F. & Young, L.J. (2005). Neuropeptides and the social brain: potential rodent models of autism. *Int J Dev Neurosci*, Vol. 23 (2-3), Apr-May, pp. (235-243)

Lintas, C. & Persico, A.M. (2009). Autistic phenotypes and genetic testing: state-of-the-art for the clinical geneticist. *J Med Genet*, Vol. 46 (1), Jan, pp. (1-8)

Liu, W.S., Pesold, C., Rodriguez, M.A., Carboni, G., Auta, J., et al. (2001). Down-regulation of dendritic spine and glutamic acid decarboxylase 67 expressions in the reelin haploinsufficient heterozygous reeler mouse. *Proc Natl Acad Sci U S A*, Vol. 98 (6), Mar 13, pp. (3477-3482)

Macri, S., Biamonte, F., Romano, E., Marino, R., Keller, F., et al. (2010). Perseverative responding and neuroanatomical alterations in adult heterozygous reeler mice are mitigated by neonatal estrogen administration. *Psychoneuroendocrinology*, Vol. 35 (9), Oct, pp. (1374-1387)

Marrone, M.C., Marinelli, S., Biamonte, F., Keller, F., Sgobio, C.A., et al. (2006). Altered cortico-striatal synaptic plasticity and related behavioural impairments in reeler mice. *Eur J Neurosci*, Vol. 24 (7), Oct, pp. (2061-2070)

McFarlane, H.G., Kusek, G.K., Yang, M., Phoenix, J.L., Bolivar, V.J., et al. (2008). Autism-like behavioral phenotypes in BTBR T+tf/J mice. *Genes Brain Behav*, Vol. 7 (2), Mar, pp. (152-163)

McKinney, W.T. (1984). Animal models of depression: an overview. *Psychiatr Dev*, Vol. 2 (2), Summer, pp. (77-96)

Medrihan, L., Tantalaki, E., Aramuni, G., Sargsyan, V., Dudanova, I., et al. (2007). Early defects of GABAergic synapses in the brainstem of a MeCP2 mouse model of Rett syndrome. *J Neurophysiol*, Vol., Nov 21,

Moessner, R., Marshall, C.R., Sutcliffe, J.S., Skaug, J., Pinto, D., et al. (2007). Contribution of SHANK3 mutations to autism spectrum disorder. *Am J Hum Genet*, Vol. 81 (6), Dec, pp. (1289-1297)

Moles, A., Kieffer, B.L. & D'Amato, F.R. (2004). Deficit in attachment behavior in mice lacking the mu-opioid receptor gene. *Science*, Vol. 304 (5679), Jun 25, pp. (1983-1986)

Mount, R.H., Hastings, R.P., Reilly, S., Cass, H. & Charman, T. (2001). Behavioural and emotional features in Rett syndrome. *Disabil Rehabil*, Vol. 23 (3-4), Feb 15-Mar 10, pp. (129-138)

Moy, S.S., Nadler, J.J., Young, N.B., Perez, A., Holloway, L.P., et al. (2007). Mouse behavioral tasks relevant to autism: phenotypes of 10 inbred strains. *Behav Brain Res*, Vol. 176 (1), Jan 10, pp. (4-20)

Nakatani, J., Tamada, K., Hatanaka, F., Ise, S., Ohta, H., et al. (2009). Abnormal behavior in a chromosome-engineered mouse model for human 15q11-13 duplication seen in autism. *Cell*, Vol. 137 (7), Jun 26, pp. (1235-1246)

Noirot, E. (1972). Ultrasounds and maternal behavior in small rodents. *Dev Psychobiol*, Vol. 5 (4), pp. (371-387)

Noirot, E. & Richards, M.P. (1966). Maternal behaviour in virgin female golden hamsters: changes consequent upon initial contact with pups. *Anim Behav*, Vol. 14 (1), Jan, pp. (7-10)

Nyby, J., Bigelow, J., Kerchner, M. & Barbehenn, F. (1983). Male mouse (Mus musculus) ultrasonic vocalizations to female urine: why is heterosexual experience necessary? *Behav Neural Biol*, Vol. 38 (1), May, pp. (32-46)

Nyby, J., Whitney, G., Schmitz, S. & Dizinno, G. (1978). Postpubertal experience establishes signal value of mammaliam sex odor. *Behav Biol*, Vol. 22 (4), Apr, pp. (545-552)

Ognibene, E., Adriani, W., Granstrem, O., Pieretti, S. & Laviola, G. (2007a). Impulsivity-anxiety-related behavior and profiles of morphine-induced analgesia in heterozygous reeler mice. *Brain Res*, Vol. 1131 (1), Feb 2, pp. (173-180)

Ognibene, E., Adriani, W., Macri, S. & Laviola, G. (2007b). Neurobehavioural disorders in the infant reeler mouse model: interaction of genetic vulnerability and consequences of maternal separation. *Behav Brain Res*, Vol. 177 (1), Feb 12, pp. (142-149)

Panksepp, J.B., Jochman, K.A., Kim, J.U., Koy, J.J., Wilson, E.D., et al. (2007). Affiliative behavior, ultrasonic communication and social reward are influenced by genetic variation in adolescent mice. *PLoS ONE*, Vol. 2 (4), pp. (e351)

Patterson, P.H. (2002). Maternal infection: window on neuroimmune interactions in fetal brain development and mental illness. *Curr Opin Neurobiol*, Vol. 12 (1), Feb, pp. (115-118)

Picker, J.D., Yang, R., Ricceri, L. & Berger-Sweeney, J. (2006). An altered neonatal behavioral phenotype in Mecp2 mutant mice. *Neuroreport*, Vol. 17 (5), Apr 3, pp. (541-544)

Pletnikov, M.V., Rubin, S.A., Moran, T.H. & Carbone, K.M. (2003). Exploring the cerebellum with a new tool: neonatal Borna disease virus (BDV) infection of the rat's brain. *Cerebellum*, Vol. 2 (1), pp. (62-70)

Pletnikov, M.V., Rubin, S.A., Schwartz, G.J., Moran, T.H., Sobotka, T.J., et al. (1999). Persistent neonatal Borna disease virus (BDV) infection of the brain causes chronic emotional abnormalities in adult rats. *Physiol Behav*, Vol. 66 (5), Jul, pp. (823-831)

Radyushkin, K., Hammerschmidt, K., Boretius, S., Varoqueaux, F., El-Kordi, A., et al. (2009). Neuroligin-3-deficient mice: model of a monogenic heritable form of autism with an olfactory deficit. *Genes Brain Behav*, Vol. 8 (4), Jun, pp. (416-425)

Rau, M.E. (1983). The open-field behaviour of mice infected with Trichinella spiralis. *Parasitology*, Vol. 86 (Pt 2), Apr, pp. (311-318)

Ricceri, L., De Filippis, B., Fuso, A. & Laviola, G. (2011). Cholinergic hypofunction in MeCP2-308 mice: Beneficial neurobehavioural effects of neonatal choline supplementation. *Behav Brain Res*, Vol., Mar 30,

Ricceri, L., De Filippis, B. & Laviola, G. (2008). Mouse models of Rett syndrome: from behavioural phenotyping to preclinical evaluation of new therapeutic approaches. *Behav Pharmacol*, Vol. 19 (5-6), Sep, pp. (501-517)

Roullet, F.I., Wollaston, L., Decatanzaro, D. & Foster, J.A. (2010). Behavioral and molecular changes in the mouse in response to prenatal exposure to the anti-epileptic drug valproic acid. *Neuroscience*, Vol. 170 (2), Oct 13, pp. (514-522)

Rubenstein, J.L. & Merzenich, M.M. (2003). Model of autism: increased ratio of excitation/inhibition in key neural systems. *Genes Brain Behav*, Vol. 2 (5), Oct, pp. (255-267)

Rutgers, A.H., Bakermans-Kranenburg, M.J., van Ijzendoorn, M.H. & van Berckelaer-Onnes, I.A. (2004). Autism and attachment: a meta-analytic review. *J Child Psychol Psychiatry*, Vol. 45 (6), Sep, pp. (1123-1134)

Sadakata, T. & Furuichi, T. (2010). Ca(2+)-dependent activator protein for secretion 2 and autistic-like phenotypes. *Neurosci Res*, Vol. 67 (3), Jul, pp. (197-202)

Sales, G.D. (1972). Ultrasound and aggressive behaviour in rats and other small mammals. *Anim Behav*, Vol. 20 (1), Feb, pp. (88-100)

Salinger, W.L., Ladrow, P. & Wheeler, C. (2003). Behavioral phenotype of the reeler mutant mouse: effects of RELN gene dosage and social isolation. *Behav Neurosci*, Vol. 117 (6), Dec, pp. (1257-1275)

Santos, M., Silva-Fernandes, A., Oliveira, P., Sousa, N. & Maciel, P. (2007). Evidence for abnormal early development in a mouse model of Rett syndrome. *Genes Brain Behav*, Vol. 6 (3), Apr, pp. (277-286)

Santucci, D., Cagiano, R. & Calamandrei, G. (1994). IGF-I and IGF-I24-41 but not IGF-I57-70 affect somatic and neurobehavioral development of newborn male mice. *Brain Res Bull*, Vol. 35 (4), pp. (367-371)

Saywell, V., Viola, A., Confort-Gouny, S., Le Fur, Y., Villard, L., et al. (2006). Brain magnetic resonance study of Mecp2 deletion effects on anatomy and metabolism. *Biochem Biophys Res Commun*, Vol. 340 (3), Feb 17, pp. (776-783)

Scattoni, M.L., Crawley, J. & Ricceri, L. (2009). Ultrasonic vocalizations: a tool for behavioural phenotyping of mouse models of neurodevelopmental disorders. *Neurosci Biobehav Rev*, Vol. 33 (4), Apr, pp. (508-515)

Scattoni, M.L., Gandhy, S.U., Ricceri, L. & Crawley, J.N. (2008). Unusual repertoire of vocalizations in the BTBR T+tf/J mouse model of autism. *PLoS ONE*, Vol. 3 (8), pp. (e3067)

Scattoni, M.L., Ricceri, L. & Crawley, J.N. Unusual repertoire of vocalizations in adult BTBR T+tf/J mice during three types of social encounters. *Genes Brain Behav*, Vol. 10 (1), Feb, pp. (44-56)

Scattoni, M.L., Ricceri, L. & Crawley, J.N. (2011). Unusual repertoire of vocalizations in adult BTBR T+tf/J mice during three types of social encounters. *Genes Brain Behav*, Vol. 10 (1), Feb, pp. (44-56)

Schaevitz, L.R., Moriuchi, J.M., Nag, N., Mellot, T.J. & Berger-Sweeney, J. (2010). Cognitive and social functions and growth factors in a mouse model of Rett syndrome. *Physiol Behav*, Vol. 100 (3), Jun 1, pp. (255-263)

Serajee, F.J., Zhong, H. & Mahbubul Huq, A.H. (2006). Association of Reelin gene polymorphisms with autism. *Genomics*, Vol. 87 (1), Jan, pp. (75-83)

Shahbazian, M., Young, J., Yuva-Paylor, L., Spencer, C., Antalffy, B., et al. (2002). Mice with truncated MeCP2 recapitulate many Rett syndrome features and display hyperacetylation of histone H3. *Neuron*, Vol. 35 (2), Jul 18, pp. (243-254)

Sheng, L., Ding, X., Ferguson, M., McCallister, M., Rhoades, R., et al. (2010). Prenatal polycyclic aromatic hydrocarbon exposure leads to behavioral deficits and downregulation of receptor tyrosine kinase, MET. *Toxicol Sci*, Vol. 118 (2), Dec, pp. (625-634)

Shi, L., Fatemi, S.H., Sidwell, R.W. & Patterson, P.H. (2003). Maternal influenza infection causes marked behavioral and pharmacological changes in the offspring. *J Neurosci*, Vol. 23 (1), Jan 1, pp. (297-302)

Silverman, J.L., Yang, M., Turner, S.M., Katz, A.M., Bell, D.B., et al. (2010). Low stress reactivity and neuroendocrine factors in the BTBR T+tf/J mouse model of autism. *Neuroscience*, Vol. 171 (4), Dec 29, pp. (1197-1208)

Singer, H.S., Morris, C., Gause, C., Pollard, M., Zimmerman, A.W., et al. (2009). Prenatal exposure to antibodies from mothers of children with autism produces neurobehavioral alterations: A pregnant dam mouse model. *J Neuroimmunol*, Vol. 211 (1-2), Jun 25, pp. (39-48)

Smotherman, W.P., Bell, R.W., Starzec, J., Elias, J. & Zachman, T.A. (1974). Maternal responses to infant vocalizations and olfactory cues in rats and mice. *Behav Biol*, Vol. 12 (1), Sep, pp. (55-66)

Spear, L.P. (1990). Neurobehavioral assessment during the early postnatal period. *Neurotoxicol Teratol*, Vol. 12 (5), Sep-Oct, pp. (489-495)

Stearns, N.A., Schaevitz, L.R., Bowling, H., Nag, N., Berger, U.V., et al. (2007). Behavioral and anatomical abnormalities in Mecp2 mutant mice: a model for Rett syndrome. *Neuroscience*, Vol. 146 (3), May 25, pp. (907-921)

Tabuchi, K., Blundell, J., Etherton, M.R., Hammer, R.E., Liu, X., et al. (2007). A neuroligin-3 mutation implicated in autism increases inhibitory synaptic transmission in mice. *Science*, Vol. 318 (5847), Oct 5, pp. (71-76)

Tams-Little, S. & Holdgrafer, G. (1996). Early communication development in children with Rett syndrome. *Brain Dev*, Vol. 18 (5), Sep-Oct, pp. (376-378)

Tecott, L.H. (2003). The genes and brains of mice and men. *Am J Psychiatry*, Vol. 160 (4), Apr, pp. (646-656)

Teitelbaum, O., Benton, T., Shah, P.K., Prince, A., Kelly, J.L., et al. (2004). Eshkol-Wachman movement notation in diagnosis: the early detection of Asperger's syndrome. *Proc Natl Acad Sci U S A*, Vol. 101 (32), Aug 10, pp. (11909-11914)

Torres, A.R. (2003). Is fever suppression involved in the etiology of autism and neurodevelopmental disorders? *BMC Pediatr*, Vol. 3, Sep 2, pp. (9)

Tsuang, M.T. (2000). Genes, environment, and mental health wellness. *Am J Psychiatry*, Vol. 157 (4), Apr, pp. (489-491)

Tueting, P., Costa, E., Dwivedi, Y., Guidotti, A., Impagnatiello, F., et al. (1999). The phenotypic characteristics of heterozygous reeler mouse. *Neuroreport*, Vol. 10 (6), Apr 26, pp. (1329-1334)

Vojdani, A., Pangborn, J.B., Vojdani, E. & Cooper, E.L. (2003). Infections, toxic chemicals and dietary peptides binding to lymphocyte receptors and tissue enzymes are major instigators of autoimmunity in autism. *Int J Immunopathol Pharmacol*, Vol. 16 (3), Sep-Dec, pp. (189-199)

Wahlsten, D., Metten, P. & Crabbe, J.C. (2003). Survey of 21 inbred mouse strains in two laboratories reveals that BTBR T/+ tf/tf has severely reduced hippocampal commissure and absent corpus callosum. *Brain Res*, Vol. 971 (1), May 2, pp. (47-54)

Weiss, L.A., Shen, Y., Korn, J.M., Arking, D.E., Miller, D.T., et al. (2008). Association between microdeletion and microduplication at 16p11.2 and autism. *N Engl J Med*, Vol. 358 (7), Feb 14, pp. (667-675)

Whitaker-Azmitia, P.M. (2001). Serotonin and brain development: role in human developmental diseases. *Brain Res Bull*, Vol. 56 (5), Nov 15, pp. (479-485)

Wolterink, G., Daenen, L.E., Dubbeldam, S., Gerrits, M.A., van Rijn, R., et al. (2001). Early amygdala damage in the rat as a model for neurodevelopmental psychopathological disorders. *Eur Neuropsychopharmacol*, Vol. 11 (1), Feb, pp. (51-59)

Yang, M., Clarke, A.M. & Crawley, J.N. (2009). Postnatal lesion evidence against a primary role for the corpus callosum in mouse sociability. *Eur J Neurosci*, Vol. 29 (8), Apr, pp. (1663-1677)

Yang, M., Scattoni, M.L., Zhodzishsky, V., Chen, T., Caldwell, H., et al. (2007a). Social approach behaviors are similar on conventional versus reverse lighting cycles, and in replications across cohorts, in BTBR T+ tf/J, C57BL/6J, and vasopressin receptor 1B mutant mice. *Front Behav Neurosci*, Vol. 1, pp. (1)

Yang, M., Zhodzishsky, V. & Crawley, J.N. (2007b). Social deficits in BTBR T+tf/J mice are unchanged by cross-fostering with C57BL/6J mothers. *Int J Dev Neurosci*, Vol. 25 (8), Dec, pp. (515-521)

Yochum, C.L., Bhattacharya, P., Patti, L., Mirochnitchenko, O. & Wagner, G.C. (2010). Animal model of autism using GSTM1 knockout mice and early post-natal sodium valproate treatment. *Behav Brain Res*, Vol. 210 (2), Jul 11, pp. (202-210)

Young, L.J. (2001). Oxytocin and vasopressin as candidate genes for psychiatric disorders: lessons from animal models. *Am J Med Genet*, Vol. 105 (1), Jan 8, pp. (53-54)

Young, L.J. (2002). The neurobiology of social recognition, approach, and avoidance. *Biol Psychiatry*, Vol. 51 (1), Jan 1, pp. (18-26)

Zaccaria, K.J., Lagace, D.C., Eisch, A.J. & McCasland, J.S. (2010). Resistance to change and vulnerability to stress: autistic-like features of GAP43-deficient mice. *Genes Brain Behav*, Vol. 9 (8), Nov, pp. (985-996)

Zhao, Y., Fung, C., Shin, D., Shin, B.C., Thamotharan, S., et al. (2010). Neuronal glucose transporter isoform 3 deficient mice demonstrate features of autism spectrum disorders. *Mol Psychiatry*, Vol. 15 (3), Mar, pp. (286-299)

19

Impaired Sociability of the Balb/c Mouse, an Animal Model of Autism Spectrum Disorders, is Attenuated by NMDA Receptor Agonist Interventions: Clinical Implications

Stephen I. Deutsch, Jessica A. Burket,
Maria R. Urbano, Amy L. Herndon and Erin E. Winebarger
Eastern Virginia Medical School, Norfolk VA
United States of America

1. Introduction

Impaired sociability is a domain of psychopathology that contributes significantly to the functional disability and poor quality of life of persons with Autism Spectrum Disorders (ASDs) (Brodkin, 2007; Crawley, 2004, 2007; Deutsch et al., 2011). Although cognitive functioning may influence the expression of impaired sociability, the relationship between cognitive deficits and impaired sociability is not a linear one; thus, for example, persons with ASDs whose IQs are in the near-normal to above normal range may manifest profound deficits of sociability that are similar to those shown by persons with ASDs and intellectual disability (Noterdaeme et al., 2010). Currently, there are no approved medications whose primary target is the domain of impaired sociability.

The N-methyl-D-aspartic acid (NMDA) receptor is an example of a glutamate-gated ion channel that is comprised of four (or possibly five) constituent polypeptide subunits; it is located both pre- and postsynaptically (Millian, 2005). Each constituent polypeptide is an integral membrane protein that has external, transmembranous and internal domains. The constituent polypeptides align themselves within the lipid bilayer of the membrane to create a potential channel, whose opening depends on the membrane potential and the binding of L-glutamate and glycine. The duration and frequency of channel opening, which results in calcium ion conductance and membrane depolarization, are highly regulated. The properties of this ligand-gated ion channel receptor are influenced genetically by the combinatorial diversity of the constituent polypeptide subunits (i.e., expression and membrane insertion of specific subunits and their splice variants can affect channel properties); allosteric modulatory ligands (e.g., neurosteroids) (Deutsch et al., 1992); the extent to which the receptor is glycosylated and nitrosylated; and the extent to which the internal domain of receptor polypeptide subunits are phosphorylated (Marino & Conn, 2002). The phosphorylation state of the internal domain is influenced by cross-talk between specific signaling pathways and the NMDA receptor; for example, stimulation of metabotropic glutamate receptors co-localized with NMDA receptors on the cell surface can influence the extent of phosphorylation (Conn et al., 2009a; Marino & Conn, 2002). When the membrane is at its resting potential, a hydrated magnesium ion occupies a binding site within the hydrophobic channel domain of the NMDA receptor; this magnesium ion blockade is removed as the receptor depolarizes, which may occur as a result of stimulating non-NMDA excitatory glutamate-gated ion channel receptors co-localized with NMDA receptors on the membrane surface (Chen et al., 1992). Once the magnesium ion blockade is removed with "depolarization" of the membrane, L-glutamate and glycine interact allosterically with each other to increase the likelihood that the channel will assume an open configuration that permits calcium ion conductance (Marino & Conn, 2002). Presynaptically, the opening of the NMDA receptor may be involved in calcium ion-dependent release of transmitters; channel opening results in the transient increase of the intraneuronal calcium ion concentration (Marino & Conn, 2002). Postsynaptically, NMDA receptors located on the surface of GABAergic inhibitory neurons contribute to regulation of the inhibitory tone of the brain (Benes, 2010). Functionally, because L-glutamate is one of the most abundant neurotransmitters in the brain, NMDA receptors are involved in many neural circuits; for example, NMDA receptors are necessary for the induction of long-term potentiation in the hippocampus and have a major role in spatial memory performance referable to the hippocampus, among many other functions (Benes, 2010).

Targeted mutations in mice that affect expression of the NR1 subunit of the NMDA receptor and its affinity for glycine, the obligatory co-agonist that binds to the NR1 subunit and contributes to regulation of channel opening, have been created (Halene et al., 2009; Labrie et al., 2008). Interestingly, in a standard sociability paradigm, these genetically-engineered mice with diminished expression of the NR1 subunit or five-fold diminished affinity of the NR1 subunit for glycine show deficits in sociability ((Halene et al., 2009; Labrie et al., 2008). Thus, altered NMDA receptor-mediated neurotransmission in mice is associated with impaired sociability (e.g., these mutant mice make fewer social approaches and spend less time in the vicinity of an enclosed or freely-moving socially-salient stimulus mouse).

The genetically inbred Balb/c mouse strain displays behavioral hypersensitivity to MK-801 (dizocilpine), a noncompetitive NMDA receptor antagonist (Billingslea et al., 2003; Burket et al., 2010a; Deutsch et al., 1997, 1998). Thus, MK-801 is more potent at antagonizing electrically-precipitated seizures in Balb/c mice than a variety of other genetically-inbred and outbred mouse strains (Billingslea et al., 2003; Deutsch et al., 1998). Additionally, Balb/c mice are more sensitive than other reference mouse strains to the elicitation of irregular episodes of intense jumping behavior, which has been referred to as "popping" (Billingslea et al., 2003; Deutsch et al., 1997). Further, relative to the outbred Swiss-Webster mouse strain, Balb/c mice engaged in more intense MK-801-elicited circling behavior (Burket et al., 2010a). The heightened behavioral sensitivity of the Balb/c mouse to MK-801 does not appear to be due to a "defect" in the receptor itself because a Western Blotting experiment revealed no differences in the immunoreactive content of six of the eight identified splice variant isoforms of the NR1 subunit, and NR2A and NR2B subunits in the hippocampus and cerebral cortex of Balb/c and NIH Swiss mice (Perera et al., 2008). Thus, the altered endogenous tone of NMDA receptor-mediated neurotransmission in the Balb/c mouse strain may be due to factors "upstream" or "downstream" of the receptor itself. In any event, the Balb/c mouse strain, like the targeted genetic mutant mouse strains described above, shows quantitative deficits of sociability in a standard mouse paradigm (Burket et al, 2010b; Brodkin, 2007; Moy et al., 2007; Sankoorikal et al., 2006). These deficits of sociability are observable when Balb/c mice are in the presence of a salient social stimulus mouse that is either enclosed or allowed to interact freely with a Balb/c mouse (Burket et al., 2010b;

Deutsch et al., 2011; Jacome et al., 2011a,b, in press). Specifically, Balb/c mice make fewer discrete episodes of social approach and spend less time exploring (sniffing) and in the vicinity of an enclosed and freely-moving social stimulus mouse (Jacome et al., 2011; Brodkin, 2007). Quite remarkably, D-cycloserine, a partial glycine agonist for the obligatory co-agonist binding site, and D-serine, a full agonist for this site that may also be the endogenous ligand, were able to attenuate the severity of the Balb/c mouse's deficits of sociability (Deutsch et al., 2011; Jacome et al., 2011a,b). These effects of NMDA receptor agonist interventions may be due to direct effects on the sociability deficit itself, as opposed to nonspecific effects resulting from increased locomotor activity in general. These preclinical results are also consistent with a pilot clinical trial of D-cycloserine administration to 10 children with ASDs; in this pilot investigation, D-cycloserine improved scores on the social withdrawal subscale of the Aberrant Behavior Checklist (Posey et al., 2004). Importantly, persons with ASDs may have deficient central inhibitory tone, consistent with the high prevalence of co-morbid seizures, which would benefit from an NMDA receptor agonist intervention.

In summary, the Balb/c mouse has emerged as a genetic mouse model of impaired sociability that is useful for screening targeted NMDA receptor agonist interventions, which may be candidates for development as medications to treat impaired sociability, a "neglected" domain of psychopathology in persons with ASDs. The topic areas introduced in this overview will be considered below in greater detail.

2. Impaired glutamatergic transmission may be a shared pathophysiological mechanism among persons with diverse etiologies of their autism spectrum disorders

Autism Spectrum Disorders (ASDs) are a heterogeneous group of disorders with respect to their clinical presentations that are highly heritable, as shown in family and twin studies (Toro et al., 2010); however, with the exception of ASDs occurring in the context of genetic disorders due to the effects of a single gene (e.g., tuberous sclerosis), the nature of what is inherited and the mode of genetic transmission are usually not known for most patients (Toro et al., 2010). Moreover, even in cases where ASDs are due to the effects of a single major mutant gene, the steps via which a single mutant gene leads to an autism syndrome are also unclear. In spite of the variability of their clinical presentations, persons with the diagnosis of an ASD manifest symptoms in three operationally-defined domains of psychopathology: "qualitative impairment in social interaction;" "qualitative impairment in communication;" and "restricted repetitive and stereotyped patterns of behavior (American Psychiatric Association 2000)." Persons with Asperger's Disorder, however, may have little or no clinically significant delays in language and cognitive development. Recent genetic investigations suggest that persons with ASDs may have "hotspots" along the genome where microdeletions or duplications of DNA, referred to as Copy Number Variations or CNVs, are more likely to occur (Bremer et al., 2011). CNVs can lead to problems related to "gene dosing effects (i.e., either absent or too much expression of genes that contribute to emergence of ASDs)" or, alternatively, can affect the coiling and higher-order structure of double-stranded DNA, which, in turn, affects transcription (Toro et al., 2010). Another possibility is that a microdeletion can lead to unmasking and unopposed expression of a "recessive" mutant gene product, whose homozygous expression may be ordinarily lethal in utero. Additionally, since the etiologies of ASDs vary but persons with ASDs share symptoms in the three discrete domains of autism psychopathology, there is interest in identifying discrete neural circuits that may serve as the substrate for impaired social-emotional cognition and other domains of psychopathology in ASDs, irrespective of etiology, and exploring the efficiency of synaptic transmission between nodes within these neural circuits in affected persons. Thus, imaging studies, such as *functional* MRI, examine activation of specific nodes, such as amygdala, fusiform gyrus, anterior cingulate cortex, among other brain areas, while subjects with ASDs view projected images of the human face displaying various facial expressions or "affects," such as fear, anger, disdain or happiness (Kleinhans et al., 2011; Ashwin et al., 2007). Moreover, disturbances within circuits may be responsible for the abnormal facial scanning strategies persons with ASDs employ (e.g., spending less time gazing at the eyes relative to typically developing normal subjects). Because pathophysiological abnormalities may represent a common final pathway that many persons with ASDs share in-common, irrespective of etiology, it may be possible to design medication strategies that target inefficient or aberrant synaptic transmission along neural circuits (e.g., the neural circuit necessary for normal social-emotional cognition) that would be beneficial for an etiologically diverse group of persons with ASDs (Table 1).

Influence Glutamate Signal Transduction by the NMDA Receptor Itself
Glutamate Reuptake Inhibitors
Glycine Reuptake Inhibitors (e.g., sarcosine and sarcosine analogues and derivatives)
Glycine Agonists (e.g., D-cycloserine, D-serine)
Allosteric Modulators of the NMDA Receptor (e.g., neurosteroids, polyamines)
Positive Allosteric Modulators of Group I Metabotropic Glutamate Receptors
Inhibitors of "Regulator of G Protein Signaling (RGS) Proteins"
Influence Downstream of "Defective" NMDA Receptor Signal Transduction Targeting GABA Inhibitory Neurons Themselves or Their Downstream Projections and Consequences
α7 Nicotinic Acetylcholine Receptor Agonist Interventions
Positive Allosteric Modulators (e.g., galantamine)
Selective Agonists (e.g., choline, anabaseine derivatives)
CB1-Cannabinoid Receptor Antagonists
Epigenetic Interventions
Histone Deacetylase Inhibitor
DNA Methyltransferase 1 Inhibitor
$GABA_A$ Receptor Agonist Interventions
Selective Benzodiazepine Agonist Interventions
Neurosteroids
Selective AMPA and Kainate Receptor (i.e., non-NMDA Excitatory Receptor) Antagonists

Table 1. Potential Pharmacological Strategies to Manipulate Endogenous Tone of NMDA Receptor-Mediated Neurotransmission

Conceivably, impairments of sociability manifested by persons with ASDs reflect disturbances within the social-emotional neural circuit (Benes, 2010). Given the quantitative importance of glutamatergic transmission in the brain and recent data suggesting that diminished or defective expression of the N-methyl-D-aspartic acid (NMDA) subtype of ionotropic glutamate receptor is causally-related to deficits of sociability in transgenic mouse strains, the NMDA receptor has emerged as a medication target to improve sociability in persons with ASDs (Halene et al., 2009; Duncan et al., 2004). More specifically, NMDA receptors are involved in regulating presynaptic release of a variety of neurotransmitters, including glutamate itself, and their postsynaptic location on the surface of GABA inhibitory neurons plays a very important role in regulating central inhibitory tone and critical oscillatory rhythms in brain (see below) (Benes, 2010, Deutsch et al., 2010). GABA inhibitory neurons project to assemblies of pyramidal neurons and it is the oscillatory firing of these latter assemblies of neurons that underlie key rhythms in the brain; the power spectra of gamma oscillations are associated with working memory (Benes, 2010; Deutsch et al., 2010). Importantly, pyramidal outflow neurons utilize glutamate as their neurotransmitter.

3. NMDA receptor – Structure and function

The NMDA receptor is a highly-regulated ligand-gated ion channel that also has features of voltage-gating; although it is a ligand-gated ion channel receptor, it does not enjoy the close homology and genetic-relatedness that nicotinic acetylcholine and $GABA_A$ receptors share with each other. However, like other ligand-gated ion channel receptors, the NMDA receptor is an oligomeric protein constructed from four constituent polypeptide subunits, each of which shares a common motif; nicotinic and $GABA_A$ receptors have five subunits (Millan, 2005). The receptor polypeptide subunits are themselves integral membrane proteins that have an N-terminal extracellular domain, four hydrophobic transmembranous domains (in fact, the third hydrophobic loop does not span the entire width of the lipid bilayer), and an intracytoplasmic loop that has consensus sequences of amino acids that serve as substrates for phosphorylation by specific kinases (Conn et al., 2009a; Marino & Conn, 2002). Phosphorylation of the intracytoplasmic loop influences the gating and channel properties of the ionophore and often occurs as a result of "cross-talk" with G-protein coupled-receptors (GPCR) located next to or near the NMDA receptor on the surface of the neuron (Conn et al., 2009a; Gregory et al., 2011). The constituent polypeptide subunits align themselves in such a manner that they form a potential pore or channel in the membrane, whose opening is dependent on the binding of glutamate and its obligatory glycine co-agonist. The filtering properties of the channel are such that calcium ions can flux through the open channel along their electrochemical gradient. At the ordinary resting membrane potential, a hydrated magnesium ion is bound within the channel; in order for the channel to become functional, this magnesium ion blockade must be relieved, which occurs as the membrane begins to depolarize. Thus, functional conductance through the NMDA receptor is dependent on membrane depolarization, which may occur through the actions of glutamate stimulating AMPA receptors, another excitatory glutamate-gated ion channel receptor that may reside in the vicinity of NMDA receptors. The functional properties of NMDA receptors themselves are influenced by the unique combinations of NR1 splice variant isoforms with NR2A and NR2B receptor subunits (Kew & Kemp, 2005). Functional receptors are dependent on inclusion of the NR1 subunit or one of its eight common splice variants; the usual combinations comprising functional NMDA receptors involve two obligatory NR1 and either two NR2A or two NR2B subunits (Kew & Kemp, 2005). Functional NMDA receptors may have two glycine binding sites, whose construction depends on the extracellular domains of NR1 subunits, and two glutamate binding sites (Kew & Kemp, 2005; Millan, 2005). Also, as noted above, the extent to which the intracytoplasmic domain is phosphorylated, and the local pH and oxidation potential surrounding the receptor influence the receptor's channel properties (i.e., the likelihood the channel will open and frequency of channel openings in response to the binding of glutamate and its obligatory glycine co-agonist to specific sites in the extracellular domain of the NMDA receptor)(Millan, 2005; Stephenson, 2006). The likelihood that glutamate and glycine will be effective in promoting channel opening is also influenced by levels of neurally-active steroids, which act as allosteric modulators (Deutsch et al., 1992). Neurally-active steroids are derived from peripheral steroid hormones and also are synthesized in situ in the brain by glial cells; the highly-regulated translocation of cholesterol across the mitochondrion is the first step in neurosteroid biosynthesis in the brain. Clearly, glutamate-gated calcium ion flux across the NMDA receptor-associated ionophore is a highly regulated process, subject to genetic influences (i.e., combinatorial diversity or the unique combination of receptor polypeptide subunits and their splice variants that comprise the receptor and influence its channel properties); post-translational modifications (e.g., the extent to which the receptor is phosphorylated and nitrosylated); and circulating levels of endogenous allosteric modulators (e.g., neurosteroids and polyamines, such as spermidine) (Conn et al., 2009a; Deutsch et al., 1992; Kew & Kemp, 2005, Millan, 2005; Stephenson, 2006).

NMDA receptors have both pre- and postsynaptic localizations on neurons. Presynaptically, NMDA receptors may participate in neurotransmitter release, a process dependent on calcium ions, whereas postsynaptically, their location on GABAergic neurons may contribute to the regulation of inhibitory tone and normal oscillatory activity in brain (Deutsch et al., 2010). Interestingly, seizures occur commonly in persons with autism spectrum disorders, consistent with diminished central inhibitory tone; also, the normal gamma oscillatory rhythm and power spectra of gamma oscillations, an important oscillatory rhythm associated with working memory and higher executive functions, are dependent on functional GABAergic projections to assemblies of pyramidal cell output neurons (Deutsch et al., 2010). Thus, the integrity of circuits necessary for normal cognition and social behavior, whose nodes include cerebral cortex, anterior cingulate gyrus, hippocampus, and amygdala, among other discrete anatomic brain regions, contain NMDA receptors (Benes, 2010). An emerging body of preclinical and clinical data suggests that NMDA receptor hypofunction at the level of the receptor itself or due to abnormalities upstream or downstream of the receptor contributes to both cognitive problems and impaired sociability (Darrah et al., 2008; Deutsch et al., 2011; Halene et al., 2009; Jacome et al., 2011b; Labrie et al., 2008).

The ability of glycine to make glutamate a more efficient neurotransmitter and, thereby, increase the likelihood the channel will transiently assume an open configuration and allow calcium ions to flux freely has aroused interest in the strychnine-insensitive obligatory glycine co-agonist binding site on the NMDA receptor as a target for medication development to address presumptive NMDA receptor hypofunction. The strychnine-insensitive glycine binding site on the NMDA receptor is also referred to as the glycine$_B$ site (Millan, 2005). Interestingly, D-serine may be the naturally-occurring and preferred ligand for the glycine binding site on the NMDA receptor; a racemase exists that converts the more commonly-occurring L-form of serine, which is incorporated into protein and extensively involved in intermediary metabolism, to the D-form, which may have a unique localization and function within brain (Jacome et al., 2011b; Long et al., 2006). Exogenously-administered D-serine and other directly acting full agonists may serve as "proofs of concept" to implicate NMDA receptor hypofunction in some aspects of the pathophysiology of autism spectrum disorders, especially in animal models studying the effects of their single dose administration on outcome measures related to sociability and cognition (Jacome et al., 2011b). However, directly-acting full $glycine_B$ agonists may have limitations with respect to their development as medication interventions, which would have to be administered chronically in disorders such as autism spectrum disorders, because of concerns about "agonist-induced" receptor desensitization and excitotoxicity (Jacome et al., 2011b). Thus, in terms of viable medication strategies, there is interest in partial glycine agonists (e.g., D-cycloserine), and influencing NMDA receptor channel properties indirectly through "cross-talk" with other receptors (e.g., strategies exploring administration of positive allosteric modulators [PAMs] of type 1 metabotropic glutamate receptors [mGluRs]). Specifically, our laboratory is interested in exploring the effect of PAMs of mGluR5 on the impaired sociability of Balb/c mice, a genetic mouse model of autism spectrum disorders, because mGluR5 stimulation leads to phosphorylation of a specific serine residue within the intracytoplasmic domain of the NR1 subunit (Takagi et al., 2010). In general, as members of class "C" G-protein coupled-receptors, mGluR5 receptors are constitutive dimers that are located postsynaptically in close functional proximity to NMDA receptors. They have a large extracellular 'venus flytrap domain (VFD)' that is the L-glutamate agonist recognition site; binding of L-glutamate leads to the propagation of a conformational change via 'cysteine-rich domains (CRD),' resulting in activation of phospholipase Cβ through its coupling to ligand-binding by a Gq, a specific GTP binding protein (Niswender & Conn, 2010). A downstream consequence of phospholipase activation includes increased phosphorylation of the NMDA receptor. There are many functional consequences of increasing the phosphorylation status of NMDA receptors, several of which may be relevant to domains of psychopathology present in ASDs. For example, MK-801 can disrupt cognitive flexibility or set-shifting ability; the severity of this disruption can be attenuated by a positive allosteric modulator of mGluR5 receptors (Darrah et al., 2008). Presumably, this positive therapeutic effect reflects the increased phosphorylation state of NMDA receptors. As will be discussed, functional NMDA receptors and "normal" tone of endogenous NMDA receptor-mediated neurotransmission are necessary for "normal" sociability in mice.

4. NMDA receptor and genetic mouse models of autism spectrum disorders

The NMDA receptor has emerged as a promising target for medication strategies designed to improve sociability (and cognition) in studies involving both genetically-engineered and inbred mouse strains, and other rodent species (Blundell et al., 2010; Deutsch et al, 2011; Darrah et al., 2008; Halene et al., 2009; Jacome et al., 2011b; Labrie et al., 2008). Importantly, the NMDA receptor is known to be involved in important aspects of electrophysiology relevant to cognition (e.g., induction of long-term potentiation in the hippocampus) and memory performance (e.g., hippocampally-dependent spatial memory). These findings were complemented with relatively recent investigations showing transgenic mice with diminished expression of the NR1 subunit of the NMDA receptor (~5 to 10% of normal levels of expression) or five-fold diminished affinity of the receptor for glycine as a result of targeted mutagenesis of the glycine binding domain on the NR1 subunit have quantitative deficits of sociability in a standard paradigm (Halene et al., 2009; Labrie et al., 2008). Perhaps, of even greater significance, a targeted NMDA receptor agonist intervention (i.e., D-cycloserine) attenuated measurable deficits of sociability in "genetically-normal" resident and intruder mice in a standardized social interaction paradigm (McAllister, 1994). Thus, even in the absence of a genetic lesion affecting the NMDA receptor itself, this receptor could serve as a target to improve sociability and cognition. Additionally, encouraging data are emerging from studies with genetic mouse models of autism spectrum disorders, which are neurodevelopmental disorders, that pharmacotherapeutic interventions can improve quantitative deficits of sociability in young adult mice (Deutsch et al., 2011; Jacome et al., 2011a,b; Sankoorikal et al., 2006). Thus, there is reason for optimism with respect to potential for effectiveness of newly-developed medications identified in standard sociability paradigms using transgenic and inbred mouse strains as subjects; unfortunately, autism spectrum disorders are not often recognized in preschool-age children and, as a result, treatment is often delayed, which is why the positive data with young adult mice are so encouraging.

5. Sociability paradigm

Our laboratory has adopted a recently established mouse behavioral procedure for the quantitative assessment of sociability (Brodkin, 2007; Burket et al., 2010b; Crawley, 2004, 2007; Deutsch et al., 2011; Jacome et al., 2011b; Moy et al., 2007; Sankoorikal et al., 2006; Silverman et al., 2010). Briefly, in the first session, a test mouse is placed in the middle compartment and allowed to acclimate to the sociability apparatus for 5 minutes. In the second 5-minute session, a stimulus mouse is enclosed in an inverted wire cup in the side designated as the social compartment, and an empty inverted wire cup is placed in the side designated as the nonsocial compartment. The side designated for the location of the enclosed stimulus mouse is randomly assigned in a counterbalanced fashion throughout the experiment. In the third 5-minute session, the stimulus mouse is released from the inverted wire cup, and the test and stimulus mice are allowed to interact freely with each other (Figure 1). All sessions are conducted in dim lighting and videotaped for future viewing and data collection.

The amount of time a test mouse spends in the social and nonsocial compartments and exploring (sniffing) the inverted wire cups is measured in session II. Locomotor activity is measured in all three sessions and is defined as the number of transitions (i.e., number of times all four extremities cross each compartment) the test mouse makes across all three compartments in each 5-min session. Other behavioral measures of the test mouse include additional measures of sociability (i.e., social approach, social avoidance, social pursuit, mounting and anogenital sniffing) and stereotypic behaviors (i.e., rearing, grooming and wall climbing), which are obtained during the 5-minute session of free interaction between test and stimulus mice (Table 2). Importantly, our laboratory showed that these behavioral measures can be reliably rated by independent observers (Jacome et al., in press).

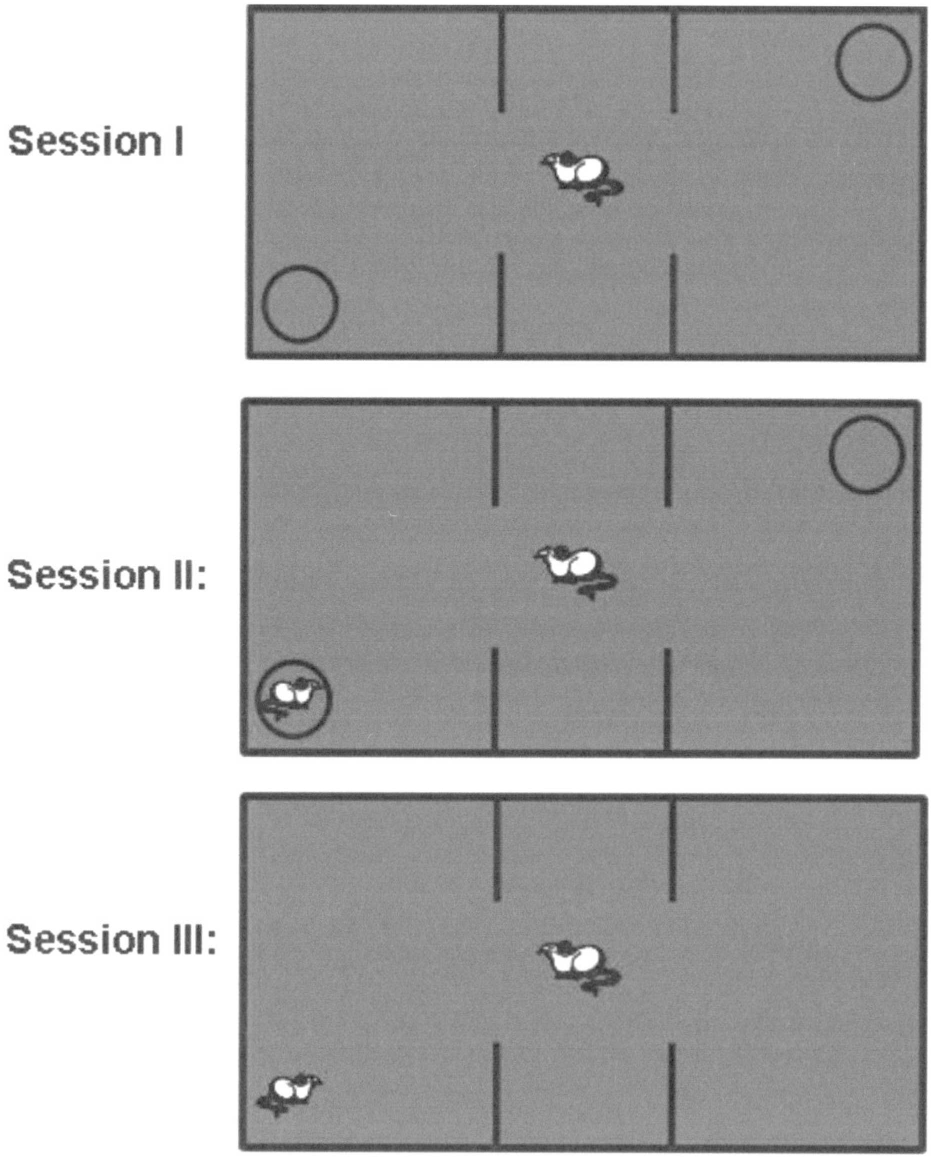

Fig. 1. Sociability paradigm

Measures of Sociability	
Social approach	A social behavior of test and stimulus mice defined as a discrete episode of their initiation of sniffing within a two-cm vicinity of each other.
Social avoidance	A nonsocial response of the test mouse defined as a discrete episode of freezing, withdrawing, or turning its head away while within a two-cm vicinity of the socially-salient stimulus mouse.
Social Pursuit	A measure of the time that the test mouse spends following or chasing the socially-salient stimulus mouse from initiation of the encounter until both mice separate by a distance of at least two cm.
Anogenital sniffing	A social behavior displayed by the test mouse defined as a discrete episode of sniffing the anogenital area of the stimulus mouse within a two-cm vicinity.
Mounting	A social behavior displayed by the test mouse defined as a discrete episode of placing the front paws on the stimulus mouse.
Measures of Stereotypic Behaviors	
Rearing	A stereotypic behavior displayed by the test mouse defined as a discrete episode of raising forelimbs and standing on hindlimbs.
Grooming	A stereotypic behavior displayed by the test mouse defined as a discrete episode of licking itself.
Wall climbing	A stereotypic behavior displayed by the test mouse defined as a discrete episode of raising forelimbs and placing front paws on walls of the sociability apparatus.

Table 2. Measures of Sociability and Stereotypic Behavior

6. The genetically-inbred balb/c mouse, a mouse strain that is behaviorally-hypersensitive to mk-801 (dizocilpine), a noncompetitive nmda receptor antagonist, shows quantitative deficits of sociability

Over the past 20 years, our laboratory has been exploring the effects of stress on the abilities of flurazepam, a benzodiazepine agonist, and MK-801 (dizocilpine), a noncompetitive NMDA receptor antagonist, to antagonize electrically-precipitated tonic hindlimb extension in mice (Billingslea et al., 2003; Burket et al., 2009; Deutsch et al., 1990; 1998). These studies showed that 24 hours after mice are forced to swim for up to 10 minutes in cold (6°C) water, the abilities of flurazepam and MK-801 to antagonize electrically-precipitated seizures are reduced. During the course of these investigations, it was observed that the genetically-inbred Balb/c mouse strain showed increased sensitivity to MK-801 administration on several behavioral measures. For example, relative to other inbred and outbred strains, the potency of MK-801 to raise the threshold voltage for elicitation of tonic hindlimb extension was greater in the Balb/c mouse (Billingslea et al., 2003; Deutsch et al., 1998). Similarly, Balb/c mice were more sensitive to the ability of MK-801 to elicit irregular episodes of intense jumping behavior, referred to as "popping," and "circling" behavior than other comparator strains (Billingslea et al., 2003; Burket et al., 2010a; Deutsch et al., 1997). The increased sensitivity to behavioral effects of MK-801 suggested to us that there is something "altered" in the endogenous tone of NMDA receptor-mediated neurotransmission in the Balb/c strain, relative to the other strains that we examined. Surprisingly, when we studied the immunoreactive protein content of six of the eight common splice variant isoforms of the NR1 subunit and NR2A and NR2B subunits in hippocampi and cerebral cortices from Balb/c and an outbred comparator strain, no significant differences were evident (Perera et al., 2008). These data suggested to us that the presumed altered endogenous tone of NMDA receptor-mediated neurotransmission in the Balb/c mouse was not at the level of the NMDA receptor itself (e.g., due to altered expression of the receptor polypeptide subunits), but, perhaps, at synapses upstream or downstream of the location of the receptor.

Because of our interest in the Balb/c mouse, we replicated reports that this mouse strain showed quantitative deficits of sociability in a standard paradigm (Brodkin, 2007; Moy et al., 2007; Sankoorikal et al., 2006), and extended these observations to include a detailed study of its locomotor activity in the presence of an enclosed salient social stimulus mouse and when Balb/c and stimulus mice are allowed to interact freely with each other. These studies showed that the locomotor activity of the Balb/c mouse strain is suppressed in the presence of a social stimulus mouse, which serves as another quantitative measure of impaired sociability (Burket et al., 2010b). The Balb/c mouse makes fewer discrete episodes of social approach, displays more social avoidance, and spends less time exploring and in the vicinity of both an enclosed and freely-behaving social stimulus mouse, than the outbred Swiss Webster comparator strain (Deutsch et al., 2011; Jacome et al., 2011b; submitted manuscript). Moreover, the impaired sociability of the Balb/c mouse affects the behavior of the social stimulus mouse when they are allowed to freely interact with each other for five minutes (Jacome et al., in press); thus, the social stimulus mouse will make significantly more discrete episodes of social approach toward the Balb/c test mouse than toward the outbred Swiss Webster comparator strain during this period of free interaction. The Balb/c mouse also demonstrates less anogenital sniffing and "mounting (i.e., placing forepaws on the stimulus mouse)" of the stimulus mouse, compared with the outbred Swiss Webster comparator strain. Another interesting behavioral feature of the Balb/c mouse is the dissociation between impaired sociability and intensity of spontaneous self-grooming behavior and other stereotypic behaviors (Jacome et al., in press). Thus, relative to the outbred Swiss Webster comparator strain, the Balb/c mouse spends less time engaged in spontaneous self-grooming and other stereotypic behaviors during the five-minute period of free interaction between test (i.e., Balb/c or Swiss Webster) and social stimulus (i.e., ICR strain) mice. This latter finding was unexpected in view of the fact that stereotypies (e.g., hand-flapping) are frequently observed among persons with autism spectrum disorders; self-grooming, rearing, and wall-climbing are examples of stereotypic behaviors measured in mice.

Because the Balb/c mouse is behaviorally-hypersensitive to MK-801, suggesting an altered endogenous tone of NMDA receptor-mediated neurotransmission, we wondered if pharmacological interventions targeting the NMDA receptor would affect its social behavior in a standard paradigm. The initial study examined D-cycloserine (320 mg/kg, intraperitoneally), a partial glycine agonist. This study confirmed that 8-week old male Balb/c mice made significantly fewer discrete episodes of operationally-defined social approach toward a 4-week old male ICR social stimulus mouse when the two were allowed to interact freely with each other, compared with the same measure of social approach of 8-week old male Swiss Webster mice in the same paradigm (Deutsch et al., 2011). Remarkably, however, the number of discrete episodes of social approach toward the social stimulus mouse made by Balb/c mice treated with D-cycloserine (320 mg/kg, intraperitoneally) did not differ from the vehicle-treated Swiss Webster mice. Moreover, the locomotor activity of D-cycloserine-treated Balb/c mice in the presence of both an enclosed and freely-behaving social stimulus mouse did not differ from the locomotor activity of vehicle-treated Swiss Webster mice under the same conditions. Thus, D-cycloserine attenuated the severity of several quantitative measures of the Balb/c mouse's deficit of sociability, restoring these measures to levels observed in vehicle-treated Swiss Webster mice, the outbred comparator strain (Deutsch et al., 2011). In further studies with D-cycloserine designed to explore possible mechanisms of its effect(s) and an explanation for the Balb/c mouse's deficit of sociability, we showed that Balb/c mice did not differ from Swiss Webster mice in terms of time spent exploring an inanimate object, whereas, as expected, Balb/c mice spent significantly less time exploring an enclosed social stimulus mouse (Jacome et al., 2011a). Moreover, the Balb/c mouse's deficit in time spent in social exploration was not an epiphenomenon of a greater basal level of "anxiety" because Balb/c mice did not spend less time in the open arms of an elevated plus maze than the Swiss Webster comparator strain. Also, D-cycloserine (320 mg/kg, intraperitoneally) significantly increased the number of open-arm entries of both strains of mice, suggesting that it causes a general increase in exploratory activity that was not strain-specific. However, there was something unique about a social stimulus mouse's ability to suppress the locomotor activity of the Balb/c strain and D-cycloserine's strain-selective ability to increase social exploration in the genetically-inbred, sociability-impaired Balb/c strain; there was no similar D-cycloserine-induced increase of social exploration in the Swiss Webster strain (Jacome et al., 2011a).

In addition to D-cycloserine, our laboratory showed that D-serine (560 mg/kg, intraperitoneally), a full glycine agonist, attenuated the severity of deficits of sociability in the Balb/c strain (Jacome et al., 2011b). The ability of D-serine to do this serves as an important "proof of concept" that targeted NMDA receptor agonist interventions can improve sociability in a genetic mouse model with presumed disturbance of endogenous NMDA receptor-mediated neurotransmission. Additionally, D-serine, like D-cycloserine, improved sociability in young adult 8-week old mice that serve as a genetic mouse model for at least some dimensions of autism spectrum disorders; these data encourage development of medication interventions in a neurodevelopmental disorder. Specifically, D-serine increased the amount of time Balb/c mice spent both in the compartment containing the enclosed social stimulus mouse and the amount of time Balb/c mice spent actually exploring and sniffing the enclosed social stimulus mouse (Jacome et al., 2011b). Importantly, the Swiss Webster comparator strain spent significantly more time in the compartment containing the enclosed social stimulus mouse and spent significantly more time exploring and sniffing this enclosed mouse even in the vehicle-treated condition.

However, as noted earlier, there are serious concerns with the development of a full agonist for the treatment of a chronic neuropsychiatric/neurodevelopmental disorder, such as an autism spectrum disorder. Specifically, a full agonist may have diminished efficacy/effectiveness over time because of agonist-induced desensitization, and a full agonist may cause excitotoxicity. Thus, D-cycloserine, a partial glycine agonist, may be expected to better retain efficacy/effectiveness upon chronic administration, while not being associated with increased risk for excitotoxicity; however, this is an empirical question that we will pursue in future studies.

As discussed, the mGluR5 receptor is functionally coupled to NMDA receptors; mGluR5 is a GPCR that is coupled to a Gq protein, whose biochemical effector is phospholipase Cβ (Borowicz et al., 2009; Niswender & Conn, 2010). Importantly, in addition to stimulating phosphorylation of a serine residue in the intracytoplasmic domain of the NR1 subunit of the NMDA receptor and, thereby, increasing the sensitivity of the NMDA receptor to stimulation by glutamate and glycine, mGluR5 receptors also play an important role in regulating translation of proteins in the basilar dendrites of pyramidal cell neurons. Stimulation of the mGluR5 receptor promotes protein synthesis (Bear et al., 2004; Dölen et al., 2010); thus, mGluR5's promotion of protein synthesis is unopposed in persons with Fragile X Syndrome, who are deficient in expression of the 'fragile X mental retardation protein." A major role of the 'fragile X mental retardation protein' is to dampen protein synthesis in basilar dendrites through its interaction and interference with the function of polyribosomes (Bear et al., 2004; Dölen et al., 2010). Because an unbalanced increase in protein synthesis in basilar dendrites is thought to contribute to the pathophysiological disturbance of Fragile X Syndrome, which has a high co-morbid prevalence of autism spectrum disorders, mGluR5 antagonism is emerging as a promising therapeutic strategy for this X-linked disorder.

The high comorbid prevalence of autism spectrum disorders among persons with Fragile X Syndrome and the beneficial effect of mGluR5 antagonism in mouse models of Fragile X Syndrome stimulated exploration of mGluR5 antagonism in another genetically-inbred mouse model of autism spectrum disorders (Silverman et al., 2010). Specifically, in a recent study, 2-methyl-6-(phenylethynyl)-pyridine (MPEP), an mGluR5 receptor antagonist that is centrally available after peripheral administration, was shown to attenuate the severity of self-grooming in BTBR T + tfj (BTBR) mice, an inbred genetic mouse model of autism spectrum disorders; the intervention did not affect locomotor activity nor did it have an effect on the impaired sociability of this mouse strain (Silverman et al., 2010). Repetitive self-grooming is thought to reflect and model the symptom domain of "restricted repetitive and stereotyped patterns of behavior," which is an important dimension of psychopathology in autism spectrum disorders. (In fact the text revision of the fourth edition of the American Psychiatric Association's Diagnostic and Statistical Manual requires that definitional criteria for at least one item/symptom in this domain must be fulfilled in order to assign a diagnosis of "autistic disorder.") Importantly, the BTBR mouse strain, in contrast to the Balb/c mouse strain, showed more intense repetitive self-grooming behavior than the comparator C57BL/6J mouse strain used in these studies (Silverman et al., 2010), the latter is a mouse strain characterized as displaying "high-sociability." Because of the interest in MPEP as a pharmacological intervention for a significant domain of autism psychopathology (i.e., "restricted repetitive and stereotyped patterns of behavior"), our group decided to study the effect of MPEP (30 mg/kg, intraperitoneally-administered) on measures of sociability and stereotypies, including spontaneous self-grooming behavior, in test mice (i.e., Balb/c or Swiss Webster) while they interacted freely with stimulus mice (i.e., ICR mice); as noted MPEP is a relatively selective, potent (IC_{50} value in the 30 nM range), blood-brain barrier permeable noncompetitive mGluR5 antagonist (Gasparini et al., 1999). Because the baseline level of stereotypies in the Balb/c strain is low, it is hard to detect drug effects on stereotypy outcome measures in this strain. However, the findings in the comparator Swiss Webster strain on reduction of stereotypies and worsening of some measures of sociability by MPEP underscore the need for caution in the development of mGluR5 antagonists as medications for the treatment of ASDs. Importantly, MPEP significantly reduced stereotypies in the Swiss Webster comparator strain, suggesting that this domain of autism spectrum disorder psychopathology may be uncoupled from sociability, reflecting, perhaps, their differences in underlying circuitry. MPEP also had socially disruptive effects in both strains (Burket et al., submitted manuscript), as well as some positive effects on sociability, thus, while MPEP attenuated stereotypies that appeared spontaneously during social interaction in both strains, it also had complex and inconsistent effects, including worsening, on sociability.

Given the role of the NMDA receptor for the display of normal sociability, these data add a cautionary note with respect to the pursuit of an mGluR5 antagonist medication strategy in autism. As a result of "cross-talk" between mGluR5 and NMDA receptors, stimulation of mGluR5 can promote phosphorylation of a serine residue in the intracytoplasmic domain of the NR1 subunit, which should result in "activation" of the NMDA receptor and its greater sensitivity to channel opening in response to glutamate and glycine (Mario & Conn et al., 2002). Moreover, MPEP is believed to exert its mGluR5 inhibitory properties by binding or interacting with a site in the seven transmembranous hydrophobic domain that is also the site of action of several positive allosteric modulators (PAMs) of mGluR5 (Conn et al., 2009b). Given the fact administration of glutamate "agonists" lack specificity and bind to a diverse variety of metabotropic and ionotropic glutamate receptors, in addition to their potential for excitotoxicity, interest has shifted to development of positive and negative allosteric modulators to selectively increase and decrease, respectively, signal transduction by metabotropic glutamate receptors (Conn et al., 2009a). Unlike the agonist recognition sites themselves that show conservation of their electronic architecture for recognition of glutamate and its analogues, allosteric modulatory sites show diversity of structure among glutamate receptors, affording "selectivity (i.e., only selected metabotropic and ionotropic glutamate receptors will be targeted)." Also, allosteric modulators are only effective in the presence of the endogenous agonist (Conn et al., 2009a); thus, they will be effective only at the precise synapse that glutamate (and glycine) is released, preserving the temporal and spatial constraints that are so critical to efficient, as opposed to "leaky," synaptic transmission. We and others are beginning to explore the potential therapeutic role of positive allosteric modulators of mGluR5 as a medication strategy to address presumptive NMDA receptor hypofunction in autism spectrum disorders.

7. Future directions and translational applications

Targeting the NMDA receptor and circuits containing and utilizing the NMDA receptor for synaptic transmission remain a promising area of future investigations. Very importantly, preclinical studies must also include chronic dosing conditions and the demonstration of sustained efficacy. Viable strategies should include manipulations both upstream and downstream of the presumed location of NMDA receptors on the surface of GABA inhibitory neurons, especially the "fast-spiking (FS)," parvalbumin-containing GABA neurons that regulate assemblies of pyramidal outflow neurons and underlie gamma oscillations (Benes et al., 2010). (In addition to NMDA receptors, specific kainate receptors, another type of ionotropic glutamate receptor, on the surface of GABA inhibitory interneurons [e.g., GluR6-containing kainate receptors] may also contribute to the generation and regulation of important oscillatory rhythms in brain.)

Thus, future studies can explore the acute and chronic consequences of both reducing (e.g., stimulating glutamate reuptake with guanosine) and increasing (e.g., via specific glutamate reuptake inhibitors) the concentration of glutamate within the synaptic cleft. Moreover, in addition to stimulation of the $glycine_B$ site with agonists, a strategy that is supported by the results of the D-serine and D-cycloserine experiments discussed in this review, interference with presynaptic reuptake of glycine via the use of glycine-1 transporter inhibitors (e.g., sarcosine and its derivatives) is another approach. We have reviewed the rationale underlying the use of PAMs of mGluR5 above; this strategy could conceivably be expanded or complemented by strategies that inhibit the activities of specific "regulators of G protein signaling (e.g., RGS4)." "Regulators of G protein signaling" promote the activities of GTPase and, thereby, dampen production of the soluble intracellular secondary messengers, whose synthesis is activated by glutamate's stimulation of metabotrobic glutamate receptors. The genetically-inbred, sociability-impaired Balb/c mouse may also be used to study the effects of neurosteroids on sociability; neurosteroids act at the level of cell surface ionotropic receptors (e.g., $GABA_A$ and NMDA receptors) to influence ion flux and membrane potential in subtle ways. Other strategies could include downstream manipulations; for example, if the GABAergic neurons containing NMDA receptors on their surface are dysfunctional, selective benzodiazepine agonist interventions could be considered (e.g., agonists that target $GABA_A$ receptors containing α3 or α5 subunits) that would promote GABAergic transmission downstream, via bypassing or compensating for the "defective" GABA inhibitory neuron. Additionally, if release of GABA is diminished, downstream glutamatergic projections could be relieved of critical GABAergic inhibition, which might be addressed by selective glutamate receptor antagonists that would block or attenuate the consequences of excessive downstream release of glutamate. Clearly, this is a highly speculative discussion, but the availability of genetic mouse models of autism spectrum disorders in general, and impaired sociability in particular, tested in a standard paradigm to assess sociability encourage and make this type of systematic examination possible.

There are provocative data suggesting that D-cycloserine improved social withdrawal in a small sample of 10 children with autism (Posey et al., 2004). Clearly, the therapeutic effect of a medication in this neurodevelopmental disorder is expected to be small and clinical trials must minimize "noise" associated with subject differences that may obscure a positive effect of treatment. Nonetheless, a medication that targets domains of sociability and cognition in the context of a well-designed interdisciplinary, individualized treatment plan that includes components of special education, speech and language therapy, occupational therapy and vocational assessment and training may contribute to significantly improved quality of life for many persons suffering with autism spectrum disorders. An outline for an integrated therapeutic strategy to address the sociability deficit of persons with autism spectrum disorders is shown in Table 3; clearly, medications will be only one component, albeit an important one, of a comprehensive individualized, interdisciplinary, multimodal treatment plan.

The NMDA receptor contributes to regulation of central inhibitory tone by influencing the firing of GABA inhibitory neurons. In addition to NMDA receptors, other receptors on the surface of the GABA inhibitory neuron may represent promising pharmacotherapeutic targets. In particular, the α_7 subunit-containing nicotinic acetylcholine receptor (α_7 nAChR), like the NMDA receptor, is a ligand-gated primarily calcium ion channel receptor on the surface of GABA inhibitory neurons that is emerging as a promising target. Recent efficient, high-throughput strategies for interrogating the human genome in large populations of referred persons with developmental disabilities showed that microdeletions of 15q13.3 (i.e., copy number variants), the locus of the α_7 nAChR, are associated with presentations of ASDs, which lend genetic support for the development of medications that target the α7nAChR. Hopefully, medication development strategies that exploit these promising genetic leads in appropriate mouse models will lead to improved treatments and outcomes for ASDs (Deutsch et al., submitted for publication).

Adjunctive Medication Strategies

Targeted NMDA Receptor Agonist Intervention

Primary defect in social motivation

Atypical Antipsychotic Medications

Stereotypies, irritability and other behaviors that interfere with learning and socialization

Anxiolytics

Social anxiety

Selective Serotonin Reuptake inhibitors

Rituals, repetitive behaviors, sadness and depression
Social anxiety

Medications are one important component of an individualized, multi-modal, interdisciplinary treatment plan that includes, but is not limited to:

Special Education
Psychosocial Skills Training
Operant/Instrumental Learning Interventions
Vocational Rehabilitation

8. References

American Psychiatric Association. (2000). *Diagnostic and statistical manual of mental disorders*, (4th ed., text revision), American Psychiatric Association, Washington, DC.

Ashwin, C., Baron-Cohen, S., Wheelwright, S., O'Riordan, M., Bullmore, E.T. (2007). Differential activation of the amygdala and the 'social brain' during fearful face-processing in Asperger Syndrome. *Neuropsychologia*, 45, 1, 2-14.

Bear, M.F., Huber, K.M., Warren, S.T. (2004). The mGluR theory of fragile X mental retardation. *Trends in Neuroscience*, 27, 370-7.

Benes, F.M. (2010). Amygdalocortical circuitry in schizophrenia: from circuits to molecules. *Neuropsychopharmacology*, 35, 1, 239-57.

Billingslea, E.N., Mastropaolo, J., Rosse, R.B., Bellack, A.S., Deutsch, S.I. (2003). Interaction of stress and strain on glutamatergic neurotransmission: relevance to schizophrenia. *Pharmacology, Biochemistry, & Behavior*, 74, 351-6.

Blundell, J., Blaiss, C.A., Etherton, M.R., Espinosa, F., Tabuchi, K., Walz, C., Bolliger, M.F., Südhof, T.C., Powell, C.M. (2010). Neuroligin-1 deletion results in impaired spatial memory and increased repetitive behavior. *Journal of Neuroscience*, 30, 2115-29.

Borowicz, K.K., Łuszczki, J.J., Czuczwar, S.J. (2009). 2-Methyl-6-phenylethynyl-pyridine (MPEP), a non-competitive mGluR5 antagonist, differentially affects the anticonvulsant activity of four conventional antiepileptic drugs against amygdala-kindled seizures in rats. *Pharmacological Reports*, 61, 621-30.

Bremer, A., Giacobini, M., Eriksson, M., Gustavsson, P., Nordin, V., Fernell, E., Gillberg, C., Nordgren, A., Uppströmer, A., Anderlid, B.M., Nordenskjöld, M., Schoumans, J. (2011). Copy number variation characteristics in subpopulations of patients with autism spectrum disorders. *American Journal of Medical Genetics Part B: Neuropsychiatric Genetics*, 156, 2, 115-24.

Brodkin, E.S. (2007). BALB/c mice: low sociability and other phenotypes that may be relevant to autism. *Behavioral Brain Research*, 176, 53-65.

Burket, J.A., Cannon, W.R., Jacome, L.F., & Deutsch, S.I. (2010a). MK-801, a Noncompetitive NMDA Receptor Antagonist, Elicited Circling Behavior in the Genetically-Inbred Balb/c Mouse Strain. *Brain Research Bulletin*, 83, 337-9.

Burket, J.A., Herndon, A.L., & Deutsch, S.I. (2010b). Locomotor activity of the genetically-inbred mouse strain is suppressed by a socially-salient stimulus. *Brain Research Bulletin*, 83, 255-256.

Burket, J.A., Mastropaolo, J., Rosse, R.B., Deutsch, S.I. (2009). Genetically inbred Balb/C mice are more sensitive to an effect of flurazepam and more resistant to an effect of stress than a genetically outbred mouse strain. *Epilepsy & Behavior*, 16, 3, 415-7.

Burket, J.A., Herndon, A.L., Winebarger, E.E., Jacome, L.F., Deutsch, S.I. (n.d.). Divergent Effects of mGluR5 Antagonism on Sociability and Stereotypic Behaviors in Mice: Possible Implications for the Pharmacotherapy of Autism Spectrum Disorders, submitted manuscript.

Chen, L. & Huang, L.Y. (1992). Protein kinase C reduces Mg2+ block of NMDA-receptor channels as a mechanism of modulation. *Nature*, 356, 521-3.

Conn, P.J., Christopoulos, A., Lindsley, C.W. (2009a). Allosteric modulators of GPCRs: a novel approach for the treatment of CNS disorders. *National Reviews Drug Discovery*, 8, 1, 41-54.

Conn, P.J., Lindsley, C.W., Jones, C.K. (2009b). Activation of metabotropic glutamate receptors as a novel approach for the treatment of schizophrenia. *Trends in Pharmacological Sciences*, 30, 1, 25-31.

Crawley, J.N. (2004). Designing mouse behavioral tasks relevant to autistic-like behaviors. *Mental Retardation and Developmental Disabilities Research Reviews*, 10, 248-258.

Crawley, J.N. (2007). Mouse Behavioral Assays Relevant to the Symptoms of Autism. *Brain Pathology*, 17, 448-59.

Darrah, J.M., Stefani, M.R., Moghaddam, B. (2008). Interaction of N-methyl-D-aspartate and group 5 metabotropic glutamate receptors on behavioral flexibility using a novel operant set-shift paradigm. *Behavioral Pharmacology*, 19, 225-34.

Deutsch, S.I., Burket, J.A., Jacome, L.F., Cannon, W.R., & Herndon, A.L. (2011). D-Cycloserine Improves the Impaired Sociability of the Balb/c Mouse. *Brain Research Bulletin*, 84, 8-11.

Deutsch, S.I., Mastropaolo, J., Hitri, A. (1992). GABA-active steroids: endogenous modulators of GABA-gated chloride ion conductance. *Clinical Neuropharmacology*, 15, 5, 352-64.

Deutsch, S.I., Mastropaolo, J., Powell, D.G., Rosse, R.B., Bachus, S.E. (1998). Inbred mouse strains differ in their sensitivity to an antiseizure effect of MK-801. *Clinical Neuropharmacology*, 21, 255-7.

Deutsch, S.I., Rosse, R.B., Huntzinger, J.A., Novitzki, M.R., Mastropaolo, J. (1990). Profound stress-induced alterations in flurazepam's antiseizure efficacy can be attenuated. *Brain Research*, 520, 1-2, 272-6.

Deutsch, S.I., Rosse, R.B., Paul, S.M., Riggs, R.L., & Mastropaolo, J. (1997). Inbred mouse strains differ in sensitivity to popping elicited by MK-801. *Pharmacology, Biochemistry & Behavior*, 57, 315-317.

Deutsch, S.I., Rosse, R.B., Schwartz, B.L., Mastropaolo, J., Burket, J.A., Weizman, A. (2010). Regulation of intermittent oscillatory activity of pyramidal cell neurons by GABA inhibitory interneurons is impaired in schizophrenia: rationale for pharmacotherapeutic GABAergic interventions. *Israel Journal of Psychiatry & Related Sciences*, 47, 1, 17-26.

Deutsch, S.I., Urbano, M.R., Burket, J.A., Herndon, A.L., Winebarger, E.E. (n.d). Pharmacotherapeutic Implications of the Association between Genomic Instability at Chromosome 15q13.3 and Autism Spectrum Disorders, submitted manuscript.

Dölen, G., Carpenter, R.L., Ocain, T.D., Bear, M.F. (2010). Mechanism-based approaches to treating fragile X. *Pharmacology & Therapeutics*, 127, 1, 78-93.

Duncan, G.E., Moy, S.S., Perez, A., Eddy, D.M., Zinzow, W.M., Lieberman, J.A., Snouwaert, J.N., Koller, B.H. (2004). Deficits in sensorimotor gating and tests of social behavior in a genetic model of reduced NMDA receptor function. *Behavioural Brain Research*, 153, 2, 507-19.

Gasparini, F., Lingenhöhl, K., Stoehr, N., Flor, P.J., Heinrich, M., Vranesic, I., et al. (1999). 2-Methyl-6-(phenylethynyl)-pyridine (MPEP), a potent, selective and systemically active mGlu5 receptor antagonist. *Neuropharmacology*, 38, 1493-503.

Gregory, K.J., Dong, E.N., Meiler, J., Conn, P.J. (2011). Allosteric modulation of metabotropic glutamate receptors: structural insights and therapeutic potential. *Neuropharmacology*, 60, 1, 66-81.

Halene, T.B., Ehrlichman, R.S., Liang, Y., Christian, E.P., Jonak, G.J., Gur, T.L., Blendy, J.A., Dow, H.C., Brodkin, E.S., Schneider, F., Gur, R.C., Siegel, S.J. (2009). Assessment of NMDA receptor NR1 subunit hypofunction in mice as a model for schizophrenia. *Genes, Brain & Behavior*, 8, 661-75.

Jacome, L.F., Burket, J.A., Herndon, A.L., Deutsch, S.I. (2011a). D-cycloserine Enhances Social Exploration in the Balb/c Mouse. *Brain Research Bulletin*, 85,3-4, 141-4.

Jacome, L.F., Burket, J.A., Herndon, A.L., Deutsch, S.I. (n.d.) Genetically-Inbred Balb/c Mice Differ from Outbred Swiss Webster Mice on Discrete Measures of Sociability: Relevance to a Genetic Mouse Model of Autism Spectrum Disorders, in press.

Jacome, L.F., Burket, J.A., Herndon, A.L., Cannon, W.R., & Deutsch, S.I. (2011b). D-serine Improves Dimensions of the Sociability Deficit of the Genetically-Inbred Balb/c Mouse Strain. *Brain Research Bulletin*, 84, 12-6.

Kew, J.N. & Kemp, J.A. (2005). Ionotropic and metabotropic glutamate receptor structure and pharmacology. *Psychopharmacology*, 179, 1, 4-29.

Kleinhans, N.M., Richards, T., Johnson, L.C., Weaver, K.E., Greenson, J., Dawson, G., Aylward, E. (2011). fMRI evidence of neural abnormalities in the subcortical face processing system in ASD. *Neuroimage*, 54, 1, 697-704.

Labrie, V., Lipina, T., Roder, J.C. (2008). Mice with reduced NMDA receptor glycine affinity model some of the negative and cognitive symptoms of schizophrenia. *Psychopharmacology*, 200, 2, 217-230.

Long, K.D., Mastropaolo, J., Rosse, R.B., Manaye, K.F., Deutsch, S.I. (2006). Modulatory effects of d-serine and sarcosine on NMDA receptor-mediated neurotransmission are apparent after stress in the genetically inbred BALB/c mouse strain. *Brain Research Bulletin*, 69, 6, 626-30.

Marino, M.J. & Conn, P.J. (2002). Direct and indirect modulation of the N-methyl D-aspartate receptor. *Current Drug Targets - CNS & Neurological Disorders*, 1, 1, 1-16.

McAllister, K.H. (1994). D-Cycloserine enhances social behavior in individually-housed mice in the resident-intruder test. *Psychopharmacology*, 116, 317-325.

Millan, M.J. (2005). N-Methyl-D-aspartate receptors as a target for improved antipsychotic agents: novel insights and clinical perspectives. *Psychopharmacology*, 179, 1, 30-53.

Moy, S.S., Nadler, J.J., Young, N.B., Perez, A., Holloway, L.P., Barbaro, R.P., et al. (2007). Mouse behavioral tasks relevant to autism: phenotypes of 10 inbred strains. *Behavioral Brain Research*, 176, 4-20.

Niswender, C.M. & Conn, P.J. (2010). Metabotropic glutamate receptors: physiology, pharmacology, and disease. *Annual Review of Pharmacology and Toxicology*, 50, 295-322.

Noterdaeme, M., Wriedt, E., Höhne, C. (2010). Asperger's syndrome and high-functioning autism: language, motor and cognitive profiles. *European Child & Adolescent Psychiatry*, 19, 6, 475-81.

Perera, P.Y., Lichy, J.H., Mastropaolo, J., Rosse, R.B., Deutsch, S.I. (2008). Expression of NR1, NR2A and NR2B NMDA receptor subunits is not altered in the genetically-inbred Balb/c mouse strain with heightened behavioral sensitivity to MK-801, a noncompetitive NMDA receptor antagonist. *European Journal of Neuropsychopharmacology*, 18, 814-9.

Posey, D.J., Kem, D.L., Swiezy, N.B., Sweeten, T.L., Wiegand, R.E., McDougle, C.J. (2004). A pilot study of D-cycloserine in subjects with autistic disorder. *American Journal of Psychiatry*, 161, 2115-7.

Sankoorikal, G.M., Kaercher, K.A., Boon, C.J., Lee, J.K., & Brodkin, E.S. (2006). A mouse model system for genetic analysis of sociability: C57BL/6J versus BALB/cJ inbred mouse strains. *Biological Psychiatry*, 59, 415-23.

Silverman, J.L., Tolu, S.S., Barkan, C.L., Crawley, J.N. (2010). Repetitive self-grooming behavior in the BTBR mouse model of autism is blocked by the mGluR5 antagonist MPEP. *Neuropsychopharmacology*, 35, 4, 976-89.

Stephenson, F.A. (2006). Structure and trafficking of NMDA and GABAA receptors. *Biochemical Society Transactions*, 34, Pt 5, 877-81.

Takagi, N., Besshoh, S., Morita, H., Terao, M., Takeo, S., Tanonaka, K. (2010). Metabotropic glutamate mGlu5 receptor-mediated serine phosphorylation of NMDA receptor subunit NR1 in hippocampal CA1 region after transient global ischemia in rats. *European Journal of Pharmacology*, 644, 96-100.

Toro, R., Konyukh, M., Delorme, R., Leblond, C., Chaste, P., Fauchereau, F., Coleman, M., Leboyer, M., Gillberg, C., Bourgeron, T. (2010). Key role for gene dosage and synaptic homeostasis in autism spectrum disorders. *Trends in Genetics*, 26, 8, 363-72.

Part 9

Sensory Motor and Visual Perspective Taking

20

Sensory Motor Development in Autism

Yesim Fazlioglu and M. Oguz Gunsen
Trakya University Deparment of Special Education Edirne, Turkey

1. Introduction

Autism is a syndrome that emerges in the first three years of life and is defined by a pattern of qualitative abnormalities in reciprocal social interaction, communication, and repetitive interests and behaviors. One of the characteristics which is most noticeable in those young children with autism who remain severely intellectually disabled is their propensity to engage in repetitive self-stimulatory actions, such as rocking, twirling objects or flapping their hand and finger. These actions appear to have no constructive use other than to provide some sensory stimulation (Attwood, 1993). Sensory and motor abnormalities commonly found in autism. These abnormalities have been described in the perception of sound, vision, touch, taste, and smell, as well as kinesthetic and proprioceptive sensations. These include reports of both hypo and hyper responsiveness to sensory input, raising the possibility that two groups of sensory responders may exist within the autism spectrum.

Comparing children with autism and children with other developmental disorders have concluded that prototypical developmental profile for children with autism is one of motor skills that are relatively more advanced than social skills, even when all delayed. Early hand-eye coordination significant predicted later vocational skills and independent functioning, while earlier fine motor skills predicted later leisure skills. Also motor development plays an important role in learning young children typically use motor skills to explore the environment, engage in social interaction, engage in physical activities, and develop basic academic skills. Unusual sensory responses are common concerns in children with autism. Given that most educational environment involve many sensorial demands, such as: noise level in classroom (O'Neill & Jones, 1997; Dawson & Watling, 2000).

These problems make the life of the child and his/her family more difficult and they prevent the child from learning new skills and having interaction with the environment. In solving sensory problems, it is important to support autistic children in gaining different sensory experiences. Sensory integration therapy program is important children with autism. Because the sensory integration therapy provides a child-centered and playful approach that is often appealing to even the most unmotivated or disengaged child (Case-Smith & Brayn, 1999; Fazlioglu & Baran, 2008).

This chapter will focus on sensory and motor development in autism, which are aimed at determining sensory problems that characterize the disorder. In addition, this chapter will comprehensive sensory integration therapy approaches, given the intensity and importance of these intervention in treatment planning.

2. Definition and development of sensory integration

Sensory integration theory was developed by Jean Ayres during 1970s. The aim of this theory is to stimulate specific locations of the body in order to ensure coordinated function of sensors. Ayres developed this theory in an attempt to better explain the relation between the sensory process, neural functions and behavior. Sensory integration treatment is used for children with autism as well as those with hyperactivity, cerebral palsy and premature birth (Fisher & Murray, 1991; Kranowitz, 1998; Bahr, 2001).

Sensory integration is a neurological process which compasses the analysis, synthesis and organization of the data received from the body and the environment. Sensory integration takes place in central nervous system. Sensory integration takes role in developing body perception, selection of concurrent stimuli, and the ability to act in convenience with the environment. Sensory receptors receive all the data from the body. Data flows through the sensory neurons in the central nervous system. Brain promptly analyses, collates associates and integrates the respective sensory signals through neurologic processing. Consequently, motor neurons send a signal to the brain. The body gives a sensory motor response to the signal. For instance; when someone says "I love you", vocal response is "I love you, too" whereas the emotional response is euphoria. Normal child is born with a perfect sensory system. Sensory integration mechanism in childhood continues through lifetime (Kranowitz, 1998).

It develops through new activities in daily life, experimenting, effort and exploring the environment. Each new piece of experience stirs the sense of achievement in the child. Developmental mechanism of sensory integration does not change and the development is constant. An example for the development of sensory integration may be a building. First, the foundation of the structure is laid which is followed by the construction of the first, second, third and fourth floor respectively. Constitution of the sensory integration is similar. Dr. Ayres defines the integration mechanism in four levels:

First Level: This level constitutes tactile, balance and movement (vestibular), deep sensory (proprioceptive), visual and auditory sensory. Babies begin to show interest in sensorial information as of second month therefore forming a basis for future learning skills. In this period, initial informative is the skin. Touch stimulus produce a fine feeling on the skin and around the mouth. The child is delighted with sucking. As a result, a strong bond is formed between the mother and the child. Thus, the baby learns to eat, hug, friendship and positive reaction. The baby is informed about vestibular and proprioceptive sensories through movement. The baby predicts and imitates the mother's facial expression with immature visual expression, beginning to develop movements including eye movement. At this time, the baby starts to recognize close objects, learns to follow the movement of his/her relatives and gains the feeling of trust in them. In the absence of the guidance of these sensories, it is difficult for the child to focus eyebeam, follow or move an object (Temel, 1992). Vestibular and proprioceptive sensories also influence the posture and muscle tone. Baby's actions in this period are automatic and situation-based. The child learns new movements. Vestibular sensations are instrumental in attaining the skill of feeling safe against the gravity by the muscles and joints. The baby learns to establish connection with the surface when lying and crawling. Therefore, the child feels safe.

Second Level: Tactile, vestibular and proprioceptive functions are essential in obtaining sensorial balance. In the emergence of distortion in the functions of these three systems, the child may provide insufficient reaction to the environment. In connection, the child may be observed to stage hyperactivity or introversion (Temel, 1992). Body perception (body awareness) consists of bilateral coordination of the body, hand preference (laterization) and motor planning (praxis). As of the first year, after achieving integration of the simple sensations in the first level, body perception and awareness start to develop. Body perception is the intellectual image of the position of body parts. Visual reactions assist in understanding how body parts move and their interactions with each others as well as developing a sense of self-identity. Developing body awareness enables bilateral integration. In this process, the child learns to use both sides of the body symmetrically. Bilateral integration is a neurologic function essential for developing bilateral coordination and behavioral skills. For instance; baby needs to develop bilateral integration in order to be able to swing or hand over the rattle.

Another function of bilateral integration is hand preference (laterization). Laterization is the detection that one side of the brain is favored. As laterization develops, the child begins to determine which hand is favored. The baby is then able to distinguish which hand is preferred. For instance, the baby may swing the rattle with one hand, while playing with his/her toes with the other hand. The child's body and neck rest above against the gravity. As head control develops, the baby's head rises and rotates around the body. Stabilizing the neck assists eye fixing. As a result, the child acquires the ability to gaze and inspect. First, the baby starts to creep, then crawls. Hands and legs act in coordination. The baby uses both sides of the brain while these movements stimulate the development of bilateral coordination, developing tactile, vestibular and proprioceptive sensories and motor planning (praxis).

Before engaging in a movement, the child thinks about how to do it. Afterwards, the baby actualizes the movement impulsively. For instance; development of motor planning is necessary for the child to roll on the ground. At first, the child practices turning and is able to roll without much effort afterwards. Thanks to the organization of the sensories, the child's activity level is better collated. Focusing duration and emotional intrepidness increases. In this period, the child may sit on the car seat and is able to distinguish between family members and foreigners.

Third Level: Sensory integration is a sustained and continuous process. Each level of integration enables the use of previous level (Temel, 1992). As the child grows, perception and understanding of the information received through the senses reaches higher levels. Expansion of the baby's environment urges the organization of sensory perception and distinguishing skills. In this level, the child has developed the ability to follow a speech completely and understand the language. Listening to a language user is the key skill in developing the ability to speak and understand the language. Hearing and language center of the brain is assisted by the vestibular system as to what is heard. Therefore, a problem in the vestibular system may lead to deficiencies in language development. Sensory integration disorder may prevent the child from feeling the position of the tongue inside the mouth as well as lip movements. Similar to speech and language, visual perception is a product of early sensory integration (Temel, 1992). In this period, visual senses convey significant importance. During this stage, the child has developed the ability to interpret visual input, understand people's and object's position in the space as well as eye-hand coordination. The child can use paints, produce simple drawings, catch a ball or pour juice into a glass. Development of eye-hand coordination contributes to the development of visual motor integration. As an example, we may point to the child's ability to place jig-saw pieces. At the age of three, the child's simple skills continue to develop and improve. The child is then ready to build a structure made of blocks.

Forth Level: The latest product of sensory integration is the academic skills. These include complex motor skills, organizing focus, organizing behavior, specialization of both sides of the body and the brain, visualizing an event, developing self-identity and self-control. These skills develop in time. Reaching the age of six, the child's brain is sufficiently proficient for such skills. Proficiency refers to the brain attaining greater efficiency in special functions while being potent and purposeful. In this level, the child's eyes and ears stand as primary teachers. Also, the child has organized the ability to distinguish concerning the touching sense.

Proprioceptive, vestibular and touching senses assist the development of motor coordination. In this period, the child can jump, run and play games with friends. The child can also button up, pull zipper and may use on hand more than the other. The child can also copy shapes and symbols using a pencil, may visualize past and future situations (for instance; we played football last night; I will have a bath tonight). Social skills are also developed in this period. The child can share ideas or toys with other people. Sensory integration is continually organized and structured throughout the life. When faced with exotic situations, the child learns to adapt and cope through sensible ways. The child holds positive feelings for him/herself and is ready for school attendance (Fisher & Murray, 1991; Kranowitz, 1998; Bahr, 2001).

3. Effects of sensory integration deficiency

Sensory integration deficiency (SID) is the inability to sufficiently perceive brain senses. SID is not considered as brain damage. This condition is named J. Ayres, "brain dyspepsia" (Royeen & Lane, 1991; Kranowitz, 1998; Bahr, 2001). The inability of the brain in processing sensory input sufficiently causes difficulties in effective management of behaviors. In cases when sensory problems are severe, the child may suffer from mental defects. Although sensory integration deficiency is a functional insufficiency, this condition does not mean total annihilation of the functions. Children with functional defects possess the same neuron count as healthy people, but the neurons cannot function cooperatively (Temel, 1992).

We may speak of four neurologic mechanism disorder considered to be related to autism in children with sensory integration deficiency. First of these is the deficiencies in registering and integration of sensory information (canalecstasia). Second are the problems concerning the proper transfer of stimulants to the right locations. The third one is anti-social behavior such as behavioral disorders and inability to initiate bilateral relations which are considered to be in connection with serotonin system disorders. The forth neurologic disorder observed in children with autism is the perceptual selectivity issue. The child may have difficulty in focusing on a specific point (Waterhouse *et al.* 1996). There are a variety of factors believed to cause sensory integration deficiency. These are:

First factor; it refers to the case when the brain has difficulty in responding to too much or too little sensory information. Excessive information input is called h*ypersensitivity*. In this case, aversion from the sensory stimulant may be observed. A low level of sensory information input is named *hyposensitivity*. In such cases, excessive self-stimulating may be needed.

Second factor; it is the neurologic organization disorder. In this case;

- Brain may not receive senses due to connection failure.
- Brain may receive sensory signals, but reception may be inconsistent.
- Brain may receive sensory signals consistently, but cannot establish the appropriate connection necessary to respond to other sensory signals.

The child's extraordinary answer to an ordinary question may reveal hypersensitivity, hyposensitivity or a combination of both. In case of hypersensitivity, the child may react with fear, irritability and protesting, negative, dissocial or introverted behavior. The child may be distracted by perceiving all the stimulants in the environment. Hypersensitive child feels disturbed when touched, avoids people and the environment. Changes in daily routine, crowd and noise are likely causes of anxiety. The child experiences difficulty understanding gestures during communication. The child may also have difficulty focusing on a purposed activity.
Recent research proposes that hypersensitivity may relate to cerebellum. Brain doesn't need the sensory signals from a movement to know the location of the body and the limbs. When limbs are moving, cerebellum predicts the consequences of the body movements and on this basis, sorts out sensory signals occurring from a touch to the body. For instance; while reaching out to grab an object afar, if we accidentally hit our other arm, we feel no anxiety or fear. In this moment, cerebellum determines the cause of the action as self or external based on predicting the results of previous motor action. It is predicted that faulty movement interpretations of sensory signals by cerebellum may be the cause of hypersensitivity (Fuentes & Bastian, 2007). In research conducted on autistic individuals, consistent cerebellar damage and Purkinje cell loss was observed which is supportive of this prediction (Bauman & Kemper, 2005).
In hyposensitivity, the child need more stimulants even to develop simple skills. Hyposensitive child is prone to touching and feeling.
Children may not demonstrate all these symptoms. For instance; the child may have a vestibular disorder while having a fine muscle tone. The child may also carry symptoms of the above mentioned disorders but may not be SID. The child may simply be undergoing emotional problems. A child may be both hypo and hypersensitive. For instance, a child may be oversensitive for a soft touch while he/she will not cry when receiving an injection (Royeen & Lane, 1991; Kranowitz, 1998; Talay-Ongan & Wood, 2000).
This factor; it is the motor, language, sensory product deficiency. Brain is inefficient in processing these signals. Therefore, it is more difficult to receive feedback. In connection with insufficient feedback, difficulty in looking and listening, failure to focus on people and objects, difficulty in processing new information, memory problems, and difficulty in learning and bilateral interaction with people will be observed.
Although sensory integration disorder has a genetic background, it is also believed that air pollution, devastating viral infections as well as chemical wastes taken into the body may cause these functional disorder (Temel, 1992). In some cases, sensory integration problems are seen intensively. These cases are:

- Autism,
- Attention deficit hyperactivity disorder,
- Difficulty in learning,
- Hearing and language problems,
- Articulation disorders,
- Visual problems,
- Nutrition problems,
- Sleeping disorders,
- Allergies.

Sensory have to function cooperatively. It is crucial that the brain receives balanced and systematic information (a well-balanced diet). Brain feeds on the functioning of many sensories. Dr. Ayres points to three important body-based sensory systems. These are tactile, vestibular and deep (proprioceptive) sensories. These sensories convey important tasks for the healthy development of a child. The functions of these sensories can be divided into three categories;

1. *Proprioceptive sense:* It is the processing of the information concerning the body position and body parts. It contains information relating to movement positions received from the muscles, joints and bonds. Proprioceptive stimulants are followed by motor response such as stimulation or inhibition.
2. *Surface sense:* Information of touch, heat, pressure and pain is seized by receptors localized in the skin. Information concerning surface sense is transmitted to corresponding areas of the central nervous system.
3. *Cortical sense:* An example for the cortical sense is the ability to recognize 3D objects by touching (stereognosis). If the child has developed stereognosis, he/she can figure out the surface shape, size or solidity of an object (Kayihan, 1989; Royeen & Lane, 1991; Kranowitz, 1998).

4. Sensory problems in autistic children

Autistic children experience a variety of problems.

4.1 Auditory problems

Autistic children may show complex reactions to sound while showing no reaction to some sounds during early childhood which leads their parents to believe that the child has hearing impairment. Children with autism may seem unable to hear. In some cases, the child may not even react to his/her own name. In light of the research conducted on this subject, it was found that autistic children cannot separate sounds in noisy environments and are disturbed by it. During the hearing tests conducted, it was revealed that autistic children possess a normal hearing ability while experiencing problems perceiving complex sounds such as speech. Children with autism do not pay attention to the speech language. They can express their wants through mimics and objects. Auditory problems in autistic children are related to speech tone and pitch (Miral *et al.,* 1994, Grandin, 1996a).

As a result of the hearing tests conducted; peripheral hearing impairment may be detected in some children, though it is generally seen that these children have no organic problems with their hearing ability (Klin, 1993). However, autistic children may fail to react to some sounds as they are not sufficiently sensitive to environmental sounds stimulants. Auditory reactions may manifest as being irritated in crowd and blocking ears in the presence of high levels of sound. In a study conducted by Rosenthall et al., hearing ability of 199 adults (153 male, 46 female) was evaluated. 7.9% of the test group showed mild hearing impairment while 1.6% had hearing problems in one side and 3.5% had hearing issues on both sides. Consequently, it is observed that hearing impairment is uncommon among autistic children (Rosenthall-Malek & Mitchell, 1997).

Autistic children may be easily irritated by high levels of sounds and stressed out by strong sound tones. Therefore, they may refuse to be present in noisy environment. In connection with extreme sensitivity to sound, autistic children may have difficulty in following intentional instructions. These children experience difficulty in oral communication which may restrain them from following simple commands which may lead to communicative problems (Attwood, 1993; Piggot & Anderson, 1993; Kavon & McLaughlin, 1995; Bettison, 1996; Hughes, 1996; O'Neill & Jones, 1997; Duchan, 1998; Grandin, 1998; Huebner & Emery, 1998; Koegel *et al.*, 1998; Gresham *et al.*, 1999; Mudford *et al.*, 2000; Anonim, 2003; Fazlioglu, 2003).

4.2 Visual problems

Some autistic individuals experience severe visual disorder. Most of autistic individuals, who cannot speak, may pretend not to see in different environments. Visual problems are caused by visual disharmony and color separation disorder. These individuals experience difficulty in spotting objects with darker colors. In addition, they may not be able to recognize shadows. Their vision may be compared to a TV with static. They also experience problems in perceiving visual signals. In autistic children, eyes and retina usually function properly. These individuals can succeed in visual evaluation tests. Their problem results from the failure to transmit visual input to the brain (Attwood, 1993; Grandin, 1996a; Senju *et al.*, 2003).

Although children with autism do not look at human face and many objects in their environment, it is known that they may view moving, rotating or shiny objects for long times. It is observed that some are irritated by light and feel more comfortable in dark rooms. It is also known that some autistic children may cover their ears when encountering light and covering eyes in the presence of high levels of noise. Visual problems in autistic children manifest as weak eye contact, sideway looking, blinking and light irritability (McConachie & Moore, 1992; Wainwright-Sharp & Brayson, 1996; Mitchell, 1997; Case-Smith & Miller, 1999).

Research conducted on controlling attention when executing an action shows that autistic children have limited skills in utilizing information received from the stimulants as well as focusing on a single determinant in selecting a stimulant. A number of researches conducted over the issue of over-selectivity revealed that mental age in autistic individuals is influential in the ability to select a stimulant from a specific distance. Autistic individuals can focus attention on a single, narrow area by distinguishing only one attribute of the stimulant in the process of determining the color and form of the stimulant in the space. This attribute is called "tunnel vision" in autistic children. In relation with this, it is prominent that failure to focus attention on a single subject and inability to focus quickly on a new subject are observed effects of this disorder (Rincover & Ducharme, 1986; Martineau *et al.*, 1992; Waterhouse *et al.*, 1996; Belmonte, 2000).

4.3 Tactile sensory problems

Tactile system is a necessary skill in daily life which ensures protection from danger and distinguishing the differences between the objects. The first of these skills is the touch sense. Normal child learns tactile individuation on the basis of how environmental elements feel. The child begins to recognize the world by feeling the warm touch of the mother, lightly grown firm beard of the father and the sound of pebble stones when walking. Children with sensory integration disorders experience difficulty in focusing on the varying attributes of people and objects as well as distinguishing between them. These children avoid touching to the point that it is possible. Since their palms are over-sensitive, they tend to inflect their fingers. Although they want to touch objects to learn, they cannot distinguish between their visuals. Thus, these children cannot develop fine senses since they cannot attain experience through tactile sensory. Movement and touching are the first teachers for a child. If the child is having problems with tactile sense, it may not be possible for them to learn through touching. Most of these problems affect the child's academic success and language development (Kranowitz, 1998).

Tactile senses allow the child to subconsciously realize body parts and their interactions with each others. The child will develop fine body awareness when tactile senses are functioning properly. Acquisition of body awareness will allow the child for easy and intentional movement. The child will know what the situation is about, as well as what he/she should do about it. In cases where the disorder manifests, the child will undergo various difficulties. For instance; the child may have difficulty directing limbs when getting dressed (Kranowitz, 1998).

Motor planning is a prerequisite for all the new movement abilities. The child will plan his/her movements with an intentional effort, will learn to successfully perform the move through continuous practice. Therefore, the child's tactile sensory is integrated. For instance, the child may feel the gymnastic ladder through hands and feet and may successfully climb it. The more objects the child discovers and touches, the better he will fare in executing different body movements, motor planning and motor skills. Attaining proficiency in a motor skill enables new experiments. For instance, after successfully climbing the ladder the child may use this skill for climbing and skinning down a tree. Children who are vulnerable tactile sense may experience dyspraxia. Dyspraxia is one of the sensory processing disorders caused by inability to coordinately execute movements. These children may not be able to execute the movement or will experience difficulty in organizing or planning the movement. Thus, they tend to avoid activities necessitating motor planning. Children with tactile disorder may develop gross motor skills late. They may also fail to learn movements and play purposeful games (Kranowitz, 1998).

Children will also experience difficulty in using simple tools (such as scissors, paint brush, fork and spoon). They also have difficulty in developing independent life skills (such as spilling food when eating). In addition, these children may have articulation issues. Since they have not matured linguistic skills, they experience insufficiency of fine motor control in the tongue and lips. Consequently, they tend to use signs rather than words (Kranowitz, 1998).

Tactile system accommodates an important role in the development of perception. Visual perception is the brain interpreting what is seen. The child will save the attributes and correlations of objects into his/her memory by touching. Therefore, most of the experience concerning tactile sense is also related to visual perception. When the child is unable to receive tactile stimulants, the brain cannot feed on basic information concerning the sense of touching, therefore experiencing difficulty in analyzing and interpreting tactile senses.

Tactile system is highly influential in child's learning skills in the school. Most objects in the world need to be hand operated (such as art materials, rhythm instruments, chalk, pencil). Tactile experience constitutes the foundation of the child's lifetime knowledge formation and guides the acquisition of new skills. Since they will avoid touching senses, children with tactile system disorder may experience difficulty in learning new skills (Kranowitz, 1998).

Tactile senses are essential in organizing relations with other people. It forms the foundation of the formation of the bond between the mother and child, touching others and enjoying being touched. When we are close to people, we learn how to communicate, how to play and how each individual's character differs from one another. Therefore, we can develop meaningful relationships. If the child has tactile vulnerability, he/she may not respond to physical connection appropriately. Children with tactile system experience problems in socializing. They may send negative signals to the environment and fail to establish friendship. Thus, the child will prefer to be alone (Parush *et al.*, 1997; Kranowitz, 1998, Halker, 2001).

Tactile system disorder occurs when signals received through the skin are not sufficiently processed in the central nervous system. Children with tactile disorder may refrain from touching objects and people or being touched. These children cannot realize the difference between dangerous and pleasing situations. They may also have difficulty in distinguishing the physical attributes of objects. Children with tactile system deficiency may manifest one or more problems concerning tactile sense integration (Royeen & Lane, 1991; Kranowitz, 1998; Bahr, 2001).

Normally developing infant will react to the mother's touch or speech in form of voice or smile. In later months, the baby will lift arms to be cuddled. The baby enjoys engaging in human relations. However, autistic children reacting to being touched or cuddled refuse physical connection and avoid having relations with the environment. Although autistic children may provide various reactions to the sensory stimulants in their environment; it is revealed that they tend to use tactile and olfaction senses when recognizing a new object. It is observed that these children may hold, smell and sometimes bite or lick an unrecognized object to learn about it. Some autistic children enjoy touching, while others prefer to be touched. In some cases however, the child may strongly refrain from both. For some children, the mildest touch is enough to be scared. These children may be scared by soft touches while showing no reaction to painful situations. This kind of case is caused by a disorder in the body's self-anaesthetizing system which is called "opiate system". Some autistic individuals may strongly refrain from self-care activities such as hair cut, washing face, nail clipping along with wearing braided cloths (Grandin, 1996b; Kientz & Dunn, 1997; Korkmaz, 2000a).

4.4 Vestibular systemic problems

Vestibular system provides information about the individual's head and body location as well as their relation in the space. This system receives sensory signals from joints, eyes and body concerning movement and balance. These signals are sent to the central nervous system to be used. Vestibular system also provides information about whether the individual is moving or stable, movements of the objects and their relation to the body as well as the direction and speed of the individual's movement. Vestibular signal receptors are located in vestibular in the inner ear. These receptors record each movement and the changes in the position of the head. These receptors are stimulated by movement and gravity.

Dr. Ayres states that the gravity has a universal power in life and plays an important role in every movement. Receptors concerning gravity are responsible for a variety of tasks such as retaining stance, ensuring the reception of movements so as to enable sufficient movement and evading hazards by perceiving vibrations in the air. Vestibular and auditory senses contain movement and acoustic vibrations. Vestibular system is a consolidative system. Activities related to this system form a basis for other experience. If the vestibular system is not functioning properly, problems may present in the interpretation of other senses.

Vestibular disorder occurs when the signals from the inner ear are not sufficiently perceived by the brain. Children with vestibular disorder are inefficient in integrating information concerning movement, gravity, balance and space. These children are oversensitive or insensitive to movement. They may also present both cases. These children may not develop postural response, may never crawl, or may be delayed from learning to walk. They may collapse on their seat and their head may fall on the hands when seated. In kindergarten activities, they will be clumsy, uncoordinated and gawky. They often fall down when walking, will hit the furniture and collapse when moving. Also, their eye movement is affected by the insufficiency of the vestibular system. In accordance they may experience visual problems. For instance, they may be inefficient in focusing sight on a moving object. These children may not develop the brain functions requisite for moving the eyes sideways. In line with this, reading issues may be observed.

Vestibular disorder may also cause difficulty in understanding a language. Linguistic issues may lead to problems in communication and learning to write and read. Children with vestibular vulnerability cannot calm down. The reason for this is the failure in the child's brain in utilizing vestibular signals properly. Children with vestibular systemic disorder experience a variety of problems concerning the integration of sensories (Fisher, 1991; Kranowitz, 1998; Bahr, 2001). These children;

1. May be oversensitive to movement. This case can manifest itself in two ways;
   - Failure to tolerate movement
   - Insecurity towards gravity.
2. May be insensitive to movement. They will have high tolerance to movement and desire to move.

Autistic children may demonstrate slow walking, unusual walking, shorter strides, increasing knee flexion as well as unusual upper extremity positions (Vilensky *et al.,* 1981). Children experiencing such difficulties may feel vulnerable when their feet are not on the ground. This insufficiency of basic sense causes the child to form gravitational insecurity. Gravitational insecurity is the abnormal reactions like stress or anxiety towards the possibility of falling. The movement is not fun, but scary for the child. When the child's head moves, he/she will respond as 'I am falling, 'I can't control myself'. The child reacts to this situation by avoiding or fighting back. The child may be nervous or angry and may avoid moving, may refuse to ride a bike or play with the slide. Children with similar problems frequently present emotional and behavioral problems. They continuously worry about falling down (Fisher, 1991; Kranowitz, 1998; O'Roidon, 2000; Bahr, 2001).

Vestibular system also provides information about how to stand. To remain standing, brain conducts a subconscious physical adaptation resulting in the balance, sustenance of this balance and easy movement. Children with vestibular systemic disorder present problems with balance and movement. It is observed that these children are uncoordinated and clumsy in activities that require movement (Gillberg, 1989; Fisher, 1991; Ghaziuddin *et al.*, 1994; Miyahara *et al.,* 1997; Brasic & Gianutsos, 2000; Rinehart *et al.,* 2001; Korkmaz, 2003).

These children experience problems when rolling a football and pressing someone during the game. Their grip is weak and need to spend a lot of energy resisting the gravity. Autistic children do not develop and preference. They occasionally use right or left hand to eat, write or hurl an object. Bilateral coordination issues may cause the child to experience problems jumping from a high place using both feet, catching a ball with both hands and clapping. They may also have difficulty holding a paper fixed when writing or using a scissor with one hand. Bilateral coordination deficiency is commonly misinterpreted as learning difficulty (Fisher, 1991; Kranowitz, 1998; Ryoichiro *et al.,* 2000; Bahr, 2001; Dewey & Hauck, 2001).

Vestibular system is essential in processing the hearing. Children with vestibular disorder commonly present language development problems. These children may experience difficulty in recognizing the differences and similarities of words. They also have problems listening or following the instructions of the teacher. They may have drawbacks asking or answering questions. After developing movement skills, they begin to speak but cannot present a fine speech craft. When balance, movement and motor planning skills are organized, language and speech craft also draw attention (Fisher & Murray, 1991; Manijiviona & Prior, 1995; Kranowitz, 1998; Bahr, 2001).

Vestibular system is greatly influential in processing the visual input. Observing the environment, moving around and active participation to sensory experience practices are necessary to attain visual-spatial processing skills. Children with vestibular disorder may experience problems with visual spatial processing skills alongside basic visual motor skills since the brain cannot efficiently integrate the signals received from the eyes and body. For instance, they may confuse or mistype the words when reading or writing. They may also confuse symbols when doing mathematics (like writing "+" instead of "x"). The movements of people and object around him/her may restrain the child. The child may experience difficulty in activities like climbing a ladder, finding jig-saw pieces, sticking stars on a paper or picturing an event. The child may fail to find the way to school cafeteria or may run in the wrong direction when playing basketball. The child acts like lost in the space (Hughes, 1996; Kranowitz, 1998).

Vestibular system also plays an important role in motor planning. Motor planning (praxis), is conceptualization, organization and realization of complex and unrecognized movements. Adapting behaviors for learning new skills may be challenging for the child with vestibular disorder. For instance, these children can skate, but cannot ice-skate. If the central nervous system cannot sufficiently process signals concerning balance and movement, brain cannot figure out how to act in these conditions. Therefore, the child cannot learn the new skills for planning (Reiss & Havercamp, 1997; Rogers *et al.*, 2003).

Vestibular system also influences the child's emotional confidence acquisition. Every child possesses emotional confidence from birth. However, children with vestibular disorder cannot feel this confidence after birth. These children suffer from gravitational insecurity in connection with hyper or hyposensitivity and cannot organize most of their lives. These children may have lower self-respect, and can experience difficulties in completing even the simplest work (Kranowitz, 1998; Bahr, 2001).

Vestibular system is related to the perception of the signals concerning the changes in the head's movement and position. Inner ear structure (semi-circular channel) upholds the task of perceiving these signals. People live unaware of the existence of this system as well as the signals it creates. However, motor coordination, eye movements and body stance require this system to function properly (Halker, 2001). Children with vestibular function disorder demonstrate insufficient motor planning (praxis). Autistic children also present certain movement disorders. Some autistic children have difficulty in accomplishing actions like climbing, standing on one foot, walking a straight line and jumping. These children may also experience difficulties in repeating an action consecutively, starting or ending the action on their own.

These disorders can vary in complex and simple movements (like flawy facial impression or body dangling). Variant movement disorders are determined for autistic individuals. These disorders can be categorized as follows;

1. *Motor function disorders:* Flexion dystonia, strained flexion in the hip and body, bizarre body posture, gnashing, making a grimace arbitrarily, anti-social facial impression, lack of eye contact, involuntary motor twitches, dyskinesia, motor stereotypes, vocal and verbal twitches, keeping arms stable when walking and other joint movement deficits can be evaluated in this category.
2. *Intentional movement disorders*: Slow moving, weakness in spontaneous movements, motor planning difficulties, consecutively repetitive spontaneous actions, examining objects by smelling, touching or tasting, walking disorders (walking slow, on tiptoes, on heel or by jumping) are in this category.
3. *Comprehensive behavior and activity disorders:* Catatonic movements, oversensitivity to environmental changes, aggression, hyperkinesis (hyperactivity), actions that include explosives and violence, indisposition to physical contact and interaction, suddenly stopping when performing an action, mutism (inability to speak), lack of ability to imitate, inability to start a movement on their own and negativism can be included in this group (Leary & Hill, 1996).

Autistic children usually provide disoriented responses to vestibular stimulants. These children generally experience visual and vestibular coordination difficulties. It is believed that vestibular systemic disorders can be related to problems in focusing or gravitating towards visual stimulants. Sensory information input disorders (modulation) are considered the first symptoms of autism. Communication and language disorders in social interactions stem from the difficulty in balancing the sensory output. These children frequently tend to engage in stereotypic actions to regulate sensory system (Case-Smith & Brayn, 1999; Korkmaz, 2000b).

Leo Kanner states that autistic children demonstrate normal motor development. These children show no abnormalities in physical appearance, but show variations in motor skill development in comparison to the contemporary. Research indicates that autistic children demonstrate difficulties in motor functions such as balance and movement, slow moving in later periods, decrease in stance consistency and oral motor disorders (Jansiewicz *et al.*, 2006; Minshew *et al.*, 2004; Page & Boucher, 1998) to distinguish from (Ozonoff *et al.* 2008).

However, researches comparing autistic children with other groups in terms of intelligence development deficiency show no difference with respect to motor skills. Reid's (1985) study determined no difference between autistic and retarded children in terms of actions like catching, jumping, hurling, running and balance. In a recent study conducted on 21-41 month old autistic children and retarded children defined no difference between the groups in terms of object manipulation, perception and visual motor integration (Provost *et al.*, 2006). Similarly, Rogers et al. found no differentiation between 2- year old autistic children and typical and atypical groups consistent in development in terms of fine motor development and motor planning. (Rogers *et al.*, 2003).

Although autistic children appear capable of developing numerous physical skills in time, some skills may develop very late. Motor skill development in autistic children is usually close to their chronologic age. These children may especially experience difficulties in executing an action in line with an instruction and consecutively. For instance; their lack in fine motor skills like paper cutting and putting cubes into a box are significant. Motor problems observed in autistic children are related to motor coordination problems. It is also expressed that their motor readiness levels for executing an action are low in comparison to the contemporary (Berninger & Rutberg, 1992; Attwood, 1998; Ryoichiro *et al.*, 2000; Beversdorf *et al.*, 2001).

It is important to include exercises supporting basic movement skills in training programs for autistic children. Attaining movement experience provides children with essential information for perceiving their own body and recognizing the environment. Also, movement training can be useful for improving the child's ability to solve problems, expressing him/herself and seeking creative solutions to problems. Movement training can also be used to develop skills such as paying attention, focusing and mediating. Children can attain emotional and social gains through movement training. Through well-planned movement training, children can develop abilities to recognize other children, act in coordination and establish cooperation (Eichstaedt & Lavay, 1992).

Studies conducted in this subject prove that it is difficult for handicapped children to discover their environment through games and movement if left alone. Therefore, it is essential to assist the child in attaining various movement experiences. Learning basic movement skills is also important for the child to learn more complex behaviors. Development of these skills constitutes a foundation for the development of other body movements and attaining complex movements. Basic movement training can be provided through simple movement experience attained from exercise programs. In later periods, the child can be diverted to sportive and recreational activities. Thus, guiding autistic children to any branch of sports (especially swimming etc.) before school age can enable a positive development (Connor, 1990; Cornish & McManus, 1996; Darıca *et al.*, 2000; Korkmaz, 2000b).

4.5 Proprioceptive systemic problems

Proprioceptive system provides information about the movements and the body position. This system assists the integration of signals concerning touching and movement. Proprioceptive signal receptors are situated in tissue connection spots in the muscles and joints. This is required for skills like catching or throwing a ball and ladder climbing.

Proprioceptive system functions; the system contributes to body awareness, motor planning and motor control. Proprioceptive system is also influential in body language and effective control of body parts. It enables abilities like straight walking, sprinting, ladder climbing, carrying a luggage, sitting, standing, and leaning upside down. It also assists in feeling emotionally safe. Proprioceptive system means the perception of unconsciously executed body actions (for instance; automatically sitting straight on a chair). In addition, conscious body positions are frequently engaged. Developing body awareness also forms the child's computative and mathematics skills (Fisher, 1991; Kranowitz, 1998; Bahr, 2001).

In the presence of proprioceptive systemic disorders, the child may not attain sufficient information concerning the body position and body parts. Proprioceptive system is also necessary in attaining the information needed for regulating the movements concerning gross and fine motor skills. Children with proprioceptive problems may have trouble in executing an action coordinately. For instance, the child may have difficulty in switching from one action to another (Kranowitz, 1998).

Proprioceptive system allows us to distinguish between the actions. Distinguishing between actions refers to feeling the magnitude of pressure that causes muscle contractions and relaxation. During an activity; we can predict the quantity and quality of muscle movements. Thus, we can adjust the amount of energy to be assigned when lifting a light ball or a heavy bucket. When this system malfunctions, the child cannot receive sufficient signals from the muscles and joints, consecutively failing to distinguish between the actions. Proprioceptive system also provides information about unconscious body movements such as sitting and standing up. Children who are experiencing problems with this system may have difficulty in adjusting their posture during daily activities. Proprioceptive system is also essential in developing emotional confidence mechanism. Children with such disorders can develop insufficient self awareness. Consequently, the child will lack the emotional confidence (Kranowitz, 1998).

Proprioceptive disorder is usually accompanied by tactile and vestibular system disorders. Children with proprioceptive disorder have difficulty in interpreting perceptions concerning the position and movements of head, arms and legs. These children receive common instinctual perceptions insufficiently. Since they have problems with fine and gross motor muscle control and motor planning, their body awareness and body position perception are also insufficient. These children may be very clumsy. They may attack everyone and everything. They may cause conflicts when walking on a street, having bath or playing in the garden. They also experience difficulties in managing objects. When gripping an object, they apply excessive or insufficient pressure (For instance, they oftly break pencil leads and their toys). They also have problems carrying a heavy object (For instance; they have difficulty when carrying a bucket). Since they lack fine body awareness, they need to follow their own body movements with eyes. They cannot complete even the simplest actions like directing the body when getting dressed, buttoning up or pulling the zipper without visual assistance. Since they lack fine postural balance, they may be afraid to move within an area. Each new movement and position may startle them, consecutively causing emotional insecurity (Kranowitz, 1998; Bahr, 2001).

Proprioceptive system constitutes joint, muscle and body awareness. Autistic children usually experience insufficiencies in fine and gross muscle skills. These skills are disorders that are included in the proprioceptive system. Most autistic children do not recognize their body position in the space. Consecutively, they may be relieved by jumping on the trampoline and riding on a swing. Some children may enjoy massage and deep pressure. These activities may assist in motivating and reorganizing the child before learning new skills (Halker, 2001).

5. Sensory integration operating scope and effects on autistic children

In sensory integration treatments prepared for autistic children, it is important to prioritize that the family understands the child's behaviors, and emotional needs so as to provide the necessary environmental regulations in the school and at home as well as allowing the child to organize and utilize the signals received from the environment (Williamson & Anzalone, 1997).

The fundamental aim of sensory integration treatment is ensure that the child controls sensory stimulants -especially inner ear balance system (vestibular)- received from the muscles, joints and skin in order to allow the child to reform the corresponding reactions that integrate these senses. Children with advanced handicaps, -especially autistic children- are likely to need more instructions than others. When conducting treatment for these children, stimulants needed by the child must be provided at the same time performing exercises to permit the child to realize his/her own emotions. The aim of this therapy is not teaching motor activities, but to assist the child in attaining motor skills, academic skills and positive behaviors necessary throughout the life (Temel, 1992).

In a case of sensory integration deficiency, the child must be evaluated before initiating treatment. When conducting the evaluation, sensory perception deficiencies, effects or sensory perception deficiencies on motor skills and the level of sensory integration development must be determined. This evaluation will provide necessary information about the child. This will ensure information about whether the child needs this kind of treatment, or on which course he/she will need intensified therapy. Evaluation should include the following courses;

- Fine and gross motor development level
- Visual motor integration (such as making jig-saw, copying figures)
- Visual perception
- Neuromuscular control (balance and posture)
- Response to sensory stimulant (tactile, vestibular, proprioceptive)
- Bilateral coordination
- Motor planning.

When it is understood that the child's problems can be explained using sensory integration theory and setting special targets, treatment can be initiated. Some children may demonstrate a lack of enthusiasm for participating in activities within the treatment course. Others may orally express reluctance to engage in an activity. Activity may be boring or too simple for the child. Therefore, the first course of action must be investigating the reason for the child's lack of motivation. If the planned activity is difficult for the child, it must be adjusted for his/her skill level. If the child thinks the activity is difficult even if it is not, he/she must be encouraged. While encouraging, the child must never be forced. If the underlying cause of the child's lack of motivation is hypersensitivity, the child must be given time to calm down.

Another important issue in the treatment is when to conclude the activity. If the child is participating in an activity that helps the child to attain adaptive skills, the activity should be sustained. The therapist should follow the child's guidance in decision-making.

In correcting problems about tactile system, the first action must be to determine whether the child is hypersensitive or hyposensitive. Consecutively, activities that can solve the problems should be selected. Examples for these activities can be; massage, hugging, pressuring, brushing or scrubbing the legs, hands and back as well as books that encourage touching, sand, beans, rice game, salt ceramics, drawing different figures using shave foam, rolling on different surfaces, playing with blowing toys, drinking juice using pipette and chewing. Through these activities, the child's hypersensitivity or hyposensitivity can be curbed. Therefore, the child can achieve different tactile experiences (Kranowitz, 1998).

Autistic children with vestibular systemic problems may demonstrate motor planning and motor coordination problems. The child must be evaluated to determine these problems. Subsequent to the evaluation, appropriate activities should be selected. Activities like standing on one foot, walking the balance plank, swinging on the balance plank and riding on a swing can be provided for the child to improve balance sensation. In addition, the child can be encouraged to extend his/her experience by imposing activities like straight walking, variant walking imitations, somersaulting and climbing. Sensory vulnerability can be treated through providence of different experiences. Therefore, the child's needs must be determined in order to plan the program correspondingly (Kranowitz, 1998).

Autistic individuals with proprioceptive vulnerability may demonstrate problems like postural dysregulation, frequent falling, failing to adjust limbs when getting dressed and inability to carry heavy objects. The child must be supported with activities to improve proprioceptive system so as to overcome these problems. Examples for these activities can be; riding the magic carpet, weight lifting (weights attached to hands, ankles and back) rope skipping, jumping on the trampoline, walking with a wheelbarrow, crawling games and dragrope game (Kranowitz, 1998).

6. Examples activities for sensory motor skill assistance

GOAL: Enabling interaction with objects of different attributes.
Expected Behavioral Gain:
1. Touching objects with different attributes.
2. Gripping objects with different attributes.
3. Walking on objects with different attributes.
4. Distinguishing between objects with different attributes.

Material: Bread paste, pudding, dry legumes, fresh fruits and vegetables, bowls.

1. *Activity:* Trainer sits the child down on a table in face to face position, places the foods in large bowls. While touching the food, trainer gives the command "touch". Trainer is to encourage the child to touch food types of different structures (bread paste, pudding, dry legumes, fresh fruits and vegetables). First, the trainer touches different types of foods, places the food on the child's palm and fingers, then asks the child to touch the food. While holding the child's hand, the trainer touches the food with the child. For the first attempt, the timeline should be limited to 2 minutes. Then, the time given for touching the child is gradually increased up to 10 minutes.

Material: Walking track.

2. *Activity:* Tracks made of different materials (e.g. rope, felting, plastic, emery, carpet, sand) are prepared. Trainer sets example for the child by walking the track. Then, the child is asked to walk the track from the start line till the finish line. Trainer assists the child by walking together while holding the child's hand. The practice is sustained until the child attains the ability to walk the track independently.

Material: Shag, velvet, flax and cotton materials.

3. *Activity:* Trainer sits down on the ground with the child in face to face position. Using gloves made of different materials (shag, velvet, flax, and cotton); trainer touches the child's limbs and face. While touching the child with the material, trainer counts from 1 to 10, later concludes the training. Trainer then uses as different material. Later, the child is directed to touch objects made of metal, wood, plastic, emery and glass. In follow up, the objects are placed in a box with all sides closed and round holes on the front side; the child is asked to reach into the box to grip and distinguish the objects (hard, ragged and soft) without looking. In the first stage of the activity, two objects (like a toy or ball) are placed in the box. These must be objects the child is familiar with.

Material: Touch box, hard, ragged and soft objects.

4. *Activity:* The child is asked to reach into the box to find and distinguish between the objects with different attributes (hard, ragged and soft). The child is orally and physically encouraged to distinguish between the objects. Trainer reaches into the box with the child, touches the objects and talks about their attributes. Trainer may point to the distinctive attributes of the objects. The child's behaviors are continuously rewarded with incentives in the first stage. In later stages, support and incentives are reduced. Incentives are only awarded when the child presents the correct answer.

Material: Sand pool, ball, toy car, cube.

5. *Activity:* Trainer sits down in the sand pool with the child in face to face position. Trainer shows an object to the child (such as toy car or cube). Then, the trainer hides the object in the sand and asks the child to find the object, encourages the child to find it. At first, the trainer finds the object and shows it to the child. Then, the object is placed in the same spot and the child is asked to find it. Trainer may hold the child's hand to pluck out the object. After attaining the ability to pluck out the object from the sand, the object is placed in different spots and the child is asked to find it. At first, the object is partially hidden so that the child can easily find it. Once the child independently finds the object, the number of objects hidden in the sand is gradually increased up to five.

Material: Heat tablets, water with different heat levels.

6. *Activity:* Trainer sits down with the child in face to face position. Plastic bottles of water with different temperatures (cold, warm, hot) are placed in front of the child. Trainer accompanies the child in touching bottles with different temperatures. Then, water with different temperature is placed in large cups. Accompanying the child, the trainer dives limbs inside the water cups with different temperatures. The trainer encourages the child orally and physically to touch the water. Then, the trainer places heat tablets with varying temperatures on the table and encourages the child to look at the tablets. While supporting the child physically, trainer touches the tables with different temperatures along with the child in order to improve touching behavior.

GOAL: Developing fine motor skills.

Expected Behavioral Gain:

1. Imitating fine motor movements.
2. Imitating objects and movements.
3. Forming shapes using blocks.
4. Stringing beads.
5. Using the scissors.
6. Placing screws on the board.
7. Copying symbols.

1. *Activity:* Trainer sits on a chair facing the child. Trainer sets an example by performing the action the child is expected to imitate. Then the child is given "do it" command (clapping, opening and closing hands, tipping with index fingers). If the child cannot perform the action, the trainer should provide physical assistance (for instance; helping the child to clap by holding his/her hands). Trainer gradually decreases the physical assistance to the child. The training is sustained until the child can independently perform the instructed action.

Material: Bell, blocks, bucket.

2. *Activity:* Trainer sits on a table with the child in face to face position. Two identical objects are placed on the table (e.g. two bells). Trainer takes one of the bells to ring it when the child is paying attention to the trainer, then asks the child to perform the same action. Trainer provides the child with "You do it" command. If the child cannot perform the action, the trainer should hold his/her hand to help doing it. Then, the action is performed repeatedly. Trainer should gradually reduce the assistance. In follow up, the trainer should direct the child to practice with different objects in a similar course of action (e.g. placing blocks in a bucket).

Material: Two triangles, two cylinders, blocks.

3. *Activity:* Trainer sits on a table with the child in face to face position. Similar blocks are placed on the table (e.g. two triangles, two cylinders). Trainer constructs a structure using blocks. Then the child is instructed to do the same using the block sets. While constructing structures using the blocks, physical guidance is provided to the child. In the first phase of the practice, one block at a time is placed (For instance; five blocks are placed on the table to the child's right). One block is brought to the middle of the table. The child is asked to select the same block and put it in the middle of the table. Trainer places different shapes of blocks and asks the child to imitate the same structure.

Material: Beads and strings.

4. *Activity:* Trainer sits on a table with the child in face to face position**.** Varying sizes of beads and strings with varying thickness are placed on the table. Training starts with big sized beads. Trainer sets an example for the child by stringing a big sized bead, then asks the child to do the same. Trainer holds the string and assists the child to place the beads by holding the child's hand. Then the bead and the string are given to the child. If the child cannot perform the stringing, physical assistance should be provided. Practice continues with different types of beads.

Material: Scissors and papers.

5. *Activity:* Trainer sits on a table with the child in face to face position. Trainer takes the scissors and sets an example for the child on how to use it, then encourages the child to do the same. When the child attains the ability to use the scissors, trainer helps the child practice using the scissors on cardboards or papers. When the child is able to use the scissors independently, the trainer instructs the child to practice straight, round, square and photo cuttings. During the practice, the child is instructed with "do it like this" command. The child is encouraged with oral and physical hints to perform the cutting. The child's actions are rewarded.

Material: Different sizes of screws and a board.

6. *Activity:* Trainer sits in front of the board alongside the child. Trainer takes a screw and places on the board, then gives the screw to the child and commands "you do it". The child is encouraged to perform the action. Then, the child is supported to place different sizes and numbers of screws on the board. When the child attains the ability to place different sizes of screws on the board, the trainer instructs the child to practice in forming patterns using the screws on the board. It is important to use big sized screws at first.

Material: Paper, shaving foam, finger paint and colored pastels.

7. *Activity:* Trainer places the drawing materials on the table where the child can see them. Using large papers, drawing practice begins. The child is encouraged to copy different patterns, digits and letters using different materials (such as working with finger paint, shaving foam and sand). Physical support should be provided as the child practices drawing and the child's drawings should be rewarded. Visual tips (e.g. dots) should be used to make the drawings easier to see. Later, the dots are removed and the child instructed to perform the correct drawing after seeing the example. The child should be encouraged to draw by holding his/her hand or giving instructions like top-down or left-to-right. Trainer practices with the child on drawing lines from simple to complex (such as horizontal drawing, vertical drawing, plus shape drawing, x shape drawing, writing letters on a straight line, drawing digits, drawing figures, drawing a child's face, drawing flowers, cars, a home, a labyrinth and human figures). Training is sustained until the child can draw the lines independently.

GOAL: Developing gross motor skills

Expected Behavioral Gain:

1. Imitating gross motor actions.
2. Participating in walking exercises.
3. Participating in running exercises.
4. Ball game.
5. Rolling.
6. Riding on a swing.
7. Climbing.

Material: The child's favorite food.

1. *Activity:* Trainer sits on a table with the child in face to face position and sets an example of the motor actions the child should perform (tipping on the table, clapping, stomping). Then, the trainer gives the child "do this" command. The child should be encouraged orally and physically to perform the action. Trainer should provide various incentives (e.g. chips, well done) for the child's effort to imitate the action and responses. Then the support in the training session should be gradually decreased. Incentives should be provided until the child's imitations become second nature.

Material: Colored adhesive tape.

2. *Activity:* The child is allowed to walk freely in a movement-free environment. A thick line is drawn on the ground (using colored adhesive tape). The trainer gives the child "walk" command. Trainer waits for the child to walk the line without stepping outside the line. Then, trainer instructs the child to practice rhythmic walking, tip-toe walking, heel-top walking, walking on the feet's outside, walking on the feet's inside and walking to a specific object (trainer commands "walk to the door"). The child should be encouraged to perform the appropriate action. The child's actions should be rewarded with incentives. In later sessions, support and incentives should be reduced to positive behaviors only.

Material: Rope, tape, chalk.

3. *Activity:* A circle is drawn on the ground with a large and thick line (using the rope, tape or chalk). The child is instructed to walk step by step and side by side before moving out of the line. The child should be encouraged to walk (trainer first sets an example for the child and provides physical and oral tips). The trainer should reward the child's actions with incentives. Later, the support and incentives should be reduced and only provided when the child achieves the goal.

Material: Rope, tape, chalk.

4. *Activity:* A zig-zag is drawn on the ground with a thick line (using rope, tape or chalk). The child is asked to walk the zig-zag without stepping out of the line. The child should be encouraged to walk and rewarded for his/her actions. In later sessions, the support and incentives should be reduced to accomplishing the track only.

Material: Ladder, different sizes of circles and boxes.

5. *Activity:* A walking band in the shape of a ladder is placed on the ground and the child is asked to walk by stepping inside the band only. The child should be encouraged to walk and rewarded for his/her actions. In later sessions, support can be gradually reduced in accordance with the child's need. Incentives should only be provided when the child completes the training. "Walk by stepping in it "practice should be extended to materials with different shapes and depths (such as colored circles, different sizes of boxes).

Material: Slalom sticks, traffic cones.

6. *Activity:* Objects are placed on the ground in a line allowing the child to walk in between (e.g. slalom sticks and traffic cones). The child is asked to walk through the objects. Trainer should set an example for the child to perform the action. The child should be encouraged to walk and rewarded for his/her actions.

Material: Ball.

7. *Activity:* Trainers stands facing the child. The child is given an object (a ball). The child is encouraged to walk the track and rewarded for his/her actions. As the amount of time the child walks decreases, support and incentives should be reduced. Later, the child should only be rewarded when he/she reaches the destination while holding an object. Then, the child is encouraged to walk with a filled object (a filled plate, a glass full of water) and rewarded for his/her actions. The support and incentives should later be reduced. The child should only be rewarded when he/she reaches the destination while holding an object.

Material: Balance plank.

8. *Activity:* The child is asked to climb up and walk the balance plank (20 cm above ground, 15cm wide and 2 mt long). The child should be supported in climbing and walking the plank. The child's actions should be rewarded. In later training sessions, the support and incentives should be reduced. Incentives should only be provided if the child can independently climb the plank and walk to the end.
9. *Activity:* Trainer sets an example for the child to imitate the walking of different animals such as; lamb walk, frog walk (jumping when crouched), duck walk (taking a step when crouching). Then the child is asked to imitate these movement patterns. The trainer should physically and orally encourage the child to perform the actions. In accordance with the child's ability to perform the actions, the support and incentives should be gradually reduced. Incentives should only be provided when the child achieves the imitated walking.

7. References

Anonim. (2003). Otizm. Otistik Cocuklari Koruma ve Yonlendirme Dernegi Yayinlari, 63 s., Izmir.

Attwood, T. (1993). Unusual behaviors associated with autism. *Health Visitor*, 66: 402-403.

Attwood, T. (1998). Asperger's sendrome: a guide for parents and professionals. Jessica Kingsley Publishers Ltd., 223 s., London and Philadelphia.

Bahr, D. (2001). Oral motor assessment and treatment: ages and stages. Allyn & Bacon, 274 s., Boston.

Bauman ML, Kemper TL. (2005). Neuroanatomic observations of the brain in autism: a review and future directions. Int J Dev Neurosci; 23:183–7.

Belmonte, M. (2000). Abnormal attention in autism shown by steady-state visual evoked potential. The International Journal of Research & Practice, 4(3); 269-286.

Berninger, V. W. and Rutberg, J. (1992). Relationship of finger function to beginning writing: application to diagnosis of writing disabilities. Developmental Medicine & Child Neurology, 34(3); 198-215.

Bettison, S. (1996). The long term effects of auditory training on children with autism. Journal of Autism and Developmental Disorders, 26(3); 361-372.

Beversdorf, D. O., Anderson, M., Manning, S. E., Anderson, S. L., Nordgren, R. E., Felopulus, G. J. and Bauman, M. L. (2001). Brief report: macrographia in high-functioning adults with autism spectrum disorder. Journal of Autism and Developmental Disorders, 31(1); 97-101.

Brasic, J. R. and Gianutsos, J. G. (2000). Noromotor assesment and autistic disorder. The International Journal of Research & Practice, 4(3); 287-281.

Case-Smith, J. and Brayn, T. (1999). The effect of occupational therapy with sensory integration emphasis on preschool-age children with autism. American Journal of Ocupational Therapy, 53(5): 489-497.

Case-Smith, J. and Miller, H. (1999). Occupational therapy with chilren with pervasive developmental disorders. American Journal of Ocupational Therapy, 53; 506-513.

Connor, F. (1990). Combating stimulus over selectivity: physical education for children with autism. Teaching Exeptional Children, 23(1); 30-33.

Cornish, K. M. and McManus, I. C. (1996). Hand prefence and hand skill in children with autism. Journal of Autism and Developmental Disorders, 26(6); 597-609.

Darica, N., Gumuscu, S. ve Piskin, U. (2000). Otizm ve otistik cocuklar. Ozgur Yayinlari, 129 s., Istanbul.

Dawson, G. & Watling, R. (2000). Intervention to facilitade auditory, visual, and motor integration in autism: a review of the evidence. *Journal of Autism and Developmental Disorders*, 30: 415-425.

Dewey, D. and Hauck, J. A. (2001). Hand preferance and motor functioning in children with autism. Journal of Autism and Developmental Disorders, 31(3); 265-277.

Duchan, F. 1998. Describing the unusual behavior of children with autism. Journal of Commun Disorders, 31(2); 93-112.

Eichstaedt, C. B. and Lavay, B. W. (1992). Physical aktivity for individuals with mental retardation, Human Kinetics Books, 463 s., Illinois.

Fazlioglu, Y. & Baran, G, R. (2008). A sensory integration therapy program on sensory problems for children with autism. *Perceptual and Motor Skills*, 106: 4115-422.

Fazlioglu, Y. 2003. Otizmli cocukla iletisim kurmanin farkli bir yontemi: PECS. Coluk Cocuk Dergisi, 6; 8-10.

Fisher, A. G. and Murray, E. A. (1991). Introduction to sensory integration theory. Sensory integration: theory and practice, Editors: A. G. Fisher, E. A. Murray, A. C. Bundy, F. A. Davis Company, s. 3-24, Philadelphia.

Fuentes C. T. & Bastıan A. J. (2007). 'Motor cognition' - what is it and is the cerebellum involved?, The Cerebellum, 2007; 6: 232–236.

Ghaziuddin, M., Butler, E., Tsai, L. and Ghaziuddin, N. (1994). Is clumsiness a marker for Asperger syndrome? Journal of Intellectual Disability Research, 38; 519-527.

Gillberg, C. (1989). Asperger syndrome in 23 Swedish children. Developmental Medicine and Child Neurology, 31; 520-531.

Grandin, T. (1996a). Thinking in pictures: and other reports from my life with autism. Random House, Inc., 222 s., New York.

Grandin, T. (1996b). Brief report: response to national institues of health report. Journal of Autism and Developmental Disorders, 26(2); 185-187.

Grandin, T. (1998). Teaching tips from a recovered autistic. Focus on Autistic Behavior, 3(1); 1-8.

Gresham, F. M., Frankenberger, B., MacMillan, E. and Donald, L. A. (1999). Selective review of treatments or children with autism: description and methodological considerations. School Psychology Review, 28(4); 559-567.

Halker, A. (2001). Otizm umudumuz: davranisci tedavi. Halker and Associates, 77 s., Bethesda, MD.

Huebner, R. A. and Emery, L. J. 1998. Social psycholical analysis of facilitated communication: implications for education. Mental Retardation, 36(4); 259-268.

Hughes, C. (1996). Brief report: planning problems in autism at level motor control. Journal of Autism and Developmental Disorders, 26(1); 99-107.

Kavon, N. M. and McLaughlin, T. F. (1995). Intervention for echolalic behavior for children with autism: a review of verbal promts and cues pause point procedure. Journal of Special Education, 19(2); 39-45.

Kayihan, H. (1989). Hemipleji'de is ve ugrasi tedavisi. Hacettepe Universitesi Fizik Tedavi ve Rehabilitasyon Yayinlari, 118 s., Ankara.

Kientz, M. A. and Dunn, W. (1997). A comparsion of the performance of children with and without autism on the sensory profile. The American Journal of Occupational Therapy, 51(7); 530-537.

Klin, A. (1993). Auditory brainstem responses in autism: brainstem dsyfunction or peripheral hearing loss? Journal of Autism and Developmental Disorders, 23(1); 15-35.

Koegel, K. L., Camarata, S. M., Valdez-Menchaca, M. and Koegel, R. L. (1998). Setting generalization of question-asking by children with autism. American Journal of Mental Retardation, 102(4); 346-357.

Korkmaz, B. (2000a). Yagmur cocuklar, otizm nedir? 2. Baski, Dogan Kitapcilik, 166 s., Istanbul.

Korkmaz, B. (2000b). Mental rötarde otistiklerde yürümenin gelişiminde gecikmenin klinik prognozla ilişkisi. Cerrahpaşa Journal of Medicine, 31(2); 66-73.

Korkmaz, B. (2003). Asperger sendromu: toplumsal ilişkilere ait bir bozukluk, yalnızlık ya da insana ait temel bir boyut. Adam Yayınları, 302 s., İstanbul.

Kranowitz, C. S. (1998). The out-of-sync child: recognizing and coping with sensory integration dysfunction, Skylight Press, 322 s., New York.

Leary, M. and Hill, D. (1996). Moving on: autism and movement distrubance. Mental Retardation, 34(1); 39-53.

Manijiviona, J. and Prior, M. (1995). Comparision of Asperger syndrome and high-functioning autistic children on a test of motor impairment. Journal of Autism and Developmental Disorders, 25(1); 23-39.

Martineau, J., Barthelemy, J., Muh, J. B. and Lelord, G. (1992). Monoamines (serotonin and catecholamines) and their derivatives in infantile autism: age related changes and drug effects. Developmental Medicine & Child Neurology, 34(7); 592-603.

McConachie, H. R. and Moore, V. (1992). Early expressive language of severly visually impaired children. Developmental Medicine & Child Neurology, 34(3); 230-239.

Miral, S., Ikiz, A. O., Gunbay, U. ve Baykara, A. (1994). Otistik cocuklarda erken ve orta latans isitsel uyarilmis potansiyeller. Cocuk ve Genclik Ruh Sagligi Dergisi, 1(2); 79-86.

Mitchell, P. (1997). Introduction to theory of mind: children, autism and apes. Arnold a member of the Hodder Headline Group, 196 s., London.

Miyahara, M., Tsujii, M., Hori, M., Nakanishi, K., Kageyama, H. and Sugiyama, T. (1997). Brief report: motor incoordination in children with Asperger's syndrome and learning disabilities. Journal of Autism and Developmental Disorders, 27; 595-603.

Mudford, O., Cross, B. and Reeves, D. (2000). Auditory integration traning for children with autism: no behavioral benefits detected. American Journal of Mental Retardation, 105(2); 118-129.

O'Neill, M. & Jones, R. P. (1997). Sensory-perceptual abnormalities in autism: a case for more research? *Journal of Autism and Developmental Disorders*, 27, 283-293.

O'Roidon, M. (2000). Superior modulation of activitivation levels of stimulus representation does not underline superior discrimination in autism. Cognition, 77(2); 81-96.

Ozonoff, S., Young, G. S., Goldring, S., Greiss-Hess, L., Herrera, A. M., Steele, J., Macari, S., Hepburn, S., Rogers, S. J. (2008). Gross Motor Development, Movement Abnormalities, and Early Identification of Autism. J Autism Dev Disord 38:644–656.

Parush, S., Sohmer, H. and Steinberg, A. (1997). Somatosensory functioning in children with attention deficit hyperactivity disorder. Develomental Medicine & Child Neurology, 39; 464-468.

Piggot, L. R. and Anderson, T. (1993). Brainstem auditory evoked response in children with central language disturbance. Journal of American Academy of Child Psychiatry, 22; 535-540.

Provost, B., Lopez, B. R., & Heimerl, S. (2006). A comparison of motor delays in young children: Autism spectrum disorder, developmental delay, and developmental concerns. Journal of Autism and Developmental Disorders, 37, 321–328.

Rapin, I. (1991). Autistic children: Diagnosis and clinical features. *Supplement to Paediatrics*, 87: 751-760.

Reiss, S. and Havercamp, S. M. 1997. Sensivity theory and mental retardation: why functional analysis is not enough. American Journal of Mental Retardation, 101(6); 553-566.

Rincover, A. & Ducharme, J. M. (1986). Variables influencing stimulus overselectivity and "tunnel vision" in developmentally delayed children. American Journal of Mental Deficiency, 91; 422-430.

Rinehart, N. J., Bradshaw, J. L., Brereton, A. V. and Tonge, D. J. (2001). Movement preparation in high-functioning autism and Asperger disorder: a serial choice reaction time task involving motor reprogramming. Journal of Autism and Developmental Disorders, 31(1); 79-88.

Rogers, S. J., Hepburn, S. L., Stackhause, T. and Wehner, E. (2003). Imitation performance in toddlers with autism and those with other developmental disorders. Journal of Child Psychology Psychiatry, 44(5); 763-781.

Rosenthal-Malek, A. and Mitchell, S. (1997). Brief report: the effects of exercise on the self-sitimulatory behaviors and positive responding of adolescent with autism. Journal of Autism and Developmental Disorders, 22(2); 193-201.

Royeen, C. B. and Lane, S. J. (1991). Tactile processing and sensory defensiveness. Sensory integration: theory and practice, Editors: A. G., Fisher, E. A. Murray. and A. C. Bundy, F. A. Davis, s. 108-133, Philadelphia.

Ryoichiro, I., Chisato, K. and Reiko, T. (2000). Brief report: comparsion of sensory-motor and cognitive function between autism and asperger syndrome in preschool children. Journal of Autism and Developmental Disorders, 30(2); 169-175.

Senju, A., Yaguchi, K., Tojo, Y. and Hasegawa, T. (2003). Eye contact does not facilitate detection in children with autism. Cognition, 89(1); 43-51.

Talay-Ongan, A. and Wood, K. (2000). Unusual sensory sensitives in autism: a possible cross roads. International Journal of Disability, Development & Education, 47(2); 201-212.

Temel, F. (1992). Duyusal kaynastirma terapisinin ozurlu cocuklarda kullanilmasi. Cocuk norolojisi gunleri ozet kitabi, s. C-28, Istanbul.

Vilensky, J. A., Damasio, A. R., & Maurer, R. G. (1981). Gait disturbance in patients with autistic behavior: A preliminary study. Archives of Neurology, 38, 646–649.

Wainwright-Sharp, J. A. and Brayson, S. E. (1996). Visual-spatial orienting in autism. Journal of Autism and Developmental Disorders, 26(4); 423-438.

Waterhouse, L., Fein, D. and Modahl, C. (1996). Neurofunctional mecanism in autism. Psyhlogical Rewiew, 103(3); 457-489.

Williamson, G. and Anzalone, M. (1997). Sensory integration: a key component of the evaluation and treatment of young children with severe difficulites in relating and comunicating. Zero to Three, 17(5); 29-36.

21

The Relationship Between Visual Perspective Taking and Imitation Impairments in Children with Autism

Yue Yu[1], Yanjie Su[1] and Raymond Chan[2]
[1]*Peking University, Department of Psychology*
[2]*Chinese Academy of Sciences, Neuropsychology and Applied Cognitive Neuroscience Laboratory, Key Laboratory of Mental Health, Institute of Psychology, Chinese Academy of Sciences*
China

1. Introduction

Perspective taking (or role taking) refers to the ability of individuals to distinguish their own perspectives from those of others, and to make correct judgments about the latter. It comprises both the visual (perceptual) level at which the individual imagines what another person can see from a contrasting vantage point (Kurdek & Rodgon, 1975) and the social-cognitive (conceptual) level at which he or she assesses another person's mental state (also referred to as the "Theory of Mind" or ToM; Baron-Cohen, Leslie, & Frith, 1985). Visual perspective taking (VPT) is further differentiated into two levels, namely, the ability to understand that people have selective visual fields (Level-1) and the ability to understand that they have different views of the *same* object (Level-2) (Flavell, Everett, Croft, & Flavell, 1981).

According to the hypothesis put forward by Baron-Cohen and colleagues (Baron-Cohen, 1988; Frith & Happé, 1999; Leslie & Frith, 1988), individuals with autism may suffer selective deficit to infer mental representations (referred to as *meta-representation*, Leslie, 1987), which may affect their ability to infer other's mental state (ToM) and their own mental state (self-consciousness). However, they can still indicate other's view in VPT tasks. Empirical evidence generally supports the hypothesis of a theory of mind deficit in autism (e.g., Baron-Cohen et al., 1985; Leslie & Frith, 1988; Perner, Frith, Leslie, & Leekam, 1989; Reed, 1994), but the results on VPT tests have been inconsistent. Some studies have demonstrated VPT deficit in autism (Hamilton, Brindley, & Frith, 2009; Reed, 2002; Warreyn, Roeyers, Oelbrandt, & de Groote, 2005; Yirmiya, Sigman, & Zacks, 1994), but others have found no such deficit (Baron-Cohen, 1989; Dawson & Fernald, 1987; Hobson, 1984; Leekam, Baron-Cohen, Perrett, Milders, & Brown, 1997; Leslie & Frith, 1988; Reed & Peterson, 1990; Tan & Harris, 1991). These contradictory findings may be due to differences in the task demands (Reed, 2002) and age of participants (Warreyn et al., 2005) among the studies, or to such methodological issues as the ceiling effect (Yirmiya et al., 1994). The first aim of the current study is thus to explore the possible reasons for these inconsistent results.

Research has also reported the imitative impairment of individuals with autism, especially with regard to the imitation of non-meaningful gestures (see Rogers & Williams, 2006; Williams, Whiten, & Singh, 2004). One specific feature of these individuals' gesture imitation is the "difficulty in correctly imitating the orientation of an action in relation to the model's body" (Rogers & Williams, 2006, pp. 281). For example, individuals with autism tend to reproduce an inward palm when the tester demonstrates an outward palm (Ohta, 1987). This "reverse" pattern has been found to prevail in both high- and low-functioning children with autism/Asperger syndrome (Vanvuchelen, Roeyers, & de Weerdt, 2007), and it is more common in children with autism than in children with other kinds of developmental disorders (Dewey, Cantell, & Crawford, 2007; Smith & Bryson, 1998; Whiten & Brown, 1998).

In imitation tasks involving self-oriented and other-oriented movements, children with autism showed a similar orientation problem. For example, in Meyer and Hobson's (2004) study, the tester moved objects either close to herself or close to the child, and the child copied the movement. Children with autism tended to copy the geometric orientations of the objects (close-to-tester move after the tester's close-to-self move), compared to non-autistic delayed children who usually mirrored the tester's action. In Carpenter, Tomasello, and Striano's (2005) study the tester demonstrated a movement either towards herself (E1 condition), towards the child (child condition), or towards another tester (E2 condition). Typically developing infants and children with developmental delay showed both self-self role reversal (self-directed movements in E1 condition) and other-other role reversal (E1-directed movements in child condition), but children with autism demonstrated neither of these role reversals.

Ohta (1987) originally interpreted this type of orientation problem as a difficulty in relating different body parts of the model as a whole in mental images. However, later studies indicated that it was more likely to be attributed to difficulty in encoding actions with reference to one's role or perspective (Barresi & Moore, 1996; Carpenter, et al., 2005; Smith & Bryson, 1998). Meyer and Hobson used the term "geometric repetition" to depict the featured response pattern in the imitation behavior observed in children with autism. Specifically, it refers to the "responding so that the physical movements and locations of the objects acted-upon were replicated" (p.237). In other words, individuals with autism seem not to view actions with reference of the demonstrator's personal perspective, instead they refer to the frame of non-personal aspects of the context (Meyer & Hobson, 2004). It is thus suggested that the orientation problem seen in imitation constitutes a perspective-taking problem.

Some empirical evidence has supported a relationship between imitation and social-cognitive abilities in individuals with autism. Imitation impairments have been reported to occur in concert with problems in joint attention (Hobson & Hobson, 2007), symbolic play (Brown & Whiten, 2000), or theory of mind (Meltzoff & Gopnik, 1993). However, we have found no study that directly compares imitation and VPT abilities in autism. We have two reasons for investigating such a connection. First, imitation and VPT share the essential element of being able to understand the correspondence between the representation of the self and that of the other. This element is supposed to be impaired in individuals with autism (Hobson & Hobson, 2007; Rogers & Williams, 2006). If individuals with autism are unable to understand the perspective of the demonstrator, they probably will not incorporate the demonstrator's stance during imitation, thus resulting in reversal error.

Second, imitation tasks capture perspective-taking skills at the perceptual level—to imitate correctly, children need to make an assumption about what the demonstrator *sees* when making a gesture or movement. More specifically, to map the demonstrator's action onto one's own action requires the ability of Level-2 VPT.

Therefore, this study further explores the controversy about VPT among children with autism and discusses the relationships between children's VPT and imitation skills. We seek to: a) explore whether children with autism show impairments in their Level-2 VPT skills; b) examine the occurrence of reversal error in these children's imitation performance; and c) investigate whether their VPT skills are related to their imitative skills. We hypothesize that both VPT and imitation skills are impaired in children with autism, and the occurrence of these two impairments are correlated.

2. Method

2.1 Participants

Fifteen children with autism and 15 typically developing children participated in the experiment. Three additional children with autism were excluded because they were not cooperative (n = 2) or because of equipment failure (n = 1). The autism group (12 boys and 3 girls) were diagnosed with either an autistic disorder (n = 13) or an atypical autism (n = 2) by experienced pediatric clinicians from the Institute of Mental Health of Peking University. These diagnoses were made according to the DSM-IV diagnostic criteria of autism (American Psychiatric Association, 1994), and were based on interview with parents, behavioral observation with children and clinical records consultation. School records showed all of the children to have an IQ below 70 at the time they entered school, as measured by the Wechsler Intelligence Scale for Children Revised (WISC-R, Chinese edition; Lin & Zhang, 1986). All showed a preference for the right hand according to the visual-motor test.

Fifteen typically developing children were recruited as controls from a local preschool. None of their parents or teachers had reported any of them to have diagnoses of medical disease or mental illness. These children were matched on a one-to-one basis with the autism group in terms of sex, verbal mental age (VMA), and handedness. The basic characteristics of the group are shown in Table 1. All of the autistic and control children received small toys or stickers after the test. Written informed consent was obtained from the children's parents or guardians prior to their participation.

2.2 General procedure

The children were tested individually in a quiet room in their own school. To achieve better engagement, the tasks were divided into two sections. The first section lasted for about 30 minutes and included the administration of the Peabody Picture Vocabulary Test Revised (PPVT-R), the visual-motor test, and the gesture imitation task. The second section lasted for about 10 minutes and included the upside-down picture task.

2.3 Measures

2.3.1 General cognitive tests

VMA was estimated using the PPVT-R (Chinese edition; Sang & Miao, 1990). We defined a VMA match between the autistic and control children as a similar PPVT-R original score (a difference of less than 3). Visual-motor integration ability was assessed by part of the geometric design task, which is a subtest of the Wechsler Preschool and Primary Scale of Intelligence (WPPSI, Chinese edition; Applied Psychology Center of Beijing Normal University, 1986). The tester asked the child to sequentially copy down four figures (a circle, a cross, a hexagon, and a diamond in a square) on a piece of paper. Their performance was scored according to the instruction booklet, out of a total of 12 points.

2.3.2 Upside-down picture task

The upside-down picture task (Guo, Wang, & Wang, 2004) was used to assess children's VPT ability. Two upside-down pictures were used in this task: a princess-granny picture (see Fig. 1A and 1B) and an elephant-swan picture (reveals an elephant from one side, and reveals a swan after rotating 180°). Both materials were printed on A4 (21 cm × 29 cm) paper. As some of the children demonstrated deficits in naming objects, they were allowed to respond by pointing out the image that resembled what they had seen from several choices (Fig. 1C). The choice images were selected from abstract cartoon sketches so that the child could not get the correct answer merely by perceptually comparing the choice images and the target. For each picture, four choice figures (two representing objects on the upside-down picture and two representing irrelevant objects) were provided and placed on a piece of A5 (15 cm × 21 cm) paper.

Children sat beside a table and the tester sat next to them. The tester showed them the elephant-swan picture first, followed by the princess-granny picture. Take the princess-granny picture as example. The frequency with which the princess or the granny was shown first was balanced between participants. The tester asked children "Who do you see in the picture?" and repeated the question if necessary. If children remained silent, then he would take out the sheet of paper with choice of images and asked them to point out the one that resembled the person they see from the picture. After children had given their answer, they were asked to point out the mouth of that person to confirm what they had seen. For the elephant-swan picture, children were asked to point out the animal's head as confirmation. After viewing the two pictures, children moved to the other side of the table and named the person or animal on the opposite side. The same confirmation process followed. The VPT test was administered only after children had identified both of the objects in at least one picture. In the VPT test, the tester asked children to go back to their original seat, and placed a bear puppet opposite to them. After making sure that children understood the puppet was looking at the picture from the opposite side of the table, the tester asked them "What do you see in the picture?" and "What would the puppet see in the picture?" Children were then asked to "point out the head/mouth" of the figure in the picture. Each child completed four such trials (two pictures in two orientations).

Each single answer was scored as correct, opposite, irrelevant, or no response. Correct answers were taken as exact or proximate naming (e.g., naming a princess as a girl or young lady) or the correct selection from the choice images. Opposite answers referred to naming or pointing to the object on the reverse side (e.g., naming the princess as granny). If children gave other answers or if their oral answers conflicted with what they had pointed to, then their response was scored as irrelevant. In the VPT test, two correct responses revealed the ability to infer another's view, whereas one correct and one opposite response (i.e., answering according to the children's view in both questions) suggested an egocentric standpoint (Piaget & Inhelder, 1963).

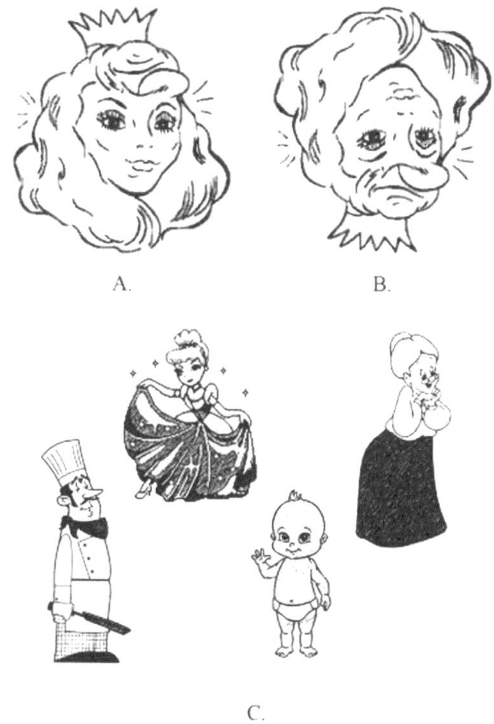

Fig. 1. Princess-granny picture and its choice figures: A. the princess; B. the granny (reverse of A); C. the choice picture, including a princess, a granny, and two irrelevant figures.

2.3.3 Gesture imitation test

The imitation test was adapted from Ohta's (1987) Gesture Imitation Test. To optimize the test for younger children, we reduced the number of trials and selected gestures that were easy to perform. Only non-meaningful gestures were included, as such gestures best capture the "reproduce the specific action" component of imitation (Williams et al., 2004). Six gestures were chosen after a pretest among typically developing 3 to 4 year olds. The unimanual gestures included a fist, a "V" posture with the index and middle fingers pointing upward, and a "bull's horn" posture with the thumb and little finger pointing upward. Each gesture could be made with the palm held either outward or inward. Three bimanual gestures were developed from Ohta's stimuli of *T* signs and were used in the test (Fig. 2).

The tester and children sat across the table facing each other. For each trial, the tester attracted children's attention by saying "watch me" before demonstrating the gesture. In the training trial, the tester held up the index finger of his left hand with the palm facing out, and asked children to "copy my action." Children who held up their right index finger facing out were considered to be correct, and those who did not make this gesture were corrected until they understood the kind of mirror copying that was expected. The main part of the test then began with the imitation of unimanual gestures, followed by bimanual gestures. The procedure was similar to the training trial except for the tester's feedback. If children did wrong, the tester would give them a verbal hint ("Are you sure?") and see if they can correct by themselves. For those who stayed wrong, the tester would demonstrate the gesture a second time, and children were given a second attempt. The order of the gestures and the direction of the palm were balanced across participants.

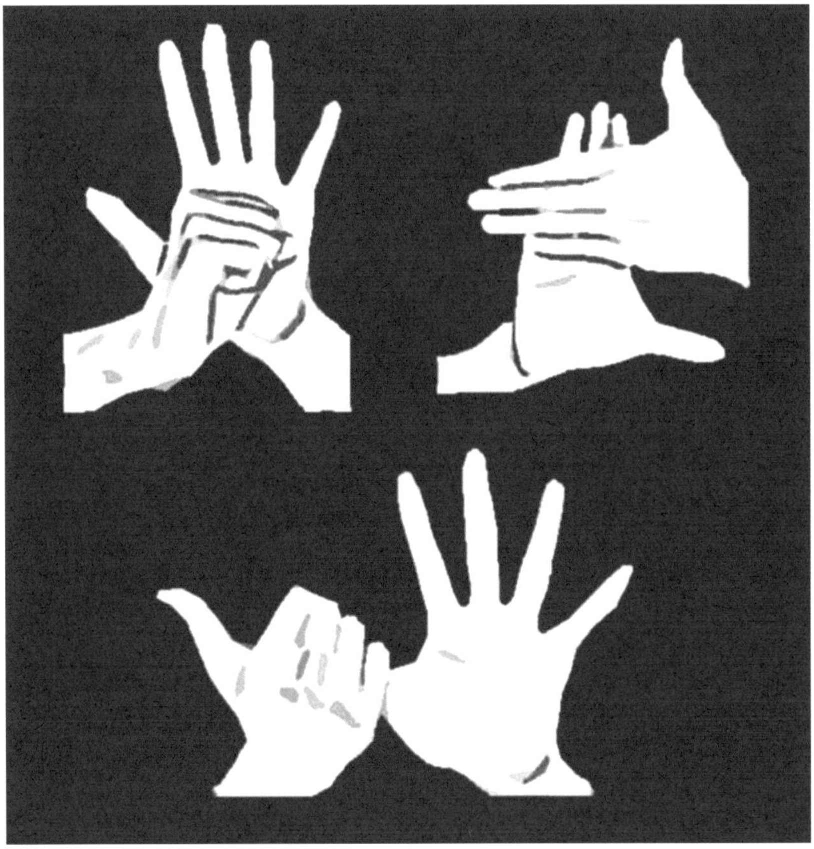

Fig. 2. Bimanual gestures used in gesture imitation.

Each child's imitation performance was videotaped and scored for correctness and error type. Correctness for each gesture was scored between 0 and 3 (3: correct in the first attempt; 2: self-corrected after the verbal hint; 1: correct in the second attempt; 0: failed). A simplified version of the six-type error system of Vanvuchelen et al. (2007) was used to determine the error types. Errors were categorized as behavioral, content, spatial, or no error. Behavioral errors referred to no response or unwilling to copy. Content error referred to using the wrong hand or fingers to perform gestures, or positioned the fingers wrongly. If the fingers were correctly positioned, but the spatial direction was wrong (rotated from the correct position), then this was regarded as a spatial error. For each gesture, error types were scored for both the first and second attempts (if children were correct at the first attempt, both attempts would be scored as "no error"). Twenty percent of the videotapes (six participants, three from each group) were randomly selected and scored by an independent observer who was blind to research hypotheses. Interrater agreement was assessed using Cohen's kappa statistic. For correctness, $\kappa = 0.76$, and for error type, $\kappa = 0.75$, both of which are above the excellent agreement level defined by Fleiss (2003).

3. Results

3.1 Data analyses

The between-group contrasts were analyzed using independent *t* tests, the Mann-Whitney U test, and mixed-design ANOVA in SPSS 13.0, with a threshold of α = .05 for statistical significance. Fisher's exact test was used to analyze the frequency data. The effect sizes of planned contrasts were assessed with Cohen's *d* and unbiased *r* (Field, 2005). A summary of results is listed in Table 1.

	Autism group (*n* = 15)			Control group (*n* = 15)			*t*-value	*p*-value
	M	*SD*	Range	*M*	*SD*	Range		
Chronological age (y; m)	8; 11	0; 7	8; 0-9; 11	3; 9	0; 8	2; 8-5; 1	21.86	< .001
Verbal metal age (y; m)	4; 10	0; 11	3; 2-6; 8	4; 9	0; 11	3; 2-6; 8	0.01	> .01
Time of training (y; m)[a]	1; 6	1; 1	0; 1-2; 7	--	--	--	--	--
Visual-motor score (max:12)	6.0	3.2	2-11	2.7	1.6	1-5	3.56	.003
Imitation score (max: 18)	7.1	3.9	2-15	11.5	2.7	5-15	-3.58	.001
Imitation error (max: 18)	10.7	3.4	3-15	5.8	2.6	3-13	4.39	< .001
VPT score (percent correct)[b]	13.9	28.3	0-75	82.8	33.7	0-100	-8.50[c]	< .001

[a] Time of training is defined as the time period of training in a special education school, and applies only to the autism group.
[b] VPT: visual perspective taking. Seven children in the autism group and nine in the control group participated in this test.
[c] Intergroup difference in the VPT score is measured by the Mann-Whitney *U* value.

Table 1. Characteristics and descriptive statistics for the autism group and the control group.

3.2 General cognitive tests

Autism group and control group were not different in the original PPVT-R score (for autism $M = 34.3$, for control $M = 34.1$, $t\ (28) = 0.04$, $p = .97$, $d = 0.01$). According to the Chinese norm (Sang & Miao, 1990), their scores were converted into VMAs of 4 years 10 months and 4 years 9 months, respectively. The children with autism exhibited better performance than did the control children in the visual-motor task, $t\ (20.5) = 3.56$, $p = .002$, $d = 1.30$.

3.3 Upside-down picture task

The results for the upside-down picture task are presented in Table 2. Six children in the autism group were excluded from this analysis because they failed the initial recognition part. Of these failures, one child failed to recognize all of the objects presented to him, and five children stuck with one object and could not figure out the competing ones (e.g., they could not recognize "granny" after they saw "princess" on the other side). The latter event also occurred to four typically developing children. Overall correctness in figuring out the competing objects did not differ between the groups ($t\ (28) = -1.08$, $p = 0.29$, $d = -0.32$). Of the nine children with autism who participated in the VPT test, only two were able to infer the puppet's view (although their performance was not consistent across the trials), and seven gave egocentric answers in 11 trials. In contrast, 10 of the 11 children in the control group were able to correctly infer the puppet's perspective (two were inconsistent), and only one gave egocentric answers. The Fisher's exact test shows an unequal distribution of the number of children capable of taking another's perspective versus the number of those taking an egocentric view between the groups (p = .003). The average VPT scores of the autism and control groups confirmed this difference (U = 8.5, $p < .001$, d = -2.18).

	Autism group (n = 15)	Control group (n = 15)
Not included in VPT test	6 (40%)	4 (27%)
fail to name either object	1 (7%)	0 (0%)
fail to recognize the alternative object	5 (33%)	4 (27%)
Included in VPT test	9 (60%)	11 (73%)
fail to take the perspective of the doll	7 (47%)	1 (7%)
inconsistently take the perspective of the puppet	2 (13%)	2 (13%)
consistently take the perspective of the puppet	0 (0%)	8 (53%)

Table 2. Percentage of each type of performance in the autism (n = 15) and control (n = 15) groups during the upside-down picture task. VPT: visual perspective taking.

3.4 Gesture imitation

The total imitation score of children with autism was significantly lower than those in the control group (t (28) = -4.40, p = .001, d = -1.31). This discrepancy was evident in both the unimanual gestures (t (14) = -2.62, p = .01, d = -0.96) and bimanual gestures (t (14) = -2.69, p = .01, d = -0.98). Fig. 3 showed the percentages of correct imitation for the first and second attempt, as analyzed in a 2 (group) × 2 (uni/bimanual) × 2 (number of attempt) repeated measures ANOVA. The results again revealed the main effect of group, F (1, 14) = 24.33, $p < .001$, $\eta^2 = .64$, the the main effect of uni/bimanual, F (1, 14) = 9.79, $p < .01$, $\eta^2 = .41$, as well as the main effect of number of attempt, F (1, 14) = 62.42, $p < .001$, $\eta^2 = .82$. Both groups performed better in unimanual gesture and in the second attempt. An interaction between group and number of attempt was also observed, F (1, 14) = 4.51, p = .05, $\eta^2 = .24$. Autism group made less improvement between the first and second attempt, t (14) = 2.12, p = .05, d = 0.54.

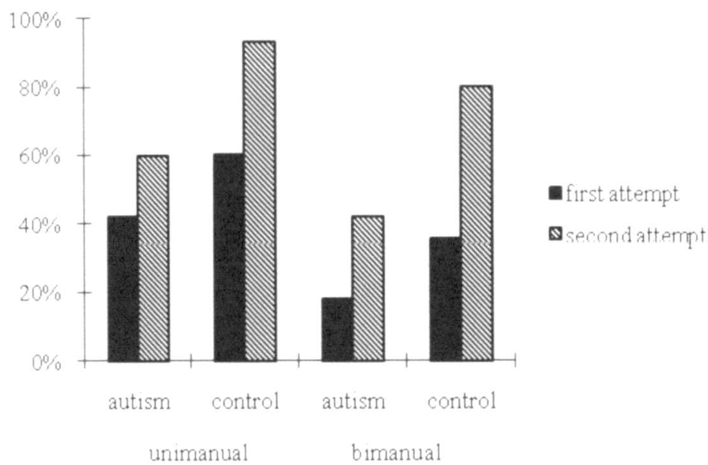

Fig. 3. Correct percentages of the first and second attempts in gesture imitation

We analyzed the types of errors in a 2 (group) × 2 (uni/bimanual) × 3 (error type) ANOVA. Results (Fig. 4) showed a main effect for all three factors. The number of errors in the autism group was significantly higher than that in the control group (F (1, 28) = 18.70, $p < .001$, r = 0.63), and the error for bimanual gestures was higher than that for unimanual gestures (F (1, 28) = 4.82, p = .02). Main effect for error type was also significant (F (2, 13) = 46.94, $p < .001$, $\eta^2 = 0.63$). A post hoc multiple-comparison Bonferroni test revealed greater spatial error than content error (MD = .32, $p < .001$) and behavioral error (MD = .30, $p < .001$), but no difference between the latter two (MD = .02, p = .28). The only interaction observed was group × error type (F (2, 56) = 5.03, p = .02). The autism group made significantly more spatial errors than the control group, t (21.6) = 2.95, p = .008, d = 1.08. There were no group differences for the behavioral and content errors.

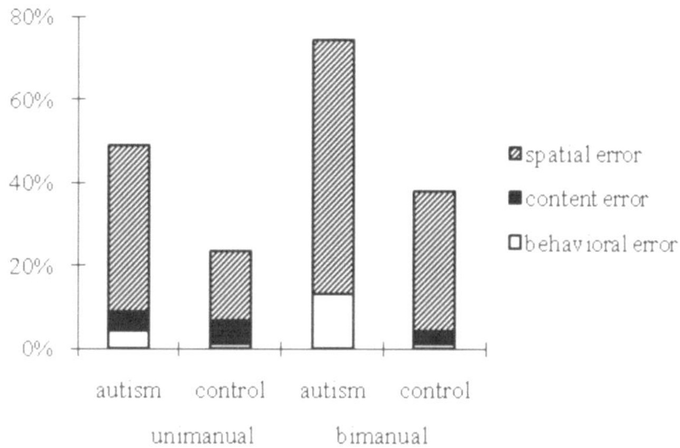

Fig. 4. Mean percentage frequency of different types of errors (+SE of total error) for the autism (n = 15) and control (n = 15) groups in unimanual and bimanual gesture imitation.

Spatial error accounted for the majority (81.4%) of total errors, so we investigated spatial error in detail. All of the observed spatial errors took the form of "reversal errors"—that is, instead of mirroring the demonstration, children rotated the hand position by 180° to replicate the actual position of the demonstration. The results showed that children with autism were more prone to this kind of error, t (21.6) = 2.95, p = .008, d = 1.08, and this was true for both the unimanual (t (28) = 2.82, p = .009, d = 1.03) and bimanual gestures (t (28) = 2.06, p = .049, d = 0.75).

3.5 Correlation analysis

We used correlation analysis to investigate the potential relationship between imitation and VPT deficiency in autism. The results of this analysis (Table 3) showed that VMA is correlated with imitation score (r = .38, p = .04); this correlation was significant for bimanual gestures (r = .41, p = .03), but not for unimanual gestures (r = .19, p = .33). Visual-motor ability and educational level showed no significant correlation with imitation performance. The VPT score was highly correlated with the imitation score (r = .74, $p < .001$), and this correlation remained significant after controlling for VMA (r = .67, p = .002). The fact that children with autism performed poorly in both VPT and imitation tasks may contribute to the correlation, so we analyzed the two groups separately. In the autism group, VMA was not associated with scores for imitation, but the VPT score showed marginal correlation with imitation score ($r = .60$, $p = .09$). Children who passed the VPT test in at least one trial scored higher in imitation than those who failed the VPT test (t (7) = 2.66, $p = .03$, $d = 2.13$). Correlation between VPT and imitation scores was also observed in the control group, but it was not statistically significant ($r = .46$, $p = .15$).

Taking the error type into account, we found that spatial error, but neither of the other two types of errors, was inversely correlated with the imitation score ($r = -.64$, $p < .001$). Moreover, while VMA, visual-motor ability, and educational level were not found to be correlated with spatial error, significant correlation was found between spatial error and the VPT score across the two groups ($r = -.59$, $p < .01$). Within the autism group, children who passed the VPT test in at least one trial made fewer spatial errors than did those who failed (t (7) = 2.82, $p = .02$, $d = 2.34$). The correlation between VPT and spatial error was not significant in the control group ($r = -.12$, $p = .73$).

		Verbal mental age	Visual-motor score	Education level	VPT score[a]	Total spatial error
Visual-motor score		0.33	--			
Education level		-0.22	-0.03	--		
VPT[a] score		0.42	-0.19	0.09	--	
Spatial error	total	-0.13	0.32	0.12	-0.59**†	--
	unimanual	-0.01	0.34	0.05	-0.49*	0.59***†
	bimanual	-0.16	0.23	0.12	-0.52*	0.92***†
Imitation score	total	0.38*	-0.15	-0.3	0.74***†	-0.64***†
	unimanual	0.19	-0.16	-0.16	0.73***†	-0.49**
	bimanual	0.41*	-0.08	-0.34	0.53*	-0.53**

[a] VPT: visual perspective taking.

*$p < .05$. **$p < .01$. ***$p < .001$.

† Significant correlations after Bonferroni correction for multiple comparisons (Abdi, 2007), $\alpha' = .05/35 = .0014$.

Table 3. Pearson correlations between individual variables and performance in gesture imitation.

4. Discussion

In this study we compared children with autism and typically developing children for their performance in a VPT task and an imitation task. The results confirmed our three hypotheses: a) children with autism showed impairment in their Level-2 VPT skills, as they were mostly unable to determine what a puppet might see in the picture that they themselves were looking at; b) these children also performed poorly in gesture imitation compared to the controls and committed more spatial errors in the form of reversal error; and c) the VPT and imitation scores and the occurrence of spatial error were correlated with one another. However, we should interpret these findings cautiously. It should be noted that the comparisons in this study are much younger typically developing children, and we did not recruit a developmental delay control with both chronological age (CA) and VMA matched. Therefore, the findings are still preliminary to suggest that the impairments are specific to children with autism.

The finding of VPT impairment in children with autism is in line with some previous studies (Hamilton, et al., 2009; Reed, 2002; Warreyn, et al., 2005; Yirmiya et al., 1994), but contradicts the findings of others (Baron-Cohen, 1989; Hobson, 1984; Leekam et al., 1997; Leslie & Frith, 1988; Reed & Peterson, 1990; Tan & Harris, 1991). One of the possible reasons for this inconsistency is the different designs of tasks. Most of the aforementioned studies had applied Level-1 VPT tasks. These include the "puppet seeing" paradigm, the "hide and seek" paradigm, and the "cube" paradigm (seminal design see Hobson, 1984). In each of these paradigms, children are required to predict whether a puppet (or the tester) would see certain object that can be either in sight/not shielded or out of sight/shielded.

The accomplishment of such Level-1 VPT tasks requires an understanding of whether there is an unbroken line-of-sight between the agent's eyes and the target. This ability is generally believed to be unaffected by the pathology of autism (Leslie & Frith, 1988). In fact, five out of the eight studies testing Level-1 VPT (Baron-Cohen, 1989; Hobson, 1984; Leslie & Frith, 1988; Reed & Peterson, 1990; Tan & Harris, 1991) found children with autism performed more than 90% correct on average. One (Leekam et al., 1997) found 66% children with autism pass the test, which is comparable to children with Down syndrome and normal children. One (Reed, 2002) found that children with autism were impaired in VPT tasks with high working memory load. One (Warreyn, et al., 2005) found Level-1 VPT deficiency in a much younger sample of autism (average CA 5;6, VMA 4;4).

The Level-2 VPT, as tested by our upside-down picture task, could not be simply solved by the line-of-sight rule. Children needed to further infer what the puppet would conclude from the properties it observed (e.g., whether the puppet would perceive a granny face with a mouth at the top or a princess face with the mouth at the bottom), which involved a mindreading component. Five studies (Dawson & Fernald, 1987; Hamilton, et al., 2009; Reed & Peterson, 1990; Tan & Harris, 1991; Yirmiya et al., 1994) had administrated Level-2 VPT tasks in children with autism, of which two (Reed & Peterson, 1990; Tan & Harris, 1991) found no impairment.

In Reed and Peterson's (1990) task, children were instructed to "turn (an object) round so I (the tester) can see the nose/tail/front/back". However, this task could be accomplished with the line-of-sight rule, if children focus on one part of the object (e.g., the nose of a teddy bear). Tan and Harris's (1991) Level-2 VPT task is susceptible to a similar problem because it required children to answer what the dolls would say that was "in front" of them. In addition, the autism sample in their study was much older than our sample in both CA (12;8 versus 8;11) and VMA (7;7 versus 4; 10), and those children performed as well as typically developing children in all of the tasks administrated.

Dawson and Fernald's (1987) study employed five perceptual perspective taking tasks, of which three (Upside down, Face and Spontaneous) resembled the tests used in our study. Sixteen children with autism (6-14 years old) scored an average of 7.8 out of 18 combining these five tasks. In comparison their average score on conceptual perspective taking was 7.4 out of 11. Unfortunately this study did not employ a control group so we do not know whether the impairment was due to delayed general intelligence or it was specific to autism.

Yirmiya and colleague's (1994) employed two turntables that have 3 or 10 items on them.

Children were requested to rotate one turntable to replicate the tester's view on the second. Children with autism (age 9;3-16;10) performed worse than the CA and IQ matched normal controls. Finally, Hamilton and colleagues (2009) included a large and well-controlled sample (23 children with autism, 60 typical children in three age groups) and tested them on a turntable-type Level 2 VPT task and a closely matched mental rotation task. The result showed that children with autism have difficulty in VPT task compared to the mental rotation task. Taken into the background of these studies, our results indicate that although children with autism can infer another's line of sight, they may suffer problem in Level-2 VPT tasks which involve a mindreading component.

In the current study, we also confirmed that children with autism display reversal error during imitation, which is consistent with previous discoveries (Ohta, 1987; Meyer and Hobson, 2004; Smith & Bryson, 1998; Vanvuchelen, et al., 2007). However, the current test differs from the previous studies in that we used a training trail where children were trained to perform mirror-image imitation. Instead of measuring instinctive response (as emphasized in Meyer & Hobson, 2004), we expected to elicit a predominant response before the main test. The results show that both groups made considerable amount of spatial error in their initial response, but autistic children were less willing to change their response style in their second attempt. Considering other studies which revealed that geometric repetition also occurred in children with learning difficulties (Meyer & Hobson, 2004) and its occurrence declined with age in typically developing children of 3-6 years old (Ohta et al., 1987), it might indicate that learning disability play a role in the imitation style of autistic children.

The current study has found the score of VPT and imitation to be correlated. Both of them also inversely correlated with the occurrence of reversal error. These findings may have implications for the mechanisms of imitative impairment in autism. According to intersubjectivity theories of autism, such as the self-other mapping theory (Rogers & Pennington, 1991) and identification theory (Hobson & Meyer, 2006), the imitative impairment in autism is rooted in difficulties in coordinating the representations of self and other, i.e., the ability to "see the other as a template of the self" or to "identify with the other." These theories explain reversal error nicely because this type of error appears to be a specific problem related to an understanding of the self-other relationship (Meyer & Hobson, 2004; Smith & Bryson, 1998), as opposed to general motivational, perceptual, or executive problems during imitation.

The current finding of a correlation between reversal error and VPT scores further supports intersubjectivity theories. The VPT and gesture imitation tasks differ in perceptual and motor requirements, but they share a common requirement to coordinate perspectives. In both tasks, children sat face to face with the tester/puppet and focused on an object (gesture/picture) placed between them. To succeed, the children needed to assume that the tester/puppet seated across from them was an agent just like themselves with a distinct perspective. In other words, children need to attribute perspectives to both the puppet in the VPT task ("he would see an upright face facing *towards him*") and the tester in the imitation task ("he held his palm facing inwards *towards himself*"). If the children failed to perceive the other as having a distinct perspective, they would probably use their own viewpoint to assume what the other would see, and at the same time perceive the demonstrator's gestures as having no personal context. The majority of our autism sample displayed such failure to appreciate the other's perspective, which fits in with intersubjectivity theories in explaining imitative and social-cognitive impairment in autism.

This study has a number of methodological limitations. Due to limited access to standard assessment tools in mainland China, the diagnoses of autism in this study were based on the checklist of symptoms from the DSM-IV, therefore lean heavily on the clinical experiences of paediatricians in daily clinical routine. We were not able to recruit a more stringent criterion for making such a diagnosis. Further study adopting more stringent diagnostic criteria according to the international standard should be conducted in the near future to cross validate the current findings.

The autism group and control group were only matched on their VMA, whereas their CA and visual-motor ability differed significantly. These differences may cause group asymmetry in many aspects, including life experience, education, etc. Therefore, the current finding is insufficient to lead to strong conclusion that the VPT and imitation impairment are specific to autism as opposed to other kinds of developmental delay. A better design would include an additional group of children with learning difficulties or a mental handicap, at the same time having similar CA and VMA with the autistic children. However, it should be noted that VMA provides a conservative estimate of mental age in an autistic sample (Reed & Peterson, 1990). Because we matched the two groups on VMA, the autism group was much older than the control group, and possessed better visual-motor skills. Therefore the lower VPT and imitation scores of the autism group is unlikely to be attributable to mental retardation or poor motor skills.

The sample size was relatively small, with only 15 participants in each group, and the sample is rather heterogeneous as the variation in VMA is large. Nevertheless, we observed consistent differences between the two groups, which resulted in acceptable statistical power despite of the adverse effect of small sample size. A replication with large sample size is needed in the future to confirm the current findings.

Notwithstanding these limitations, the current findings suggest the deficiency in Level-2 VTP in children with autism may be related to their imitative impairment, which supports intersubjectivity theories. These results point to the possibility that autistic children's impairments in social cognition and imitation may be rooted in the lack of awareness to see other people "as a template of the self" (Rogers & Pennington, 1991). If future studies could confirm the current findings, several practical implications may be derived. First, the fact that children with autism were more prone to reversal errors and that the number of reversal errors correlated with VPT and imitation performance may contribute to the identification of autism. Since imitation starts in early infancy (Meltzoff & Gopnik, 1993), reversal error in imitation or other kinds of turn-taking play may serve as an indictor in the screening of infants at risk for autism and in the early diagnose of autism. Second, the current results also suggested that fostering intersubjective engagement in children with autism might enhance both their imitation skills and their ability to appreciate events in the world from multiple points of view. Further studies are needed to explore the underlying mechanisms that cause VPT and imitation impairments in children with autism, and to examine the feasibility of improving these skills through fostering intersubjectivity experience.

5. Conclusion

This study compared the performance of 15 children with autism and 15 matched typically developing children on a Level-2 VPT task and a gesture imitation task. The children with autism performed worse in both tasks compared to control group, and the scores for the two tests correlate with each other and with the amount of reversal error during imitation. These findings suggest a problem in coordinating the perspective of self and others underlies both the imitation and VPT impairments of children with autism.

6. Acknowledgment

This study was supported by a grant from the Natural Science Foundation of Beijing (7072036) and the NSFC (30770728, 30970907) to Dr. Yanjie Su and grants from the Project-Oriented Hundred Talents Programme (O7CX031003) and the Knowledge Innovation Project of the Chinese Academy of Sciences (KSC X2-YW-R-131 & KSCX2-EW-J-8) to Dr. Raymond Chan. We are also indebted to the children and their parents and the teachers of the Haidian Peizhi Central School for the Mentally Retarded and the Preschool Center affiliated to Peking University.

7. References

Abdi, H (2007). Bonferroni and Sidak corrections for multiple comparisons, In: *Encyclopedia of Measurement and Statistics,* N. J. Salkind (Ed.), 103–107, Sage, ISBN 978-141-2916-11-0, Thousand Oaks, California, USA, October 13, 2006

American Psychiatric Association (1994). *Diagnostic and Statistical Manual of Mental Disorders* (4th ed.), American Psychiatric Publishing, ISBN 978-089-0420-25-6, Washington DC, USA

Applied Psychology Center of Beijing Normal University. (1986). *Wechsler Pre-school and Primary Scale of Intelligence* (Chinese ed.) [in Chinese], Beijing Normal University Press, Beijing, China

Baron-Cohen, S. (1988). Social and pragmatic deficits in autism: Cognitive or affective? *Journal of Autism and Developmental Disorders,* Vol. 18, No. 33, (September 1988), pp. 379–402, ISSN 0162-3257

Baron-Cohen, S. (1989). Perceptual role taking and protodeclarative pointing in autism. *British Journal of Developmental Psychology,* Vol. 7, No. 2, (June 1989), pp. 113–127, ISSN 0261-510X

Baron-Cohen, S.; Leslie, A. M. & Frith, U. (1985). Does the autistic child have a "theory of mind"? *Cognition,* Vol. 21, No. 1, (October 1985), pp. 37–46, ISSN 0010-0277

Brown, J. & Whiten, A. (2000). Imitation, theory of mind and related activities in autism: An observational study of spontaneous behaviour in everyday contexts. *Autism,* Vol. 4, No. 2, (June 2000), pp. 185-204, ISSN 1362-3613

Carpenter, M.; Tomasello, M. & Striano, T. (2005). Role reversal imitation and language in typically developing infants and children with autism. *Infancy,* Vol. 8, No. 3, (November 2005), pp. 253–278, ISSN 1532-7078

Dawson, G. & Fernald, M. (1987). Perspective-taking ability and its relationship to the social behavior of autistic children. *Journal of Autism and Developmental Disorders,* Vol. 17, No. 4, (December 1987), pp. 487–498, ISSN 0162-3257

Dewey, D.; Cantell, M. & Crawford, S. G. (2007). Motor and gestural performance in children with autism spectrum disorders, developmental coordination disorder, and/or attention deficit hyperactivity disorder. *Journal of the International Neuropsychological Society,* Vol. 13, No. 2, (March 2007), pp. 246-256, ISSN 1355-6177

Field, A. P. (2005). *Discovering statistics using SPSS for Windows: Advanced techniques for the beginner* (2nd ed.), Sage, ISBN 978-076-1957-55-3, London, UK

Fleiss, J. L. (2003). *Statistical Methods for Rates and Proportions* (3rd ed.), Wiely, ISBN 978-047-1526-29-2 New York, USA

Flavell, J. H.; Everett, B. A.; Croft, K. & Flavell, E. R. (1981). Young children's knowledge about visual perception: Further evidence for the Level 1-Level 2 distinction. *Developmental Psychology,* Vol. 17, No. 1, (January 1981), pp. 99–103, ISSN 0012-1649

Frith, U. & Happé, F. (1999). Theory of mind and self consciousness: What is it like to be autistic?. *Mind and Language,* Vol. 14, No. 1, (March 1999), pp. 1-22, ISSN 0268-1064

Guo, L.; Wang, X. & Wang S. (2004). An investigation of cognitive development with upside-down pictures [in Chinese]. *Psychological Science,* Vol. 27, No. 4, (July 2004), pp. 850–854, ISSN 1671-6981

Hamilton, A. F.; Brindley, R. & Frith, U. (2009). Visual perspective taking impairment in children with autistic spectrum disorder. *Cognition,* Vol. 113, No. 1, (October 2009), pp. 37-44, ISSN 0010-0277

Hobson, R. P. (1984). Early childhood autism and the question of egocentrism. *Journal of Autism and Developmental Disorders,* Vol. 14, No. 1, (March 1984), pp. 85–104, ISSN 0162-3257

Hobson, J. A. & Hobson, R. P. (2007). Identification: The missing link between joint attention and imitation? *Development and Psychopathology,* Vol. 19, No. 2, (April 2007), pp. 411–431, ISSN 0954-5794

Hobson, R. P. & Meyer, J. (2006). Imitation, identification, and the shaping of mind: Insights from autism, In: *Imitation and the social mind: Autism and typical development,* S. J. Rogers, & J. H. G. Williams (Eds.), 198–226, The Guilford Press, ISBN 978-159-3853-11-2, New York, USA

Kurdek, L. A. & Rodgon, M. M. (1975). Perceptual, cognitive, and affective perspective taking in kindergarten through sixth-grade children. *Developmental Psychology,* Vol. 11, No. 5, (September 1975), pp. 643–650, ISSN 0012-1649

Lin, C. D. & Zhang, H. C. (1986). *The Chinese Revision of WISC-R* [in Chinese], Beijing Normal University Press, Beijing, China

Leekam, S.; Baron-Cohen, S.; Perrett, D.; Milders, M. & Brown, S. (1997). Eye-direction detection: A dissociation between geometric and joint attention skills in autism. *British Journal of Developmental Psychology,* Vol. 15, No. 1, (March 1997), pp. 77–95, ISSN 0261-510X

Leslie, A. M. (1987). Pretense and representation: The origins of "theory of mind". *Psychological Review,* Vol. 94, No. 4, (October 1987), pp. 412–426. ISSN 0033-295X

Leslie, A. M. & Frith, U. (1988). Autistic children's understanding of seeing, knowing and believing. *British Journal of Developmental Psychology,* Vol. 6, No. 4, (November 1988), pp. 315-324, ISSN 0261-510X

Meyer, J. A. & Hobson, R. P. (2004). Orientation in relation to self and other: The case of autism. *Interaction Studies,* Vol. 5, No. 2, (Summer 2004), pp. 221–244. ISBN 1572-0373

Meltzoff, A. N. & Gopnik, A. (1993). The role of imitation in understanding persons and developing a theory of mind. In: *Understanding other minds: Perspectives from autism,* S. Baron-Cohen, H. Tager-Flusberg, & D. J. Cohen (Eds.), 335-366, Oxford University Press, ISBN 978-019-2620-56-9, New York, USA

Ohta, M. (1987). Cognitive disorders of infantile autism: A study employing the WISC, spatial relationships, conceptualization, and gestural imitation. *Journal of Autism and Developmental Disorders,* Vol. 17, No. 11, (March 1987), pp. 45–62, ISSN 0162-3257

Piaget, J. & Inhelder, B. (1963). *The Child's conception of space.* Routledge & Kegan Paul, ISBN 978-039-3004-08-3, London, UK

Perner, J.; Frith, U.; Leslie, A. M. & Leekam, S. R. (1989). Exploration of the autistic child's theory of mind: Knowledge, belief, and communication. *Child Development,* Vol. 60, No. 3, (June 1989), pp. 689–700, ISSN 1467-8624

Reed, T. (1994). Performance of autistic and control subjects on three cognitive perspective-taking tasks. *Journal of Autism and Developmental Disorders,* Vol. 24, No. 1, (February 1994), pp. 53–66, ISSN 0162-3257

Reed, T. & Peterson, C. (1990). A comparative study of autistic subjects performance at two levels of visual and cognitive perspective taking. *Journal of Autism and Developmental Disorders,* Vol. 20, No. 1, (December, 1990), pp. 555–567, ISSN 0162-3257

Reed, T. (2002). Visual perspective taking as a measure of working memory in participants with autism. *Journal of Developmental and Physical Disabilities,* Vol. 14, No. 1, (March 2002), pp. 63–76, ISSN 1056-263X

Rogers, S. J. & Pennington, B. F. (1991). A theoretical approach to the deficits in infantile autism. *Development and Psychopathology,* Vol. 3, No. 2, (April, 1991), pp. 137–162. ISSN 0954-5794

Rogers, S. J. & Williams, J. H. G. (2006). Imitation in autism: Findings and controversies. In: *Imitation and the social mind: Autism and typical development,* S. J. Rogers, & J. H. G. Williams (Eds.), 377–309, The Guilford Press, ISBN 978-159-3853-11-2, New York, USA

Sang, B. & Miao, X. (1990). The revision of trail norm of Peabody picture vocabulary test revised (PPVT-R) In Shanghai proper [in Chinese]. *Psychological Science,* Vol. 13, No. 5, (September 1990), pp. 22–27, ISSN 1671-6981

Smith, I. M. & Bryson, S. E. (1998). Gesture imitation in autism I: Nonsymbolic postures and sequences. *Cognitive Neuropsychology,* Vol. 15, No. 6, (September 1998), pp. 747–770, ISSN 0264-3294

Stieglitz Ham, H.; Corley, M.; Rajendran, G.; Carletta, J. & Swanson, S. (2008). Imitation of meaningless gestures in individuals with Asperger syndrome and high-functioning autism. *Journal of Autism and Developmental Disorders,* Vol. 38, No. 3, (March 2008), pp. 569–573, ISSN 0162-3257

Tan, J. & Harris, P. L. (1991). Autistic children understanding seeing and wanting. *Development and Psychopathology,* Vol. 3, No. 2, (May 1991), pp. 163–174, ISSN 0954-5794

Vanvuchelen, M.; Roeyers, H. & de Weerdt, W. (2007). Nature of motor imitation problems in school-aged males with autism: How congruent are the error types? *Developmental Medicine and Child Neurology,* Vol. 49, No. 1, (January 2007), pp. 6–12, ISSN 0012-1622

Warreyn, P.; Roeyers, H.; Oelbrandt, T. & de Groote, I. (2005). What are you looking at? Joint attention and visual perspective taking in young children with autism spectrum disorder. *Journal of Developmental and Physical Disabilities,* Vol. 17, No. 1, (March 2005), pp. 55–73, ISSN 1056-263X

Whiten, A. & Brown, J. D. (1998). Imitation and the reading of other minds: Perspectives from the study of autism, normal children and non-human primates. In: *Intersubjective communication and emotion in ontogeny,* S. Bråten (Ed.), 260–280, Cambridge University Press, ISBN 978-052-1029-89-6, Cambridge, UK

Williams, J. H. G.; Whiten, A. & Singh, T. (2004). A systematic review of action imitation in autistic spectrum disorder. *Journal of Autism and Developmental Disorder,* Vol. 34, No. 3, (June 2004), pp. 285–299, ISSN 0162-3257

Yirmiya, N.; Sigman, M. & Zacks, D. (1994). Perceptual perspective-taking and seriation abilities in high-functioning children with autism. *Development and Psychopathology,* Vol. 6, No. 2, (Spring, 1994), pp. 263–272, ISSN 0954-5794

Part 10

The Education and Statistical Analysis

22

Embodied Conversational Agents for Education in Autism

Marissa Milne, Martin Luerssen, Trent Lewis,
Richard Leibbrandt and David Powers
*Flinders University,
Australia*

1. Introduction

Individuals with high-functioning autism and Asperger Syndrome find everyday social interactions very challenging due to their impairments in language, communication and social skills (Rapin & Tuchman, 2008). As their IQ scores are in the average and above range, they are typically placed into mainstream schools and face complex social interactions with their peers and educators daily. Individuals with autism have a strong preference for sameness and so often feel more comfortable interacting with computers and robots than their peers (Putnam & Chong, 2008). A computer program providing a virtual human tutor that teaches social skills can capitalise on this preference for technology, while working towards improved social competence. Such an approach is expected to provide a motivating, non-judgemental environment in which to develop social skills, while offering a tool that can be used independently by the individual, relieving pressure from carers, educators and therapists working with the learner. While little existing research has focussed on using embodied conversational agents (ECAs) for teaching children with autism, what has been done has led to promising outcomes (see Bosseler & Massaro, 2003; Tartaro & Cassell, 2006). In developing an ECA for improving social competence in children with autism, the particular needs of these individuals must be taken into account. Very importantly, this means that the tutor must present content in a way that suits the learning style and sensory needs of the learner, provide assessment tasks that are both appropriate and relevant and interpret the results of these assessments in a meaningful manner.

2. Embodied conversational agents

Embodied Conversational Agents (ECAs) are autonomous, animated virtual agents, typically human in appearance, that interact with users in real-time dialogue, recognising and performing both speech and gesture, much akin to real human-to-human interaction (Cassell, 2001). To implement a virtual embodied conversational agent requires use of a range of cutting edge technologies and significant computational power. Thus, most agents referred to as ECAs are not truly embodied in the sense of the given definition, with many relying on heuristics to give the appearance of embodiment while being computationally efficient enough to run on standard personal computers. In this chapter, we use the term 'virtual agent' to refer to a virtual entity with some autonomous decision making capabilities. Virtual agents can be broadly categorised as being 'authorable' or 'autonomous', with authorable agents requiring someone to observe the user and select from a control panel actions for the agent to take, much like a virtual puppet, and autonomous agents being self-contained and usable without such outside interaction. Examples of both authorable and autonomous agents are discussed in Section 2.2.

2.1 Virtual tutors and why they can benefit children with autism

ECAs are used in a range of applications. When used in an educational context, they are often referred to as virtual tutors or pedagogical agents. There are a multitude of reasons why virtual tutors are well suited to use with individuals with autism, including the affinity that many report having with technology (Putnam & Chong, 2008). A technology based intervention for improving social competence appeals to children with autism and allows them to progress through material at their own pace rather than being subjected to the constraints of a classroom. Nothing should aim to replace interaction with peers and others when learning about social interaction, however, an independent learning tool, such as one including a virtual tutor, can be a valuable tool in developing these complex social skills.

Autonomous virtual tutors can complement other interventions and allow learners to practice their developing skills independently, reducing pressure on those who work with the student and allowing them to focus on more complex aspects of the learner's education, while general topics are covered by the software. The anxiety connected with interacting with real humans is absent when using a virtual tutor, which can be programmed to ensure that only positive and guiding feedback is provided, rather than the criticism that peers may give. Additionally, using a virtual tutor means that the learner can practice their skills without interfering with others or learning inappropriate responses from incidental people in the environment (Kerr, 2002). Another advantage is that the virtual tutor will never get tired or impatient (Massaro, 2004) and it is available for practice at any time of the day, which may particularly suit those who experience abnormal sleep patterns (Limoges et al., 2005). Virtual tutors provide consistent feedback and behaviours, again helping to control anxiety in sufferers who feel more at ease in predictable situations (Parsons et al., 2000).

Virtual tutors can be highly customizable, allowing them to be tailored to suit an individual learner's needs. For example, for a learner who finds looking at faces uncomfortable, the tutor's face could start out cartoon-like and, as the learner becomes accustomed to it and their confidence grows, the complexity can be increased. Likewise, the lesson content can be modified to meet the learner's current level of interest and need. Being software-based, a variety of media can be incorporated into the learning material, for example photos, videos, animations and more, which can help to support generalisation of skills to novel situations.

In the context of developing nonverbal skills, animated virtual tutors can be particularly useful as they can model behaviours for the learner, such as facial expressions and gaze. This is akin to video modelling, which has had success with many individuals with autism (Marcus & Wilder, 2009; Sherer et al., 2001). Multiple tutor 'personas', with differing appearances and voices, can be used to model the behaviours, encouraging generalisation to novel situations. The flexibility and customisation that virtual tutors offer makes them a cost effective and potentially highly beneficial intervention tool.

2.2 Examples of existing virtual tutors

Several virtual tutors have been developed for a variety of educational applications, some with embodied agents. Two well-known examples that do not incorporate an embodied agent are Project LISTEN (Mostow, 2005), a reading tutor aimed at neurotypical primary school students and Carnegie Mellon's Cognitive Tutor (Ritter et al., 2007), aimed at neurotypical secondary school students who are low-achieving in mathematics. Virtual tutors with embodied agents include Wayang Outpost (Woolf et al., 2010) and iSTART (McNamara et al., 2004), which both have multiple agents and target neurotypical secondary school students, Wayang Outpost focussing on mathematics and iSTART on reading comprehension. All of these tutors are autonomous and have been empirically evaluated with very positive results; however, none were designed for or evaluated with learners with autism and all deal with domain knowledge where questions have clear-cut correct answers. Two examples of ECA tutors for children with autism are Baldi (Bosseler & Massaro., 2003), an autonomous agent originally designed to increase the vocabulary of hearing-impaired children but found to be highly successful in trials with children with autism, and Sam (Tartaro & Cassell., 2008) a virtual peer used to improve social interaction skills, including turn-taking and gaze behaviour. Unlike the previous tutors, Sam is an authorable agent and requires a researcher or the learner to select behaviours to display via a control panel. Results of the evaluations of both Sam and Baldi were positive, particularly exciting being that both interventions resulted in skills generalising to novel contexts. A month after the intervention with the embodied agent, children were still using their newly acquired vocabulary in everyday situations (Bosseler & Massaro., 2003). After interaction with Sam, children improved their scores on the Test of Early Language Development and displayed increased social behaviours, such as improved gaze (Tartaro & Cassell., 2008). The results from these evaluations are very encouraging, and it is hoped that an autonomous social skills tutor aimed at children with autism will likewise lead to improved social outcomes.

3. Teaching methods

When developing a virtual tutor, it is imperative that the teaching methods employed are carefully selected to best support the target group in achieving success with the content being taught. To make an informed decision regarding teaching social skills through software, we must first understand what methods are typically used to teach social skills and what can be achieved in a software context. In this section, a range of approaches are briefly addressed including those used by human educators and those used in software.

3.1 Approaches used by human educators for learners with autism

A range of approaches are available for teaching children with autism, and typically a variety of methods will be used. Here, focus is given to approaches with established effectiveness in addressing the needs of children with autism including the techniques of direct teaching, modelling, scenario-based learning and role playing, tutoring, exploratory and naturalistic play, conceptual mapping, and reflective practice.

3.1.1 Direct teaching

Learners with autism have difficulty learning from experience and typically need new ideas specifically taught to them. In contrast to student-directed approaches, direct teaching involves explicitly teaching skills and knowledge to learners and providing reinforcement for desired responses. Taking such a direct approach is often effective for this learner group.

Applied Behaviour Analysis (ABA) is one of the best known techniques for altering behaviours in children with autism. Developed in the 1960s by Ivar Lovaas, ABA involves a therapist providing direct consequences for behaviours, for example providing toys or food that the learner finds reinforcing when desirable behaviours occur (for details see Keenan et al., 2005). There are a number of shortcomings to this approach, one being the time consuming nature of it. It also requires trained professionals, which becomes very expensive over multiple sessions, and requires the child to interact socially in an intense fashion which can be confronting, at least initially (Hailpern, 2007). Many similar programs have been developed and the core principles of prompting and positive reinforcement are widely used in a range of settings (Reichow & Volkmar, 2010). While the ABA approach is effective for many and is widely used, there are now options available that gently prepare the child for intense social interaction before exposing them to it in all its complexity.

Another commonly used program is the Treatment and Education of Autistic and Communication Handicapped Children (TEACCH) program. Panerai et al. (2002) investigated the effectiveness of the TEACCH program as compared to a control group who were in typical classrooms with support teachers. They found that students in the experimental group made significant gains across the duration of the evaluation. TEACCH provides continuous, structured intervention, has a strong focus on the use of visual aids to make abstract concepts more concrete and provides for environmental adaptation and training in alternative communication (for more information see Panerai et al., 2002). As autism is a pervasive disorder, TEACCH is designed to be used in all aspects of the learner's life, not just school activities. The use of visual aids, adaptations in the learner's environment and the focus on providing methods of communication are all important general principles for educating children with autism.

One theory that attempts to explain some of the social difficulties that children with autism encounter suggests that they lack a fully developed 'Theory of Mind' (Leslie, 1987). This means they struggle to understand that other people have separate thoughts and feelings to their own. Carol Gray's Social Stories™, Comic Strip Conversations and the thought bubble approach used by Wellman et al. (2002) aim to address this deficit. Social Stories™ are instructional stories that explain to the learner how to behave in particular social situations. They are written following a set of guidelines developed by Carol Gray, that state that sentences should be short and explicit and accompanied by simple, informative images that support understanding. Social Stories™ are very visual and provide explicit instructions specific to the situation, suiting the common learning style of children with autism. Several studies found significant improvements to social behaviours from using Social Stories™ (Quirmback et al., 2008; Sansosti & Powell-Smith, 2008), while other studies suggest that the effectiveness of a Social Story™ is reliant on a variety of factors, including the quality of the story itself and the behaviour it is targeting (Lorimer et al., 2002; Reynhout & Carter 2006). Carol Gray has also developed Comic Strip Conversations, which are developed following similar rules to the stories, but in comic strip format. The use of these comic strips has led to similarly positive results. Wellman et al. (2002) also use a pictorial approach, but start with concrete objects and gradually work towards abstract images. Initially, Wellman et al. (2002) used dolls with cardboard thought bubbles above their heads and gradually reduced the concrete supports until images alone were sufficient for the learners. In all of these approaches focus is given to providing visual supports along with clear and concise step-by-step information, as suits the typical learning style of individuals with autism. The same guidelines can be incorporated into software developed for this user group, whenever visual, written or spoken information is presented.

3.1.2 Modelling, scenarios and role playing

Many people, those with autism included, learn better by performing a skill than they do only reading or hearing about it. Modelling desired behaviours and then having learners act them out in artificial but sufficiently natural scenarios can be highly beneficial in assisting them to perform the targeted behaviours in real situations.

The Social Use of Language Program (SULP) approach is used with small groups of students. Initially, a story addressing the target behaviour is shared, similar to the Social Stories™ approach discussed earlier. Next, adults model the desired behaviours for learners to observe before they practice the behaviours themselves and play games with their group that facilitate skills practice. Finally, activities are performed in new situations to encourage generalisation. Children who undertook the SULP intervention made significant improvements in comparison to the control group (Owens et al., 2008).

Video modelling is a technique where the learner is shown a video of themselves or a peer performing a skill that they are intended to acquire. Video modelling has many advantages. Minimal expertise and expense is required to implement the intervention, it is repeatable, it can be conducted in a standardised manner and it is portable. A recent review into best practices for social skills interventions found numerous studies supporting the effectiveness of video modelling, but suggest that video modelling alone may not be sufficient to maintain long term behavioural changes (Reichow & Volkmar, 2010). Marcus and Wilder (2009) compared the effectiveness of self-video modelling and peer-video modelling with three children with autism and found that in the self-modelling condition, all participants reached the mastery condition whereas only one did in the peer-modelling condition. Anecdotally, the authors reported that children enjoyed the self videos more and wanted to watch them even after the study was concluded. However, this study involved a text based task, not a socially oriented one. Sherer et al. (2001) compared self and video modelling for teaching conversation skills to five children and found no significant difference between the two, with some learners performing better in one condition and some in the other. Thus it seems that video modelling is an effective teaching tool, but as with most approaches, should be optimised to suit the individual learner.

3.1.3 Tutoring

One-on-one tutoring has been found to produce greater conceptual understanding and a higher level of motivation in students than traditional classroom situations, with students even progressing through topic content at a faster rate. The average performance of students when working individually with a tutor was found to be up to 2.3 standard deviations above that of students in a typical classroom situation (Chi et al., 2001; Graesser et al., 1999), providing strong evidence for the benefits that a personal tutor can provide a student.

Human tutors typically follow a set pattern. First, the tutor asks a question, to which the student provides an answer. The tutor provides immediate feedback and performs scaffolding across a number of turns with the student in order to help the learner develop their understanding. It is this process that is thought to contribute most to the increased benefits of tutoring over traditional classroom situations. Finally the tutor assesses the learner's comprehension of the taught content (Chi et al., 2001). Scaffolding is an essential aspect to learning, particularly for individuals with autism who need concepts to be explicitly taught. Scaffolding involves breaking down concepts and procedures into smaller, more manageable tasks (Jackson et al., 2010). Tutors encourage learning by helping students to master these small tasks, gradually working towards the final goal. Throughout this process the tutor monitors the learner for confusion and frustration and provides assistance where needed. This is critical as deeper and more rapid learning is achieved when misunderstandings are addressed immediately (Chi et al., 2001; Kerr, 2002; Silver & Oakes, 2001). As opposed to a classroom setting, where the learner often passively receives information from a teacher addressing the entire class simultaneously, tutoring encourages students to interact with their new knowledge through predicting, justifying, criticising and otherwise engaging with the material (Chi et al., 2001). Scaffolding is an essential educational technique that can also be implemented via a virtual tutor.

3.1.4 Explorative and naturalistic play

Less structured, naturalistic approaches that utilise innately motivating and reinforcing everyday activities and materials have been shown to support generalisation of skills in children with autism. However, care must be taken when using exploratory approaches. While they facilitate students with existing skills to expand their knowledge by encouraging them to engage in observational and experiential learning, as well as trial and error, they are typically less effective with lower skilled learners who need more structure (Conati, 2002). It is expected that learners with autism will often need more structure, due to their preference for sameness and difficulty learning without explicit explanations.

LEGO™ therapy is one example of a successful play-based therapy for children with autism. In LEGO therapy, children in small groups are given roles and must work together to build a LEGO construction. The group can also include neurotypical peers and adults. The construction task provides group members with an opportunity to practice many social behaviours including joint attention, verbal and nonverbal communication, collaboration and problem solving skills. LEGO is predictable and systematic, catering for the preference for consistency many learners with autism display. A study by Owens et al. (2008) contrasted two peer group therapies for 6-11 year olds, LEGO therapy and SULP (discussed earlier). It was found that the children in both groups outperformed the control group and those in LEGO therapy outperformed those in SULP. The researchers note that the two therapies may be best for different sets of social skills, with more research required. However, this is a good example of how naturalistic play, when guided to encourage social skills, can improve the social behaviours of children with autism.

3.1.5 Conceptual mapping

Existing work has shown that drawn and written graphic organisers, such as concept maps, can lead to strong learning gains in children with high functioning autism (Roberts & Joiner, 2007) and when used in conjunction with peer group instruction, can lead to improvements in social skills (Laushey et al., 2009). Concept maps are graphical representations of concepts, typically consisting of labelled nodes interconnected by directional arrows representing the relationships between the nodes. These are very visual and thus make clear otherwise abstract ideas and the connections between these ideas. Existing research by

Kinchin et al. (2000) suggests that concept mapping allows us to discover what students really know and how their knowledge is interconnected, rather than trying to make judgements and informed guesses. It also helps to emphasise the importance of synthesising and integrating ideas and concepts, rather than simply repeating isolated facts and expecting students to make meaning from this. It is hoped that by using concept mapping to teach social skills, it will help students understand the cause and effect relationships connected to our behaviours, rather than just being taught rigid rules, and will therefore help them apply their skills in novel situations.

3.1.6 Reflective practice

Meyer and Land (2010) recommend the use of speak aloud self-explanations, where the learner describes the ideas they are learning in their own words, as a reflective practice to enhance learning. Meta-cognitive skills and reflective practice such as this have been demonstrated to lead to better problem solving skills and the construction of deeper, more meaningful conceptual connections as they encourage students to consider the processes they use when learning instead of focussing only on the content itself (Mitrovic, 2001). Black and William (2009) also emphasise the importance of reflective practice for deep and long term learning. They suggest that reflection can assist students to make the processes they use unconsciously explicit and concrete, making them easier to understand and implement in future. It is suggested that discussion with peers and others improves the outcomes of reflective practice, in following with Vygotsky's principle that ideas are initially constructed in social interactions, and then internalised by the learner (Black & William, 2009). Additionally, challenging students to identify other situations where they can use the same thinking processes, to compare and contrast ideas and to critically analyse them can help learners improve their problem-solving and cognitive skills in general and to apply their skills to other areas.

3.2 Approaches used by virtual educators

Tartaro and Cassell (2006) and Silver and Oakes (2001) provide guidelines specifically for developing software for individuals with autism, derived from their own experiences doing so. One of the key points is the importance of scaffolding, which as we have already seen is an important general educational consideration. Herrera et al. (2008) developed a virtual environment that used an explicit scaffolding approach to gradually take children from functional interaction to imaginative play. In this manner, abstract ideas can be made concrete. Use of this software led to improved skills and evidence of generalisation. In the following sections key educational approaches taken in virtual tutoring software are briefly discussed, including static and dynamically sequenced activities, explorative activities, teaching a virtual peer, conceptual mapping and reflective practices.

3.2.1 Statically sequenced activities

Human teachers are capable of adapting their lesson sequences on the fly. This is a challenging task for a computer and so many software tutors present the learner with a set sequence of tasks. Such an approach can still lead to positive outcomes, as evidenced by The Junior Detective game (Beaumont & Sofronoff, 2008). This software was evaluated as part of a social skills group therapy program, where students were also given opportunities to role play the skills taught. This combination led to significant improvements in participants' social skills and their ability to suggest strategies to manage emotions. In a follow up session months later, participants maintained their skills (Beaumont & Sofronoff, 2008). Emotion Trainer is software designed to improve facial expression recognition in learners (Silver and Oakes 2001). It simply presents scenarios and photos as a multiple choice quiz, repeating the same section until the learner gets a certain number correct. Emotion Trainer was evaluated in a randomised control trial with eleven pairs of children with autism. One child in each pair used the software. All children who used the software improved their skills to varying degrees. Additionally, children were able to generalise their skills to a similar paper based task, but their ability to apply their skills to real social situations was not investigated (Silver & Oakes, 2001). These examples demonstrate how software, even with a static activity sequence, can be used as a step in the scaffolding process that leads to the development and maintenance of sophisticated social behaviours and problem solving skills.

Another example of statically sequenced educational software leading to positive outcomes is the social skills virtual tutor developed and evaluated in the pilot study by Milne et al. (2010). Two modules were developed, both with significant positive outcomes. In the module addressing strategies for dealing with bullying participants exhibited an average improvement of 54% from pre- to post-testing and in the conversation skills module improved on average 32%. Participants reported the experience to be an overall positive and non-threatening way to improve their social competence. Future plans for this tutor are to implement automated assessment to facilitate dynamic sequencing of learning activities.

3.2.2 Dynamically sequenced activities

To tailor experiences and activities to suit individual learning styles, a student model for the individual is required (Wittwer et al., 2010). A number of factors influence a students' learning style at a given moment, including their pre-existing preferences (for example children with high-functioning autism tend to be very visual learners) and their level of experience with the current concept. It has been shown that inexperienced and experienced learners display different styles, with inexperienced learners gaining more from following worked examples and experienced learners benefitting more from solving problems (Wittwer et al., 2010). Automated software that can determine and implement a favourable method of instruction for the student's current situation, as human educators naturally do, would be a valuable component for an autonomous tutoring system.

Shute and Towle (2003) present a generic framework for intelligent tutoring systems that takes into account individual learner differences, the learner's current state of knowledge and best practices for instruction. It is based on aptitude-treatment interaction (ATI) research, which uses a range of learner profiles to predict the user's needs and allow for lesson content and presentation to be adapted appropriately. Content presentation can range from step-by-step, highly structured instruction to exploratory presentation where the student has much control over the lesson sequence. Shute and Towle (2003) propose the use of small, self-contained and reusable components that can be combined into lesson sequences. Each unit should be limited to one of the three types of knowledge: basic knowledge (such as facts or formulas), procedural knowledge or conceptual knowledge. Sets that teach a single skill or idea can then be defined, with relationships between units influencing the sequence that tasks are presented in. This framework provides the flexibility required for a social skills tutor given the diverse range of user needs.

In the development of the Carnegie Mellon Cognitive Tutor, the Adaptive Control of Thought - Rational (ACT-R) theory of human cognition was central to its design (Anderson,

1990). The ACT-R theory, one of the more strongly supported and well established theories of human cognition, suggests that for educational materials to be most effective they must present concepts along with procedures, allowing students to understand what they are doing and why, new knowledge must build upon existing knowledge so that stronger and longer lasting connections can be made, students must be presented with a variety of opportunities to learn and practice their skills, and students' knowledge must be assessed regularly to ensure that the educational materials presented are focussing on what the individual needs, rather than providing unnecessary instruction in areas where the student is already proficient (Ritter et al., 2007). Thus, the ACT-R theory emphasises the importance of students building conceptual knowledge and cognitive skills, not just procedural skills and disconnected facts, and provides a framework to achieve this.

3.2.3 Explorative activities

Crystal Island and Gaining Face are examples of software designed to teach through a primarily explorative approach, where learners work through the software at their own pace without any goals being set explicitly by the program (Robison et al., 2009). Gaining Face provides learners with resources that they can use to investigate which nonverbal cues match with which emotions. Both detailed written information and diagrams are presented, and learners are able to compare two emotions at once. It also has an inbuilt self-test and covers a wide range of facial expressions. Crystal Island is a narrative-based learning environment that encourages self-reflection. Users explore the game environment and when they interact with game characters, they are prompted to self-report their affective state. This information is used to inform what feedback the user is given. More research is needed to evaluate the effectiveness of using an explorative approach in educational software.

3.2.4 Teaching a virtual peer

A recent approach that is gaining interest is that of a teachable agent, where the student teaches the agent as a means of learning new concepts themselves. This idea is motivated by the observation that many teachers find they have a better understanding of a concept or skill after they have taught it. In this scenario, the student takes responsibility for their own learning, a valuable life skill, and tests their understanding by trying to pass on their knowledge to a virtual agent. Betty's Brain is an example of such an agent (Blair et al., 2007). Using a concept map interface, students teach Betty concepts by adding nodes and connections between the nodes. Betty can then answer questions using the concept map and can tell students when she detects missing information. Betty's Brain has been incorporated into a number of appealing video game fronts, including a quiz where students put their virtual agents against one another to see which has learnt the concepts most thoroughly. The Betty's Brain system was tested with fifth grade students on a task requiring them to develop concept maps about river ecosystems and eight weeks later used the same systems but applied to a new topic, the land-based nitrogen cycle. Three versions of Betty's Brain were tested, one in which students taught the system, one in which they taught the system and received prompts from Betty and one in which they built a concept map for themselves but with coaching from the system. It was found that students in the first two conditions performed better than in the last, providing evidence that learning by teaching is a valuable technique (Biswas et al., 2009).

3.2.5 Conceptual mapping

Conceptual mapping, as mentioned earlier, is a beneficial and well-supported educational tool. Meyer and Land (2010) recommend conceptual mapping as a method of making misunderstandings and barriers to knowledge observable and hence manageable for educators. Many software systems exist for building concept maps, an example being Kidspiration (Inspiration Software, 2011). As a learning and formative assessment tool, concept maps can be created collaboratively between peers or the learner and educator. In software, a virtual tutor may assist the student by adding a node or reversing the direction of a connection that the student has placed. Concept maps are particularly applicable to autonomous tutoring software as, when structured appropriately, they can be automatically assessed and are valuable for use with children with autism as they are highly visual.

3.2.6 Reflective practice

As discussed earlier, reflective practice is a valuable tool that leads to richer educational outcomes and can be readily facilitated in a software context. Mitrovic (2001) conducted a study with university level computer science students to evaluate their self-assessment capabilities. Students used SQL-tutor, an application for practicing programming in the SQL database language. If students abandon a problem before completion, they are asked to specify a reason why - too hard, too easy or want a different type of question. It was found that more able students displayed better understanding of their own educational needs, rarely abandoning questions, and typically selecting wanting a different type of question as the reason when they did. Less able students abandoned many more questions, often citing that the problem was too easy even when evidence suggested otherwise. This suggests that a system that visualises interaction history and perhaps prompts students to more carefully consider the reasons for their difficulties may help to nurture meta-cognitive skills and improve educational outcomes. It has also been found that discussion with peers nurtures reflective practice, as the learner must justify and clarify their own understanding. This may appear impossible with individually-used social tutoring software, however, a possibility is to have the virtual agent play the role of a peer and activate these same learning benefits.

4. Assessment methods

Assessment is a broad term and can include assessing a student's learning style or their level of motivation. While these are relevant areas to investigate, here we focus on assessing content mastery. While many people automatically think of an "end of topic" test as a key assessment task, it is important to understand that assessment serves several purposes and must be conducted at multiple points throughout the learning process. Black and William (2009) emphasise the need for ongoing assessment, as it provides three key functions: establishing what students already know, what they need to know and determining what to do to reach these goals. If this is done regularly, the educational process is managed so that misunderstandings, repetition of already mastered content and other difficulties are minimised. To accurately assess a student's needs, the reason behind their difficulty must be determined. This could be a range of reasons, including misunderstanding the language used, the purpose of the task or the task itself, being misled by an unimportant element of the task, using ineffective strategies or simply not providing a clear or sufficiently detailed response (Black & William, 2009). It is also possible that the student does in fact have the targeted skills or knowledge mastered, but simply misunderstood what was required of them. Thus, ongoing assessment conducted in a manner that allows for effective analysis of student needs is essential for effective teaching and learning. In the context of developing a virtual social skills tutor for children with autism, ideas from two key areas must be synthesised: assessment of social skills and computer automated assessment techniques.

4.1 Assessment of social skills

There are a range of techniques used by therapists, teachers and others to assess the social skills of children, both neurotypical and those on the autistic spectrum. Here we provide a brief overview of techniques that can potentially be integrated into a virtual tutoring context, including observations, interviews, self-reports, checklists and scales.

4.1.1 Observations

Observations, both in real-time and from pre-recorded video, are often used when assessing social competency of children with autism. This is typically combined with a checklist or other rigorous method of systematically recording children's behaviours. Unfortunately, assessment through observing real social situations is not a viable technique in a computer based system intended for independent use and thus determining whether an issue reflects an underlying skill deficit or performance deficit is difficult. Having the learner interact with virtual humans in role play situations and recording learner behaviours in these situations may help to determine such differences. Another way of potentially integrating observations into a software program would be to provide a mechanism through which adults working with the learner can input their observations into the software system.

4.1.2 Interviews and self-reports

Sansosti (2010) recommends interviews as a useful assessment tool able to provide a picture of the student's needs and states that asking parents, teachers and the student themselves about the learner's typical behaviours and antecedents to desirable and undesirable behaviours will give the best overall indication of a learner's social competence. Interviews are difficult to reliably conduct in a natural, open-ended way in software; however, asking a question and allowing the interviewee to respond using multiple choice check boxes or sliding scales may be a viable option. Such a technique could also be used for self-reporting by the student, however care must be taken when using self-reports for judging social competency, as discrepancies can exist between what a student knows they should do and what they actually do. It can also be a challenge to determine whether a difficulty stems from a skills deficit or a performance deficit, however, the distinction impacts strongly on the educational tasks required to overcome the difficulty (Bellack, 1983). Carefully constructed and clearly worded questions can provide a valuable starting point for social skills education and are simple to implement in software.

4.1.3 Checklists and scales

A number of established social skills assessment tools exist, however, currently there is no one tool that is universally preferred and so only a small sample is discussed here (Gresham et al., 2010). Two examples of existing scales are the Matson Evaluation of Social Skills with Youngsters (MESSY) and the Social Skills Rating System (SSRS) (Wilkins, 2010). In both MESSY and SSRS, evaluation items are presented in Likert-style scale and forms exist for the individual, parent and teachers to respond. This process can be automated and thus incorporated into an autonomous social tutor. MESSY and SSRS are valid for use with school age children. MESSY has sound psychometric properties and has been validated for use with individuals with autism, whereas the SSRS was designed for use with neurotypical children, thus the MESSY assessment tool appears preferable for implementation in tutoring software for children with autism (Wilkins, 2010; Williams White et al., 2007).

The Behavioural Assessment of Social Interaction in Young Children (BASYC) is a recently developed tool that may be useful for high level assessment in a social tutoring application, as it is designed for teachers to administer and thus does not require psychology training, and can be used for goal planning and progress monitoring (Gillis et al., 2010). The BASYC provides a list of interactions as a guide and a checklist of behaviours, so the influence of examiner subjectivity is minimised and the task of automating assessment is simplified. The BASYC requires behavioural observation in a naturalistic, semi-structured setting so it remains to be seen whether adaptation to a software context is viable.
Measuring social competence by observing displayed behaviours has been suggested as insufficient and assessing social problem-solving and critical thinking skills, identification of a key idea and interpretation of abstract language may in fact give a better indication of a learner's social competence (Garcia Winner, 2002). The development of an assessment tool that is reliable, valid, appropriately sensitive to change, and reflects the learner's overall performance is still an active research area in itself (Gresham et al., 2010).

4.2 Computer automated assessment

Common computerised methods of evaluating concept mastery, for example achieving a particular percentage or a certain number of consecutive assessment tasks correct, are generally insufficient for providing a realistic picture of student understanding (Shute & Towle, 2003). Traditional approaches with closed-end answers, for example multiple choice questions and fill in the blanks, do not allow the learner to adequately demonstrate their knowledge. In many cases a learner can explain what behaviours are expected of them, but fail to demonstrate these behaviours in the situations we intend them to be performed in. Thus, more sophisticated methods of computer automated assessment are required.

4.2.1 Approaches based on psychology research

Sehaba et al. (2005) developed a system for use with lower functioning children with autism, to assist them to develop their motor skills and spatial and temporal understanding. The system continually collects information about user interactions with the system, including keyboard input, mouse actions and camera feed, and uses this to understand the child's behaviour and respond to it in real time. The system consists of a number of agent modules with differing roles. The User Observation Agent (UOA) records and associates user actions with terms that characterise the behaviour, notifies other agent modules when required and controls access to system resources. The UOA was inspired by the Theory of Affordances and Theory of Procedural Semantics. The Tutor Agent selects the current teaching strategy based on its knowledge of the user needs and profile, which includes preferences, general information, history and domain knowledge. It stores experiences and updates the user history and profile where applicable, making the overall system adaptable to individual needs. The Exceptions Management Agent (EMA) monitors interactions between the system and the user and makes modifications when it detects special cases needing unique treatment, for example with avoidance behaviour the EMA can intervene to engage the user again. The software employs a memory system based on Schank's Dynamic Memory Model, where Generalised Episodes are extracted from similar events, allowing for past episodes applicable to the current one to be rapidly found. System behaviours are determined using case-based reasoning, where past solutions and behaviours are applied to current ones. Preliminary evaluation of the system is said to be promising (Sehaba et al., 2005).

Gao and Xu (2007) also developed a model for assessing student needs and delivering applicable content based on Herbert A. Simon's classic decision-making process model. The four stages of the model are the intelligence stage, where information is gathered and the problem identified, the design stage where success criteria and alternative solutions are proposed, the choice stage where the best alternative is chosen and the review stage where the outcome is analysed. The review stage can help influence the intelligence stage for future decisions, improving outcomes over time and ensuring the system is adaptable. The system developed is similar to that of Sehaba et al. (2005) and is a prototype.

4.2.2 Probabilistic approaches

Probabilistic approaches can be used to identify gaps or misunderstandings in learners' knowledge that would not necessarily be found using traditional approaches to computerised assessment, while providing flexibility for dealing with the variety of answers students can provide. Shute and Towle (2003) recommend the use of Bayesian inference networks (BINs) or student mental modelling to provide probabilistic values which can be used to identify such issues within learners' knowledge. Martin and VanLehn (1995) implemented a Bayesian network approach to assess student understanding of university level physics. The network takes student behaviours as input and calculates the probability that they know and are using the appropriate rule for the given question. Bayesian networks allow for the system's hypotheses about student knowledge to be ranked rather than just classified, providing a flexible approach to assessment and better informing the sequence of tasks presented to the student.

Conati (2002) proposes a method for implementing a decision-theoretic agent, that is, one where the agent makes decisions based on maximising the likelihood of a desired outcome. In the decision-theoretic model, world states are assigned a value indicating their desirability and agents provide a value indicating their belief that the particular state will lead to the desired outcome. Using this information, actions are selected with the aim of bringing the system closer to the desired goal. Conati (2002) suggests using Decision Networks (DNs), an extension of Bayesian Networks allowing for this behaviour. By combining DNs with the Five Factor Model of Personality and the OCC model of emotion and cognition, predictions about the user's emotional state can also be made (Ortony, Clore and Collins, 1988). The OCC model explains that emotional reactions are the result of the desirability of a given outcome, the desirability being influenced by the goals and preferences of the user. Thus, if the user goals and preferences can be determined, the OCC theory provides a clear basis for predicting emotional outcomes and thus allows the agent to manage and adapt to situations taking user emotions into account. Negative emotional states are not conducive to learning and it is the job of the tutor to guide learners through these states and into a positive affective state, as human teachers do (Kort et al., 2001)

4.2.3 Latent semantic analysis

In autonomous tutoring applications, a common approach to judging student knowledge is to use latent semantic analysis (LSA) to judge the semantic similarity of student responses to a provided 'ideal' response. This is the approach taken in the iSTART tutoring system discussed earlier (Jackson et al., 2010). LSA is used for higher-level assessment and provides a judgement about the student's overall understanding. Hu and Xia (2010) also use latent semantic techniques in their automated assessment system, first performing pre-processing of student answers to generate a document of relevant words then comparing this to the similarly processed expected response. Hu and Xia (2010) found no significant difference between the grades provided by their system and those provided by teachers, suggesting that this is an educationally valid technique. Latent semantic techniques such as these rely on comparisons between blocks of text; however, as autism is partly characterised by impairment in communication and language skills, it is unreasonable to expect these children using the system to be able to provide sufficient written responses for LSA techniques to be applicable. While some form of statistical similarity measures may be applicable for assessment in this context, it will be dependent on the tasks presented.

4.2.4 Conceptual mapping

Concept mapping is a beneficial training tools that can be used for both summative and formative assessment purposes. A number of concept map types exist, and the type used should be considered carefully in relation to the desired outcome, as no dominant or recommended method currently exists (Park & Calvo, 2008). Spontaneous maps can be challenging to automatically assess, as students are free to use any terms and interconnections they wish, however, the richness of assessment is immense, with map hierarchy indicating knowledge depth (Kinchin et al., 2000; Park & Calvo 2008). One of the simplest concept maps to assess is the "fill in the blanks" style map and if terms to fit the blanks are provided, the task of assessment is simplified even further (Cline et al., 2010; Park & Calvo 2008). Concept map styles can fit anywhere between these two extremes, however, care must be taken in structuring the concept map appropriately to ensure outcomes are representative of actual knowledge and not just 'good guessing' and yet assessable in a consistent and valid way. Depending on the map type, measures may include raw and weighted counts of connections, node and proposition matching and the proportion of valid student connections over total or student-made connections (Park & Calvo 2008).

Cline et al. (2010) developed an automated system for constructing and assessing concept maps known as the Concept Mapping Tool (CMT). The CMT is a web-based tool that allows teachers to build criterion concept maps and for students to build their own maps, in the form of directed graphs, which are then compared to produce a grade. CMT uses a rule-based evaluation system to compare the nodes, direction of connections between nodes and other aspects of the map to determine a final grade. The system provides students with immediate feedback, which has been repeatedly demonstrated to be beneficial to the learning process (Cline et al., 2010). Students are presented with the central concept, concept nodes and distractor nodes based on the criterion map provided by the teacher, and are required to use these to demonstrate their knowledge by providing connections between appropriate concept nodes. This is highly structured, as students cannot provide their own terms for concepts, however, it is also flexible as distractor nodes are present and no hints are given regarding the connections between the concept nodes.

To increase the flexibility of this approach and allow students to provide their own terms, it is suggested that CMT and similar programs could be integrated with online thesauri and tools such as WordNet (Harrison et al., 2004). However, great care must be taken to maintain the correct meaning when using synonyms as many words have multiple meanings with subtle differences. This approach is taken in the automated concept map assessment program Robograder, developed by Luckie et al. (2004), and further research is looking at marking maps in a holistic manner as many human markers do. The validity of the holistic approach is questionable, as existing educational research has shown that using a rational approach when assessing concept maps provides more consistent and accurate results than holistic approaches (Cline et al., 2010). When map structure and assessment approach are carefully selected, concept mapping techniques can provide strong educational benefits to learners while being reliably and rapidly automatically assessed.

4.2.5 Scenario-based techniques

Scenario-based techniques are valuable training tools that can also be used for assessment purposes. These involve the learner working through a fictional scenario. Periodically, the system presents the student with a situation within the scenario, for which the learner selects the response they would take, and the system then informs them of the consequences of their choice. The Pedagogical Psychology Computer Assisted Assessment project (PePCAA) developed a computer automated tool to assess trainee teachers' pedagogical knowledge (Crisp & Ward, 2008). Trainee teachers were presented with scenarios based on realistic classroom situations and required to apply their problem solving skills and knowledge of best practice. The scenarios had multiple steps, with subsequent questions being based on the trainee's earlier choices. Trainees were asked to give a confidence rating and to justify their choices. Feedback for open ended tasks involved presenting the trainee with a list of points that should have been included and asking them to select which ones were covered in their answer. This scenario-based technique is constrained enough to be analysed by a computer, while providing deeper insight into learners' understanding than most traditional methods could.

In evaluation of the 'Fear Not!' software, designed to teach users how to constructively deal with bullying, Hall et al. (2009) evaluated neurotypical children's social awareness through Theory of Mind (ToM) questions. Children were presented with bullying scenarios acted by virtual characters and were asked by the 'victim' character for advice. At the conclusion of the program, children were asked to judge how different characters felt at various points throughout the story. The questions required learners to make judgements about mental states, emotions and intentions of the characters. Students were asked a combination of short-answer and multiple choice style questions, which were accompanied by visual prompts to help them remember the role-play. Hall et al. (2009) found this technique provided valuable insight into the children's social awareness of the presented situations; however, application of this insight was not discussed. Assessing social awareness is a challenge as even socially competent adults often disagree on the interpretation of a social situation, thus there is often no definite distinction between 'right' and 'wrong', with answers falling on a continuum of acceptability.

Jarrold (2007) attempts to address the problem of judging whether a learner's social assessment is valid or not in comparison to neurotypical adults' assessments by analysing adult responses and developing a rule-based system that can make judgements on par with humans. The system must allow for a wide variety of plausible social judgements, while still being able to identify inappropriate responses. This system will be used to generate Theory of Mind style questions commonly used with learners with autism. To achieve this goal, three related studies were performed. In the first study a small set of items from Teaching Children with Autism How to Mind Read (Howlin et al., 1998) were selected and neurotypical adults asked to provide responses, as is done for children with autism when judging their ToM skills. The responses were used to inform a model of adult inferences. The second study validated the outcome of the first, by asking raters to assess the believability of statements generated using the new model. The third study used data from the previous two to build a model and expert system that includes background knowledge about the world, allowing for a wider range of realistic scenarios to be generated. The expert system uses general goals and rules that can be applied to many situations, and was found to perform almost as well as humans in creating affective evaluations. Such a tool would be very valuable in both generating scenarios for learning and for assessing responses given by students in an autonomous tutoring application, as it is both flexible and automated.

5. Developing an ECA for social skills teaching

All learners have varying preferences and needs, so it is unlikely that a static, one-size-fits-all approach can be taken in any educational program. In an ECA-based social skills tutor, the ability to adapt to the learner's needs, coupled with a range of customisation capabilities, is desirable. In the existing work by Milne et al. (2010) a highly customisable ECA, Head X (Luerssen et al., 2011), is at the heart of the autonomous social skills tutoring software. This ECA can be readily customised to have varying appearances, voices and facial expressions, and work is being conducted to allow parents, teachers and others to create their own lesson units and to easily modify existing ones, for example replacing the images provided with images that the particular learner finds more stimulating or understands better. It is believed that ECA methods will offer caregivers and educators an engaging and worthwhile educational tool that can be applied to a wide range of learning requirements.

5.1 Developing software for users with autism

When designing for a particular group the traits and needs particular to that group must be thoughtfully catered for. For software users with autism, communication challenges and sensory challenges are particularly important to take into consideration, as is the need to support generalisation of skills to other contexts.

5.1.1 Sensory challenges

Sensory tolerance can be a significant issue for some individuals with autism. To minimise the risk of sensory overload, it is advisable to omit unnecessary visual or aural material. In practical terms, this means avoiding animations and sound effects unless they add significant educational value. This simplifies the interface and avoids causing distraction or fixation (Davis et al., 2005). Some sufferers have low tactile tolerance, making mouse and keyboard use challenging, while others have low aural tolerance, making speech-recognition and text-to-speech interfaces confronting (American Psychiatric Association, 2000). To meet such diverse needs, providing multiple input and output options, such as letting the user choose between speech recognition and keyboard input, can be beneficial.

5.1.2 Communication impairment

Impairment in communication skills is a significant aspect of autism. Children with autism are often visual learners, so it is recommended to provide a visual prompt, such as an icon, along with any verbal or written information given (Quill, 1997; Shane et al., 2009). Icons should be simple and clear and used only when they add meaning without contributing to sensory overload. Provision of multiple input and output modes is also important in the context of the communication difficulties. For example, expecting a learner with communication difficulties to write lengthy sentences when language skills are not the lesson focus only serves to discourage and distract from the social skills concepts being taught. Instead, point and click interfaces and other simple interaction modes may better allow students to express and explore their knowledge without communication barriers. Following this idea, written information should be in the form of simple, concise sentences. Learners with autism can miss subtle cues and become confused or distressed by ambiguity, so instructions must be in clear, simple steps and scaffolding used to move learners from basic concepts to more complex ones as their skills improve (Brown et al., 2001; Parsons et al., 2000; Silver & Oakes, 2001). Self-paced lessons are ideal as they give learners control and ownership of the learning process, lowering anxiety and helping with content retention.

5.1.3 Generalisation to novel contexts

It is not unusual for learners with autism to improve at an intervention task, but fail to exhibit the same improvements in their everyday interactions (Bosseler & Massaro, 2003; Silver & Oakes, 2001). One tactic to facilitate generalisation is to embed tasks in real world situations, allowing the learner to understand its social value. Another is to expose the learner to sufficient variety within a task, in an effort to assist with generalising to novel contexts (Bosseler and Massaro 2003). In the case of a software-based intervention, this means exposing the learner to a range of media, for example when teaching recognition of emotions, instead of using only photographs, also include videos and drawings. With an animated virtual tutor, the ability to change the tutor's appearance and voice may also be beneficial as it is analogous to having a student role play situations with a variety of peers instead of just one. This avoids the learner associating the task with a single presenter and helps them identify common elements across multiple situations. Additionally, presenting predictable tasks does not mean identical tasks, as variety encourages generalisation. Instead, tasks should follow a predictable pattern, warn the learner prior to major deviations, but be somewhat different with each presentation.

5.1.4 Supporting learning

When teaching individuals with autism, Silver and Oakes (2001) emphasise the importance of providing opportunities to repeat tasks in order to reinforce the concepts within them, and stress the need to provide timely and accurate feedback so learners understand where they went wrong, why and what to do next time. Children with autism have difficulty learning from their own mistakes, so such feedback is vital. Tartaro and Cassell (2006) and Silver and Oakes (2001) both state that providing tasks that are inherently reinforcing and rewarding leads to the richest outcomes. Tartaro and Cassell (2006) add that social skills interventions should provide a safe environment for children to practice their skills in, as neurotypical peers can be critical of the learner, and that the use of roles can help children understand the dynamics and social conventions involved in social situations. Children with autism, just like their neurotypical peers, are individuals and thus interventions should be customisable to their personal needs and skills. In the case of virtual tutors, much can be adapted to the child including, but not limited to, the appearance and voice of the virtual tutor and the content and format of the lessons provided.

5.2 Identifying a social skills curriculum

Selecting a suitable curriculum for implementation in social tutoring software is important, thus we propose a set of guidelines for this process. First, the curriculum should cover an appropriate skill set at an appropriate level of difficulty for the software's target audience.

Lower functioning and younger students are likely to require a simpler curriculum, while older and higher functioning students may require a curriculum that covers more subtle aspects of social competency. Ideally, a curriculum will be accompanied by specifically designed assessment tools. The next major consideration is that the chosen curriculum should be formally evaluated with positive experimental results. Evaluations should include data on generalisation and maintenance of taught concepts, as these are areas where many existing interventions fall short (Bosseler & Massaro, 2003; Silver & Oakes, 2001). Ideally, a curriculum developed specifically for children with autism, or at a minimum one with experimental support as to its appropriateness for this learner group, should be used. This can be challenging, as many of the social skills curricula available have been developed for neurotypical students. To remain as true to the original curriculum as possible, it is important that activities can be translated into a software context with minimal changes. Too many deviations from the original curriculum and they are no longer comparable. Finally, cultural appropriateness should be considered, thus a locally developed curriculum or one being used with success in local schools is preferred.

5.3 Training methods

When selecting training methods for implementation in social tutoring software, we propose that the approaches must meet several criteria. First, it must be possible to robustly implement the chosen training method in a software context, for example having a speech-recognition based conversation on an open-ended topic is not a viable option given the current state of the art (Schuller et al., 2009). However, having the learner speak answers to questions using key words, for example yes or no, is achievable. Another criterion to be met is that there should be existing evidence of the value of the chosen method for use with children with autism. Methods must be suited to teaching the concept or procedure at hand, for example video modelling a very abstract concept is unlikely to be effective, however, using diagrams or concept maps may be. Where possible, a range of approaches should be offered to the learner, particularly if they are having difficulty. It is often seen that where one approach fails, another will succeed.

Training methods previously discussed that have been identified as fitting the criteria for social tutoring software include modelling, including video modelling shown as media clips on-screen and tutor modelling, where the animated tutor acts out behaviours, for example facial expressions (Reichow & Volkmar, 2010). Simulated role-plays and scenarios are also possibilities, although these must be structured in such a way as to be robust to unexpected user responses and behaviours. For example, a completely open-ended scenario may not be viable, but one where the user can select from a large range of presented options is both flexible and easily implemented in software. Direct teaching is a commonly used technique in educational software; while sometimes criticised as not challenging learners to construct their own knowledge, with communication-challenged learners it is a valuable tool. To effectively use direct teaching, emphasis must be put on providing clear steps and explanations for the learner and presenting content in a scaffolded manner (Kerr, 2002). Concept maps are another valuable technique, shown to be effective in paper-based form for teaching social skills to children with autism (Laushey et al., 2009). When structured appropriately concept maps can be automatically analysed in software, are highly visual, suiting the common learning style of those with autism, and help learners to identify connections between concepts, and cause-and-effect relationships. Wherever possible, a range of these methods that meet the selection criteria should be used to teach each concept, as the variety will assist in maintaining learner interest and motivation as well as increasing the chances of exposing the learner to a task that they find best explains the new concept.

5.4 Assessment methods

In order to present students with learning tasks suited to their current needs, it is essential to continually assess their state of knowledge in a robust and accurate manner. It is often seen that students learn how to complete a task or pass a topic without gaining any deep understanding of the topic material covered (Conati, 2002). It is thus essential to assess student knowledge continually so that needed adjustments to learning tasks can be made.

It is proposed that selection criteria for assessment methods reflect the criteria proposed for training methods, in that the approach chosen must be robustly implementable in a software context, established as both valid and effective for use with children with autism, and provide an accurate picture of mastery of the targeted concept or skill. One example is the use of established social skills scales and checklists, such as MESSY or SSRS (Wilkins, 2010; Williams White et al., 2007). Some list items may be assessable as part of the software, for example sequencing and reasoning tasks, while others, such as those requiring observation, are not suitable for automatic assessment, however, the software could provide an option for these items to be manually entered. Being open-ended, management of these entries must be conducted carefully. Information from scales, checklists and observations will assist in continually updating the student model held by the software and thus used to inform decisions regarding what content to present and how to present it.

Two approaches that can be used for both training and assessment are scenario-based approaches and concept mapping (Crisp & Ward, 2008; Park & Calvo, 2008). In a software environment there is a concern that learners will be able to respond to learning activities correctly without truly understanding the ideas being taught. Scenarios and concept mapping attempt to address this. With concept maps, learners must demonstrate their understanding of relationships between concepts in a visual manner. Participants are typically provided with labelled nodes and must arrange and connect these appropriately. To accurately complete a concept map without fully understanding the concepts involved is unlikely and so concept mapping provides us with better look at a learner's understanding than many traditional assessment approaches (Park & Calvo, 2008). With scenario-based approaches, learners are presented with a situation and are required to select a response. This list can include distractor items with varying subtlety and similarity to the desired answer. Additionally, learners can be requested to select or provide a justification for their choice, and be presented with self-reflection questions (Crisp & Ward, 2008). Carefully structuring the assessment task ensures it is a flexible and rich experience, while providing suitable information for computer automation. As with the training approaches implemented, the assessment tasks chosen depend heavily on the content being taught, and similarly it is often advisable to assess content using multiple techniques. Doing so results in a more accurate picture of student understanding.

6. Conclusion

Tools to assist children with autism to develop their social competence are in demand, according to a recent survey (Putnam & Chong, 2008). ECAs as virtual tutors appear to be a promising avenue for addressing this need, as children with autism report an affinity for technology, feel more comfortable interacting with it than with peers, and existing work in similar areas is thus far producing encouraging results (Bosseler & Massaro, 2003; Tartaro & Cassell, 2006). ECAs, such as Head X (Luerssen et al., 2011), are highly customisable and, when coupled with an appropriately computerised social skills curriculum, have much potential to provide a flexible, stress-free and self-paced learning tool for individuals with high functioning autism and Asperger Syndrome. To achieve this, the social skills curriculum, training methods and assessment tools must be carefully chosen. Selection criteria for these include that they must be implementable in a computerised context, must have established effectiveness and applicability to learners with autism and must be suited to the social skills concepts targeted. Additionally, the learning style of the individual must be supported, visual learning is dominant for the target user group, and other particular challenges, such as sensory issues, must be addressed effectively. By addressing these considerations it is envisioned that a valuable ECA-based learning tool, that is one that is adaptable, motivating and suited to independent use, can be successfully developed.

7. References

American Psychiatric Association (2000). *Diagnostic and statistical manual of mental disorders: DSM-IV-TR*. Washington, DC, American Psychiatric Association.

Anderson, J.R. (1990). *The Adaptive Character of Thought*, Lawrence Erlbaum Associates, ISBN-0-8058-0419-6, Hillsdale, New Jersey.

Beaumont, R. & Sofronoff, K (2008). A multi-component social skills intervention for children with Asperger syndrome: The Junior Detective Training Program. *Journal of Child Psychology and Psychiatry*, Vol. 49, No. 7, pp. 743-753, ISSN-0021-9630.

Bellack, A. (1983). Recurrent problems in the behavioral assessment of social skill. *Behaviour Research and Therapy*, Vol. 21, No. 1, pp 29-41, ISSN- 0005-7967.

Biswas, G.; Roscoe, R.; Jeong, H. & Sulcer, B. (2009). Promoting Self-Regulated Learning Skills in Agent-based Learning Environments. *Proceedings of the 17th International Conference on Computers in Education*, Hong Kong, December 2009.

Black, P. & William, D. (2009). Developing the theory of formative assessment. *Educational Assessment, Evaluation and Accountability*, Vol. 21, No. 1, pp. 5-31, ISSN-1874-8597.

Blair, K.; Schwartz, D.; Biswas, G. & Leelawong, K. (2007). Pedagogical agents for learning by teaching: teachable agents. *Educational Technology*, Vol. 47, No. 1, pp. 56-61,.

Bosseler, A. & Massaro, D. (2003). Development and Evaluation of a Computer-Animated Tutor for Vocabulary and Language Learning in Children with Autism. *Journal of Autism and Developmental Disorders*, Vol. 33, No. 6, pp 653-672, ISSN- 1573-3432.

Brown, D. J.; Standen, P. J.; Proctor, T. & Sterland, D. (2001). Advanced Design Methodologies for the Production of Virtual Learning Environments for Use by

People with Learning Disabilities. *Presence: Teleoperators and Virtual Environments,* Vol. 10, No. 4, pp. 401-415, ISSN-1054-7460.

Cassell, J. (2001). Embodied conversational agents: representation and intelligence in user interfaces. *AI Magazine,* Vol. 22, No. 3, pp. 67-83, ISSN-0738-4602.

Chi, M.; Siler, S.; Jeong, H.; Yamauchi, T. & Hausmann, R. (2001). Learning from human tutoring. *Cognitive Science,* Vol. 25, No. 4, pp. 471-533, ISSN- 0364-0213.

Cline, B.; Brewster, C. & Fell, R. (2010). A rule-based system for automatically evaluating student concept maps. *Expert Systems with Applications,* Vol. 37, No. 3, pp. 2282-2291, ISSN-0957-4174.

Conati, C. (2002). Probabilistic Assessment of User's Emotions in Educational Games. *Applied Artificial Intelligence,* Vol. 16, No. 7, pp. 555-575, ISSN-0883-9514.

Crisp, V. and Ward, C. 2008. The development of a formative scenario-based computer assisted assessment tool in psychology for teachers: The PePCAA project. *Computers and Education.* Vol. 50, No. 4, pp. 1509-1526, ISSN-0360-1315.

Davis, M.; Robins, B.; Dautenhahn, K.; Nehaniv, C. & Powell, S. (2005). A Comparison of Interactive and Robotic Systems in Therapy and Education for Children with Autism. In *Assistive Technology: From Virtuality to Reality.* A. Pruski and H. Knops (Eds.), pp. 353-357, IOS Press, ISBN-158-6035-43-6, Oxford.

Gao, S. & Xu, D. (2007). Intelligent agent-assisted decision support for personalised virtual learning environment. *The 9th International DSI and the 12th Asisa-Pacific DSI Joint Meeting,* pp. 1-11, ISSN-1539-1191, Bangkok, Thailand, July 11-15, 2010.

Garcia Winner, M. (2002). Assessment of Social Skills for Students with Asperger Syndrome and High-Functioning Autism. *Assessment for Effective Intervention,* Vol 27, No. 1-2, pp. 73-80, ISSN-1534-5084.

Gillis, J., M.; Callahan, E. H. & Romanczyk, R. G. (2010). Assessment of social behavior in children with autism: The development of the Behavioral Assessment of Social Interactions in Young Children. *Research in Autism Spectrum Disorders,* Vol. 5, No. 1, pp. 351-360, ISSN-1750-9467.

Graesser, A.; Wiemer-Hastings, K.; Wiemer-Hastings, P. & Kreuz, R. (1999). AutoTutor: A simulation of a human tutor. *Cognitive Systems Research,* Vol. 1, No. 1, pp. 35-51.

Gresham, F.; Cook, C.; Collins, T.; Dart, E.; Rasetshwane, K.; Truelson, E. & Grant, S. (2010) Developing a Change-Sensitive Brief Behaviour Rating Scale as a Progress Monitoring Tool for Social Behaviour - An Example Using the Social Skills Rating System - Teacher Form, *School Psychology Review,* Vol. 39, No. 3, pp. 364-379.

Hailpern, J. (2007). Encouraging speech and vocalization in children with autistic spectrum disorder. *SIGACCESS Accessibility and Computing,* Vol. 89, pp. 47-52.

Hall, L.; Woods, S. & Hall, M. (2009). Lessons Learned Using Theory of Mind Methods to Investigate User Social Awareness in Virtual Role-Play. *Human Technology,* Vol. 5, No. 1, pp. 68-89, ISSN-1795-6889.

Harrison, S.; Wallace, J. (2004). C-TOOLS Automated Grading for Online Concept Maps Works Well with a Little Help from "WORDNET", *Proceedings of the First International Conference on Concept Mapping,* pp. 211-214, A. J. Cañas, J. D. Novak, & F. M. González (Eds.), Pamplona, Spain 2004.

Herrera, G.; Alcantud, F.; Jordan, R.; Blanquer, A.; Labajo, G. & De Pablo, C. (2008). Development of symbolic play through the use of virtual reality tools in children with autistic spectrum disorders: Two case studies. *Autism*, Vol. 12, No. 2, pp. 143-157, ISSN-1362-3613.

Howlin, P.; Baron-Cohen, S. & Hadwin, J. (1999). *Teaching children with autism to mind-read : a practical guide for teachers and parents*. John Wiley & Sons, Inc, ISBN-978-0-471-97623-3, Bristol.

Hu, X. & Xia, H. (2010). Automated Assessment System for Subjective Questions Based on LSI, *Third International Symposium on Intelligent Information Technology and Security Informatics*, pp. 250-254, ISBN-978-1-4244-6730-3, Jinggangshan, China, April 2010.

Inspiration Software (2011). Kidspiration, 8.3.11, Available from: http://www.inspiration.com/

Jackson, G.; Guess, R. & McNamara, D. (2010). Assessing cognitively complex strategy use in an untrained domain. *Topics in Cognitive Science*, Vol. 2, No. 1, pp. 127-137.

Jarrold, W. L. (2007). Treating Autism with the Help of Artificial Intelligence: A Value Proposition. *Proceedings of Agent-Based Systems for Human Learning and Entertainment Workshop at AAMAS*, Menlo Park, CA, USA.

Keenan, M.; Kerr, K. & Dillenburger, K. (2005). *Parents' Education as Autism Therapists*. Jessica Kingsley Publishers, ISBN-978-1-85302-778-9, Great Britain.

Kerr, S. J. (2002). Scaffolding: design issues in single & collaborative virtual environments for social skills learning. *Proceedings of the Workshop on Virtual Environments 2002*, pp. 81-92, ISBN-1581-135-35-1, Barcelona, Spain, May 2002.

Kinchin, I.; Hay, D. & Adams, A. (2000). How a qualitative approach to concept map analysis can be used to aid learning by illustrating patterns of conceptual development. *Educational Research*, Vol. 42, No. 1, pp. 43-57, ISSN-0013-1881.

Kort, B.; Reilly, R. & Picard, R.W. (2001). An affective model of interplay between emotions and learning: Reengineering educational pedagogy-building a learning companion, *Proceedings of the IEEE International Conference on Advanced Learning Technology: Issues, Achievements and Challenges*, pp. 43-48. ISBN- 0-7695-1013-2, Madison, USA, August 6-8, 2001.

Laushey, K.; Heflin, L.; Alberto P.A.; Fredrick L. & Shippen M. (2009). Concept Mastery Routines to Teach Social Skills to Elementary Children with High Functioning Autism. *Journal of Autism and Developmental Disorders*, Vol. 39, No. 10, pp. 1435-1448, ISSN- 0162-3257.

Leslie, A. (1987). Pretense and Representation: The Origins of "Theory of Mind". *Psychological Review*, Vol. 94, No. 4, pp. 15, ISSN-0033295X.

Limoges, E.; Mottron, L.; Bolduc, C.; Berthiaume, C. & Godbout, R. (2005). Atypical sleep architecture and the autism phenotype. *Brain*, Vol. 128, No. 5, pp. 1049-1061.

Lorimer, P.; Simpson, R.; Smith Myles, B. & Ganz, J. (2002). The Use of Social Stories as a Preventative Behavioral Intervention in a Home Setting with a Child with Autism. *Journal of Positive Behavior Interventions*, Vol. 4, No. 1, pp. 53-60, ISSN-1098-3007.

Luckie, D.; Harrison, S. & Ebert-May, D. (2004). *Introduction to C-Tools: Concept mapping tools for online learning*, pp. 261-264, A. J. Cañas, J. D. Novak, & F. M. González (Eds.), Pamplona, Spain 2004.

Luerssen, M.; Lewis, T. & Powers, D. (2011). Head X: Customizable Audiovisual Synthesis for a Multi-purpose Virtual Head, *AI 2010: Advances in Artificial Intelligence*, Vol. 6464, pp. 486-496, ISSN-0302-9743.

Marcus, A. & Wilder, D. (2009). A comparison of peer video modeling and self video modeling to teach textual responses in children with autism. *Journal of applied behavior analysis*, Vol. 42, No. 2, pp. 335-341, ISSN-0021-8855.

Martin, J. & VanLehn, K. (1995). Student assessment using Bayesian nets. *International Journal of Human Computer Studies*, Vol. 42, No. 6, pp. 575-592, ISSN-1071-5819.

Massaro, D. (2004). Symbiotic Value of an Embodied Agent in Language Learning. *Proceedings of the 37th Hawaii International Conference on System Sciences*, pp. 1-10.

McNamara, D.; Levinstein, I. & Boonthum, C. (2004). iSTART: Interactive strategy training for active reading and thinking. *Behavior Research Methods, Instruments, & Computers*, Vol. 36, No. 2, pp 222-233, ISSN-0743-3808.

Meyer, J. & Land, R. (2010). Threshold concepts and troublesome knowledge: Dynamics of assessment, pp. 61-79, ISBN-978-94-6091-207-8, *Proceedings of the 2nd International Conference on Threshold Concepts*, Kingston, Ontario, Canada; June 25 - 27 2008.

Milne, M.; Luerssen, M.H.; Lewis, T.W.; Leibbrandt, R.E. & Powers, D.M., (2010). Development of a Virtual Agent Based Social Tutor for Children with Autism Spectrum Disorders. *Proceedings of the International Joint Conference on Neural Networks*, pp. 1555-1563, ISBN-978-1-4244-6916-1, Barcelona, Spain, July 2010.

Mitrovic, A. (2001). Investigating students' self-assessment skills. *User Modeling*, No. 2109, pp. 247-250, ISSN-0302-9743.

Mostow, J. (2005). Summary, In *Project LISTEN: A Reading Tutor that Listens*. 2.08.2010, Available from http://www.cs.cmu.edu/~listen/research.html.

Ortony, A.; Clore, G. & Collins, A. (1988). *The Cognitive Structure of Emotions*, Cambridge University Press, ISBN-0521353645, Cambridge.

Owens, G.; Granader, Y.; Humphrey, A. & Baron-Cohen, S. (2008). LEGO® Therapy and the Social Use of Language Programme: An Evaluation of Two Social Skills Interventions for Children with High Functioning Autism and Asperger Syndrome. *Journal of Autism and Developmental Disorders*, Vol. 38, No. 10, pp. 1944-1957, ISSN-0162-3257.

Panerai, S.; Ferrante, L. & Zingale, M. (2002). Benefits of the Treatment and Education of Autistic and Communication Handicapped Children (TEACCH) programme as compared with a non-specific approach. *Journal of Intellectual Disability Research*, Vol. 46, No. 4, pp. 318-327, ISSN-0964-2633.

Park, U. & Calvo, R. (2008). Automatic concept map scoring framework using the semantic web technologies. *Eighth IEEE International Conference on Advanced Learning Technologies*, pp. 238–240, ISBN-978-0-7695-3167-0, Santander, Cantabria, July 2008.

Parsons, S.; Beardon, L.; Neale, H.; Reynard, G.; Eastgate, R.; Wilson, J.; Cobb, S.; Benford, S.; Mitchell, P. & Hopkins, E. (2000). Development of social skills amongst adults with Asperger's Syndrome using virtual environments. In *Proceedings of the 3rd International Conference on Disability, Virtual Reality and Associated Technologies*, pp. 163-170, ISBN-0-7049-11-42, Sardinia Italy, September 2000.

Putnam, C. & Chong, L. (2008). Software and technologies designed for people with autism: what do users want? *Proceedings of the 10th International ACM SIGACCESS Conference on Computers and accessibility*, pp. 3-10, ISBN-9781605605630, Halifax, Nova Scotia, Canada, ACM.

Quill, K. A. (1997). Instructional Considerations for Young Children with Autism: The Rationale for Visually Cued Instruction. *Journal of Autism and Developmental Disorders*, Vol. 27, No. 6, pp. 697-714, ISSN-0162-3257.

Quirmbach, L.; Lincoln, A.; Feinberg-Gizzo, M.; Ingersoll, B. & Andrews, S. (2008). Social Stories: Mechanisms of Effectiveness in Increasing Game Play Skills in Children Diagnosed with Autism Spectrum Disorder Using a Pretest Posttest Repeated Measures Randomized Control Group Design. *Journal of Autism and Developmental Disorders*, Vol. 39, No. 2, pp. 299-321, ISSN-0162-3257.

Rapin, I. & Tuchman, R. (2008). Autism: Definition, Neurobiology, Screening, Diagnosis. *Pediatric Clinics of North America*, Vol. 55, No. 5, pp. 1129-1146, ISSN-0031-3955.

Reichow, B. & Volkmar, F. (2010). Social Skills Interventions for Individuals with Autism: Evaluation for Evidence-Based Practices within a Best Evidence Synthesis Framework. *Journal of Autism and Developmental Disorders*, Vol. 40, No. 2, pp. 149-166, ISSN-0162-3257.

Reynhout, G. & Carter, M. (2006). Social Stories™ for Children with Disabilities. *Journal of Autism and Developmental Disorders*, Vol. 36, No. 4, pp. 445-469, ISSN-0162-3257.

Ritter, S.; Anderson, J.; Koedinger, K. & Corbett, A. (2007). Cognitive Tutor: Applied research in mathematics education. *Psychonomic bulletin & review*, Vol. 14, No. 2, pp. 249-255, ISSN-1069-9384.

Roberts, V. & Joiner, R. (2007). Investigating the efficacy of concept mapping with pupils with autistic spectrum disorder. *British Journal of Special Education*, Vol. 34, No. 3, pp. 127-135, ISSN-0952-3383.

Robison, J.; McQuiggan, S. & Lester, J. (2009). Modeling Task-Based vs. Affect-based Feedback Behavior in Pedagogical Agents: *An Inductive Approach. International conference on artificial intelligence in education*, pp. 25-32, ISBN-9781607500285, Amsterdam; Lancaster, July 2009.

Sansosti, F. (2010). Teaching social skills to children with autism spectrum disorders using tiers of support: A guide for school-based professionals. *Psychology in the Schools*, Vol. 47, No. 3, pp. 257-281, ISSN-0033-3085.

Sansosti, F. J. & Powell-Smith, K. A. (2008). Using Computer-Presented Social Stories and Video Models to Increase the Social Communication Skills of Children With High-

Functioning Autism Spectrum Disorders. *Journal of Positive Behavior Interventions*, Vol. 10, No. 3, pp. 162-178, ISSN-1098-3007.

Schuller, B.; Wöllmer, M.; Moosmayer, T. & Rigoll, G. (2009). Recognition of noisy speech: a comparative survey of robust model architecture and feature enhancement. *EURASIP Journal on Audio, Speech, and Music Processing*, Vol. 2009, pp. 1-17, ISSN-1687-4714.

Sehaba, K.; Estraillier, P. & Lambert, D. (2005). Interactive Educational Games for Autistic Children with Agent-Based System. *4th International Conference on Entertainment Computing*, pp. 422-432, ISBN-3540290346, Sanda, Japan, September 19-21 2005.

Shane, H.; O'Brien, M. & Sorce, M. (2009). Use of a Visual Graphic Language System to Support Communication for Persons on the Autism Spectrum. *Perspectives on Augmentative and Alternative Communication*, Vol. 18, No. 4, pp. 130-136,.

Sherer, M.; Pierce, K.; Paredes, S.; Kisacky, K.; Ingersoll, B. & Schreibman, L. (2001). Enhancing Conversation Skills in Children with Autism Via Video Technology: Which Is Better, "Self" or "Other" as a Model? *Behavior Modification*, Vol. 25, No. 1, pp. 140, ISSN- 1552-4167.

Shute, V. & B. Towle (2003). Adaptive e-learning. *Educational Psychologist*, Vol. 38, No. 2. pp. 105-114, ISSN-0046-1520.

Silver, M. & P. Oakes (2001). Evaluation of a New Computer Intervention to Teach People with Autism or Asperger Syndrome to Recognize and Predict Emotions in Others. *Autism*, Vol. 5, No. 3, pp. 299-316, ISSN-1362-3613.

Tartaro, A. & J. Cassell (2006). Authorable Virtual Peers for Autism Spectrum Disorders. *Proceedings of the 17th European Conference on Artificial Intelligence*, ISBN-978-1-59593-642-4, Riva del Garda, Italy.

Tartaro, A. & J. Cassell (2008). Playing with Virtual Peers: Bootstrapping Contingent Discourse in Children with Autism. *Proceedings of International Conference of the Learning Sciences*. Utrecht, Netherlands, June 24-28 2008.

Wellman, H. M.; Baron-Cohen, S.; Caswell, R.; Gomez, J.; Swettenham, J.; Toye, E. & Lagattuta, K. (2002). Thought-Bubbles Help Children with Autism Acquire an Alternative to a Theory of Mind. *Autism*, Vol. 6, No. 4, pp. 343-363, ISSN-1362-3613.

Wilkins, J. (2010). The Relationship Between Social Skills and Challenging Behaviors in Children with Autism Spectrum Disorders, PhD Thesis, Louisiana State University.

Williams White, S., Koenig, K., & Scahill, L. (2007). Social skills development in children with autism spectrum disorders: A review of the intervention research. *Journal of Autism and Developmental Disorders*, Vol. 37, No. 10, pp. 1858-1868, ISSN-0162-3257.

Wittwer, J.; Nückles, M. & Renkl, A. (2010). Using a Diagnosis-Based Approach to Individualize Instructional Explanations in Computer-Mediated Communication. *Educational Psychology Review*, Vol. 22, No. 1, pp. 9-23, ISSN-1040-726X.

Woolf, B.; Arroyo, I.; Muldner, K.; Burleson, W.; Cooper, D.; Dolan, R. & Christopherson, R. (2010). The Effect of Motivational Learning Companions on Low Achieving Students and Students with Disabilities. *Intelligent Tutoring Systems*, Vo. 6094, pp. 327-337.

23

Statistical Analysis of Textual Data from Corpora of Written Communication – New Results from an Italian Interdisciplinary Research Program (EASIEST)

Lorenzo Bernardi and Arjuna Tuzzi
University of Padua
Italy

1. Introduction

Autism spectrum disorder (ASD) is a form of pervasive developmental disorder characterized by complex communication needs and early onset. The "triad" of symptoms for diagnosing ASD includes three areas: (a) social interaction; (b) language and communication; (c) behavior, activities, and interests (American Psychiatric Association, 2000). Complex qualitative and quantitative language and communication needs are acknowledged among the specific characteristics of this disorder, though defining and identifying these "needs" often proves a difficult task (Boucher, 2003; Sikora, Hartley, Mccoy, Gerrard-Morris, & Dill, 2008; Snyder, Miller, & Stein, 2008). Enhancing effective communication in everyday life and investigating new ways to help individuals with ASD (IWA) to communicate are fundamental issues (Tager-Flusberg & Caronna, 2007; Ostryn, 2008; Koegel & Brown, 2007) and, more in general, recent results (Rapin & Tuchman, 2008) stress the growing need for special services and treatments for an increasing number of children (and adults).

1.1 The EASIEST project

The EASIEST project ("Espressione Autistica. Studio Interdisciplinare con Elaborazione Statistico-Testuale" [*Autistic expression. An interdisciplinary study based on statistical and textual analysis*]) is an Italian interdisciplinary research program (Bernardi, 2008) aiming to study the linguistic features of texts written by IWA and facilitators (without disabilities).

The acronym giving the project its name refers to three terms coinciding with the three research areas characterizing the study, i.e.

1. *Autistic expression*: the program focuses on a particular form of communication used by IWA, achieved by means of a dedicated commitment to facilitated communication (FC), a method adopted and taught by specially-trained personnel in the course of a lengthy process requiring a great deal of effort. We are therefore dealing with a practice that is useful for taking action on just one of the three conditions that have to be met to establish a diagnosis of ASD, i.e. the qualitative impairment of an individual's capacity for communication and imagination (Wing & Gould, 1979);

2. *Statistical and textual analysis*: methodological advances made in recent years in the statistical methods for analyzing qualitative materials (and text in particular) afford new opportunities for studying materials generated in the FC setting; in many ways, this provides the load-bearing support for any analyses conducted using complementary disciplinary approaches in this project;
3. *Interdisciplinary study*: expertise in analytical methods is not enough in itself to ensure that the analyses of texts generated in the FC setting are relevant, or to suggest at least one roughly appropriate interpretation of the results that does not seem either pointless or even misleading; hence our recourse to different types of expert, who contributed to defining the theoretical grounds for our research, and subsequently prompted and arranged the considerations that emerged in the appropriate and pertinent scientific contexts (linguistics, neuropsychiatry, psychology, sociology, statistics, text mining and computer-aided text processing).

In this frame, the EASIEST research group made every effort to develop a plan of action that would lead to the production of consistent quantitative references and could thus serve as a precious archive, also providing materials relating to more or less lengthy periods of participation in FC schemes. The general founding assumption was as follows: with adequate (albeit laborious) training on the shared use of a "mechanical" medium (the computer), IWA can unleash their often only potential expressive skills to best effect, somehow "formalizing", or rather "encoding" the very core of their way of thinking.

The analysis focused along three lines:

- first of all, to ensure that we started by building grounds as solid as possible for the subsequent stages, we needed to prepare a lexical analysis designed to bring out the frequency and nature of the words and compounds (multiwords) contained in the texts examined: this statistical approach precedes consequential qualitative lines of research and, to some degree, it provides the necessary input and it can orient subsequent syntactic and semantic assessments;
- to examine the syntactic structure of expressions written by IWA, i.e. to start identifying and recognizing any regularities in sentence structure for comparison with that of their respective facilitators, and also more in general with the structure of their language (Italian in this case), and written language in particular;
- to examine the semantic specificities of their language, pinpointing any regularities in the frequent use of metaphor (often referring to concrete elements) seen in the more "creative" texts.

To ensure the best conditions for managing these research goals, several methodological coordinates had to be imposed on the process for producing the materials to analyze, i.e.

i. a large number of subjects had to be considered;
ii. a large amount of material had to be collected;
iii. several centers needed to be involved, where FC is a well-established and accredited practice;
iv. it was essential to rely on expert, habitual facilitators;
v. the IWA involved had to have reached a good level of independence;
vi. the IWA-facilitator relationship had to be demonstrable and well-established, and capable of generating a good degree of fluidity in the written word;
vii. steps had to be taken so that each pair would produce texts meeting the minimum requirements in terms of quality (variety of content and topics considered) and quantity

(volume of pages and words), while the material generated by particularly fecund subjects had to be contained;

viii. it was advisable for more than one facilitator to work with the same IWA, partly to check for any influence of the former, and partly to ascertain the expressive stability of the latter even in the presence of several facilitators;

ix. subjects and materials useful for longitudinal studies should also be included.

With these aims and behavioral rules, the work plan were characterized by:

a. reference to four accredited centers;

b. the collection of texts from three different groups of subjects, giving rise to three corresponding corpora:

b1) 13 subjects with a known history of FC training, from the introductory phase to full and independent control of the method; these subjects were supported by 33 facilitators and the mass of material available for analysis consisted of approximately 400 pages, corresponding to 130,142 word tokens;

b2) 37 subjects who had reached a high level of independence, whose texts were collected during the course of the present project under conditions of "reduced facilitation" (beyond arm/shoulder level) with at least three different facilitators. In all, 92 facilitators were involved (some of them worked with more than one IWA) and about 900 pages were generated, corresponding to 290,496 word tokens;

b3) a case-control experiment was arranged, involving 6 IWA and 6 individuals without disabilities, comparing their performance in a given essay. The corpus obtained in this case was naturally much more limited (14 pages containing 4,360 word tokens).

c. In short, the project's methodological coordinates can be summarized as follows:

c1) construction of a very large database;

c2) three analytical approaches, i.e.

c2.1) transversal on 37 cases;

c2.2) longitudinal on 13 cases;

c2.3) experimental on 6 cases versus 6 controls;

and more specifically, from the point of view of the knowledge goals:

c3) a study on the stylistic and lexical characteristics of homogeneous groups:

c3.1)IWA versus facilitators;

c3.2)IWA versus controls;

c4) a study on particular individual traits:

c4.1) chronological analysis of language development;

c4.2) comparison between texts written by the same IWA with different facilitators.

Finally, to achieve these study goals, different types of text were used, differing in nature and origin, i.e. the texts were drawn from:

a. conversations in daily life;

b. questioning about school-related experiences and topics;

c. training interviews;

d. text composition proper (essays, prose, etc.).

In conclusion, the fundamental goals of the research project are briefly recalled below:

- *on the problem of using written language*: to identify the semantic and syntactic characteristics of texts produced by IWA and by their facilitators;

- *on the learning problem*: to analyze the temporal development of linguistic structures from the point of view of learning theories;
- *on the problem of the statistical method adopted*: to ascertain the applicability of lexical-textual methods and the interpretative capacity of the indicators derivable therefrom;
- *on the debate concerning the authenticity of texts generated using FC*: to retrace the issues in the discussion between convinced supporters of its utility as a method capable of facilitating the free expression of IWA, on the one hand, and scholars who firmly deny its efficacy or even its appropriateness), sometimes based on solid experimental assessment methods.

1.2 Facilitated communication

Facilitated communication (FC) is a form of augmentative and alternative communication that first attracted attention in Australia at the end of the 1970s, thanks to Rosemary Crossley (Crossley & McDonald, 1984); it was introduced in the United States by Douglas Biklen (1993), who helped popularize the method. Proponents of FC (Crossley, 1997; Crossley & Remington-Gurney, 1992) claim that it is an alternative means of expression for people with complex communication needs who are unable to speak (or whose speech is seriously limited) and cannot point reliably owing to developmental disabilities or other significant neuromotor impairments. FC entails learning to communicate by typing on a keyboard and requires a combination of physical and emotional support measures. People resorting to FC may need to be supported in various ways: to contain their emotional reactions, coordinate their movements (pointing), help them focus on activities, etc.

Support is provided according to the specific needs of individual FC users and depends on habits they develop in years of practice. The person providing such support is called a facilitator and may be a teacher, a professional trainer, a relative, a friend, etc. Facilitators provide emotional support because they are trained to manage possible reactions from the individuals with whom they write. They also encourage and stimulate FC users both orally and in writing. Facilitators may touch different parts of the FC user's body. During the first sessions, the facilitator's hand usually touches the FC user's hand or wrist, then moves up towards the elbow, upper arm, shoulder, and so on. This upward movement depends on how well FC users can type unassisted. The facilitator's aim is to encourage them to write as autonomously as possible, sometimes up until they can do so alone (Rossetti, Ashby, Arndt, Chadwick, & Kasahara, 2008). Both facilitators and other people who use FC need extensive, individualized training and the support of professional trainers before they can start using the method. FC can be used by people with a variety of communication needs, and many IWA are candidates for this augmentative and alternative form of communication.

1.3 The debate on FC

FC has met with sharp criticism and its usefulness as an alternative means of communication is still an extremely controversial issue. Researchers have yet to agree on a validation method and the scientific controversy on the validity of FC remains unsettled (Beck & Pirovano, 1996; Biklen & Cardinal, 1997; Bomba, O'Donnell, Markowitz, & Holmes, 1996; Braman, Brady, Linehan, & Williams, 1995; Jacobson, Mulick, & Schwartz, 1995; Montee, Miltenberger, & Wittrock, 1995; Mostert, 2001; Probst, 2005; Sbalchiero & Neresini, 2008; Sheehan & Matuozzi, 1996; Simpson & Myles, 1995; Weiss, Wagner, & Bauman, 1996). Biklen and Cardinal (1997) attempted to explain why some controlled studies support FC while others do not. According to Biklen (2005), naturalistic settings foster positive results, while more controlled settings lead to negative results. Sbalchiero and Neresini (2008) endeavored to pinpoint the basic elements of this scientific controversy from the viewpoint of the sociology of science.

FC has presented scholars with an ethical dilemma: either to run the risk of denying FC users the right to communicate, or to adopt a method that has yet to be fully validated by scientific studies. The crucial issue concerns the number of individuals with complex communication needs who may or may not benefit from an alternative means of communication. Given the fundamental role of expert practitioners in providing people with treatment, rehabilitation and education for the life-long management of their disorders, some proponents of this method - rather than focusing on the scientific controversy over the validity of FC - stress the importance of "how", "why" and "when" FC training should be implemented, identifying "best practices" and developing practice guidelines (Calculator, 1999; Duchan, 1993; Duchan, 1999; Duchan, Calculator, Sonnenmeier, Diehl, & Cumley, 2001; Koegel, 2000).

Since the facilitator's support is liable to influence the movements and pointing of an IWA, whether it is the facilitator who is communicating or the IWA remains debatable (for a review, cfr. Jacobson et al. 1995; Mostert, 2001). The issue of authorship attribution in the context of written conversations produced during FC sessions derives from two contrasting views: communication may be the outcome of a facilitator's cueing (Green, 1994, Wheeler, Jacobson, Paglieri, & Schwartz, 1993), or it may be the genuine, intentional output of an IWA; for the latter to be true, the IWA must presumably have the necessary competence (Biklen & Burke, 2006; Biklen, Saha, & Kliewer, 1995; Cardinal, Hanson, & Wakeham, 1996; Mirenda, 2008). Controlled studies have established that the facilitator does have an influence (Mostert, 2001) and proponents of FC have acknowledged that cueing (be it deliberate or subconscious) does occur, but controlled studies have also established authentic authorship (Weiss et al. 1996; Cardinal et al. 1996). Certain texts produced in specific settings prove genuine, even though the same person may be influenced by the facilitator in different settings (Emerson, Grayson, & Griffiths, 2001). Further studies and observation of cases of independent typing demonstrated that FC may be effective, but it is impossible to establish how often and in which cases (Beukelman & Mirenda, 1998; Mirenda & Beukelman, 2006). Based on the analysis of texts retrieved on-line and written by IWA, Davidson (2008) even goes so far as to take authorship for granted and claim the existence of distinctive autistic styles of communication as part of an emerging "autistic culture".

Few studies aiming to solve the authorship issue have focused directly on texts written during FC sessions (Niemi & Kärnä-Lin, 2002; Niemi & Kärnä-Lin, 2003; Saloviita & Sariola, 2003; Scopesi, Zanobini, & Cresci, 2003; Zanobini & Scopesi, 2001), and few considered large corpora (i.e. exceeding a hundred thousand words) and several individuals. The studies conducted so far nonetheless stress the need to identify the distinctive linguistic (lexical and morpho-syntactical) features of texts written by IWA, and they tend to support the case for their authenticity.

1.4 Ongoing research

The EASIEST Project collected large corpora of texts written at four accredited FC centers in Italy. It is of paramount importance to consider a large body of words, i.e. a large corpus of texts, in order to analyze the distinctive language features of a group of writers. Written conversations retrieved from material produced during FC sessions enable researchers to collect large corpora of texts written by several individuals. The fact that the research is conducted in a setting of spontaneous written conversation and a semi-controlled environment is a major advantage (Rutter, 2005; Tager-Flusberg, 2004).

A recent study developed in the frame of the EASIEST Project had already shown that the lexis used by IWA only partially overlapped with that of facilitators (Tuzzi, 2009). When lexical richness, i.e. the number of different words (NDW) (Duràn, Malvern, Richards, & Chipere, 2004; McKee, Malvern, & Richards, 2000; Watkins, Kelly, & Harbers, 1995) was measured, it emerged that the group including IWA used more different words and therefore had a greater lexical richness than the group of facilitators (Tuzzi, 2009).

The present study was designed as a natural continuation of the mainstrain EASIEST research, involving a detailed analysis of several specific lexical features of a large corpus of texts and measuring to what extent the words used by IWA differ from those used by facilitators. A novel approach was used, based on the concept of intertextual distance, i.e. the strategy chosen to implement text clustering (texts that are lexically homogeneous within clusters and non-homogeneous between clusters). The aim of this study was to show that even mere quantitative lexical data (word frequency) can draw a clear distinction between texts written by IWA and those written by facilitators. We also expected to identify two distinct clusters that could support text authorship.

2. Method: Textual data analysis

The main focus of this further study was a quantitative analysis of textual data from a corpus of texts written during FC sessions by IWA and facilitators (without disabilities). The aim was to analyze the writers' lexicon and contribute to the debate on the authorship issue. The analysis was conducted on 91 texts comprising 1,000 words sampled from the corpus of written conversations produced by 37 IWA who had reached a high level of independence. The ideal situation would include only IWA who had already mastered independent typing, but they are very rare and we preferred to involve a large number of individuals.

2.1 Participants

The 37 IWA involved in this study were diagnosed by neuropsychiatrists and assessed according to the DSM-IV-TR (2000) at the four accredited FC centers involved in the project. The group included 29 males and 8 females (table 1). At the beginning of the EASIEST project their age ranged between 9 and 32 years; 59.4% of the IWA were between 11 and 20 years old. The majority had started using FC by the age of 15 (84.8%), 35.1% by the age of 7. Their verbal communication was absent (21 out of 37) or severely impaired (16 out of 37). The group included no individuals diagnosed with Asperger syndrome or high-functioning autism.

All these IWA had reached a good degree of self-sufficiency in written communication and were capable of writing with little facilitation, i.e. the support provided by facilitators was limited to contact between the facilitator's hand and the individual's upper arm, shoulder, neck, head, back or leg; contact was intermittent, occasional or absent in some cases. The facilitators involved were professionals, supervisors, teachers or parents specifically trained in this technique at the four accredited Italian FC centers. For each IWA there were three different facilitators (typically a professional facilitator, a parent and a teacher), for a total of 92 (some professional facilitators worked with more than one IWA at the same center). All IWA involved in the EASIEST project had used this communication method regularly in different settings (with teachers at school, with parents at home, etc.).

IWA and facilitator selection was based on their "familiarity" with FC with a view to obtaining texts that would be satisfactory in terms of their length and complexity, and to reducing the "noise" in the initial training period (facilitators have to learn to manage physical and emotional reactions; IWA are unfamiliar with keyboards; both need to refine their coordination, etc.).

Variable	n	%
Gender		
Male	29	78.4
Female	8	21.6
Age (years)		
Up to 10	3	8.1
11 to 15	11	29.7
16 to 20	11	29.7
21 to 25	7	18.9
Over 25	5	13.5
Age of starting FC		
Before 7 years old	13	35.1
8 to 15 years old	18	48.6
Over 15 years old	6	16.2
Years of FC training		
Up to 5	10	27.0
6 to 10	23	62.2
More than 10	4	10.8

Table 1. Distribution of study variables for IWA involved in producing the corpus

2.2 Corpus

The texts produced during FC sessions were open-ended, non-structured, non-standardized, non-compulsory conversations between an IWA and a facilitator, written on PCs. These exchanges were partly educational in nature and partly for communicating day-to-day routine information. The topics concerned private matters, school activities, essays, etc.

For the purposes of the statistical analysis on the textual data, each FC session produced a very short text and lasted a very long time. To obtain large corpora, some of the texts collected during the EASIEST project in 2005-2006 were considered and additional texts were retrieved from the FC centers' archives. The texts produced by each IWA were the result of several sessions, written at different ages and with different levels of ability, but all with a good degree of self-sufficiency; by the time the sessions took place, all the IWA were able to write with little facilitation and had already been using FC for years (62.2%

for 6-10 years and 10.8% for over a decade). The texts written as part of the project and those retrieved from the archives both met the requirements of our research protocol, having been collected at the four accredited FC centers according to guidelines that suited our needs.

Corpus analysis can focus on letters, syllables, words, word groups or lexemes, as well as phonemes, morphemes, etc. For the statistical analysis of textual data, the statistical units are generally word tokens (or tokens), which are identified and treated by software. Tokens are defined as sequences of letters taken from the alphabet and isolated by means of blanks and punctuation marks. The size N of a corpus is the total number of tokens. A token is a particular occurrence of a word type (e.g. the word type *the* has many tokens in any English text) and the list of word types constitutes the vocabulary of a corpus.

The whole corpus included 290,496 tokens: 159,243 (54.8%) written by facilitators and 131,253 (45.2%) by IWA; both these sub-corpora were large (over 100,000 tokens) and they were well balanced in terms of their size. The tokens written by IWA were distributed by level of facilitation as follows: upper arm, 27.0%; arm, 16.2%; shoulder, 35.0%; neck/head, 5.2%; back, 5.5%; leg, 4.6%; independent typing, 2.3%.

2.3 Text chunk selection

First, all conversational turns within the whole corpus written by the same writers were grouped to obtain 129 sub-corpora (37 IWA and 92 facilitator). Sub-corpora composed of less than 1,000 tokens were discarded to avoid working on texts that were too short, and consequently unsuitable for a quantitative-lexical approach. The analysis thus involved 91 (of the 129) writers who had produced sub-corpora including at least 1,000 tokens (table 2), i.e. all 37 IWA and 54 facilitators (out of 92).

Center	Before selection			After selection		
	IWA	*FAC*	Total	*IWA*	*FAC*	Total
1	9	18	27	9	18	27
2	9	25	34	9	10	19
3	10	25	35	10	10	20
4	9	24	33	9	16	25
Corpus	37	92	129	37	54	91

Table 2. Number of participants before and after selection

In any text, consecutive words produce clauses, sentences, paragraphs, etc. This study considered text chunks resulting from the combination of whole segments or sentences written by the same author. Segments and sentences were selected by random sampling without replacement. Text chunks are the result of a random sampling not of words but of whole sentences and segments, so their original structure is maintained. The resulting 91 text chunks included a mean 1,003 tokens, with minor variations because the conversational turns were not cut. The text chunks ranged between 990 and 1,010 tokens for each writer, with an approximately 5-token standard deviation (table 3).

	Min	Max	Mean	Std.Dev.
IWA	991	1,010	1,004	5.02
FAC	990	1,010	1,003	4.96
Corpus	990	1,010	1,003	5.02

Table 3. Size of text chunks in word tokens

2.4 Lemmatization

A word type can be defined as a higher-rank unit called a lemma type (e.g. *tooth* and *teeth* are both associated with the lemma *tooth* and the category "noun"; *go, goes, went, gone* are associated with the lemma *to go* and the category "verb", etc.) and the list of lemma types constitutes the lemma vocabulary of a corpus. The frequency of each lemma type is given by the number of corresponding tokens. The lemma vocabulary with frequencies produces the lexical profile of the corpus and reflects its lexicon. The lexical profile includes all information about the type and number of lemmas and their frequency in the corpus.

Since the study was conducted on texts written in Italian and its aim was to analyze lexical features, the statistical unit chosen was the lemma type, so a preliminary lemmatization of the corpus was needed. Lemmatization generally has an important role in Italian (more so than in other languages) because it overcomes the limitation imposed by the contingent nature of some lexical choices (e.g. tenses) and variations (masculine, feminine and plural forms, six different persons, verb conjugations, clitic pronouns, etc.), which do not depend on an individual's lexical features. The lemmatization process associated each token with a pair including a lemma and a grammatical category; for instance, in Italian the token *faccia* is associated with either the lemma *fare* [to do] and the grammatical category "verb" or the lemma *faccia* [face] and the category "noun". Lemmatization was conducted on the whole corpus using a partly manual, partly automatic process. The researchers' manual intervention is necessary when the software fails to disambiguate or identify a lemma or grammatical category. For example, Italian adjectives and past participles can often only be distinguished after a qualitative/semantic evaluation of the context in which they occur (they are homographs), which cannot always be translated into an algorithm and the state-of-the-art software tools currently available cannot ensure the full and accurate lemmatization of Italian texts.

2.5 Measures

The frequency of a lemma type in the corpus was given by the sum of its occurrences in the 91 text chunks comprising the sample. The frequency of each lemma type in each text chunk was given by the number of corresponding tokens in the text chunk. The lemma vocabularies of the text chunks with frequencies produced 91 lexical profiles, i.e. a lexical profile for each writer. Each lexical profile reflected its writer's lexical range, including all information about the lemmas and their frequency in the text chunks.

The concept of the intertextual distance between texts can be used to compare lexical profiles and ascertain to what extent they may be similar (or dissimilar). To position the 91 text chunks in terms of reciprocal proximity, we adopted the concept of intertextual distance based on lexical connection, first introduced by Brunet (1988) and recently developed by Labbé (Labbé, 2007; Labbé & Labbé, 2001; Tuzzi, Popescu, Altmann, 2010). Following the

mentioned studies and consistently with the strategy described in the previous paragraph, our calculations were lemma-based (Pauli & Tuzzi, 2009).
Given a pair of texts A and B of size N_A and N_B with $N_A \le N_B$, the frequency $f_{l,B}$ of each lemma type l in the larger text B was reduced according to the size of the shorter text A in estimating the mathematical expectancy $f^*_{l,B}$ of the frequency of the lemma type l in A by means of a simple proportion:

$$f^*_{l,B} = f_{l,B} \frac{N_A}{N_B} \tag{1}$$

thus $N^*_B = N_A$. The distance d between text A and text B was obtained as follows:

$$d(A,B) = \frac{\sum_{l \in L_{A \cup B}} \left| f_{l,A} - f^*_{l,B} \right|}{2N_A} \tag{2}$$

where $L_{A \cup B}$ was the lemma vocabulary of text A and text B, i.e. all the lemmas present in at least one of the texts.
If two texts were identical, they contained the same words with the same frequency and their distance amounted to zero. If two texts had no words in common, they were separated by a distance amounting to 1 (maximum theoretical distance). The generic element of the matrix D is such that $d_{ij} = d_{ji}$ since the distance between A and B is the same as the distance between B and A. The generic element of the main diagonal is $d_{ii} = 0 = d(A,A)$ because the distance between each writer and him/herself amounts to zero.
Briefly, the intertextual distance was obtained by calculating the difference between the frequency of any lemma in text A and its (estimated) frequency in text B. In our case, the calculation concerned the distance between a pair of text chunks approximately including 1,000 tokens each and no $f^*_{l,B}$ correction was necessary. The intertextual distance was calculated according to the lexical profiles of all possible text chunk pairs (i.e. all pairs of writers). The distances between text pairs was expressed by a square matrix of dimensions $n \times n$ ($n = 91$) with rows and columns assigned to writers. The total number of pairs to consider was 4,095, as expressed through $n(n-1)/2$.
From a statistical standpoint, the writers' lexicon was measured by means of simple indicators of the presence, absence or (more generally) the frequency of lemmas in their written texts. The intertextual distance is a composite indicator that reflected the lexical distance between two writers (texts).

2.6 Comparisons

Labbé and Labbé (2001) have provided a standardized scale of intertextual distance. According to the authors, an intertextual distance below 0.20 suffices for a reliable attribution of authorship, whereas distances beyond 0.30 point to different authors, text genres and topics. We preferred to proceed according to a comparative approach within our matrix because we were not interested in the absolute values of intertextual distances; we focused instead on all pairs of writers to establish who was more or less close to whom. The intertextual distances contained in the matrix provided information on similarities and differences between all text chunk pairs. These distances also enabled us to represent the 91 text chunks in a dendrogram typical of cluster analysis. Clustering depends on the type of metrics used, so we considered the results of different types of agglomeration.

A first cluster analysis of the 91 text chunks was performed using a square matrix of distances and an agglomerative hierarchical cluster algorithm with complete linkage (Everitt, 1980), i.e. the distance between pairs of clusters was obtained as the maximum distance between all pairs of elements in the two clusters; pairs of clusters with a minimum distance were aggregated. We first used a complete linkage because we expected to find clearly separate, tight (convex-shaped) clusters.

A second agglomerative hierarchical cluster analysis was performed on the same data using Ward's method, where the distance between cluster pairs was Euclidean; cluster pairs minimizing the deviance between centroids were aggregated (Ward, 1963; Ward & Hook, 1963).

Textual data were processed with the Taltac2 dedicated software (Bolasco, Baiocchi, & Morrone, 2009) and statistical analyses were conducted with the R (R Development Core Team, 2009). Taltac2 is a program developed by a research team from "La Sapienza" University in Rome using statistical and linguistic resources for the purposes of textual data analysis (Cortelazzo & Tuzzi, 2008; Lebart, Salem, & Berry, 1998; Tuzzi, 2003) and text mining (Bolasco, Canzonetti, & Capo, 2005; Sirmakessis, 2004). R is a language and environment for statistical computing and graphics available as free software under the terms of the Free Software Foundation's GNU General Public License in source code form.

3. Results

Table 4 shows the main summaries of the data in the matrix of intertextual distances between all 4,095 text chunk pairs. Distances ranged between 0.37 and 0.82 and the mean distance was 0.55. Interpreted according to Labbé and Labbé (2007), these figures point to different authors writing on different topics. Analyzing the matrix blocks showed that the distances between pairs of facilitators were slightly smaller than the mean and the distances between pairs of IWA were more variable.

Pairs	n	Min	Max	Mean	Std.Dev.
IWA versus *IWA*	666	0.45	0.80	0.58	0.059
FAC versus *FAC*	1,431	0.37	0.71	0.50	0.055
IWA versus *FAC*	1,998	0.42	0.82	0.58	0.050
Corpus	4,095	0.37	0.82	0.55	0.067

Table 4. Intertextual distances between pairs of writers

The first dendrogram (fig. 1) shows the mutual positions of the 91 text chunks according to the agglomerative hierarchical cluster algorithm with complete linkage. For the sake of clarity, the letter "a" marks all 37 text chunks written by IWA and "f" the 54 text chunks written by facilitators. Cutting the dendrogram at a height of approximately 0.66 gave rise to five clusters (numbered from 1 to 5) and one singleton (number 6). Cluster No. 1 was composed of text chunks written by IWA and, together with singleton No. 6, produced a cluster including text chunks written exclusively by IWA (20 out of 37) and clearly different from all the others in lexical terms. Cluster No. 3 was also composed almost entirely of text chunks written by IWA (13 out of 37) with the exception of one written by a facilitator.

The central part of the dendrogram contained cluster No. 4, 100% of which consisted of text chunks written by facilitators. Cluster No. 5 was also almost wholly composed of text chunks written by facilitators. Clusters No. 5 and No. 4 formed a homogeneous group of 50 out of 54 facilitators, the only exception being a text chunk written by an IWA. No. 2 was the only cluster that may be described as mixed, since it included text chunks written by 3 facilitators and 3 IWA.

The second dendrogram (fig. 2) shows the mutual positions of the 91 text chunks according to the agglomerative hierarchical cluster algorithm based on Ward's method. This second representation of the matrix of distances identified two clusters: one (A) almost entirely composed of text chunks written by IWA, the other (B) containing two sub-clusters, the vast majority of which consisted of text chunks written by facilitators (B1 and B2). After cropping the dendrogram at an approximate height of 1.45, cluster A included 33 IWA (out of 37), plus one facilitator (cluster A represented the same text chunks as in clusters No. 1 and No. 3 and singleton No. 6 in the previous dendrogram); cluster B included 53 facilitators (out of 54) and 4 IWA, the latter all belonging to cluster B2 (clusters B1 and B2 together represented the same text chunks as in clusters No. 2, 4 and 5 in the previous dendrogram).

To sum up, the combination of the two cluster analyses differentiated between the group of IWA and the group of facilitators, with only 5 out of 91 text chunks misclassified (4 written by IWA, and 1 by a facilitator). Retrieving the original texts might enable further comment on these 5 cases and on the members of the clusters classified as similar in terms of intertextual distance.

In figure 3, the 5 writers are identified by a black dot and alphanumerical codes are used to identify adjacent writers (in the code, the numbers 1 to 4 after the letters "a" or "f" refer to the FC center to which the IWA or facilitator belonged).

Some remarks might be made on the misclassification of four IWA in cluster B2 and one facilitator in cluster A. The IWA a2AL was included in cluster B2, which also contained many facilitators, but only two of the latter belonged to the same FC center (No. 2) as the IWA and neither of them had been among the IWA's facilitators (who were in B1). The IWA a4GG was much closer to facilitator f4RS, who belonged to the same FC center (No. 4), but was not one of the IWA's facilitators (who were in B1); the facilitator f4RS worked with one IWA included in cluster A.

There were only two cases showing a certain proximity between members of the pair (facilitator and IWA) writing together. The IWA a4DN was near facilitator f4LC, who wrote only with that particular IWA, whereas a4DN also wrote with two other facilitators included in B1. In all the analyses, a2AF was isolated in a small group of facilitators that also included one of the IWA's facilitators (f2BG) and another facilitator from the same FC center. The facilitator was included among the IWA in cluster A, near a4CO, for whom f4GF acted as facilitator; f4GF only wrote with a4CO, however, whereas a4CO also wrote with another two facilitators included in cluster B.

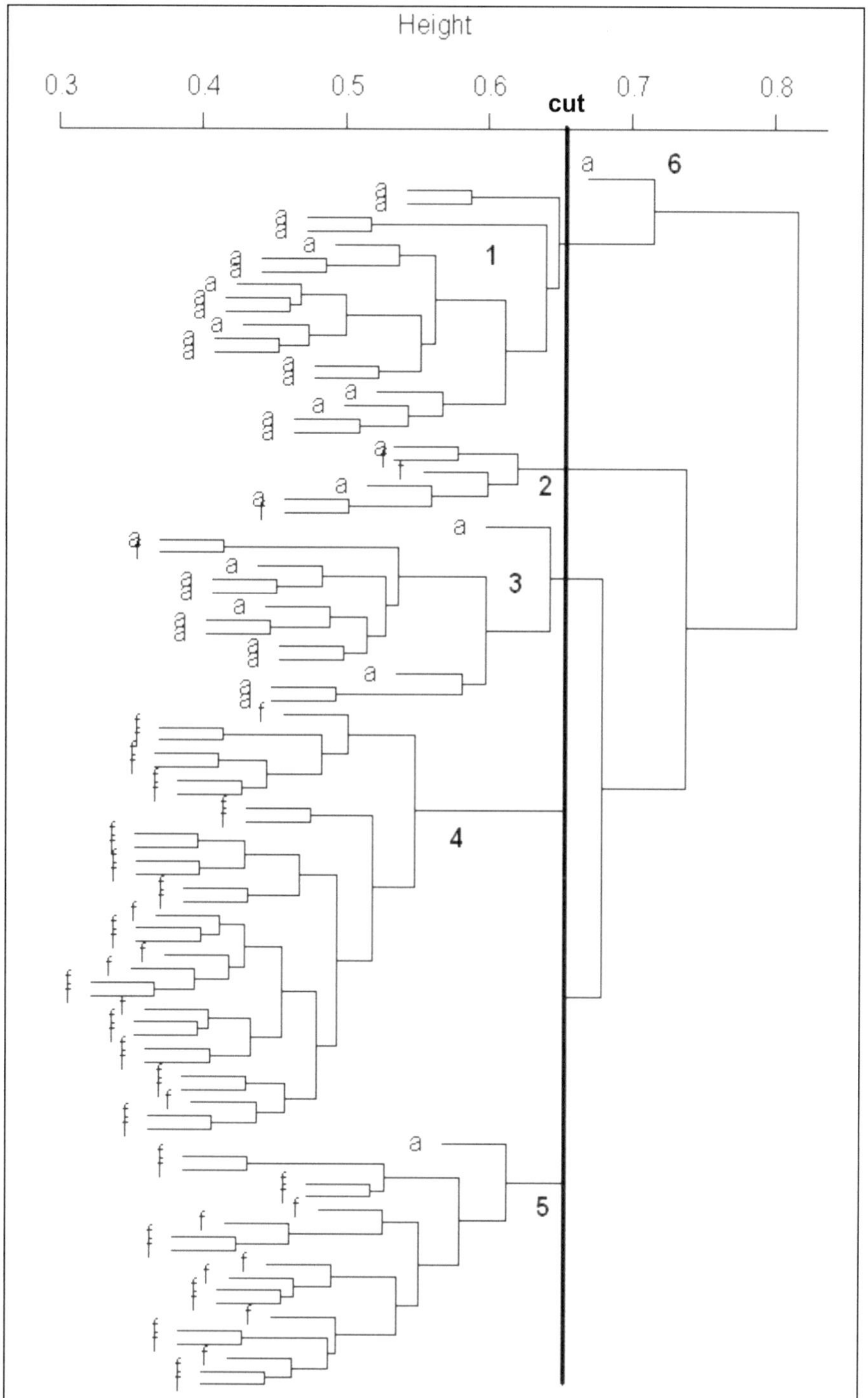

Fig. 1. Agglomerative hierarchical cluster algorithm with complete linkage. Dendrogram and clusters.

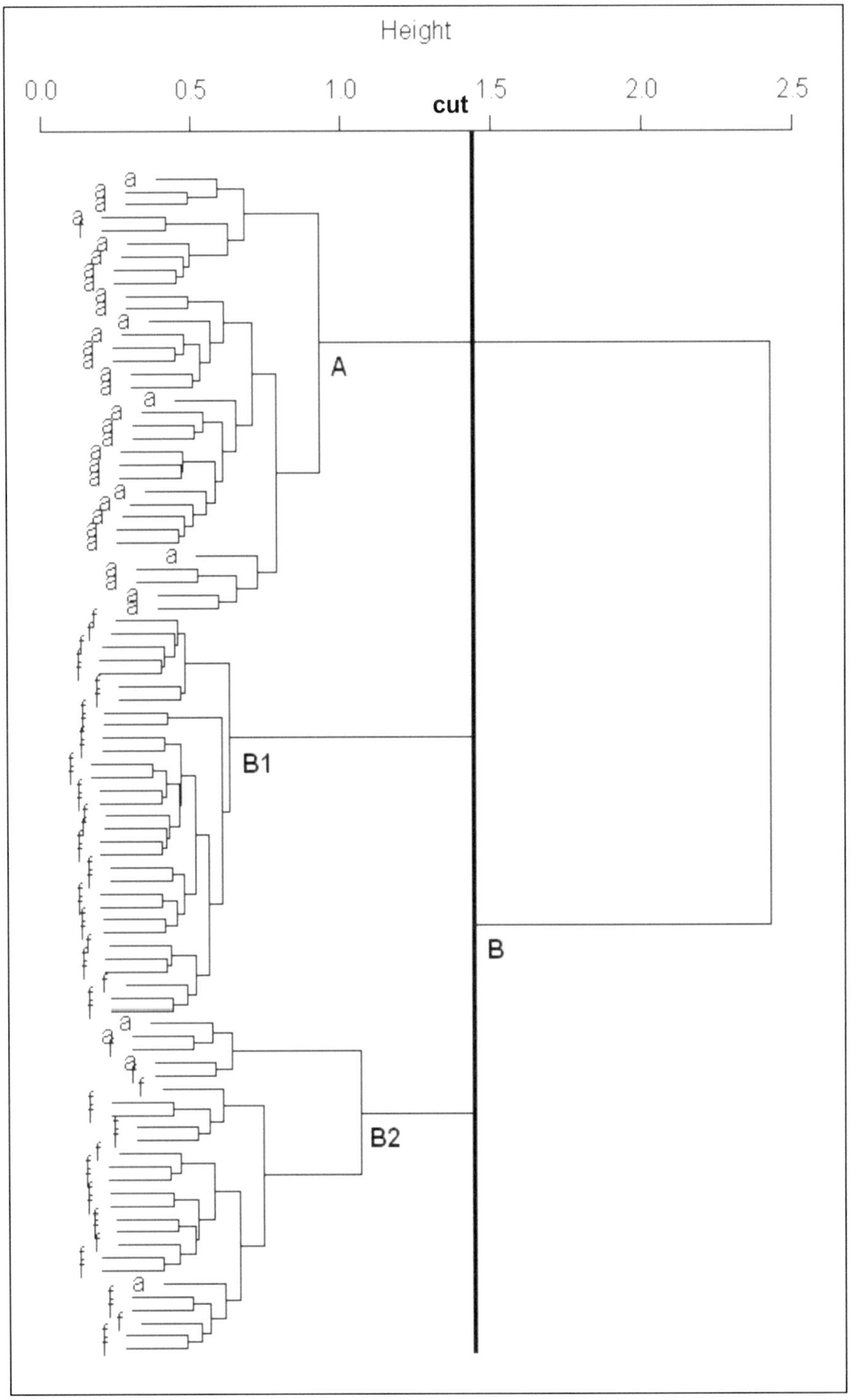

Fig. 2. Agglomerative hierarchical cluster algorithm according to Ward's method. Dendrogram and clusters.

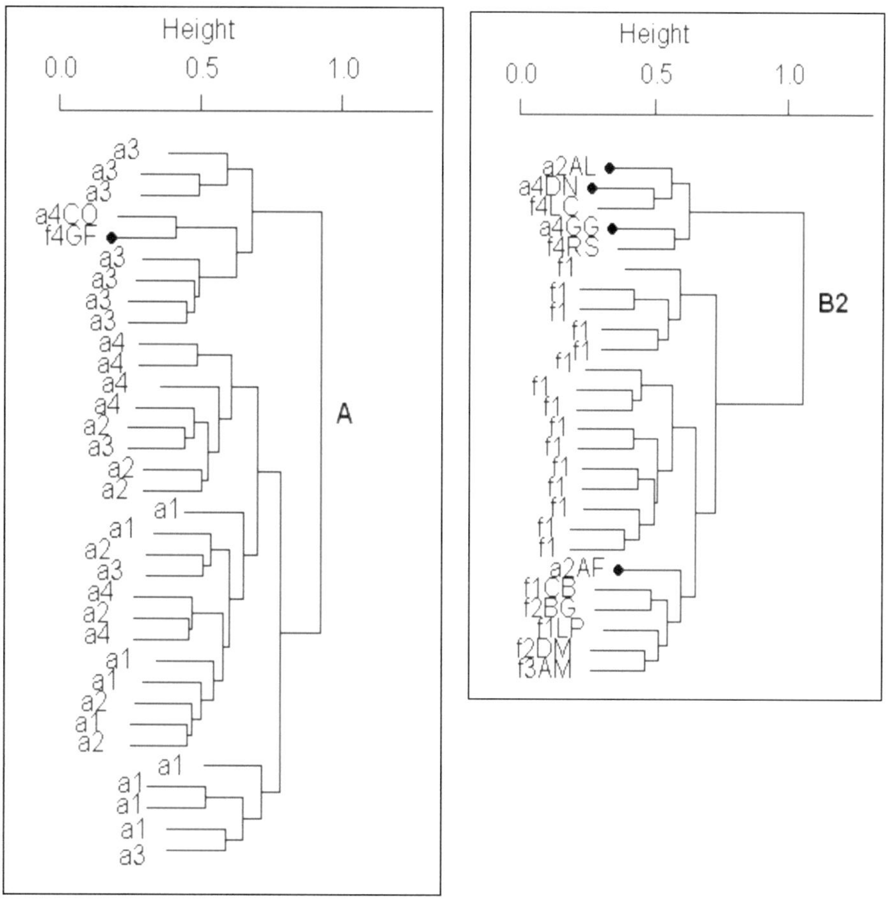

Fig. 3. Agglomerative hierarchical cluster algorithm according to Ward's method. Zoom on clusters A and B2.

4. Discussion and conclusion

The present study analyzed samples of texts generated at FC sessions to see whether distinctive lexical features emerged that could clearly differentiate between IWA and facilitators. The outcome of cluster analysis (dendrogram) graphically showed that the texts written by IWA were similar to each other and differed from the texts produced by their facilitators, which also resembled each other. These findings support the hypothesis that texts written by IWA are characterized by distinctive and consistent lexical features. As already explained by Tuzzi (2009) and Niemi and Kärnä-Lin (2003), the hypothesis that the majority of facilitators managed to imitate such a specific style while remaining consistent would be difficult to support. Our findings are also in favor of distinct authorship, since it is unlikely that such a large number of facilitators could produce texts characterized by two different lexicons (giving rise to two distinct and homogenous clusters) in a real-time dialogical context. In our analysis, the misclassified cases did not support the hypothesis of non-authenticity because no proximity emerged between the parties involved in the conversations (the facilitator and IWA writing together during the same FC sessions). There were only three cases of people writing in pairs and proving very similar in terms of intertextual distance. Two of the three cases involved a facilitator who wrote only with one particular IWA and in one of the two the facilitator seemed to adopt communication modes less like those of facilitators and more like those of IWA. The third case concerned an IWA displaying communication modes similar to those characterizing one group of facilitators.

The distinctive linguistic features identified by the statistical analysis of lexical data derive from the greater complexity of the texts written by the IWA in terms of both lexis and morphological and syntactic structures. Grammatical categories (nouns, adjectives, verbs, adverbs, etc.) show a particular distribution (Tuzzi, 2009) and particular syntactic structures tend to emerge in texts written by IWA (Fratter, 2008). For example, IWA tend to resort more frequently than facilitators to modifiers (Benelli & Cemin 2008; Ursini, 2008): adverbs (e.g. *ti sono autisticamente vicino* [I am autistically close to you], *finisco l'anno scolastico vitalmente e filmicamente* [I complete the school year vitally and filmically]) and adjectives (*mio rotto gretto perduto corpo* [my broken coarse lost body], *miei incoerenti prodi prodigati provetti Lucia lenti fetenti maledetti oscuri professori* [my inconsistent brave generous experienced Lucy slow stinky damned obscure teachers]; note the alliteration in the Italian version). They also tend (Di Benedetto, 2008) to omit grammatical words (prepositions, conjunctions, articles, pronouns) when this does not hamper the understanding of the sentence's meaning (e.g. *non ho parole bocca* [I have no words mouth], or the definition of a volcano as *montagna rotta lava fuori* [broken mountain lava out]).

As stressed in other studies, the lemmas used by IWA were qualitatively different from those used by facilitators (Cortelazzo, 2008). High-register words that do not belong to a basic vocabulary (Marconi, Ott, Pesenti, Ratti, & Tavella, 1993) were used by children under 10 years of age (e.g. *asserire* [to affirm], *auspicare* [to foretell], *bramare* [to yearn], *diffidare* [to mistrust], *inibire* [to inhibit], *stereotipo* [stereotype]). Stylized language also emerges from creative expressions (e.g. *diverbio generazionale* [generational row], *sondare le persone* [to probe people]) and the creation of neologisms (e.g. *ditodipendente* [fingerdependent], *iperrumore* [hypernoise]).

4.1 Future directions

One of the advantages of intertextual distance lay in that it is a very simple comparative tool and, with a few exceptions, it led to a clear differentiation between the groups of IWA and facilitators. The values obtained cannot be compared with theoretical thresholds to assess the results, however, because intertextual distance has been widely tested in the French language, but further investigations are needed to develop a standardized scale for the evaluation of Italian texts.

The results of this study are encouraging and suggest that we are moving in the right direction, but further studies based on large corpora are needed for an overall comparison between the written language of IWA and the language of people without disabilities. Moreover, because textual data analysis calls for large corpora, our study fails to consider the effect of other variables because grouping texts by writer's age, FC training, facilitation level, etc. would make the resulting sub-corpora too small for significant comparative analyses. Further studies are needed to establish which factors can help describe the written language of IWA.

5. Acknowledgments

The present study was part of the activities conducted within the frame of the EASIEST Project, which focused on the written language of IWA and involved an interdisciplinary study covering linguistics, neuropsychiatry, psychology, sociology, statistics, and computer-aided text processing (Bernardi, 2008), funded by the University of Padua (Scientific Coordinator: Lorenzo Bernardi, Department of Statistical Sciences, University of Padua). Text collection was coordinated by Vittoria Cristoferi Realdon, child neuropsychiatrist, and conducted at four accredited FC centers in Italy, i.e. the Centro Studi e Ricerca in Neuroriabilitazione CNAPP in Rome, the Centro Studi sulla Comunicazione Facilitata - W.O.C.E. in Zoagli (GE), the Istituto M.P.P. Padri Trinitari A. Quarto di Palo in Andria (BA), and the Centro Sperimentale per i Disturbi dello Sviluppo e della Comunicazione in Padua.
The present study is now included among the activities conducted within the frame of the GIAT, the Interdisciplinary Group on Text Analysis (www.giat.org).

6. References

American Psychiatric Association (2000). *Diagnostic and Statistical Manual of Mental Disorders DSM-IV text revision.* (4th ed.). Washington, DC: American Psychiatric Association.

Beck, A.R., & Pirovano, C.M. (1996). Facilitated communicators' performance on a task of receptive language. *Journal of Autism and Developmental Disorders*, 26, 5, 497-512.

Benelli, B., & Cemin, M. (2008). Rappresentazioni semantiche nel linguaggio degli autistici: il caso degli avverbi [Semantic Representations of the Language of Individuals with Autism: the Case of Adverbs]. In: L. Bernardi (Ed), *Il delta dei significati* (pp. 105-124). Rome: Carocci.

Bernardi, L. (Ed.) (2008). *Il delta dei significati.* [The Delta of Meanings]. Rome: Carocci.

Beukelman, D. R., Mirenda, P. (1998). *Augmentative and Alternative Communication: Management of Severe Communication Disorders in Children and Adults.* Baltimore: Paul H Brookes Pub Co.

Biklen, D. (1993). *Communication unbound: how facilitated communication is challenging traditional views of autism and ability/disability*. New York: Teachers College Press.

Biklen, D. (2005). *Autism and the myth of the person alone*. Cambridge: University Press.

Biklen, D., & Burke, J. (2006). Presuming competence. *Equity and Excellence in Education*, 39, 166-175.

Biklen, D., & Cardinal, D. (Eds.) (1997). *Contested words, contested science: unraveling the facilitated communication controversy*. New York: Teachers College Press.

Biklen, D., Saha, N.; & Kliewer, C. (1995). How teachers confirm the authorship of facilitated communication: a portfolio approach. *Journal of the Association for Persons with Severe Handicaps*, 20, 1, 45-56.

Bolasco, S., Baiocchi, F., & Morrone, A. (2009). *TaLTaC²: Trattamento automatico Lessicale e Testuale per l'analisi del Contenuto di un Corpus* (rel. 2.9) [Software: *Lexical and Textual Automatic Treatment for Content Analysis of a Corpus*]. Rome, Italy. Retrieved (July 2008) from http://www.taltac.it

Bolasco, S., Canzonetti, A., & Capo, F. M. (Eds) (2005). *Text Mining*. Rome: CISU.

Bomba, C., O'Donnell, L., Markowitz, C., Holmes, D.L. (1996). Evaluating the impact of facilitated communication on the communicative competence of fourteen students with autism. *Journal of Autism and Developmental Disorders*, 26, 1, 43-58.

Boucher, J. (2003). Language development in autism. *International Journal of Pediatric Otorhinolaryngology*, 67, S159-S163.

Braman, B.J., Brady, M.P., Linehan, S.L., & Williams, R.E. (1995). Facilitated communication for children with autism: an examination of face validity. *Behavioral Disorders*, 21, 1, 110-118.

Brunet, E. (1988). Une mesure de la distance intertextuelle: la connexion lexicale. Le nombre et le texte. *Revue informatique et statistique dans les sciences humaines*, Université de Liége.

Calculator, S.N. (1999). Facilitated communication - Look who's pointing now: cautions related to the clinical use of facilitated communication. *Language Speech and Hearing Services in Schools*, 30, 4, 408-414.

Cardinal, D. N., Hanson, D., & Wakeham, J. (1996). Investigation of authorship in facilitated communication. *Metal Retardation*, 34, 4, 231-242.

Cortelazzo, M., & Tuzzi, A. (2008). *Metodi statistici applicati all'italiano*. [Statistical Methods Applied to Italian]. Bologna: Zanichelli.

Cortelazzo, M.A. (2008). Ricchezza del lessico nel corpus EASIEST. [Lexical richness in the EASIEST corpus]. In: L. Bernardi (Ed), *Il delta dei significati* (pp. 66-79). Rome: Carocci.

Crossley, R., & McDonald, A. (1984). *Annie's Coming Out*. New York: Viking Penguin.

Crossley, R. (1997). *Speechless: facilitating communication for people without voices*. New York: Dutton.

Crossley, R., & Remington-Gurney, J. (1992). Getting the words out: facilitated communication training. *Topics in Language Disorders*, 12, 29-45.

Davidson, J. (2008). Autistic culture online: virtual communication and cultural expression on the spectrum. *Social & Cultural Geography*, 9, 7, 791-806.

Di Benedetto, C. (2008). Isole semantiche nell'emotivo mare: un'analisi lessicale, retorica e sintattica. [Semantic islands in the emotional sea: a lexical, rhetorical and syntactic analysis]. In: L. Bernardi (Ed), *Il delta dei significati* (pp. 80-96). Rome: Carocci.

DSM-IV-TR (2000). American Psychiatric Association, *Diagnostic and Statistical Manual of Mental Disorders*, 4th ed., text revision, APA, Washington D.C. (trad. it. DSM-IV-TR Manuale diagnostico e statistico dei disturbi mentali - text revision, Masson Editore, 2001).

Duchan, J.F. (1993). Issues raised by facilitated communication for theorizing and research on autism. *Journal of Speech and Hearing Research*, 36, 6, 1108-1119.

Duchan, J.F. (1999). Facilitated communication - views of facilitated communication: what's the point? *Language Speech and Hearing Services in Schools*, 30, 4, 401-407.

Duchan, J.F., Calculator, S., Sonnenmeier, R., Diehl, S., & Cumley, G.D. (2001). A framework for managing controversial practices. *Language Speech and Hearing Services in Schools*, 32, 3, 133-141.

Duràn, P., Malvern, D., Richards, B., & Chipere, N. (2004). Developmental trends in lexical diversity. *Applied Linguistics*, 25,2, 220-242.

Emerson, A., Grayson, A., & Griffiths, A. (2001). Can't or won't? Evidence relating to authorship in facilitated communication. *International Journal of Language & Communication Disorders*, 36 (Supp), 98-103.

Everitt, B. (1980). *Cluster Analysis*. New York.

Fratter, I. (2008). «Palombaro ero in fondo al mare»: uno studio di caso sull'analisi diacronica dei costituenti nella CF. ["Diver I was on the sea floor": a case study of facilitated communication factors in time]. In: L. Bernardi (Ed), *Il delta dei significati* (pp. 97-104). Rome: Carocci.

Green, G. (1994). Facilitated communication: mental miracle or sleight of hand? *Skeptic*, 2, 3, 68-76.

Jacobson, J.W., Mulick, J.A., & Schwartz, A.A. (1995). History of facilitated communication - science, pseudoscience, and antiscience - Science Working Group on Facilitated Communication. *American Psychologist*, 50, 9, 750-765.

Koegel, L.K. (2000). Interventions to facilitate communication in autism. *Journal of Autism and Developmental Disorders*, 30, 5, 383-391.

Koegel, L.K., & Brown, F. (2007). Autism spectrum disorders: trends, treatments, and diversity. *Research and Practice for Persons with Severe Disabilities*, 32, 2, 87-88.

Labbé, C., & Labbé D. (2001). Inter-textual distance and authorship attribution. Corneille and Moliére. *Journal of Quantitative Linguistics* 8, 213-231.

Labbé, D. (2007). Experiments on authorship attribution by intertextual distance in English. *Journal of Quantitative Linguistics* 14, 33-80.

Lebart, L., Salem, A., & Berry, L. (1998). *Exploring Textual Data*. Dordrecht: Kluwer-Academic Pub.

Marconi, L., Ott, M., Pesenti, E., Ratti, D., & Tavella, M. (1993), *Lessico Elementare. Dati statistici sull'italiano letto e scritto dai bambini delle elementari*, Bologna: Zanichelli. [Elementary lexicon. Statistical data on how Italian pupils read and write in primary school].

McKee, G., Malvern, D., & Richards, B. (2000). Measuring vocabulary diversity using dedicated software. *Literary and Linguistic Computing*, 15, 3, 323-337.

Mirenda, P. (2008). A back door approach to autism and AAC. *Augmentative and Alternative Communication*, 24, 3, 220-234.

Mirenda, P., Beukelman, D. (2006), *Augmentative & Alternative Communication: Supporting Children & Adults With Complex Communication Needs*. Baltimore: Paul H Brookes Pub Co.

Montee, B.B., Miltenberger, R.G., & Wittrock, D. (1995). An experimental-analysis of facilitated communication. *Journal of Applied Behavior Analysis*, 28, 2, 189-200.

Mostert, M.P. (2001). Facilitated communication since 1995: A review of published studies. *Journal of Autism and Developmental Disorders*, 31, 3, 287-313.

Niemi, J., & Karna-Lin, E. (2002). Grammar and lexicon in facilitated communication: a linguistic authorship analysis of a Finnish case, *Mental Retardation*, 40, 5, 347-357.

Niemi, J., & Kärnä-Lin, E. (2003). Four vantage points to the language performance and capacity of human beings: response to Saloviita and Sariola. *Mental Retardation*, 41, 5, 380-385.

Ostryn, C. (2008). Autism spectrum disorders and AAC. *Research and Practice for Persons with Severe Disabilities*, 33-34, 273-274.

Pauli, F., & Tuzzi, A. (2009). The end of year addresses of the Presidents of the Italian Republic (1948-2006): discoursal similarities and differences, Glottometrics, 18, 40-51.

Probst, P. (2005). Communication unbound - or unfound? An integrative review on the effectiveness of facilitated communication (FC) in non-verbal persons with autism and mental retardation. *Zeitschrift fur Klinische Psychologie Psychiatrie und Psychotherapie*, 53, 2, 93-128.

R Development Core Team. (2008). *R: A language and environment for statistical computing* (Ver. 2.8.1) [Software]. Vienna, Austria: R Foundation for Statistical Computing. Retrieved [December, 2008] from http://www.R-project.org.

Rapin, I., & Tuchman, R.F. (2008). What is new in autism? *Current Opinion in Neurology*, 21, 2, 143-149.

Rossetti, Z., Ashby, C., Arndt, K., Chadwick, M., & Kasahara, M. (2008). I like others to not try to fix me: agency, independence, and autism. *Intellectual and Developmental Disabilities*, 46, 5, 364-375.

Rutter, M. (2005). Autism research: lessons from the past and prospects for the future. *Journal of Autism and Developmental Disorders*, 35, 2, 241-257.

Saloviita, T., & Sariola, H. (2003). Authorship in facilitated communication: a re-analysis of a case of assumed representative authentic writing. *Mental Retardation*, 41, 5, 374-379.

Sbalchiero, S., & Neresini, F. (2008). La scienza e l'eresia: il controverso caso della Comunicazione Facilitata. [Science and heresy: the controversial case of facilitated communication]. In: L. Bernardi (Ed), *Il delta dei significati* (pp. 125-135). Rome: Carocci.

Scopesi, A., Zanobini, M., & Cresci, L.R. (2003). Aspetti semantici e stilistici della produzione di un bambino autistico in situazione di Comunicazione Facilitata. [Semantic and stylistic aspects of the production of a child with autism in a facilitated communication environment]. *Rivista di psicolinguistica applicata*, 2-3, 83-105.

Sheehan, C.M., & Matuozzi, R.T. (1996). Investigation of the validity of facilitated communication through the disclosure of unknown information. *Mental Retardation*, 34, 2, 94-107.

Sikora, D.M., Hartley, S.L., Mccoy, R., Gerrard-Morris, A.E., & Dill, K. (2008). The performance of children with mental health disorders on the ADOS-G: a question of diagnostic utility. *Research in Autism Spectrum Disorders*, 2, 1, 188-197.

Simpson, R.L., & Myles, B.S. (1995). Effectiveness of facilitated communication with children and youth with autism. *Journal of Special Education*, 28, 4, 424-439.

Sirmakessis, S. (Ed.) (2004). *Text Mining and its Applications*. Berlin: Springer.

Snyder, D.M., Miller, K., & Stein, M.T. (2008). It looks like autism: caution in diagnosis. *Journal of Developmental and Behavioral Pediatrics*, 29, 1, 47-50.

Tager-Flusberg, H. (2004). Strategies for conducting research on language in autism. *Journal of Autism and Developmental Disorders*, 34, 1, 75-80.

Tager-Flusberg, H., & Caronna, E. (2007). Language disorders: autism and other pervasive developmental disorders. *Pediatric Clinics of North America*, 54, 3, 469.

Tuzzi, A. (2003). *L'analisi del contenuto. Introduzione ai metodi e alle tecniche di ricerca*, [Content analysis. An introduction to research methods and techniques], Rome: Carocci.

Tuzzi, A. (2009). Grammar and lexicon in texts written by individuals with autism: a statistical analysis of a large Italian corpus. *Intellectual and Developmental Disabilities*, 47, 5, 373-385.

Tuzzi A., Popescu I.-I., Altmann G. (2010). *Quantitative Analysis of Italian Texts*. Lüdenscheid, Germany: RAM-Verlag.

Ursini, F. (2008). Le parole tra noi leggère cadono. [Words between us lightly fall]. In: L. Bernardi (Ed), *Il delta dei significati* (pp. 56-65). Rome: Carocci.

Ward, J.H. (1963). Hierarchical grouping to optimize an objective function. *Journal of the American Statistical Association*, 58, 236-244.

Ward, J.H., & Hook, M.E. (1963). Application of an hierarchical grouping procedure to a problem of grouping profiles. *Educational Psychological Measurement*, 23, 69-81.

Watkins, R.V., Kelly, D. J., & Harbers, H.M. (1995). Measuring children's lexical diversity. Differentiating typical and impaired language learners. *Journal of Speech and Hearing Research*, 38, 1349-1355.

Weiss, M.J.S., Wagner, S.H., & Bauman, M.L. (1996). A validated case study of facilitated communication. *Mental Retardation*, 34, 4, 220-230.

Wheeler, D.L., Jacobson, J.W., Paglieri, R.A., & Schwartz, A.A. (1993). An experimental assessment of facilitated communication. *Mental Retardation*, 31, 49-60.

Wing L., Gould J. (1979), Severe impairments of social interaction and associated anormalities in children: epidemiology and classification. *Journal of Autism and Developmental Disorders*, 9, 11-29.

Zanobini M., Scopesi A. (2001). La comunicazione facilitata in un bambino autistico. [Facilitated communication: the case of a child with autism]. *Psicologia clinica dello Sviluppo*, 3, 395-421.

Part 11

An Integrated Approach and Transition to Adulthood

24

The Body of the Autistic Child: An Integrated Approach

Fabien Joly
Centre Ressources AUTISMES de Bourgogne
Conseil Scientifique de l'ANCRA
« CORPS & PSYCHE », C.R.A. Bourgogne
France

1. Introduction

The question of the infantile autism was mistreated for such a long time in partisan reductions and blindnesses "of chapels". According to us, it is a question of measuring today the real stakes in a conception developmental complex and multidimensional of the disorders of the autistic spectrum.

A real plea for a developmental psychopathology will deduct which, of the research and the hypotheses of etiology until the modalities of interventions and accompaniments (educational as much as psychotherapeutics), should consider just as much the substrata of equipment and the genetic, neurobiological and cognitive reasons in the peculiarity of the autistic functions, that the reasons of stories of life and the other psychic and emotional stakes (*intra-* as *inter-*subjective) which inextricably mixed prematurely the development of the young autistic to color, to direct, to subvertir sometimes, to repair the other times, the initial data, and the instrumental peculiarities and of equipment.

The body - and the singular way "to live in it" - is probably the first presentation of the person with autism both in its difficulties, specificities and in its sometimes extraordinary potentialities; the first one as the ultimate datum of this specific development. We suggest here approaching this issue developmental multi-dimensional by the question of the body.

If we notice all that the persons with autism treat rather the details than a global seizure of things, we immediately have to notice the autistic "contamination" which makes that the specialists never consider the global apprehension of the person with autism but only a collection of functions and singular difficulties... And for example towards the body, we decline all the perceptivo-driving difficulties, praxies and instrumental, ever the global apprehension of the body, the singular way of the subject to live in its body, the representation of one and the images of the body which are his, dimension of its *body-in-relation* to evoke J. de Ajuriaguerra. By this integrated approach (the global nature of the body) we find a more complete and more complex vision of the pervasive developmental disorder of autistic spectrum.

Based on the historic teachings of "*the French school of psychomotricity*" we shall develop:

a. *the physical stake in the development* : a body lived as place of articulation order between the data of equipment and the historic data and developmental of the successive investments of the instrumentation of the autistic child ;
b. the early psychomotor signs at the babies at autistic risks ;
c. *the physical and psychomotor dimension of the specificities of functioning of the person with autism* turned out at all the ages of the life (singular autistic way of living and of instrumenting its body and its sensori-motricity or its psychomotricity;
d. finally, we shall *reconsider the variety of the therapeutic approaches and the diverse modalities of accompaniment of the autistic.*

To conclude, we remind that any unambiguous reduction of our understandings as our interventions is a mutilation and *in fine* an ill-treatment of the autism, and above all the person with autism; and we propose that the physical and psychomotor stakes are thought as epistemology and theory clinical fundamental positions for the respect and for the best understanding of the autism.

2. The body and the psyche: An integrated approach

The body and the psyche are in one complex intricacy and permanent interactive process ; and in fact a clinical psychology, whatever is her theoretical option it is not still more or less a psychology of the body, a psychopathology of an embodied subject existing only by and in its body. The body is permanently crossed, in its emotional stakes, in its developmental, cognitive and instrumental stakes, in its feature and in its investment, by the psychic ; infested, modified, drained by the quality specifically emotional of his being *intra-* as *inter-*subjective and historic. While the psyche is, as for her, drained continuously by its physical, sensory and perceptive anchoring; better, than she finds her foundation and her lively source in the impulsive and interactive stakes taken in and on the body. More exactly according to the canonical formula of Ajuriaguerra [1] than she is *body-in-relation. It is nothing in the spirit which is not passed in the senses and the motricity.* The body is at the same time our carnal evidence without which we are nothing: instigation of the equipment and the visible somatic evidence (*res extensa* of Descartes) this "place of me" the most intimate, around which the psychic subjectivity and the most personal identital-narcissist establish, feel and imagine themselves. Our body it is the place source, the party and the whole of our being, our grip on the reality, broadcasting and receiving of one towards the world and the others and mutually.

It is precious to remember itself at once that it is by the body that we think, that it is by the body that we recognize: different there from all other people, from all the animals as much as the various forms of artificial intelligences; that it is about our most intimate ID card and most fundamentally embodied there. And nevertheless, in spite of this evidence, it is not excess to remember itself how much the philosophy, the religion, the psychoanalysis even, and the learned speech generally, tried desperately to force the body, to reduce it, to forget him, to send back him to the trivial or to the evanescent in the unspeakable, even in the suspect or imperceptible. Preferring by far a modelling of a spiritual, neuronal or IT being untied from its physical anchoring, from flesh, from tried, from hand-to-hand fight. This solitude of the body, reduced then to the somatic and to the delegation of therapeutics and theorization in the only hard sciences or in the medicine, leaves according to us the human body to the state of corpse or machinery, putting aside the subjective thickness of the body, its tried, its vitality, its actions on the world and on the others.

But if the body insists, difficult to avoid, it is not of the soma about which it is a question; rather of an already "double" body: at the same time relational material and subject object. A resumption infiltrated psychic of the stakes and data of equipment of the soma; the sum of the relational experiences of the physical machinery. In fine, the problem of the body interests us in psychology and in clinical psychopathology through the question of what we could call *the way "to live in its body"*. We shall never insist maybe enough on the function which holds this body as mediator and relational stake principal between two subjects on one hand, and between the psyche of the subject and the world on the other hand. From this point of view there, the body is just as much a sensory body than an impulsive body, and just as much a body psychomotor agent, an instrument of action on the world that permanent receptacle of tried and of information ; a neuro-cognitive body of management, storage and treatment of this information as much as a body represented in the mental life (body image); just as much a body of thickness, flesh and tonus, which a body wraps and sphincter interesting the specialist of the psychic only leaves its holes or its surfaces!
We shall observe here the question of the autistic child towards the way of living in its body and its psychomotricity. And by way of introduction in this present reflection, we would again like to remind that the psychomotricity of an individual is exactly the way of a subject to live in its body. It is strangely, according to the principal definition of Ajuriaguerra [1], the *body-in-relation* of a subject whatever his age and his pathology. It is obviously in this respect, at the same time and inextricably mixed, the imaginary and eminently psychic dimension of the representations of itself and the investment of its physical state, and the more cognitive, neurological, developmental and functional dimension of its body in its relationship to the world: the "instrumentation" in the sense of Bullinger [3,4] private individual (praxies, physical plan and spatiotemporal organization of the appropriate body, tonic and postural registers, quality of the movement, sensory-motricity, etc.) for a given individual. Better maybe, it is the place crossroads of articulation of this double dimension inferred by our *body-in-relation*: at once in the psychic pole and in the neurological pole, inextricably braided together. So understood, we can envisaged the psychomotricity through the question of the development, towards of the psychopathology (specific psychomotor disorders or psychomotor colors of any functioning); as she can decline in multiple theoretical viewpoints; or open finally to a praxis and in this particular case in a set of techniques and therapeutics *(cf.* Joly [11]).

3. The body of the autistic child

The body of the autistic child, in the diverse theorizations and the descriptions of the autistic problems and the other similar disorders, is maybe the least looked, the least described in the psychopathologic plan, different of specificities of cognitive, perceptive and socio-communicational functioning, or still fears and psychic, emotional and relational peculiarities. Nevertheless, the body of the autistic child is doubtless the first one and the ultimate witness of an autistic specificity. Better, it is the meshing and the crossroads lived on knotting between the reasons of equipments and the developmental reasons which make the autistic syndrome. The approaches physical and mediatized by the persons with autisms are, of their sides, maybe the least studied, the least elaborated, and the least evoked in the current debates and within the diverse studies and the recommendations of treatments and methods of accompaniment; when they are not the most attacked in the same way as the strategies of nursing accompaniments (cf. the *pack* or the *paddling pool* for example).

Nevertheless, they appear to all the practitioners as essential tools of the therapeutic of the autistic suffering; and they are among the most invested and most declined within institutions and mostly by the parents.

The autism (in the singular as a paradigm) and the declension of the various pictures (in the plural) of the autistic states or pervasive disorders of the development represent a singular clinical prototype which questions primarily the adversities of the psychomotor development, and a so particular psychomotor way of being to the world. The body of the autistic child is maybe - if we consider at it good - its first difference, its first and singular presentation. Better maybe it is doubtless in the place of the body of the autistic that the data of equipment (genetic and neurobiological), the cognitive, perceptive and sensori-motor peculiarities, with the emotional, relational, psychic stakes, and historic cross themselves in the development of the child. The psychomotricity of the autistic countered so central: since the performances (rather global psychomotor delay, and psychomotor disharmonies in most of the pictures of autism), until the particular autistic lines in the most obvious of the body (driving stereotypes, whirling, singular postures, physical rhythms, etc.), and more determining maybe still the tension perms between the various sensitivity and motor sectors in *hypo-* or *hyper-* functioning. Functional specificities pulling inevitably a very particular way for the autistic to perceive his own body, as much as the surrounding world and the other subject, in his body and in his psychic apparatus.

Next to the pathognomonic set of three of the autism in the CIM-10 now DSM-IVR the suffering children of autistic disorders also present numerous peculiarities expressing himself at the physical level. We do not think here of the possible neurological infringements or the possible genetic of dysmorphies witnesses of pathologies frequently associated with the autism, but many peculiarities of the functioning, the investment and the use of their body.

I proposed [7] - by borrowing the canonical formula "*our body is nothing without the body of the other one*" to Julian de Ajuriaguerra [1] - to think that: the autism could be, in fact understood, throughout the development, as the prototypic representation of the fact what would be our body without the body of the other one, in its subjective dimensions as the instrumental and functional registers. It is the exploration of this psychomotor approach of the autism that I propose here briefly as an integrated precious perspective.

The body of the autistic child is an imperative axis of reflection, at least in the evidence of the psychomotor signs almost of the turned out autistic state, of the psychopathological paradigm that is the syndrome of early infantile autism for the sense of Kanner. Psychomotor elements (and psychomotor disharmonies) in the autistic clinical, through which we shall see so much the essential aspect of the disorders of the body (in the way of living in its body and the harmony of the psychomotor sphere) and the perverse drift as for paradoxical skills and disharmonies, towards the closed circuit self-sensuality, towards the bankruptcy of the representation and the psycho-affective interaction, which usually makes, in the commonplace development, the bed of our human being's specifically psychic quality. It is just as much precious for me to study the future of these psychomotor signs of the autism, in the fate of the patients affected by the syndrome of A.I.P. and the variety of the fact that we call states comment autistic, as much as in the way of research rapidly expanding which refers to the other end of the early signs of interactive drift and developmental of the babies at autistic risk.

In the turned out autistic clinical picture, it thus seems to me good to specify at first the intrusive dimension of the body signs.
That we think first of all of the generic set of three specific signs of the autism (whatever are schools and obediences) because we agree to hold around the diagnosis of autism: *1/ the isolation or the deficiency of the social interaction* (it is the *aloneness* of Kanner), *2/ aspects always restricted by the activities and the centres of interests* (was it towards the islands of strange and paradoxical capacities) *and desire of stability* (it is the *sameness* by Kanner), 3/ finally *the quantitative and qualitative deficiency of the verbal and not verbal communication, and the imagination.* A set of this three specific signs of the autism which gets organized - and we could say first of all in the early ages where the autistic picture takes shape - around a mode to be psychomotor very singular.
At the level 1/ of the *aloneness*, the considerable retreat and the social bankruptcy autistic, the obvious indicators are, indeed, the aversion for the contact or the simple physical moved closer, the tonic shell, the defects of joint attentions, the oddities and the other tonic and emotional conflicts, the disorders of the perceptive behaviours there (hypothesis of deafness or blindness at children whose additional examinations testify nevertheless of the integrity of the neuro-sensitivity circuits), the behaviours of clinging to the body or to the percept, and the demonstrations of dismantling, the emotional detachment and the defect of ability to react to quote only these physical principals indicators.
Of the side 2/ of the limitation of the activities and the *sameness*, the main signs are exactly: the psychomotor indifference to the world, the lack of desire and initiative or reset in the driving and sensory games, the search for stability in repeated complex rites compulsive, the stereotypical self-focus behaviour, the strange manipulations of objects, the inactivity and the absence of interest for toys, little of desire in the requests of a *body-in-relation* even the agonistic disorganization when we come to provoke the meeting of bodies.
On the register 3/ of the qualitative and quantitative deficiency of the communication, the first indicators upstream even of the language (of his absence, his adversities or his oddities when he happens) are, actually, the disorders of the not linguistic social behaviours and the defect of non-verbal communication there (defect of tonic adjustment, absence of checking, dullness of a babble which when it appears is neither interactive, nor "affected", defect of contact eye with eye, absent, fickle, crossing glance, or stuck in suburb, etc.).
I would like, as for me, to insist even more specifically on six essential very points double or to say the least paradoxical.

- Towards the driving and rhythmic stereotypes, the behaviours of body or percept clinging, and the attachment for the "*autistic sensations-objects*" or the "*autistic sensations-forms*" (in the sense of Frances Tustin [14]) of these patients, we shall notice a first level of psychomotor conflict of which shows the paradox of such a permanent auto-sensual centre on the sensory and the engine, at the same time as these behaviours testify, in fact and to look at it well, of a real autistic dam in the perception. The sensitivity is here, in the autistic syndrome, not at all the usual link to the world, to the objects and to the others, the vector link of a permanent psychic translation, and a work of representation appropriation and emotional through the tried of a subject, but rather exact opposite of a movement anti-psychic and avoiding with regard to the world in what we can call a psychomotor "perversion" (and a failure) of this sensori-motor investment.

- On another plan (very proximal) we could linger more for a long time over the evolutionary, functional and instrumental disharmony and over the area of the conflicts in the psychomotor sphere: I shall evoke here, in passing, only the only paradoxical skills of the autistics in the global driving development, the delays and the abnormalities in the cognitive development with very long prevalency of the sensori-motor plans; the stunning addresses in some autistic manipulations opposed by one almost debilitated engine in the other sectors; the disorders of the image of the body; atypical postures and reduced tonic harmony; the driving initiatives globally so insufficient; the so poor or non-existent graphics etc.; as so many witnesses of a dramatic failure of the psychomotricity as fundamental link between body and psyche, between subject and object, between affect and representation via the experience of the *body in relation.*
- The sentimentality aggravated by these children as "tormented souls" and reacting to tiny perceptions (visual, sound, tactile, etc.), in tiny changes or modifications is, at the same time as (or set paradoxically in) frost of the affect and against the emotional not ability to react even, more extreme still, the not ability to react in the pain, the third paradoxical aspect of the autistic body of the subject on which we would like to insist.
- The autistic dismantling and its price to pay in desperate clinging and absolved in a not-consensual single sensory channel is another characteristic of the autistic clinical with a type of dismantled (or more exactly not-mantled) in a single sensory channel to the detriment of any tuning, of any trans-modality and of any driving relation in the object with the paradoxical fixation of an attention of survival, an cling to this only one sensory canal absorption, to the detriment of quite other attention on the world and on the other one.
- Towards the "physical terrors" and the other primitive death-agonies if copies of the autism (cf. Tustin [14]: premature phobias, crises to *temper tantrum*, archaic frights sometimes organized in real massive and atypical phobia of the contact, etc.), of these very acute emotional states with alternation of hypertonic states and big hypotonies of lived on fall even of liquefaction. I wish to point out here the bipolarity of the native and autistic pre-emotional life *(cf.* Joly [7-11]) that is the existence of a native immoderation, an excess, a traumatic overflowing in all the forms of autistic emotional life - as well in death-agonies and terrors not event presentables as in ecstatic excitements so little divisable - below a some emotional qualification, that is below a primary shape of psychic representation.
- At the level of the disorders of the spatial-temporality and the relationship in objects finally, the exploration of the space and the objects which populate him testifies, in these clinical parts of the country, of the trend to remain in a close (one or two-dimensional) space, in adhesive clinging or by swirling around a point, while the time seems as for him always unidirectional, motionless or circular in stabbing one repetition.

4. The autistic psychomotricity

Let us resume at the moment this question of the body in the autism; of the body, its way to live in it, and its psychic destiny, its experiences and its adversities, so omnipresent in the heart of the autistic clinical. Since the observation of the early psychomotor signs of the babies at autistic risk, until the major educations of the mobilizations and the physical

requests appropriate for the psychomotor praxis so essential in the accompaniment of the autistic children; we defend - we said it above -, the idea according to which the psychomotor development and the experiences of the *body in relation* would be good, in a psychopathologic and complex vision, the *missing link* of our theories and the link missed by the young child in the autistic process.
Which one, in a real *psychomotor subversion* would give us to see, throughout a singular development, *what would be our body without the body of the other one*! If we want to specify these remarks and fundamental observations on the place of the psychomotricity in the infantile autism, there is certain number of points on which we shall quickly agree!

4.1 The peculiarity of the tonic and postures adjustments

We notice all and always a bad tonic regulation (tonic and emotional conflicts in the interaction, the defect of interactive patterns - to stretch out arms, tonic adaptation - poverty of the mimes and the gestural and preverbal communications, etc.). In the difference for example of "damaged" babies neurologically, we are going to spot at baby's at autistic risks of the alternations between hypertonic moments and a more hypotonic bottom; but especially permanent seesaws between *hypo-*and *hyper-* tonic effect; a tonico-emotional not adaptation during the grips in arms; a dys-regulation becomes generic from the tonic relation to the other one and in the stimulations of the world. We so observe on a general bottom of hypotonie, dystonics attitudes, even hypertonic brightness, and little harmonious movements hampered by this bad regulation of the tonus. The tonic dialogue is also rather atypical with these children, either totally indifferent to the touch and the laborers of relaxation, either hyper-reagent withdrawing as "tormented souls" in a defensive attitude. In every case, this tonico-emotional conflict is as contagious, and the clinician has difficulty decoding, in him, the affects of the child, his state of well-being or on the contrary his faintness. In the same way the incapacities and the peculiarities of the postural control in the autistic states are almost systematically found by all the practitioners.

4.2 The specific driving behaviour

Later in the development, appear atypical steps, affectations, stereotypes, or postures of balance. And even if all this is enough little invading in the first 18 months of the life, it is the sector which we can investigate obviously the more before, and the more upstream; and we can then see premises of specific driving behaviour, strange, already clashing, possibly repetitive driving sets and mostly self-centred, always preferred to the interactive movements, to the psychomotor play in connection with the other one.

4.2.1 The disorders of the regulation of the motricity are constant

the children present or an extreme excitement or on the contrary a general slowing down of their activity, and mostly a rather perpetual passage and without visible logic of the first state to the second without intermediate level.

4.2.2 The general coordinations are affected almost always

We see very often abnormal movements accompanying the movements, and the replacing the usual coordinations of stabilization and accompaniment. The finer manual coordinations and the oculo-manual coordinations are also very damaged and of praxic and gestural adaptations, as because of some hyper or *hypo*-sensibilities. We meet disorders inferred by the occulo-manual coordination (absence of visual control during the movements), difficulty reproducing gestures, difficulties of grapho-perceptive organization, and globally difficulties in the spatial and temporal apprehension.

4.3 A defect of packagings and physical envelopes

non-existent or very fragile envelopes, with a conflict inferred in the way of investing and of living in its body, and a bankruptcy of the images of the body are always observed by all the clinicians.

4.4 The other peculiarity, it is the sensitivity and the sensori-motricity of the autistic

We can only underline, indeed, the pathognomonic stakes of the sensory and the sensori-motricity (search for sensory flows aggravated without intermodal coordinations, and without interactive regulations, etc.). The abnormalities of the sensory modes of integration are so important at the young child's autistics as Michel Lemay suggests as for him [12] considering them as principals markers of the first years. There is indeed an autistic constant living in the enigmatic alternation at the same time of hypo-and of hyper sensibility towards the hearing, visual, tactile stimulations, labyrinthics, and gustative; and in the joint failure of the usual modalities of integration, gathering and sensory co-modalities.

4.5 The rarity or the poverty then (even the extreme difficulty) playful driving activities, driving games, body experiences in the relation with other

Empty of desire or curiosity in the spontaneous exploration and especially in the emotional and interactive shared experiences.That we can move closer to a defect of to investing the diverse functions as playful driving experiences in the relation to the other one. It is necessary to insist on this determining aspect: little of spontaneous, affected and shared psychomotor explorations, or almost systematic choice of the self-centred and auto-sensual stimulation rather than from the relation to the other one and the playful exchange. This bankruptcy of the *playful motricity in relation* before being perceived in the observation of the spontaneous behaviour and the initiative appears as difficulty for the interlocutor to find and to maintain this type of early exchange with the child in the autistic process. Finally, the disturbances maybe the most characteristic of the autism affect the non-verbal communications of the child: the peculiarities of the glance (running away), the poverty of the mime, the absence of use of gestures to communicate, misses him general expressiveness, the defect of synchronization.

4.6 The intensity of the physical fears

Is another clinical evidence on which we hardly need to extend (cf. [7][14]).

4.7 Finally, in a more generic order, we find *psychomotor disharmonies* and rather *specific developmental disorders*

For a long time in the history of the autism, we were maybe filled by physical and driving skills in sectors but really rather clashing for these children sometimes fascinating us of their strange functioning and leading us to leave aside the authentic and cleanly psychomotor difficulties. Really, the detailed examination shows that many psychomotor functions are acquired, but that a global disharmony is found almost always with conflicts in the various sectors, invested or not, by the psychomotricity.

The difficulties of control of the equilibration are recurring: sometimes surprising, even paradoxical, the stake of equilibration and in harmony is in the majority of the disturbed, delayed cases or perturbed ; there are unusual movements, tiptoe, bizarre steps, search perms of flow of equilibration, breaks of the rhythms of the step.

All these physical and psychomotor disturbances in the autism that must be seen - i join Mr Lemay on this essential point: "at once as overdrawn phenomena (the subject "get" not), and as hypertrophied processes (the subject too much seems to receive without being able to abandon the stimulus for the other one) ". More essential and singular still we have to take the measure that "excepted certain subjects, the neurological or genetic infringements of which are recognized (...) The body is intact (but) everything takes place as if the body not altered in the point of departure, in its way of being, languished if he could not get, experiment, and create a personal identity" [12]. This evidence deducts which the careful evaluation of the psychomotricity in the primary development constitutes an essential stage of the differential diagnosis and the premature care.

For André Bullinger [3,4] and his school, it does not make doubt that the body and its various expressions occupy a dominating place at the autistic children; that to be always singular, of course, to every child, these physical peculiarities appear as determining elements of understanding the world of the autistics and their specific difficulties and their felt. Rather close to perspectives deployed somewhere else by Jean Ayres [2] in conformance with "*the sensory integration*", the *sensori-motor perspective* developed by Bullinger, at once instrumental or functional, neuropsychological, cognitive and developmental, knew how to measure and light certain number of physical and psychomotor autistic peculiarities of the child.

The children presenting an autistic or disorders of the P.D.D. series seem in this sensori-motor reading sharpened by Bullinger [4][6] always to present incapacities of sensori-motor integration and being made an instrumentation always very particular which are going to produce or to accompany one certain numbers of difficulties:

- at the sensory level, the persons with autism "maximize" the archaic sensations to maintain a tonic mobilization rather than to use in exploratory or manipulator purposes sense organs, in particular to the detriment of the spatial representations;
- while at the postural level, we observe a tonic regulation in extension with a defect of équilibration between the flexion and the extension, the difficulties in the coordination of the various physical spaces straight ahead / left and top / bottom (stocking, bottoms, stockings).
- We find pathological postures, disorders of the suction, and the problematic tonic regulations, the possibilities of insatiable incorporations and ascendancies of the archaic systems, in particular explorations, disorders were inferred by praxies oculomotrices; tonic recruitments in extension around a pneumatic tonus; tonic regulations of lower limbs by all or none; fixations(bindings) on the oral space, and difficulties of coordinations of spaces right and left with an important limitation of the activities elaborated praxiques.

The autistic child often resorts(turns) to compulsive behaviours and discharges driving as stereotypies. Really, he has difficulty in reaching a representation untied(removed) from the action(share). As says it Bullinger: "*the image of the body is maintained present by the very sensations; but as soon as the sensations stop the image of the body becomes blurred*" [4]. All these drivings(behaviors) have, in the end(final), a role of gathering; and repeated in so atypical a way them become of real (necessary but intrusive) modalities of agrippements or " prostheses of gathering ".

They appear when the situation pulls(entails) an emotional overflowing further to a sensory stimulation which they cannot check(control). Evident incidences deduct in the therapeutic plan, because it will be a question for example, in a work in psychomotricity, of aiming globally at a better integration of the physical envelope (from experience(experiment) shared by relational porterages with various mediators seeking and enriching capacities of representations of various levels).

5. The early psychomotor signs of the autism

Towards the early signs of an autistic risk and a commitment of an autistic process, we can notice that certain number of clinical signs allows to suspect (and warn maybe prematurely) the eventuality otherwise of an already established autism, to say the least a developmental adversity at very high psychiatric risk, a autistic risk, of a possible forecast of later autistic evolution. We have to add at once that the parents and mostly the professionals of the early childhood track down generally the first signs of conflict, rather during the second year of life of the child, and, for the main part, signs of the communicational series (which are always the most obvious and the most worrisome for them); much less to say almost never upstream the signs of the nevertheless essential physical and psychomotor series. The qualitative specificities of the global delay of development and the earlier indicators of the tonic and postural side, playful and emotional very early, are in fact only little moderate, even ignored by the specialists of the early childhood, often still badly formed in this extremely fine screening the subtlety of which is confused with the neurological items and the only acquisition of the big driving functions (motive units for example). From this point of view, it seems to me important to proclaim quite a reverse the importance to observe the psychomotor development and tonic-postural at the child generally, and strangely at that at autistic risk [4,9,10,13]; but farther to seize in the early psychomotor development the principal stakes of the later deployments in germs so much socio-communicational side, as cognitive and emotional. It is what to what we would like to become attached, as for us, in this present reflection.

We have, as for us, to develop - in the *C.R.A. of Burgundy* [1] [9] - a prospect of psychomotor research on *the signs of alert of an early autism;* a research eminently developmental and complex articulating *a)* a positive and negative methodology at the same time (specific signs, presence or absence of indicators of normal development and perceptible and singular abnormalities of these developmental processes), and *b)* a plural perspective around a developmental early major axis of the child at risk: the psychomotor sphere [tonus, postural, sensori-motricity, development of the playing and the psychomotor interactions, the desire in the interactive driving and physical exploration, the deployment of the executive functions, the perceptive and the praxies, etc.] ...

With an underlying hypothesis which would be that the defect and the principal abnormality in the very early development of the future autistics (and before even the appearance of the differentials signs that they decline in a way turned out in the cognitive or psycho-affective sphere) this native defect would indeed deceive in the psychomotor

[1] Every region in *France* have of a "*Resources Autisms Center*" where the persons with autism, the family as the professionals can find helps, advice, information, technical and practical trainings, and where differential diagnoses or functional evaluations can be proposed, led researches, work of network and organized partnership, and colloquiums and study days organized.

register, more exactly in the failure, the failure or the specific abnormality of the crossroads and the early psychomotor knotting.

The first elements of the research (collected during on 2009 and to seem: meta analysis of the national and international literature; perusal of a investigation with the French-speaking professionals of the psychomotor approach of the babies "to risks"; elements of a first analysis of the inaugural stage of the research on family movies from a railing of observation elaborated by our team) go to the direction of:

- a confirmation of the developmental and multi-factorial hypothesis of a autistic process deployed from a compost of equipment at risk, and more or less realized and fixed as the case may be singulars and the fates, in the developmental process driving to the autistic picture;
- a location of points of alerts, sufferings early developmental or of pre-autistic peculiarities testifying every time in the fall of the evolution of the malleability of the early signs: who seem through the development little as a "*extinction of lights*". To be early, they are neither permanent nor immediate and become more marked in the fall of the development; while go out quite the reverse of more positive elements, still present in the first months;
- a confirmation of the critical period of fixation or unlike developmental, strangely decisive processing between 6 and 18 months (golden age of the psychomotricity of the young child);
- the report that in the difference of all the parental and professional centred alerts (during the second year) on the not appearance of the linguistic items and socio-communicational it is many items of the psychomotor, sensori-motor and physical series that appear in the first year of life as the first indicators of a failure or a developmental drift at high risk;
- the measure that these signs of the psychomotor series (tonic, postural and sensori-motor) are first and not only in the time but maybe as precursors and organizers of the later significant signs of the cognitive series (defect of *theory of the spirit*, the defect of *central coherence*, peculiarity of the perception, the memory, and the *executive functions* etc.) as of the psychic and emotional series (singular quality of the fears, the specificities of the identifications, the splits and the poverty of the psychic play - being made, that before the signs of the specific cognitive and functional series [6,14] or that the clinical quality tried by the autistic peculiarities (specific fears, operating procedure in dismantling and adhesivity [7,14]) these psychomotor items should be systematically studied and detected);
- a demonstration that these early signs are marked at first in the negative series (all which is not set up and does not appear as usual in the interactive flight of the early development) before to create specific and "positive" autistic signs of the series;
- All these indicators, finally, are increased in the interactions and the environmental situations of relational stimulations and interactive appeals, and underestimated in time more solitary and less inter-subjective.

6. By way of conclusion: The French psychomotor prospect in the disorders of development

All in all, sensori-motor and psychomotor all these disorders of the autistic body, these adversities in the P.D.D. is almost specific of the autistic problem, and should be added as such maybe to the set of three of the fundamental signs (socio-emotional difficulties, delays and peculiarities of the communication and the language, the repetitive and restricted behaviour. These signs of the body indicate, within the framework of this prototypic disorder of the development, a disharmony developmental major the psychomotor and physical elements of which can hardly appear as simple additional effects of accompaniment, or as a kind of secondary and inescapable co-morbidity, but according to me must be well included as an aspect obviously central and primary of this singular development.

Better, maybe, we can make here the hypothesis that it is this shunt of the development and the psychomotor harmony that is the substratum and the source of the autistic cognitive "styles" or the later executive and functional difficulties in an understanding developmental complex.

Therapeutic psychomotor and the other therapeutic and educational physical mediations constitute consequently, and according to us, paradigm of a privileged treatment of the autism: *1/* of a "regime" rich in social games or so difficult for the autistic child; *2/* of a support and a relaunching for the subjective appropriation of the development with a playful transformation of the difficulties of functioning (or an ironing on developmental failures adults of the autistic); *3/* an original and mediatized business with the object, facilitating "the taming" and the meeting experiences of the patient autistic, supporting permanently the play, the creativity and the psychic drive since the survival inhabited with the therapist and since its playful creativity, in its body and in its psyche, weaving preferentially symbolizations, representations and affects, in the link in the other one; *4/* favoring as a matter of fact that a young patient conquers himself through the objectal meeting. It is indeed all in all about an approach privileged by the construction of the person and by the feeling of identity, as well as consistently by the opening in an authentic work of the thought which favors the development of the playful interactions, the representation and the processes of so outstanding symbolizations usually in the early infantile autism.

The therapeutic work at the sensory and psychomotor level with the autistic children is one of better opportunities to introduce them even to the emotional language, to the communication with the other one as with itself, and to the social and relational desire. There is a large number of actions led to the psychomotor plan which are susceptible to act on certain psychic, social and cognitive functions so disrupted in the autism, and susceptible also to transform autistic behavior so crippling.

If the body of the autistic child illustrates regrettably in a exemplary way it *anything that would be*, according to Julian de Ajuriaguerra, *our body, without the body of the other one*; the psychomotor meeting of these young patients besides being a playful taming and mediatized rubbing up the wrong way in a way backwards intrusive strategies of autistic avoidance; farther still than to be a situation experiential favoring as few other numbers of even cognitive socio-cultural, playful, emotional, instrumental learning; this psychomotor meeting appears to me more decisively as an relational business knotted around *the playful motricity in connection with this body of the other one* exactly, and being made a singular and, to say the bottom of my unique thought, inter-subjective developmental experience who is invested by drive ...

In the end of this reflection, this exploration, this "plowing" of the question of *the body of the autistic child*: we shall have understood that this autistic body is leads imposes upon the understanding, imposes upon the coverage and upon the daily and sometimes very pragmatic and behavioural consideration, but also stands out as object of thought as question to think in theory. Better he obliges us to leave farthest possible our blindness of school and our fragmented little points of view, our narrow quarrels to impose a complex and multidimensional vision so much development as the pathology and all the more of an authentic developmental psychopathology which tries to report the autism and the disorders allies of the family of Pervasive Developmental Disorders ...

This body - which interests us here and which is imperative in the clinical of the autism as somewhere else in the other psychopathological regions - is not indeed the only soma and its reasons of equipments, its neuro-cognitive, functional and instrumental stakes it is not more for the psychic pole the only dimension of the images of the body it is exact intertwining of these two registers forming the subjectivity of every human being, crossing and articulating for each the peculiarities so essential developmental here for the persons with autism?

The *French school of psychomotricity* - next to the other numerous additional perspectives - is one of theoric and clinical perspectives, developmental and psychopathologic but also therapeutics and readaptation which rethinks the problem of the autistic spectre in a complex vision of the development which integrates effectively all these registers into the place of the body living of the small subject in development. The problem of the body of the autistic child requires from us a thought complex and integrated by these psychomotor stakes. The young patients and their families wait at the bottom of us that we do not mutilate this complex dimension in excessive simplifications that they were for a long time in France only psycho-analytic that they are international only neuro-cognitive, educational and behavioural today. Any unambiguous thought is an ill-treatment of the autism as any unambiguous care, an ill-treatment of the person with autism.

We arrive, there as for us, (between clinical experiences, theoretical conceptualizations and look for psychopathologic) to think that on the background of a compost of equipment "at risk", hindering for multidimensional reasons the premature interactions and the tension of the baby towards the other human being, and making difficult the immediate use of the propositions of the essential psychic partner, settles then, in the first 6 months of the life, the bases of a interactive spiral pathogenic auto-going out little by little in vicious circles of avoidance and autarkic confinement. Vicious circles where the autistic contamination quickly plays a not insignificant role on the paradoxical answers of the interactive partner. Pathogenic bases at high risk which lead to the second half-year of life in an autistic potentiality, that is in a "perversion" or in a developmental twisting and in an acceleration of the autistic processes towards the clinical picture little by little specific and so resistant, of the syndrome of early infantile autism.

I would thus like to propose here - originally multifactorial and integrated model of the autistic fates - the idea of a major adversity of the *motricity-play in relation*, as real *missing link* of the autistic fates (before the advent of the *reflexive capacity* of P. Fonagy and of the *theory of the spirit* according to cognitive Baron-Cohen, Frith, Leslie) in the place of "*the primary intersubjectivity*" (Trevarthen) and first "*emotional tunings*" on the background of which (Stern) a subject appears in the harmonious development of the structures and the relation in the object. This principal axe of the psychomotricity for become a subject at this young age, and for engine the impulsive circuit and the psychic destiny. An adversity even a perverse drift of the psychomotricity of the babies at autistic risks which do not use any

more this potentiality of interactive playful and psychic experiences in the meeting of the world, the objects, and the other one, than in the withdrawal of investment and a mechanical and instrumental use. A shunt of the psychomotricity which - at best! - allows some paradoxical performances and an appearance of good functional and body living, but watch really the practitioner who meets at these levels these patients a conflict and a radical psychomotor strangeness.
It is good by the *motricity in relation*, what the autistic peculiarity appears to the interlocutor, because it is by the same *motricity in relation* that the drive meets the object in the drive principal trajectory of which a psychic subject source usually!
A large-scale conclusion deducts of all this: the psychomotricity of any young is at once a precursor and a central organizer of the later functioning of the personality (so cognitive as perceptive and psycho-affective); and the failure of these early psychomotor stakes is a point of maximum alert of later shady intrusive of the development: strangely of the typical autism. We do not have more than to let it know and to hope that the community of the autism mobilizes to investigate these principal stakes.

7. References

[1] Ajuriaguerra (J. de) : *J. de Ajuriaguerra et la naissance de la psychomotricité* Ed. F. Joly et G. Labes - Paris, Ed. du Papyrus 2008.
[2] Ayres (J.) : *The development of sensory integrative theory and practice* Kendall, Hunt Pub co, 1974
[3] Bullinger (A.) : *Le développement sensorimoteur* Ramonville Ste Agne, Erès, 2004.
[4] Bullinger (A.) : « Le dialogue sensori-moteur avec l'enfant : les particularités du bébé à risque autistique » In P. Delion et coll. *Les bébés à risques autistiques* Toulouse, Erès 2008, pp.47-59
[5] Curcio (F.) : « Sensorimotor functionning and communication in mute autistic children » *J. Autism Child Schizo.* 1978 / 8 pp.281-292
[6] Demyer (M. K.) : « Motor, perceptual-motor and intellectual disabilities of autistic children » In L. Wing ed. : *Early Cildhood Autism* – London Pergamon Press, 1976.
[7] Joly (F.) : « Notre corps n'est rien sans le corps de l'autre » *Thérapie Psychomotrice* 2003 n°134 pp.40-58
[8] Joly (F.) : « Le corps en question : psychopathologie des troubles instrumentaux » *Le Carnet Psy* oct.2009 n°138 pp.39-49
[9] Joly (F.) : « Les signes psychomoteurs précoces de l'autisme » *Contrastes* 2008 n°28-29 pp.179-198
[10] Joly (F.): «Des troubles psychomoteurs précoces dans l'autisme à une vision psychomotrice de l'autisme infantile » *A.N.A.E.* 2009 n°104-105 pp.407-416
[11] Joly (F.) : « Le sens des thérapeutiques psychomotrices en psychiatrie de l'enfant » *Neuropsychiatrie de l'Enfant et de l'Adolescent* 2007 Vol.55 n°2 pp.73-86
[12] Lemay (M.) : « L'enfant face au dialogue avec lui-même et avec autrui » In *L'autisme aujourd'hui* pp.53-86 Paris, O. Jacob, 2004.
[13] Teitelbaum (P.), Teitelbaum, O., Nye, J., Fryman, J. & Maurer, R. G. . *Movement analysis in infancy may be useful for early diagnosis of autism, Proc. Natl. Acad. Sci.* U S A – 1988 / 95, 23, 13982-7
[14] Tustin (F.) : *Autistic States in Children* Routledge and Kegan Paul, London U.K., 1981.

25

Transition to Adulthood for High-Functioning Individuals with Autism Spectrum Disorders

Steven K. Kapp, Alexander Gantman and Elizabeth A. Laugeson
University of California, Los Angeles
United States of America

1. Introduction

Adolescence and young adulthood appear to form the most difficult period in the lives of high-functioning individuals with autism spectrum disorders (ASD; Tantam, 2003). The challenges often faced by those without intellectual disabilities appear to result from the demands of social relationships, academics, employment, and independent living in those with ASD, which may exacerbate core ASD deficits or co-occurring conditions (Barnhill, 2007; Howlin, 2000). The features of these developmental periods, combined with the general challenges with transitions in this population, may explain why the reduction in ASD symptoms that individuals experience throughout life (Seltzer et al., 2003) tend to slow in the transition to adulthood (Taylor & Lounds, 2010). This population appears to be growing despite a shortfall in services and knowledge about these individuals, posing the need for more attention to this area (Barnard et al., 2001; Gerhardt & Lainer, 2011; Shattuck et al., 2011).

Adulthood marks a transfer of legal responsibility for individuals with ASD from parental support to self-advocacy. Young adults are often faced with needs to make decisions about their lives, yet they may not fully understand their own unique profile of strengths and weaknesses, or how to advocate for services to meet their needs (Geller & Greenberg, 2010; Townson et al., 2007). In addition, these young adults often feel socially alienated during this period of transition, as though they do not belong or fit in with their peer group (Portway & Johnson, 2003; Ryan & Raisanen, 2008; Simmeborn Fleischer, in press), while sensing others' may be underestimating their competences (Ashby & Causton-Theoharis, 2009). These struggles may not only relate to social deficits, but may also be associated with cognitive, emotional, and sensory information processing deficits (Chamak et al., 2008). For example, sensory overload may compromise the cognitive performance of individuals with ASD or lead to withdrawal or absence of participation from various social situations (Madriaga, 2010).

Yet for adults with ASD, quality of life or subjective wellbeing appears positively related to perceived informal support and inversely related to unmet formal support needs. Disability characteristics such as ASD symptoms and IQ appear to be unrelated to subjective wellbeing (Renty & Roeyers, 2006). These findings have implications for the provision of accommodations and formal support for relationships and daytime activities for adults with ASD. Yet services tend to decline for individuals with ASD after they leave high school, which appears related to reduced abatement of ASD symptoms, the frequent absence of daytime activities such as higher education or work, and strains on the mother-child relationship (Shattuck et al., 2011; Taylor & Seltzer, 2011, in press). This gap in services suggests the need for strong coping skills, yet the strategies adults with ASD employ in their daily lives vary widely in types and degrees of success (Simmeborn Fleischer, in press; Müller et al., 2008; Sperry & Mesibov, 2005). Given the importance of quality of life during transition to adulthood and beyond, this chapter focuses on areas that encompass environmental components related to wellbeing, such as: social relationships, mental health, education, employment, and independent living.

2. Outcomes in adolescence and adulthood

The core symptoms found in ASD include deficits in communication, impaired social interaction, and restricted interests and repetitive behavior (American Psychiatric Association [APA], 2000). These core deficits are further highlighted by poor social cognition or lack of theory of mind, a hallmark feature in ASD. For example, those with ASD often demonstrate deficits in the ability to understand another person's perspective, the demonstration and expression of empathy, or the understanding of emotions, all of which may be related to deficits in imagination and ability to engage in meaningful social interactions (Baron-Cohen & Wheelwright, 2004; APA, 2000). Such impairments in adults with ASD may include deficits in inferring point of view from language, explaining thoughts or feelings, or relating them to behavior and events, especially when provided with less apparent social cues (Colle et al., 2008).

Adults with ASD also have a tendency for selective attention that allows them to take in a high amount of information, but also display difficulties in integrating information or applying it in context (Bogte et al., 2009; Remington et al., 2009), resulting in a trend toward systematic, exhaustive decision making despite the ability to process information at a typical speed (Johnson et al., 2010). This type of idiosyncratic information processing (Minshew et al., 1997) can prove challenging in a variety of social contexts. While the tendency toward restricted, repetitive behaviors can be enhanced through selective attention and may even prove useful for scientific or professional endeavors (Yechiam et al., 2010), idiosyncratic information processing may actually impede reciprocity and spontaneity in social conversations and interactions (APA, 2000). Similarly, lack of cognitive flexibility and executive function deficits in individuals with ASD (Kleinhans et al., 2005) may relate to the greater unpredictability of social norms and contexts (Geurts, et al., 2009; Kenworthy, et al., 2008), making social interactions even more challenging.

Social deficits and low cognitive flexibility lie at the root of many challenges faced by individuals with ASD, particularly with regard to social relationships, education, mental health, education, employment, and independent living (Barnhill, 2007; Farley, 2009; Howlin et al., 2004). The following chapter will highlight the challenges experienced by transitional youth and young adults with ASD in these five key areas, all of which encompass transition into adulthood (Geller & Greenberg, 2010; Hendricks & Wehman, 2009; Lawrence et al., 2010).

2.1 Social relationships

Not surprisingly, autism spectrum disorders (ASD) are characterized by impairments in the ability to develop peer relationships like friendships (American Psychological Association, 2000). Adolescents with ASD, relative to their neurotypical peers, tend to have low friendship quality, if they have any friends, and to be on the periphery of social networks at their school, if not isolated (Locke et al., 2010). Although adolescents with ASD sometimes describe friendships in terms suggesting social and emotional reciprocity, such as mutual caring, responsiveness, and forgiveness, they often focus on concrete areas like common interests (Daniel & Billingsley, 2010; Howard et al., 2006; Carrington et al., 2003). This tendency does not appear to reflect lack of caring or poor emotional empathy, but rather deficits in understanding others' perspective (Blair, 2005; Dziobek et al., 2008; Jones et al., 2010; Poutska et al., 2010; Rogers et al., 2007). Individuals with ASD may identify making friends as their greatest social challenge, which may relate not only to knowing how to make appropriate choices regarding compatible social status groups or personalities, but also failing to initiate social interactions, and passively waiting for others to approach in order to avoid social rejection (Daniel & Billingsley, 2010).

One critical challenge in forming and maintaining relationships lies in conversational skills. Many, if not most, adolescents and adults with ASD have a pedantic speaking style (Ghaziddin & Gerstein, 1996). They also often have difficulty with articulation in areas such as phrasing, stress, and tone when speaking (Shriberg et al., 2001). Other difficulties include inappropriately formal, irrelevant or inappropriate detail, out-of-sync content and unannounced topic shifts, topic perseveration, unresponsiveness to others' cues, little reciprocal exchange, and absent or inappropriate intonation or gaze (Paul et al., 2009). Children with ASD may show deficits in resolving ambiguity, understanding inferential language, and using linguistic flexibility to produce speech acts limited by the communicative context. Adults with ASD may demonstrate difficulties in interpreting figurative language and producing relevant speech acts (Lewis et al., 2007). Moreover, linguistic impairments appear mostly related to specific pragmatic deficits rather than general linguistic abilities, as individuals with ASD may not demonstrate impairments in general narrative abilities like story length and syntactic complexity, but may not use the gist well to organize the story cohesively (Colle et al., 2008).

Perhaps due to deficits in conversational skills and difficulty relating to peers, many adolescents with ASD identify adults and school staff as their friends (Daniel & Billingsley, 2010; Humphrey & Symes, 2010b), even though they enjoy or desire friendships with peers (Daneil & Billingsley, 2010; Howard, Cohen, & Orsmond, 2006; Carrington, Templeton, & Papinczak, 2003). In turn, these adolescents often report comparable social support from teachers relative to typical peers, but low social support from classmates and friends (Humphrey & Symes, 2010b; Lasgaard et al., 2010). These adolescents may also view peers as unpredictable (Humphrey & Symes, 2010b) or disagree with the services for which their parents are advocating (Humphrey & Lewis, 2008), but think of teachers as reliable, helpful resources and sometimes as confidantes or "friends" (Humphrey & Symes, 2010b). For instance, in response to ridicule, adolescents with ASD will usually tell a teacher or another trusted adult (Connor, 2000), even though this strategy has limited effectiveness (Humphrey & Symes, 2010a).

Similarly, many adolescents and young adults with ASD have no friends, or only one or two casual friends, and rarely participate in social and recreational activities like making phone calls, having get-togethers, and attending clubs or social activities (Liptak et al, 2011; Orsmond et al., 2004). Friendships in both adolescents and adults with ASD often lack rich quality regarding intimacy, empathy, and supportiveness (Baron-Cohen & Wheelwright, 2003). Already challenged by poor social skills in such basic areas as using social cues and entering, engaging in, and exiting two-way conversations, many young adults with ASD further limit their opportunities for social success by making few social initiations or withdrawing from social interactions or settings altogether (Shatyermann, 2007). Yet adults with ASD do not necessarily prefer to be alone and may spend as much time in social company as their neurotypical peers, but tend to do so with people more familiar to them (Hintzen et al., 2010). Not surprisingly, many parents play an active role in social coaching or facilitating friendships for their adolescents and young adults with ASD (Howard et al., 2006; Orsmond et al., 2004), and parental advocacy tends to improve social participation (Liptak et al, 2011). For example, parents may encourage get-togethers and help their adolescent or young adult identify potential sources of friends in part by suggesting clubs that emphasize their child's interests and strengths (Gantman et al., in press; Geller & Greenberg, 2010; Laugeson & Frankel, 2010, Laugeson et al., 2009, Laugeson et al., in press).

Many adolescents and adults with ASD describe their social challenges or deficits as barriers to their goal of fitting in (Humphrey & Lewis, 2008; Jones & Meldal, 2001) and often view their differences related to ASD as an underlying problem or obstacle to social acceptance (Humphrey & Lewis, 2008). For example, adolescents and young adults with ASD may rigidly adhere to moral or social rules or norms (e.g., "lying is bad") even at the expense of self-presentation gains, which suggests a need for tact and flexibility (Scheeren et al., 2010). Restricted styles of information processing may explain why adolescents and young adults with ASD may refuse to deceive even when they show understanding of how to make a good impression (Scheeren et al., 2010). Moreover, they may make a similar degree of positive self-statements when they want a peer to like them, but also make more references to honesty or truth than neurotypical peers that can interfere with the goal of a positive social impression. For instance, they may appear less strategic in adjusting to audience preferences and demands, in part because of a choice to not lie (such as pretending that one shares an interest in a neighbor's new pet; Scheeren et al., 2010). By adulthood, some individuals with ASD adopt diverse strategies in how they present themselves in public, with some trying to "pass" or apply additional effort to manage impairments related to ASD, and others openly self-disclosing their diagnosis for educational and advocacy purposes (Davidson & Henderson, 2010). Adults may also tend to be more open and less strategic around loved ones and friends, who tend to be more understanding.

Not surprisingly, the presence of poor social skills also appears to impact the development of romantic relationships and further affect the social independence of adolescents and young adults with ASD. Most neurotypical individuals develop close friendships and romantic relationships by young adulthood (Collins & Madsen, 2006), during which time romantic relationships are associated with achieving norms of adulthood like independence from parents, identity development, and commitment to long-term social relationships (Barry et al., 2009). The social and romantic functioning of individuals with ASD compares unfavorably to neurotypical peers, with social skills predicting the ability to form romantic relationships (Stokes et al., 2007). Even though both groups report sharing similar interests in forming intimate relationships, those with ASD often lack the social skills knowledge to appropriately pursue and engage in romantic relationships (Hellemans et al., 2007; Ousley & Mesibov, 1991),For example, they may not understand norms of social boundaries and naively behave in an intrusive manner with potential romantic partners, which may even be perceived as stalking behavior (Stokes et al., 2007). Other behavior possibly perceived as abusive includes inappropriate violent or sexual comments to peers of either sex, touching peers without invitation, and pursuing younger children because of their greater compliance (Ray et al., 2004).

While many adults with ASD recognize that they need more education regarding romantic relationships and would benefit from receiving it a younger age (Mehzabin & Stokes, 2011; Müller et al., 2008), parents of youth with ASD often have concerns about their adolescent's sexuality or dating that surpass his or her social deficits and may not feel ready to have their child address this topic (Stokes & Kaur, 2005). Perhaps for all these reasons, romantic relationships appear to be infrequent (Stokes et al., 2007) and marriages are even rarer (Barnhill, 2007) for adults with ASD.

Nevertheless, while individuals with ASD may encounter great challenges establishing romantic relationships, some of those who do marry may enjoy successful relationships in part because of ASD-related qualities. Some men with ASD have happy, decades-old marriages in which informal support from family and friends, but not necessarily formal support or other coping styles, predict individual and marital well-being for both spouses (Renty & Roeyers, 2007). Marriage may provide more satisfaction to women than men with ASD; in marriages in which one spouse has high ASD traits, having high ASD traits may lower marital satisfaction for husbands but not wives. In both cases, the spouse's high ASD traits do not appear to affect the martial satisfaction of the spouse without high ASD traits (Pollmann et al., 2010). Strengths and weaknesses among the marital relationships between ASD husbands and neurotypical wives do exist. For example, young adult men with high ASD traits in romantic relationships show less interest in sex and less extravagant courtship than men with low ASD traits, but higher commitment to specific partners and long-term romantic relationships and greater investment of the allocation of resources toward a career and potential marriage (Del Guicide et al., 2010). Suggesting further complexity of romantic relationships, college students with high ASD traits may experience more romantic loneliness compared to their counterparts with low ASD traits, but ultimately may experience longer relationships (Jobe & Williams White, 2007). The ASD traits of attention to detail and difficulties with attention switching or need for sameness seem to instill a hyperfocus on loyalty to a specific partner that can lead to a committed relationship (Del Guicide et al., 2010; Jobe & Williams White, 2007).

Likely related to low self-awareness of social impairment, adolescents and young adults with ASD rate themselves more positively on measures of social functioning than do their parents, teachers, and clinicians, regardless of IQ (Cederlund et al., 2010; Green et al., 2000; Johnson et al., 2009; Koning & Magill-Evans, 2001). For example, many adolescents with ASD have poor self-awareness and report no differences between themselves and neurotypical peers (Green et al., 2000). Furthermore, many adolescents and young adults with ASD go through life never imagining that they have a disability until their parents disclose their ASD diagnosis to them, which often does not happen until at least adolescence (Huws & Jones, 2008). Even if their diagnosis had been shared at an earlier age, many adolescents seem unaware or unaccepting of their ASD diagnosis by not talking about their disability despite being asked about it (Camarena & Sarigiani, 2010). Perhaps earlier disclosure about ASD in a developmentally and socially sensitive manner, that takes into account the whole person and both the strengths and weaknesses associated with ASD, would help many individuals with ASD have a better understanding of themselves and their differences. In this way, these individuals might have a greater self-knowledge and self-awareness on which to build their social skills so that they may develop stronger and more meaningful friendships and romantic relationships.

2.2 Mental Health

The social deficits just described often co-occur and interact with psychiatric conditions such as anxiety and, perhaps especially, depression (Ghaziuddin et al., 2002). Adolescents who feel different from their peers are more likely to endorse depressive symptoms (Hedley & Young, 2006). A complicating factor may be that the depressed adolescent with ASD may not fully understand the role their ASD diagnosis or social deficits play in their challenges, consider themselves misunderstood and mistreated, and consequently feel depressed. Similarly, adolescents with ASD may develop a passive, failure-prone attributional style consistent with learned helplessness and depression (Abramson et al., 1978). Perceiving themselves as having made many great efforts at friendship in various settings, many make low ability attributions for social failure, thereby causing depression (Barnhill, 2001). They may generalize this social attribution, explaining negative events with internal, stable, and global causes and attributing external, unstable, and specific causes to negative events. This low-ability attribution to pervasive, outside forces beyond their control suggests a poor coping style, rather than more adaptively attributing failure to lack of effort or chance and task difficulty factors (Barnhill & Myles, 2001). Self-doubt, low self-esteem, and other depressive symptoms may intensify during the transition to adulthood, sometimes externalized as oppositional, irritable, or aggressive behaviors, or internalized as isolation and profound sadness (Ghaziuddin et al., 2002).

In adulthood, depression co-occurs more commonly in those who are older, have higher IQ, and less severe ASD symptoms, possibly reflecting greater self-awareness and harsher attitudes by others who have higher expectations (Sterling et al., 2008). For example, adolescents and young adults with less severe ASD symptoms are more likely to be victimized by peers, perhaps because they appear odd, rather than impaired by disability, making them more vulnerable to anxiety, depression, suicidal ideation, and avoidant behavior (Shtayermman, 2007). Adolescents and young adults with ASD often suffer from social stigma (Shtayermann, 2009). This social stigma relates not so much to disclosure of a label like Asperger's Disorder , but more to the presentation of atypical behaviors associated with ASD (Butler & Gillis, 2011).

Having a good friend or even physical companionship can form a strong shield against peer victimization (Hodges et al., 1999), and ultimately depression or anxiety. Perhaps due to the social naïveté and social isolation experienced by many with ASD, these adolescents and young adults may be seen as easy targets for teasing and bullying (Humphrey & Symes, 2010). Loneliness, low-quality best friendships (Whitehouse et al., 2009) and social withdrawal (White & Roberson-Nay, 2009) contribute to depression in adolescents and likely adults with ASD. Furthermore, social disability, poor social motivation, and negative affect have negative social impacts for adolescents with ASD (Schwartz et al., 2009; White & Roberson-Nay, 2009; Whitehouse et al., 2009). Furthermore, social rejection such as bullying may lead to a cycle of more bullying, because for most victims with ASD, the experience of bullying weakens social relationships and creates or exacerbates mental health problems like anxiety, low self-esteem, and loneliness, resulting in more asocial behavior like withdrawal (Humphrey & Symes, 2010).

Feelings of loneliness about relationships with peers often contribute to depression and social withdrawal in adolescents and adults with ASD. Usually in inclusive settings, adolescents with ASD interact mainly with and make regular social initiations toward neurotypical peers, but their social difficulties often result in social neglect and thus loneliness (Bauminger et al., 2003). Indeed, low perceived social support from classmates and friends contributes to the experience of loneliness in this population (Lasgaard et al., 2010; Whitehouse et al., 2009) and possibly relates to low centrality and connectedness in social networks with peers (Locke et al., 2010). Adults with ASD describe experiencing a profound sense of isolation and related depression, with low-quality social relationships because of not knowing how to initiate and sustain conversations and relationships (Müller et al., 2008). For many adults with ASD, the highest level as existing friendships are "acquaintanceships" (Müller et al., 2008). Similarly, writings and interviews with people with ASD commonly include intense descriptions of loneliness and alienation related to social difficulties (Causton-Theoharis et al., 2009; Jones et al., 2001). Furthermore, because many individuals with ASD lack the social skills to appropriately engage in romantic relationships (despite having similar interests in these relationships compared to neurotypical peers), adolescents and adults with ASD often experience romantic loneliness (Mehzabin & Stokes, 2011; Ousley & Mesibov, 1991). Young adults with ASD report high concerns that they may never find a life partner (Mehzabin & Stokes, 2011) and adults with ASD in romantic relationships report longing for greater intimacy (Müller et al., 2008).

Like depression, anxiety appears to increase over time in people with ASD. Specifically, social anxiety and withdrawal increase throughout adolescence in this population, even though these symptoms tend to decrease during this period of development for neurotypical peers (Kuusikko et al., 2008). Anxiety appears to reflect concerns about peer relationships for adolescents and young adults with ASD, but may have a deeper root, as ASD symptoms may overlap with generalized anxiety and social anxiety (Cath et al., 2008). Restricted interests and general rigidity may cause anxiety about unfamiliar or unstructured experiences, as individuals with ASD often display obsessive behavior but are much less likely to seek out or feel rewarded by new stimuli (Anckarsäter et al., 2006; Ozonoff et al., 2005; Soderstrom et al., 2002). Although many want to establish and maintain social relationships, transitional youth with ASD may feel so anxious about the possibility of rejection that they feel compelled to avoid social situations and the possible risk of rejection or social failure. This avoidance may be so severe that these individuals do not even exhibit the initiative and self-directedness to give themselves the necessary exposure to peers or a significant chance to succeed (Anckarsäter et al., 2006; Ozonoff et al., 2005; Soderstrom et al., 2002).

Low social functioning and anxiety in social relationships tends to carry over to romantic relationships in adolescents and adults with ASD (Stokes et al., 2007). Romantic relationships appear more challenging and infrequent for young adults with ASD than other social relationships (Jennes-Coussens et al., 2006). Reports indicate significant concern and worry that others may misinterpret their behavior as sexual, possibly related to a lack of understanding about privacy and social boundaries, and sometimes a lack of understanding about their own sexual physical responses such as arousal (Mehzabin & Stokes, 2011). Having had less sex education and fewer sexual experiences than neurotypical peers, adolescents and young adults with ASD learn from themselves, peers, or friends, even though the information gleaned may be less accurate than that coming from an authoritative source.

Related to comorbid depression and anxiety, the low ability to self-regulate emotions at a physiological level may also render individuals with ASD especially vulnerable to stress in their social interactions (Bellini, 2006). Instead of trying to adaptively manage intense emotions, adolescents and adults may try to avoid them and associated interactions (Corden et al., 2008). The high prevalence of a cognitive form of alexithymia in adults with ASD (Berthoz & Hill, 2005), a personality trait that poses barriers for the recognition, description, and interpretation of one's own emotional states (Silani et al., 2008), presents further obstacles for the ability of adolescents and adults with ASD to understand and regulate difficult emotions that impair psychosocial functioning (Hill et al., 2004). Alexithymia positively correlates with depression in adults with ASD (Hill et al., 2004), in part because it limits their ability to dissociate the emotions of others from their own. It may occur in at least 85 percent of the ASD population, but only 15 percent of the general population, suggesting that an inability to recognize and interpret emotional states may be a core feature of ASD (Hill et al., 2004). Alexithymia may also significantly reduce empathy in both the ASD (Bird et al., 2010) and general (Grynberg et al., 2010) population.

Poor emotion regulation abilities appear related to anxiety, possibly not only linking to emotional reactivity but also playing a role in the etiology of anxiety disorders (Cisler et al., 2010). While generalized anxiety relates more closely to poor emotion regulation strategies and intensity of emotions, social anxiety relates to poor emotional understanding (Mennin et al., 2009), all of which appear significant in ASD. Furthermore, many people with ASD refer to impairments in emotion regulation as sources of distress, fear, and anxiety and caused by sensory and information overload (Chamak et al., 2008). Indeed, sensory processing difficulties can cause anxiety for those with ASD across the lifespan, but they manifest heterogeneously within the population (Crane et al., 2009; Lane et al., 2010). Hypersensitivity to sensory input, such as sensitivity to noise and touch, can also impact physical health through discomfort and behavioral dysregulation, affecting energy, sleep, and exercise (Jennes-Coussens et al., 2006).

Co-occurring conditions may exacerbate core ASD social deficits (Barnhill, 2007), yet comorbid symptoms often go overlooked or lack treatment priority because they fall outside the hallmark aspects of ASD (Sterling et al., 2008). Accordingly, psychiatric disabilities like psychosis, schizophrenia, and bipolar disorder often viewed as less related to ASD than anxiety and depression may not receive sufficient clinical attention, even though adults with ASD present with all these conditions in higher proportions than the general population (Spek & Woulters, 2010; Stahlberg et al., 2004). While adolescents and adults with ASD often experience clinically significant distress, the extent to which it relates to self-evaluations or the social environment compared to biology remains unclear. Therefore, threats to mental health abound in adolescents and young adults with ASD and may occur more pervasively and at a more basic level than largely recognized.

2.3 Education

While adolescents and adults with ASD who have average to high intelligence have the potential to perform well academically, many still underachieve. Many individuals with ASD lack the motivation to succeed academically, perhaps in part because of the wide range of subjects covered outside of restricted interests (Koegel et al., 2010). Others argue that adolescents with ASD regard school as an overstimulating and stressful environment for social and sensory reasons (Humphrey & Lewis, 2008), making it difficult to achieve academically. Thus, many individuals with ASD underachieve relative to their intellectual abilities (Estes et al., in press), a problem that intensifies with age, as primary grade children with ASD usually fare as well as their neurotypical peers, but fall behind in secondary school (Goldstein et al., 1994). Moreover, many individuals with ASD drop out of college or never pursue post-secondary education despite their intelligence and focused interests (Cederlund et al., 2008).

Accordingly, while many with ASD can and aspire to succeed in college, they often require continued accommodations and services to do so (Van Bergeijk et al., 2008). The less structured nature and increasing independence of academics and life in college, and the exposure to peers in new environments, pose significant challenges for transitioning to and performing well in higher education (Adreon & Durocher, 2007). Large colleges and universities tend to have larger classes and a more impersonal nature than secondary schools, while smaller colleges usually lack the opportunities for students with ASD to find programs that match their interests and strengths (Van Bergeijk et al., 2008). Moreover, students with disabilities can no longer receive accommodations modifying academic content, but must personally navigate the service delivery system because at age 18, students with ASD and other disabilities become legal self-advocates who must self-disclose and identify their needs (Adreon, & Durocher, 2007). Unfortunately, campus disability offices, historically designed for veterans and still more suitable for students with physical and learning disabilities, usually lack the resources to meet the needs of students with ASD (Van Bergeijk et al., 2008). Sadly, many college students with ASD may lack the initiative or self-advocacy skills needed to seek these resources because of social deficits, anxiety, immaturity, and sometimes passive-dependent temperament (Anckarsäter et al., 2006; Soderstrom et al., 2002).

Although a growing number of colleges offer support programs for students with ASD (Zager & Alpern, 2010), some students may view supports as stigmatizing or unhelpful and prefer not to enroll in special programs despite their parents' wishes (Camarena & Sarigiani, 2009). Conflicting priorities arise from the trend that parents often consider their child's skill deficits most salient in college planning considerations, such as availability of social support and mentoring, while transitional youth with ASD may place greater value on environmental concerns such as the coursework and campus disability awareness (Camarena & Sarigiani, 2010).

The academic difficulties adolescents with ASD often exhibit may relate to Minshew and colleagues' (1997) description of ASD as a disorder of complex information processing that features uneven, idiosyncratic profiles of intelligence that show deficits in social contexts (Goldstein et al., 2008). A review of academic achievement among individuals with ASD found that upper grades require higher-order thinking that may place high demands on the cognitive styles of those with ASD, who struggle with organizational skills, switching attention, problem solving, and comprehension of complex operations (Whitby & Mancil, 2009). Adolescents and adults with ASD show deficits in judging the passage of time (Martin et al., 2010) and in cognitive flexibility (Bogte et al., 2009).

Although deficits which may impede academic success do exist, research also suggests that individuals with ASD may also possess several cognitive strengths. According to empathizing-systemizing theory (Baron-Cohen, 2009), individuals with ASD have deficits in empathizing, but selective advantages in systemizing, a personality characteristic concerned with the understanding of rules, the inner workings of objects, and the organization of systems. Systemizing involves a preference for systems that change in predictable, rule-based ways, and high "systemizers" attempt to find lawful patterns in data and discover the "truth" (Baron-Cohen, 2008). As an example, scientists as a group have high autistic traits and are better "systemizers" (Baron-Cohen et al., 2001). In addition, people with ASD tend to have a meticulous decision-making style regardless of IQ that appears related to a heightened capacity for information load. However, operating on this higher level to filter out distracting, irrelevant stimuli may be required in order to be productive (Remington et al., 2009). Therefore, while ASD may relate to focused abilities that can produce talent (Asperger, 1944/Frith 1991; Baron-Cohen et al., 2009; Happe´ & Vital, 2009), sustained effort toward quality work may require great motivation and a conducive environment.

Despite the high potential of the more intellectually able students with ASD, many possible obstacles may hinder success and make the prospect of higher education a stressful experience (Glennon, 2001). The increasingly complex nature of assignments and course expectations in secondary school and then post-secondary higher education is just the beginning of these challenges. The transfer of responsibility from parents to individuals for disability-related needs and general independence imposes demands on decision-making and daily adaptive functioning that can become burdensome. Even those students who make wise choices that resiliently accentuate their strengths and compensate as much as possible for their deficits may struggle in group projects or otherwise with the attitudes of peers in classes and on campus, who often do not respond positively to ASD-like behavior (Campbell, 2007; Nevill & White, in press). Nevertheless, colleges and universities offer many social opportunities such as with student organizations and campus events; involvement in college life often complements academic success and may provide a buffer against risks to mental health (Wolf-Wendel et al., 2009). In addition, individuals with ASD may consider taking a "gap year" before starting college to work on social, academic, or independent living skills and to become more certain and motivated about their plans for college (Martin, 2010).

2.4 Employment

Perhaps more so than in education, individuals with ASD tend to fare much worse in employment settings than the potential suggested by their abilities (Geller & Greenberg, 2010). This is particularly true for those with at least average intelligence. While restricted interests may lead to hyperfocus and exceptional talent in a specialized area that can offer a foundation for a successful career (Grandin & Duffy, 2004), unfortunately, deficits in social skills often lead to employment failures despite task-related qualifications or performance. Core deficits in social interaction, communication, and sensory regulation; poor self-understanding of matching a personal profile of strengths, weaknesses, and interests to the work environment; and misperceptions by coworkers or supervisors have meant that many technically able people with ASD have failed to maintain appropriate employment or any employment whatsoever (Müller et al., 2003; Simone, 2010).

Adolescents with ASD already begin to fall behind their neurotypical peers in work experience, when ideally one would want them to get an early start to prepare for the intense challenges likely to come (Geller & Greenberg, 2010). Many neurotypical adolescents obtain summer or part-time jobs as a fast food worker, movie ushers, or camp counselors, but these jobs require social skills adolescents with ASD may lack. Many adolescents with ASD spend summers unoccupied, mostly staying home to play video games or keep to themselves, often lacking work experiences of even visiting their parent's work for a day or equivalent exposure (Bashe & Kirby, 2001). Moreover, high schools often no longer offer vocational classes like auto shop, woodworking, or drafting, which could offer useful experience for students with ASD, who often have creative or mechanical talents. To compensate for this gap in teaching, students could instead take classes in community college, technical school, or online; however, they may not have the time and energy amid their other secondary school activities (Grandin & Duffy, 2004). Other opportunities may include extracurricular school activities related to career interests, internships, service learning, or occupational mentoring to learn and practice work behaviors and gain awareness of a potential professional niche. Additional support on the job during the first few weeks of employment may help adults with ASD, as a mentor or job coach may provide advice about office politics or assist with the facilitation of flexible schedules or job sharing (Hurlbutt & Chalmers, 2004; Nesbitt, 2000; Portway & Johnson, 2005). Such support more easily takes place through the provision of supported employment, but few high-functioning academically included students with ASD receive such services (Higgins et al., 2008).

Indeed, employment needs often far exceed supports available for adolescents and adults with ASD (Gerhardt & Lainer, 2011). This phenomenon especially applies to those without intellectual disability or more severe symptoms of ASD (Liptak et al., 2011). Young adults with ASD and at least average intelligence are several times more likely to not have a daytime activity outside the home, such as higher education or work, than young adults with ASD and intellectual disability, who sometimes attend sheltered workshops or day activity centers (Taylor & Seltzer, 2011). Although adults with ASD without intellectual disability served by vocational rehabilitation centers incur lower costs to the system, these individuals are actually employed at lower percentages and for shorter periods of time than those with ASD and intellectual disabilities (Cimera & Cowan, 2009). Usually lacking formal support and various skills generally necessary for the workplace, even highly intelligent individuals with ASD at any one time are generally, if not unemployed, underemployed throughout adulthood (Howlin et al., 2004; Jennes-Cousens et al., 2006; Simone, 2010).

Several hypotheses have been offered to explain difficulties in employment for those with ASD. An initial challenge is the interview. Prospective employers expect a reciprocal conversation that requires quick thinking and responses to questions, posing a large hurdle for many adolescents and adults with ASD (Berney, 2004). Without knowledge of the ASD diagnosis, the interviewer may quickly conclude that the person with ASD has difficulty communicating and may erroneously think of him or her as intellectually incompetent or mentally unsuitable for the task (Portway & Johnson, 2005; Lawrence et al., 2010). However, disclosing one's diagnosis of ASD at an interview also poses risks to the hiring process (Meyerding, 2006). Individuals with ASD may need to have much higher skills and quality work than other applicants to get the job, and need to sell their portfolio, resume, or talents rather than their personality (Grandin & Duffy, 2004). For these reasons, some adults with ASD never get a job in their field of study (Hurlbutt & Chalmers, 2004).

As difficult as the hiring process may be, perhaps the greatest challenge individuals with ASD experience lies in maintaining employment. Related to the core deficits of ASD, these individuals may dominate conversations, perseverate on topics of personal interest, talk about inappropriate topics or make other social blunders, be misunderstood or feel disrespected, become exhausted by social demands, or think of small talk as phony (Grandin & Duffy, 2004; Simone, 2010). They may not know how to engage in office politics or refrain from doing so for ethical reasons so as not to compromise their integrity. They may get bullied, scapegoated, or deceived by coworkers, which can be a humiliating experience that weakens mental health or even physical health, and can be difficult to move past because of difficulty regulating emotions (Simone, 2010). They may try to react to victimization by being polite, but if seen as naïve and defenseless, co-workers' victimizing behavior may escalate (Hurlbutt & Chalmers, 2004). They may unknowingly violate other workers' personal space, causing discomfort, or cause stigma for other odd behaviors that do not demonstrate empathy or good listening skills, such as a pedantic speaking style coupled with poor reading of nonverbal cues that can cause them to be perceived as arrogant (Higgins et al., 2008). Or they may lack social tact and sound blunt in sensitive situations (Hurlbutt & Chalmers, 2004; Simone, 2010). As a method to combat these difficulties, coworkers who act as mentors or coaches may provide great help for these individuals in handling the challenges of the workplace (Hurlbutt & Chamlers, 2004; Simone, 2010). This informal support could reduce the need to disclose the ASD diagnosis on the job for accommodations or adjusted expectations, which, while possibly not as risky as doing so during the application or interview process, involves complicated considerations because of poor understanding or information about ASD in the workplace (Meyerling, 2000; Nesbitt, 2000).

Cognitive and sensory characteristics associated with ASD can also make completing work itself difficult. Employees with ASD may want to stress the need for explicit expectations with clear, written instructions, such as an outline (Hurlbutt & Chalmers, 2004; Simone, 2004). These individuals often struggle with multitasking, but perform well when they can focus on one task at a time (Higgins et al., 2008; Simone, 2010). As perfectionists without good perspective taking abilities, they may offer unsolicited advice or constructive feedback, or become immersed in a task or project of interest beyond the needs of the assignment (Simone, 2010). They may need autonomy to work at their own pace or flexible arrangements like working from home (Simone, 2010), but may have trouble asking for help or advocating for their needs (Hurlbutt & Chalmers, 2004; Simone, 2010). Moreover, sensory issues like sensitivity to noise, odor, sound, and lights may cause workers with ASD to become irritable or withdraw (Grandin & Duffy, 2004; Higgins et al., 2008; Simone, 2010). Some employees with ASD require total silence to concentrate and may even experience loud noises as traumatizing. They may be especially physically uncomfortable with the dress code or air conditioning and need to take frequent breaks to get natural lighting from overstimulation by fluorescent lights (Simone, 2010).

Despite the desire and ability of intellectually capable adolescents and adults with ASD, they tend to have poor job experiences. They typically have many positive characteristics related to ASD that can be assets at work, such as attention to detail, honesty, integrity, focus, diligence, taking pride in their work, a desire to please, independent and creative thinking, perseverance, and the ability to handle high amounts of data (Grandin & Duffy, 2004; Meyerling, 2006; Simone, 2010). Yet most do not disclose their ASD diagnosis at work, and those who do usually only tell a few supportive coworkers, for fear they will be suspicious, hostile, or patronizing from misunderstanding (Meyerling, 2006; Simone, 2010). This creates a higher need for workers with ASD to try to compensate by learning their field and building skills exceptionally well beyond the social challenges of marketing themselves and networking. If they do so, and find a field that values their strengths and tolerates their eccentricities and weaknesses, they have a much better opportunity of maintaining a suitable career (Grandin & Duffy, 2004).

2.5 Independent living

As a pervasive developmental disability, ASD typically affects the ability to live independently. While individuals with ASD and intellectual disability generally do not achieve typical outcomes such as independent living in adulthood, the performance varies widely in those with ASD and at least average intelligence (Howlin et al., 2004). Instead, daily living skills - perhaps more so than other types of adaptive behaviors - play a significant role in having friendships, employment or education typical of one's cognitive abilities, and general independence (Farley et al., 2009). Many adolescents and adults with ASD have difficulties with life skills such as cleaning, cooking, and hygiene (Balfe & Tantam, 2010) or other aspects of daily living such as sleeping (Limoges et al., 2005; Oyane & Bjorvatn, 2005), healthy or flexible eating, managing money, shopping, and driving or taking public transportation (Geller & Greenberg, 2010) . Poor physical quality of life appears common and may contribute to this phenomenon beyond social naïveté or lack of motivation, as many report dependence on medical treatment or pain and discomfort that can limit energy, work capacity, and other activities of daily living (Jennes-Coussens et al., 2006). Poor mental health can also reduce independence, as young adults with ASD who live with their parents endorse more depressive symptoms than those who live independently (Cederlund et al., 2010).

Individuals with ASD vary in their ability to live independently from an almost typical level of functioning in general to requiring constant supervision (Frith, 2004). It remains unclear how many adults with ASD live independently. In countries like Sweden, where more formal support is provided, it appears that the majority lives independently but still may depend on services (Cederlund et al., 2008; Engström et al., 2003). Yet independent living involves taking responsibility for one's day-to-day affairs such as managing personal finances, gainful employment, and buying clothes for oneself, and in these respects a large minority, if not majority, of adults with ASD in Britain (Howlin, 2000; Howlin et al., 2004) and the United States (Farley et al., 2009) attain at least a moderate degree of independence. Generally, adults with ASD achieve adulthood milestones such as steady employment and living by oneself or with a partner or children later than neurotypical adults, and are unlikely to achieve independence during the traditional college-going years (Marriage et al, 2009).

This high dependence of individuals with ASD on their parents during young adulthood appears to place additional stress on the family during this period. For young adults with ASD, the parent-child relationship is generally positive and may protect against distress from poor peer relationships or the demands of daily living across the autism spectrum; parents tend to display positive affect and lack significant emotional expressivity or criticism toward their child (Greenberg et al., 2006; Wasserman et al., 2010). Yet, while the relationship generally improves as the child progresses through high school, and may continue to maintain or improve during the transition to adulthood for those with intellectual disability (Lounds et al., 2007), gains in the relationships (such as maternal warmth) may slow or reverse during the transition to young adulthood for those with at least average IQ (Taylor & Seltzer, in press). Since those without intellectual disabilities tend to experience a greater loss in services and are more likely to not have a daytime activity, increasing caregiving burdens and unmet needs for services or high expectations for development may strain parents (Taylor & Seltzer, 2011; Taylor & Seltzer, in press).

Adults with ASD tend to exert little responsibility for themselves relative to their peers. Individuals with ASD generally feel more comfortable with rigid routines and restricted interests, and may resist change (Frith, 2004; Ozonoff et al., 2005). From childhood and throughout adulthood they may remain averse to seeking new experiences and, unlike neurotypical peers, become more motivated by fear of failure or other dangers than approaching the possibility of success or another reward (Anckarsäter et al., 2006; Schwartz et al., 2009; Soderstrom et al., 2002; South et al., 2011). By adolescence they may blame themselves for social or other disappointments and develop learned helplessness (Barnhill, 2001; Barnhill & Myles, 2001). Alternatively, they may become perfectionists (Greenaway & Howlin, 2010), such that those who are more intelligent or self-aware may continue to work on tasks that have a greater chance of failure despite having greater anxiety than others with ASD or neurotypical peers (South et al., 2011). These patterns reflect poor coping that can manifest in passive, avoidant behavior or obsessive, explosive behavior rather than flexibility and balanced risk-taking (Anckarsäter et al., 2006; Soderstrom et al., 2002).

Part of the challenge may lie in poor understanding of the self and others. People with ASD experience deficits in inferring others' emotional or mental states from social cues, sometimes referred to as *theory of mind* or *mindreading*, especially when they are subtler or numerous (Koning & Magill-Evans, 2001). They may sometimes compensate in understanding others' perspective through the use of logic and conscious effort (Beeger et al., 2010; Ponnet et al., 2004, 2005), but their judgments may still show impaired accuracy in more dynamic or unfamiliar, less structured contexts (Ponnet et al., 2008; Roeyers & Demurie, 2010). This ASD hallmark of poor social cognition may stem from introspective deficits about one's own thoughts and emotions (Lombardo & Baron-Cohen, 2011), although adults with ASD appear to have an intact sense of agency, or understanding themselves as the generators of their actions (David et al., 2008; Zwickel et al., in press). Therefore, individuals with ASD may have poor awareness of their various challenges in general, which may affect strategies of working toward goals of independent living.

Moreover, adolescents and adults with ASD may have subtle difficulties or deficits in executive functions like planning and making decisions, other goal-directed thinking, and self-regulation (Hill, 2004), which would make independent living challenging at best. Although these abilities show improvement into young adulthood (Berger et al., 2003; Luna et al., 2007), nevertheless, adults with ASD continue to fare best with predictability and may not know how to apply exceptions to rules (Pijnacker et al., 2009) during independent living. They tend to experience difficulties making valid inferences from prior knowledge (McKenzie et al., 2010; Bowler, et al., 2008), and thinking flexibly. They also may not understand the gist of things and instead attend to details, or when they have the opportunity, take longer to gather and choose between information before making confident decisions (Johnson et al., 2010; Yechiam et al., 2010).

The difficulties adolescents and adults with ASD may have making decisions for themselves suggests the pervasive nature of potential obstacles to independence that transcend difficulties with peer relationships (Channon et al., 2001). Transition planning teams during high school need to prepare adolescents with ASD for life and work skills toward independent living, but often fail to include age-appropriate goals (Kurth & Mastergeorge, 2010). Even so, more services are needed in adulthood. Meanwhile, parents need to strike a balance between providing support and facilitating a transition to social and general independence so that their children learn to advocate for themselves, whether through formal systems or informally.

3. Conclusion

This chapter suggests that individuals with ASD usually experience significant challenges in typical milestones or expectations in adulthood (Geller & Greenberg, 2010). While they tend to desire them, adolescents and adults with ASD usually lack or struggle to establish a peer support network, friendships, or romantic relationships. Social disappointments or failures often harm self-esteem and contribute to mental health problems that reduce motivation for growth opportunities like constructive risk-taking. Despite the prevailing focus in transition planning on academic achievement, even adults with advanced degrees in relevant fields often fail to secure suitable employment. Difficulties with creating self-disciplined structure and routines, and communicating personal needs, create challenges in higher education and work beyond following instructions from professors or employers and cooperating with classmates or coworkers. Adults with ASD often remain highly dependent on their family of origin, sometimes limited in the development and expression of separate values, preferences, and goals. While well-meaning parents sometimes become overly protective, the lack of sufficient professional support through transition planning and social, job, or life coaches means that strategic use of support from parents can help individuals with ASD acquire the skills to become more independent. Transitioning youth and adults with ASD must learn to exert control over their lives and undertake as much responsibility as possible. Clearly much work lies ahead in helping individuals with ASD become more socially connected, emotionally secure, educated, productive, and independent into adulthood. The descriptions in this chapter suggest continuity as well as change in the ASD phenotype; and more investigation into the development of ASD across the lifespan, which has traditionally focused on early and middle childhood (Matson & Neal, 2009).With more and better research and provision of services for adolescents and adults with ASD, perhaps supports can help to strike an appropriate balance between adaptation and accommodation (Barnhill, 2007). This may be especially true for employment, as the same restricted interests and attention to detail that can become disabling in social contexts can produce talent in the workforce (Happé & Vital, 2009). Indeed, Hans Asperger noted this phenomenon in the original paper on the disability named after him that the special interests and abilities of individuals with ASD can lead to success in professions such as the scientific or artistic fields (Asperger, 1944/Frith, 1991). With the right support, more adults with ASD can achieve success like Temple Grandin (2006), whose interests in science and animals led her to develop many of the humane livestock facilities in the world, and Tim Page (2009), whose early interests in music and media pointed him to a Pulitzer Prize-winning career as a music critic.

To maximize outcomes, the identification of and provision of services for adults with ASD need significant expansion. Most adults who meet criteria for ASD in the general population lack a clinical diagnosis, and among them, most lack personal awareness of ASD (Brugha et al., 2011, 2007; White et al., 2011). The amount of adults who meet diagnostic criteria for ASD appears comparable to the current diagnosed prevalence of ASD in children, or about one percent (Brugha et al., 2011, 2007).

Evidence suggests that the prevalence of ASD in the general population does not vary by age within adulthood, suggesting a long history of neglect for the clinical and support needs of many individuals in this population (Brugha et al., 2011). Undiagnosed individuals with ASD tend to lack intellectual disability, but the absence of a diagnosis does not reflect achievement of potential or lack of need for services. Compared with the general population, these individuals have less likelihood of marriage or owning property, lower educational qualifications and income, and higher dependence on government support (Brugha et al., 2011). Lack of a diagnosis may exacerbate distress and make accessing appropriate mental health services, among other forms of help, more difficult. For example, symptoms in undiagnosed ASD in adults often relate to social anxiety, depression, and aggression, yet such adults do not appear to have greater use of the mental health system than the general population (Brugha et al., 2011; White et al., in press).

Providing appropriate support to adults with ASD will not only help them achieve a higher quality of life, but the increased productivity that may result from this investment can also ultimately save social economic costs. While adults with ASD tend to be unemployed or underemployed, they often do not receive supported employment programs to help integrate them into the workforce. When provided, they tend to help adults with ASD move toward competitive employment that reduces or eliminates their need for welfare and also contribute more to the economy and society (Howlin et al., 2005; Ja¨rbrink et al., 2007). Beyond social services, clinical interventions also have the potential to significantly help adults with ASD. Not only must research on interventions for adults continue, but also the ASD field would benefit from longitudinal research on early intervention to understand long-term implications for commonly used and evidence-based programs for children with ASD.

Continuing to gain and disseminate knowledge about the ASD population may help individuals with ASD, their families, and professionals better understand their challenges and help them accomplish a high quality of life. As attention to the range of practical issues facing individuals with ASD and public understanding of ASD increases, tolerance for ASD may grow and current misperceptions of behaviors associated with ASD as character flaws may decline (Geller & Greenberg, 2010). Such progress, along with more understanding of how to legally accommodate individuals with ASD in higher education and especially the workplace, may encourage more adults with ASD to self-disclose to become more comfortable and proactive toward advocating for their needs and achieving greater success.

4. Acknowledgements

The first author gratefully acknowledges the generous support of the Philip & Aida Siff Educational Foundation toward work on this book chapter.

5. References

Abramson, L.Y., Seligman, M.E.P., & Teasdale, J.D. (1978). Learned helplessness in humans: Critique and reformulation. *Journal of Abnormal Psychology,* Vol. 87, No. 1, pp. 49-74

Adreon, D. & Durocher, J. S. (2007). Evaluating the college transition needs of individuals with high-functioning autism spectrum disorder. *Intervention in School and Clinic,* Vol. 42, No. 5, (May 2007), pp. 271-279

American Psychiatric Association. (2000). Diagnostic and statistical manual of mental disorders (4th ed., text revision). Author, IBN 978-0890420256, Washington, DC

Anckarsäter, H., Stahlberg, O., Larson, T., Hakansson, C., Jutblad, S .B., Niklasson, L., Rastam, M. (2006). The impact of ADHD and autism spectrum disorders on temperament, character, and personality development. *The American Journal of Psychiatry,* Vol. 163, No. 7, (July 2006), pp. 1239-1244

Ashby, C.E., & Causton-Theoharis, J.N. (2009). Disqualified in the human race: a close reading of the autobiographies of individuals identified as autistic. *International Journal of Inclusive Education,* Vo. 13, pp. 501-516

Asperger, H. (1944). Autistic personality disorders in childhood. In U. Frith (Ed.), *Autism and Asperger syndrome* (pp. 147– 183). Cambridge University Press, ISBN 978-0521386081, London.

Balfe, M., & Tantam, D. (2010). A descriptive social and health profile of a community sample of adults and adolescents with Asperger syndrome. *BMC Research Notes,* V. 3, pp. 300-306

Barnard, J., Harvey, V., Potter, D., & Prior, A. (2001). Ignored or ineligible? The reality for adults with autism spectrum disorders. National Autistic Society, ISBN 1-899280-61-8, London.

Barnhill, G. P. (2007). Outcomes in adults with Asperger syndrome. *Focus on Autism and Other Developmental Disabilities,* Vol. 22, No. 2, (Summer 2007), pp. 116-126

Barnhill, G. P. (2001). Social attributions and depression in adolescents with Asperger syndrome. *Focus on Autism and Other Developmental Disabilities,* Vol. 16, No. 1, (Spring 2001), pp. 46–53

Barnhill, G. P. & Myles, B. (2001). Attributional style and depression in adolescents with Asperger syndrome. *Journal of Positive Behavioral Intervention,* Vo. 3, No. 3, (July 2001), pp. 175-190

Baron-Cohen, S. (2009). Autism: The empathizing-systemizing (E-S) theory. *Annals of the New York Academy of the Sciences,* Vol. 1156, (March 2009), pp. 68-80

Baron-Cohen, S. (2008). Autism, hypersystemizing, and truth. *The Quarterly Journal of Experimental Psychology,* Vol. 61, No. 1, pp. 64-75

Baron-Cohen, S., Ashwin, E., Ashwin, C., Tavassoli, T., & Chakrabarti, B. (2009). Talent in autism: hyper-systemizing, hyper-attention to detail and sensory hypersensitivity. *Philosophical Transactions of the Royal Society B Biological Sciences,* Vol. 364, No. 1522, (May 2009), pp. 1377-1383

Baron-Cohen, S., & Wheelwright, S. (2004). The Empathy Quotient: An investigation of adults with Asperger's disorder or high functioning autism, and normal sex differences. *Journal of Autism and Developmental Disorders*, Vol. 34, No. 2, pp. 163-175

Baron-Cohen, S., & Wheelwright, S. (2003). The Friendship Questionnaire: An investigation of adults with Asperger syndrome or high-functioning autism, and normal sex differences. *Journal of Autism and Developmental Disorders,* Vol. 33, No. 5, (October 2003), pp. 509-517

Baron-Cohen, S., Wheelwright, S., Skinner, R., Martin, J., & Clubley, E. (2001). The Autism Spectrum Quotient (AQ): Evidence from Asperger syndrome/high functioning autism, males and females, scientists and mathematicians. *Journal of Autism and Developmental Disorders,* Vol. 31, No. 1, pp. 5-17

Barry, C. M., Madsen, S. D., Nelson, L. J., Carroll, J. S., & Badger, S. (2009). Friendship and romantic relationship qualities in emerging adulthood: Differential associations with identity development and achieved adulthood criteria. *Journal of Adult Development*, Vo. 16, No. 4, pp. 209-222

Bashe, P.R., & Kirby, B.L. (2001). *The O.A.S.I.S. guide to Asperger syndrome: Advice, support, insight, and inspiration.* Crown, IBSN 978-0609608111, New York.

Begeer, B., Malle, B.F., Nieuwland, M.S., & Keysar, B. (2010). Using theory of mind to represent in social interactions: Comparing individuals with high-functioning autism and typically developing controls. *European Journal of Developmental Psychology*, Vol. 7, No. 1, pp. 104-122

Bellini, S. (2006). The development of social anxiety in high functioning adolescents with autism spectrum disorders. *Focus on Autism and Other Developmental Disabilities*, Vol. 21, pp. 138-145

Berger, H.J.C., Aerts, F.H.T.M., Spaendonck, K.P.M., Cools, A.R., & Teunisse, J.P. Central coherence and cognitive shifting in relation to social improvement in high-functioning young adults with autism. *Journal of Clinical and Experimental Neuropsychology*, Vol. 25, No. 4, (June 2003), pp. 502-511.

Berney, T. (2004). Asperger syndrome from childhood into adulthood. *Advances in Psychiatric Treatment*, Vol. 10, pp. 341–351

Berthoz, S. & Hill, E.L. (2005). The validity of using self-reports to assess emotion regulation abilities in adults with autism spectrum disorder. *European Psychiatry*, Vol. 20, pp. 291-298

Bird, G., Silani, G., Brindley, R., White, S., Frith, U., & Singer, T. (2010). Empathic brain responses in insula are modulated by levels of alexithymia but not autism. *Brain*, Vol. 133, pp. 1515-1525

Blair, R.J.R. (2005). Responding to the emotions of others: Dissociating forms of empathy through the study of typical and psychiatric populations. *Consciousness and Cognition*, Vol. 14, No. 4, (December 2005), pp. 698-718.

Bogte, H., Flamma, B., Van der Meere, J., & Van Engeland. (2009). Divided attention capacity in adults with autism spectrum disorders and without intellectual disability. *Autism*, Vol. 13, pp. 229-243

Bowler, D. M., Gaigg, S. B., & Gardiner, J.M. (2008). Subjective organization in the free recall learning of adults with Asperger's syndrome. *Journal of Autism and Developmental Disorders*, Vol. 38, pp. 104-113

Brugha, T.S., McManus, S., Bankart, J., Scott, F., Purdon, S., Smith, J., et al. (2011). Epidemiology of autism spectrum disorders in adults in the community in England. *Archives of General Psychiatry*, Vol. 68, No. 5, pp. 459-465

Brugha, T.S., McManus, S., Meltzer, H., Smith, J., Scott, F.J., Purdon, S., et al. (2009). Autism spectrum disorders in adults living in households throughout England: Report from the adult psychiatric morbidity survey 2007. Leeds: The NHS Information Centre for Health and Social Care.

Buller, D.B., & Burgoon, J.K. (1996). Interpersonal deception theory. *Communication Theory*, Vol. 6, pp. 203-242

Butler, R.C., & Gillis, J.M. (2011) The impact of labels and behaviors on the stigmatization of adults with Asperger's disorder. *Journal of Autism and Developmental Disorders*, Vol. 41, No. 6, pp. 741-749

Camarena, P.M., & Sarigiani, P.A. (2009). Postsecondary educational aspirations of high-functioning adolescents with autism spectrum disorders and their parents. *Focus on Autism and Other Developmental Disabilities*, Vol. 24, pp. 115-128

Campbell, J.M. (2007). Middle school students' response to the self-introduction of a student with autism: Effects of perceived similarity, prior awareness, and educational message. *Remedial and Special Education*, Vo. 28, no. 3, pp. 163-173

Carrington, S., Templeton, E., & Papinczak, T. (2003). Adolescents with Asperger syndrome and perceptions of friendship. *Focus on Autism and Other Developmental Disabilities,* Vol. 18, pp. 211-218

Cath, D.C., Ran, N., Smit, J.H., van Balkom, A.J.L.M., & Comijs, H.C. (2008). Symptom overlap between autism spectrum disorder, generalized social anxiety disorder, and obsessive-compulsive disorder in adults: A preliminary case-controlled study. *Psychopathology,* Vol. 41, pp. 101-110

Causton-Theoharis, J., Ashby, C., & Cosier, M. (2009). 'Islands of loneliness': Exploring social interaction through the autobiographies of individuals with autism. *Intellectual and Developmental Disabilities,* Vol. 47, pp. 84-96

Cederlund, M., Hagberg, B., Billstedt, E., Gillberg, I.C., & Gillberg, C. (2008). Asperger syndrome and autism: A comparative longitudinal follow-up study more than 5 years after original diagnosis. *Journal of Autism and Developmental Disorders,* Vol. 38, No. 1, pp. 72-85

Cederlund, M., Hagberg, B., & Gillberg, C. (2010). Asperger syndrome in adolescent and young adult males. Interview, self- and parent assessment of social, emotional, and cognitive problems. *Research in Developmental Disabilities,* Vol. 31, pp. 287-298

Chalmers, L., & Hurlbutt, K. (2004). Employment and adults with Asperger syndrome. *Focus on Autism and Other Developmental Disabilities,* Vol. 19, no. 4, pp. 215-222

Chamak, B., Bonniau, B., Jaunay, E., & Cohen, D. (2008). What can we learn about autism from autistic persons? *Psychotherapy and Psychosomatics,* Vol. 77, pp. 271-279

Channon, S., Charman, T., Heap, J., Crawford, S., & Rios, P. (2001). Real-life-type problem-solving in Asperger's syndrome. *Journal of Autism and Developmental Disorders,* Vol. 31, pp. 461-469

Cimera, R., & Cowan, R. (2009). The costs of services and employment outcomes achieved by adults with autism in the U.S. *Autism,* Vol. 13, No. 3, pp. 285-302

Cisler, J.M., Olatunji, B.O., Feldner, M.T., & Forsyth, J.P. (2010). Emotion regulation and the anxiety disorders: An integrative review. *Journal of Psychopathology and Behavioral Assessment,* Vol. 32, pp. 68-82

Colle, L., Baron-Cohen, S., Wheelwright, S. & van der Lely, H.K.J. (2008). Narrative discourse in adults with high-functioning autism or Asperger syndrome. *Journal of Autism and Developmental Disorders,* Vol. 38, pp. 28-40

Collins, W. A., & Madsen, S. D. (2006). Personal relationships in adolescence and early adulthood. In A. L. Vangelisti & D. Perlman (Eds.). *The Cambridge handbook of personal relationships* (pp. 191-209). Cambridge University Press, IBN 978-0521533591, New York.

Connor, M. (2000). Asperger syndrome (autistic spectrum disorder) and the self-reports of comprehensive school students. *Educational Psychology in Practice,* Vol. 16, pp. 285-296

Corden, B., Chilvers, R., & Skuse, D. (2008). Avoidance of emotionally arousing stimuli predicts social-perceptual impairment in Asperger's syndrome. *Neuropsychologia,* Vol. 46, No. 1, pp. 137-147.

Crane, L., Goddard, L., & Pring, L. (2009). Sensory processing in adults with autism spectrum disorders. *Autism,* Vol. 13, No. 3, pp. 215-228

Daniel, L.S., & Billingsley, B.S. (2010). What boys with an autism spectrum disorder say about establishing and maintaining friendships. *Focus on Autism and Other Developmental Disabilities,* Vol. 25, pp. 220-229

David, N., Gawronski, A., Santos, N.S, Huff, W., Lehnhardt, F.G., Newen, A., & Vogeley, K. (2008). Dissociation between key
processes of social cognition in autism: Impaired mentalizing but intact sense of agency. *Journal of Autism and Developmental Disorders,* Vol. 38, pp. 593-605.

Davidson, J., & Henderson, V.L. (2010). 'Coming out' on the spectrum: Autism, identity and disclosure. *Social & Cultural Geography,* Vol. 11, No. 2, pp. 155-170

Del Giudice, M., Angeleri, R., Brizio, A., & Elena, M.R. (2010). The evolution of autistic-like and schizotypal traits: A sexual selection hypothesis. *Frontiers in Psychology,* Vol. 1, (August 2010), pp. 1-18

DePaulo, B.M., & Kashy, D.A. (1998). Everyday lies in close and casual relationships. *Journal of Personality and Social Psychology,* Vol. 74, No. 1, (January 1998), pp. 63-79

Dziobek, I., Rogers, K., Fleck, S., Bahnemann, M., Heekeren, H.R., Wolf, O.T., & Convit, A. (2008). Dissociation of cognitive and emotional empathy in adults with Asperger syndrome using the multifaceted empathy test (MET). *Journal of Autism and Developmental Disorders,* Vol. 38, No. 3, pp. 464-473

Engstrom, I., Ekstrom, L., & Emilsson, B. (2003). Psychological functioning in a group of Swedish adults with Asperger syndrome or high-functioning autism. *Autism,* Vol. 7, No. 1, (March 2003), pp. 99–110.

Estes, A., Rivera, V., Bryan, M., Cali, P., & Dawson, G. (In press). Discrepancies between academic achievement and intellectual ability in higher-functioning school-aged children with autism spectrum disorder. *Journal of Autism and Developmental Disorders.*

Farley, M.A., McMahon, W.M., Fombonne, E., Jenson, W.R., Miller, J., Gardner, M., Block, H., Pingree, C.B., Ritvo, E.R., Ritvo, R.A., & Coon, H. (2009). Twenty-year outcome for individuals with autism and average or near-average cognitive abilities. *Autism Research,* V.2, No. 2, (April 2009), pp. 109-118

Frith, U. (2004). Emanuel Miller lecture: confusions and controversies about Asperger syndrome. *Journal of Child Psychology and Psychiatry,* Vol. 45, No. 4, (May 2004), pp. 672–686

Gantman, A., Kapp, S.K., Orenski, K., & Laugeson, E.A. (In press). Social skills training for young adults with high-functioning autism spectrum disorders: A randomized controlled intervention study. *Journal of Autism and Developmental Disorders.*

Geller, L., & Greenberg, M. (2010). Managing the transition process from high school to college and beyond: Challenges for individuals, families, and society. *Social Work in Mental Health,* Vol. 8, No. 1, pp. 92-116

Gerhardt, P.F., & Lainer, I. (2011). Addressing the needs of adolescents and adults with autism: A crisis on the horizon. *Journal of Contemporary Psychotherapy,* Vol. 41, No. 1, pp. 37-45

Geurts, H.M., Corbett, B., & Solomon, M. (2009). The paradox of cognitive flexibility in autism. *Trends in Cognitive Sciences,* Vol. 13, No. 2, (February 2009), pp. 74-82

Ghaziuddin, M., & Gerstein, L. (1996). Pedantic speaking style differentiates Asperger syndrome from high-functioning autism. *Journal of Autism and Developmental Disorders,* Vol. 26, No. 6, pp. 585–595

Ghaziuddin, M., Ghaziuddin, N., & Greden, J. (2002). Depression in persons with autism: Implications for research and clinical care. *Journal of Autism and Developmental Disorders,* Vol. 32, No. 4, pp. 299-306

Glennon, T.J. (2001). The stress of the university experience for students with Asperger syndrome. *Work,* Vol. 17, No. 3, pp. 183-190

Goldstein, G., Allen, D.N.,, Minshew, N.J., Williams, D.L., Volkmar, D.L., & Klin, A. (2008). The structure of intelligence in children and adults with high functioning autism. *Neuropsychology,* Vol. 22, No. 3, pp. 301-312

Goldstein, G., Minshew, N. J., & Siegel, D. J. (1994). Age differences in academic achievement in high- functioning autistic individuals. *Journal of Clinical and Experimental Neuropsychology,* Vol. 16, No. 5, pp. 671–680

Grandin, T. (2006). *Thinking in Pictures: My Life with Autism.* Vintage Books, ISBN 978-0-307-27565-3, New York.

Grandin, T., & Duffy, K. (2004). Developing talents: Careers for individuals with Asperger syndrome and high functioning autism. Autism Asperger Publishing Company, ISBN 978-1931282567, Shawnee Mission, KS.

Green, J., Gilchrist, A., Burton, D., & Cox, A. (2000). Social and psychiatric functioning in adolescents with Asperger syndrome compared with conduct disorder. *Journal of Autism and Developmental Disorders,* Vol. 30, No. 4, pp. 279-293

Greenaway, R., & Howlin, P. (2010). Dysfunctional attitudes and perfectionism and their relationship to anxious and depressive symptoms in boys with autism spectrum disorders. *Journal of Autism and Developmental Disorders,* 40, No. 10, pp. 1179-1187

Greenberg, J.S., Seltzer, M.M., Hong, J., & Orsmond, G.I. (2006). Bidirectional effects of expressed emotion and behavior problems and symptoms in adolescents and adults with autism. *American Journal of Mental Retardation,* Vol 111, No. 4, (July 2006), pp. 229-249

Grynberg, D., Luminet, O., Corneille, O., Grèzes, J., & Berthoz, S. (2010). Alexithymia in the interpersonal domain: A general deficit of empathy? *Personality and Individual Differences,* Vol. 49, No. 8, (December 2010), pp. 845-850

Happé, F., & Vital, P. (2009). What aspects of autism predispose to talent? *Philosophical Transactions of the Royal Society B,* Vol. 364, No. 1522, (May 2009), pp. 1369-1375

Hellemans, H., Colson, K., Verbraeken, C., Vermeiren, R., & Deboutte, D. (2007). Sexual behavior in high-functioning male adolescents and young adults with autism spectrum disorders. *Journal of Autism and Developmental Disorders,* Vol. *37,* No. 2, pp. 260-269

Hendricks, D.R., & Wehman, P. (2009). Transition from school to adulthood for youth with autism spectrum disorders:Review and recommendations. *Focus on Autism and Other Developmental Disabilities,* Vol. 24, No. 2 (June 2009), pp. 77-88.

Higgins, K. K., Koch, L. C., Boughfman, E. M., & Vierstra, C. (2008). School-to-work transition and Asperger syndrome. *Work,* Vol. 31, pp. 291-298

Hill, E.L. (2004). Executive dysfunction in autism. *Trends in Cognitive Sciences,* Vol. 8, No. 1 (January 2004), pp. 26-32

Hill, E., Berthoz, S., & Frith, U. (2004). Brief report: Cognitive processing of own emotions in individuals with autistic spectrum disorder and in their relatives. *Journal of Autism and Developmental Disorders,* Vol. 34, No. 2, (April 2004), pp. 229-235

Hintzen, A., Delespaul, P., van Os, J., & Myin-Germeys, I. (2010). Social needs in daily life in adults with pervasive developmental disorders. *Psychiatry Research,* Vo. 179, No. 1, pp. 75-80

Hodges, E. V. E., Boivin, M., Vitaro, F., & Bukowski, W.M. (1999). The power of friendship: Protection against an escalating cycle of peer victimization. *Developmental Psychology,* Vol. 35, No. 1, pp. 94-101

Howard, B., Cohn, E., & Orsmond, G. (2006). Understanding and negotiating friendships: Perspectives from an adolescent with Asperger syndrome. *Autism,* Vol. 10, No. 6, (November 2006), pp. 619-627

Howlin, P. (2000). Outcome in adult life for more able individuals with Asperger syndrome. *Autism,* Vol. 4, No. 1, (March 2000), pp. 63–83

Howlin, P., Alcock, J., & Burkin, C. (2005). An 8 year follow-up of a specialist supported employment service for high-ability adults with autism or Asperger syndrome. *Autism,* Vol. 9, No. 5, (December 2005), pp. 533-549

Howlin, P., Goode, S., Hutton, J., & Rutter, M. (2004). Adult outcome for children with autism. *Journal of Child Psychology and Psychiatry, and Allied Disciplines,* Vo. 45, No. 2, (February 2004), pp. 212–229

Humphrey, N, & Lewis, S. (2008). Make me normal: The views and experiences of pupils on the autistic spectrum in mainstream secondary schools. *Autism,* Vol. 12, No. 1, pp. 1362-3613

Humphrey, N. & Symes, W. (2010). Perceptions of social support and experience of bullying among pupils with autistic spectrum disorders in mainstream secondary schools. *European Journal of Special Needs Education,* Vol. 25, No. 1, (February 2010), pp. 77-91

Humphrey, N., & Symes, W. (2010). Responses to bullying and use of social support among pupils with autism spectrum disorders (autism) in mainstream schools: a qualitative study. *Journal of Research in Special Educational Needs,* Vol. 10, No. 2, (June 2010), pp. 82-90

Huws, J.C., & Jones, R.S.P. Diagnosis, disclosure, and having autism: An interpretative phenomenological analysis of the perceptions of young people with autism. *Journal of Intellectual & Developmental Disability,* Vol. 33, No. 2, pp. 99-107

Ja¨rbrink, K., McCrone, P., Fombonne, E., Zande'n, H., & Knapp, M. (2007). Cost-impact of young adults with high-functioning autistic spectrum disorder. *Research in Developmental Disabilities,* Vol. 28, pp. 94-104

Jennes-Coussens, M., Magill-Evans, J., & Koning, C. (2006). The quality of life of young men with Asperger syndrome: A brief report. *Autism,* Vol. 10, No. 4, (June 2006), pp. 511-524

Jobe, L.E., & Williams White, S. (2007). Loneliness, social relationships, and a broader autism phenotype in college students. *Personality and Individual Differences,* Vol. 42, No. 8, (June 2007), pp. 1479-1489

Johnson, S.A., Blaha, L.M., Houpt, J.W., & Townsend, J.T. (2010). Systems factorial technology provides new insights on global-local information processing in autism spectrum disorders. *Journal of Mathematical Psychology,* Vol. 54, No. 1, (February 2010), pp. 53-72

Johnson, S.A., Filliter, J.H., & Murphy, R.R. (2009). Discrepancies between self- and parent-perceptions of autistic traits and empathy in high functioning children and adolescents on the autism spectrum. *Journal of Autism and Developmental Disorders,* Vol. 39, No. 12, pp. 1706-1714

Jones, A.P., Happe´, F.G.E., Gilbert, F., Burnett, S., & Viding, E. (2010). Feeling, caring, knowing: Different types of empathy deficit for boys with psychopathic tendencies and autism spectrum disorder. *Journal of Child Psychology and Psychiatry,* Vol. 51, No. 11, (November 2010), pp. 1188-1197

Jones, R.P., & Meldal, T.O. (2001). Social relationships and Asperger's syndrome: A qualitative analysis of first-hand accounts. *Journal of Intellectual Disabilities,* Vol. 5, No. 1 (March 2001), pp. 35-41

Jones, R.S.P., Zahl, A., & Huws, J.C. (2001). First-hand accounts of emotional experiences in autism: A qualitative analysis. *Disability & Society,* Vol. 16, No. 3, pp. 393-401

Kenworthy, L., Yervs, B.E., Gutermuth Anthony, L., & Wallace, G.L. (2008). Understanding executive control in autism spectrum disorders in the lab and in the real world. *Neuropsychology Review,* Vol. 18, No. 4, pp. 320-338

Kleinhans, N., Akshoomoff, N., & Delis, D.C. (2005). Executive functions in autism and Asperger's disorder: Flexibility, fluency, and inhibition. *Developmental Neuropsychology,* Vol. 27, No. 3, pp. 379-401

Koegel, L.K., Singh, A.K., & Koegel, R.L. (2010). Improving motivation for academics in children with autism. *Journal of Autism and Developmental Disorders,* Vol. 40, No. 9, pp. 1057-1066

Koning, C., & Magill-Evans, J. (2001). Social and language skills in adolescent boys with Asperger syndrome. *Autism,* Vol. *5,* pp. 23-36.

Kurth, J., & Mastergeorge, A.M. (2010). Individual education plan goals and services for adolescents with autism: Impact of age and educational setting. *Journal of Special Education,* Vol. 44, No. 3, (November 2010), pp. 146-160

Kuusikko, S., Pollock-Wurman, R., Jussila, K., Carter, A.S., Mattila, M.L., Eberling, H....Moilanen, I. (2008). Social anxiety in high-functioning children and adolescents with autism and Asperger syndrome. *Journal of Autism and Developmental Disorders,* Vol. 38, No. 9, pp. 1697-1709

Lane, A.E., Young, R.L., Baker, A.E.Z., & Angley, M.T. (2010). Sensory processing subtypes in autism: Association with adaptive behavior. *Journal of Autism and Developmental Disorders,* Vol. 40, No. 1, pp. 112-122

Lasgaard, M., Nielsen, A., Eriksen, M.E., & Goossens, L. (2010). Loneliness and social support in adolescent boys with autism spectrum disorders. *Journal of Autism and Developmental Disorders,* Vol. 40, No. 2, pp. 218-226

Laugeson, E.A., & Frankel, F. (2010). *Social Skills for Teenagers with Developmental and Autism Spectrum Disorders: The PEERS Treatment Manual.* Routledge, ISBN 978-0-415-87203-4, New York

Laugeson, E. A., Frankel., F. Gantman, A., Dillon, A. R., & Mogil, C. (in press). Evidence-based social skills training for adolescents with autism spectrum disorders: The UCLA PEERS Program. *Journal of Autism and Developmental Disorders.*

Laugeson, E.A., Frankel, F., Mogil, C., & Dillon, A.R. (2009). Parent-assisted social skills training to improve friendships in teens with autism spectrum disorders. *Journal of Autism and Developmental Disorders,* Vol. 39, No. 4, pp. 596-606

Lawrence, D.H., Alleckson, D.A., & Bjorklund, P. (2010). Beyond the roadblocks: Transitioning to adulthood with Asperger's disorder. *Archives of Psychiatric Nursing*, Vol. 24, No. 4, (August 2010), pp. 227-238

Lewis, F.M., Murdoch, B.E., & Woodyatt, G.C. (2007). Communicative competence and metalinguistic ability: Performance by children and adults with autism spectrum disorder. *Journal of Autism and Developmental Disorders*, Vol. 37, No. 8, pp. 1525-1538

Limoges, E., Mottron, L., Bolduc, C., Berthiaume, C., & Godbout, R. (2005). Atypical sleep architecture and the autism phenotype. *Brain*, Vol. 128, No. 5, (May 2005), pp. 1049-1061

Liptak, G.S., Kennedy, J.A., & Dosa, N.P. (2011). Social participation in a nationally representative sample of older youth and young adults with autism. *Journal of Developmental & Behavioral Pediatrics*, Vol. 32, No. 3, pp. 1-7

Locke, J., Ishijima, E.H., Kasari, C., & London, N. (2010). Loneliness, friendship quality and the social networks of adolescents with high-functioning autism in an inclusive school setting. *Journal of Research in Special Educational Needs*, Vol. 10, No. 2, pp. 74-81

Lombardo, M.V., & Baron Cohen, S. (2011). The role of the self in mindblindness in autism. *Consciousness and Cognition*, Vol. 20, No.1, (March 2011), pp. 130-140

Lounds, J., Seltzer, M.M., Greenberg, J.S., & Shattuck, P.T. (2007). Transition and change in adolescents and young adults with autism: Longitudinal effects on maternal well-being. *American Journal on Mental Retardation*, Vol. 112, No. 6, (November 2007), pp. 401-417

Luna, B., Doll, S.K., Hegedus, S.J., Minshew, N.J., & Sweeney, J.A. (2007). Maturation of executive function in autism. *Biology Psychiatry*, Vol. 61, No. 4, (15 February 2007), pp. 474-481

Madriaga, M. (2010). "I avoid pubs and the student union like the plague': Students with Asperger syndrome and their negotiation of university spaces. *Children's Geographies*, Vol. 8, No. 1, pp. 39 - 50

Marriage, S., Wolverton, A., & Marriage, K. (2009). Autism spectrum disorder grown up: A chart review of adult functioning. *Journal of the Canadian Academy of Child & Adolescent Psychiatry*, Vol. 18, No. 4, pp. 322-328

Martin, A.J. (2010). Should students have a gap year? Motivation and performance factors relevant to time out after completing school. *Journal of Educational Psychology*, Vol. 102, No. 3, pp. 561-576.

Martin, J.S., Poirier, M., & Bowler, D.M. (2010). Brief report: Impaired temporal reproduction performance in adults with autism spectrum disorder. *Journal of Autism and Developmental Disorders*, Vol. 40, No. 5, 640-646

Matson, J. L., & Neal, D. (2009). Diagnosing high incidence autism spectrum disorders in adults. *Research in Autism Spectrum Disorders*, Vo. 3, No. 3, (January-March 2009), pp. 581-589

McKenzie, R., Evans, J. S. B. T., & Handley, S. J. (2010). Conditional reasoning in autism: Activation and integration of knowledge and belief. *Developmental Psychology*, Vo. 46, No. 2, (March 2010), pp. 391-403

Mehzabin, P., & Stokes, M.A. (2011). Self-assessed sexuality in young adults with high-functioning autism. *Research in Autism Spectrum Disorders*, Vol. 5, (January-March 2011), pp. 614-621

Mennin, D.S., McLaughlin, K.A., & Flanagan, T.J. (2009). Emotion regulation deficits in generalized anxiety order, social anxiety, and their co-occurrence. *Journal of Anxiety Disorders*, Vo. 23, No. 7, (October 2009), pp. 866-871

Meyerding, J. (2004). Coming out autistic at work. In D. Murray (Ed.), *Coming out Asperger: Diagnosis, disclosure, and self-confidence* (pp. 245-247). Jessica Kingsley, ISBN 978-184310-240-3, London.

Minshew, N. J., Goldstein G., & Siegel, D. J. (1997). Neuropsychologic functioning in autism: Profile of a complex information processing disorder. *Journal of the International Neuropsychological Society*, Vol. 3, pp. 303–316

Müller, E., Schuler, A., Burton, B.A., & Yates, G.B. (2003). Meeting the vocational support needs of individuals with Asperger syndrome and other autism spectrum disabilities. *Journal of Vocational Rehabilitation*, Vol. 18, No. 3, pp. 163-175

Müller, E.; Schuler, A., & Yates, G.B. (2008). Social challenges and supports from the perspective of individuals with Asperger syndrome and other autism spectrum disabilities. *Autism*, Vol. 12, No. 2, pp. 173-190

Nesbitt, S. (2000). Why and why not? Factors influencing employment for individuals with Asperger syndrome. *Autism*, Vol. 4, No. 4, (December 2000), pp. 357-369

Nevill, R.E.A, & White, S.W. (In press.) College students' openness toward autism spectrum disorders: Improving peer acceptance. *Journal of Autism and Developmental Disorders*.

Orsmond, G. L., Krauss, M. W., & Selzter, M. M. (2004). Peer relationships and social and recreational activities among adolescents and adults with autism. *Journal of Autism and Developmental Disorders*, Vol. 34, No. 3, pp. 245–256

Ousley, O.Y., & Mesibov, G.B. (1991). Sexual attitudes and knowledge of high-functioning adolescents and adults with autism. *Journal of Autism and Developmental Disorders*, Vol. 21, No. 4, pp. 471-481

Oyane, N. M. F., & Bjorvatn, B. (2005). Sleep disturbances in adolescents and young adults with autism and Asperger syndrome. *Autism*, Vol. 9, No. 1, pp. 83–94

Ozonoff, S., Garcia, N., Clark, E., & Lainhart, J.E. (2005). MMPI-2 personality profiles of high-functioning adults with autism spectrum disorders. *Assessment*, Vol. 12, No. 1, pp. 86-95

Page, T. (2009.) *Parallel Play: Growing Up with Undiagnosed Asperger's*. Doubleday, ISBN 978-0385525626, New York

Paul, R., Orlovski, S.M., Marcinko, H.C., & Volkmar, F. (2009). Conversational behaviors in youth with high-functioning ASD and Asperger syndrome. *Journal of Autism and Developmental Disorders*, Vol. 39, No. 1, pp. 115-125

Pijnacker, J., Geurts, B., van Lambalgen, M., Kan, C.C., Buitelaar, J.K., & Hagoort, P. (2009). Defeasible reasoning in high-functioning adults with autism: Evidence for impaired exception-handling. *Neuropsychologia*, Vol. 47, No. 3, pp. 644-665

Pollmann, M. M. H., Finkenauer, C., & Begeer, S. (2010). Mediators of the link between autistic traits and relationship satisfaction in a non-clinical sample. *Journal of Autism and Developmental Disorders*, Vol. 40, No. 4, pp. 470–478

Ponnet, K., Buysse, A., Roeyers, H., & De Clercq, A. (2008). Mind-reading in young adults with ASD: Does structure matter? *Journal of Autism and Developmental Disorders*, Vol. 38, pp. 905-918.

Ponnet, K., Buysse, A., Roeyers, H., & De Corte, K. (2005). Empathic accuracy in adults with a pervasive developmental disorder during an unstructured conversation with a typically developmentally stranger, Vol. 35, No. 5, (October 2005), pp. 585-600.

Ponnet, K.S., Roeyers, H., Buysse, A., De Clercq, A., Van Der Heyden, E. (2004). Advanced mind-reading in adults with

Asperger syndrome. *Autism,* Vol. 8, No. 3, (September 2004), pp. 249-266.

Portway, S.M., & Johnson, B. (2005). Do you know I have Asperger's syndrome? Risks of a non-obvious disability. *Health, Risk and Society,* Vol. 7, No. 1, pp. 73-83

Portway, S. & Johnson, B. (2003). Asperger syndrome and the children who 'don't quite fit in'. *Early Child Development and Care,* Vol. 173, pp. 435-443

Ray, F., Marks, C., & Bray-Garretson, H. (2004). Challenges to treating adolescents with Asperger's syndrome who are sexually abusive. *Sexual Addiction & Compulsivity,* Vol. 11, No. 4, pp. 265-285

Remington, A., Swettenham, J., Campbell, R., & Coleman, M. (2009). Selective attention and perceptual load in autism spectrum disorder. *Psychological Science,* Vol. 20, No. 11, pp. 1388-1393

Renty, J., & Roeyers, H. (2007). Individual and marital adaptation in men with autism spectrum disorder and their spouses: The role of social support and coping strategies. *Journal of Autism and Developmental Disorders,* Vol. 37, No. 7, pp. 1247–1255

Renty, J.O., & Roeyers, H. (2006). Quality of life in high-functioning adults with autism spectrum disorder: The predictive value of disability and support characteristics. *Autism,* Vol. 10, No. 5, pp. 511-524

Roeyers, H., & Demurie, E. (2010). How impaired is mind-reading in high-functioning adolescents and adults with autism? *European Journal of Developmental Psychology,* Vol. 7, No. 1, pp. 123-134

Rogers, K., Dziobek, I., Hassenstab, J., Wolf, O. T., & Convit, A. (2007). Who cares? Revisiting empathy in Asperger syndrome. *Journal of Autism and Developmental Disorders,* Vol. 37, No. 4, pp. 709-715

Ryan, S., & Raisanen, U. (2008). "It's like you are just a spectator in this thing": Experiencing social life the 'aspie' way. *Emotion, Space and Society,* Vol. 2, pp. 135–143

Schwartz, C.B, Henderson, H.A., Inge, A.P., Zahka, N.E., Coman, D.C., Kojkowski, N.M., et al. (2009). Temperament as a predictor of symptomotology and adaptive functioning in adolescents with high-functioning autism. *Journal of Autism and Developmental Disorders,* Vol. 39, No. 6, pp. 842-855

Scheeren, A.M., Begeer, S., Banerjee, R., Terwogt, M.M., & Koot, H.M. (2010). Can you tell me about yourself? Self-presentation in children and adolescents with high-functioning autism spectrum disorder in hypothetical and real life situations. *Autism,* Vol. 14, No. 5, (September 2010), pp. 457-473

Seltzer, M.M., Krauss, M.W., Shattuck, P.T., Orsmond, G., Swe, A., & Lord, C. (2003). The symptoms of autism spectrum disorders in adolescence and adulthood. *Journal of Autism and Developmental Disorders,* Vol. 33, No. 6, (December 2003), pp. 565–581

Shattuck, P.T., Wagner, M., Narendorf, S., Sterzing, P., & Hensley, M. (2011). Post-high school service use among young adults with an autism spectrum. *Archives in Pediatrics and Adolescent Medicine,* Vol. 165, No. 2, (February 2011), pp. 141-146

Shriberg, L.D., Paul, R., McSweeny, J.L., Klin, A., & Cohen, D.J. (2001). Speech and prosody characteristics of adolescents and adults with high-functioning and Asperger syndrome. *Journal of Speech, Language, and Hearing Research,* Vol. 44, (October 2001), pp. 1097-1115.

Shtayermman, O. (2009). An exploratory study of the stigma associated with a diagnosis of Asperger's Syndrome: The mental health impact on the adolescents and young adults diagnosed with a disability with a social nature. *Journal of Human Behavior in the Social Environment,* Vol. 19, No. 3, pp. 298–313

Shtayermman, O. (2007). Peer victimization in adolescents and young adults diagnosed with Asperger's syndrome: A link to depressive symptomatology, anxiety symptomatology and suicidal ideation. *Issues in Comprehensive Pediatric Nursing,* Vol. 30, No. 3, pp. 87-107

Silani, G., Bird, G., Brindley, R., Singer, T., Frith, C., & Frith, U. (2008). Levels of emotional awareness and autism: An fMRI study. *Social Neuroscience,* Vol. 3, No. 2, pp. 97-112

Simmeborn Fleischer, A. (In press). Alienation and struggle: Everyday student-life of three male students with Asperger syndrome. *Scandinavian Journal of Disability Research.*

Simone, R. (2010). *Asperger's on the Job: Must-Have Advice for People with Asperger's or High Functioning Autism and their Employers, Educators, and Advocates.* Future Horizons, ISBN 978-1935274094, Arlington, TX.

Soderstrom, H., Rastam, M., & Gillberg, C. (2002). Temperament and character in adults with Asperger syndrome. *Autism,* Vol. 6, No. 3, (September 2002), pp. 287-297

South, M., Dana, J., White, S.E., & Crowley, M.J. (2011.) Failure is not an option: Risk-taking is moderated by anxiety and also by cognitive ability in children and adolescents diagnosed with an autism spectrum disorder. *Journal of Autism and Developmental Disorders,* Vol. 41, No. 1, pp. 55-65

Spek, A.A., & Wouters, S.G.M. (2010). Autism and schizophrenia in high functioning adults: Behavioral differences and overlap. *Research in Autism Spectrum Disorders,* Vol. 4, No. 4, (October-December 2010), pp. 709-717.

Sperry, L.A., & Mesibov, G. B. (2005). Perceptions of social challenges of adults with autism spectrum disorder. *Autism,* Vol. 9, 362–376

Stahlberg, O., Soderstrom, H., Rastam, M., & Gillberg, C. (2004). Bipolar disorder, schizophrenia, and other psychotic disorders in adults with childhood onset AD/HD and/or autism spectrum disorders. *Journal of Neural Transmission,* Vol. 111, No. 7, pp. 891-902.

Stokes, M., & Kaur, A. (2005). High-functioning autism and sexuality: A parental perspective. *Autism,* Vol. 9, No. 3, (August 2005), pp. 266-289

Stokes , M., Newton, N., & Kaur, A. (2007). Stalking, and social and romantic functioning among adolescents and adults with autism spectrum disorder. *Journal of Autism and Developmental Disorders,* Vol. 37, No. 10, pp. 1969-1986

Tager-Flusberg, H. (2007). Evaluating the theory-of-mind hypothesis of autism. *Current Directions in Psychological Science,* Vol. 16, No. 6, pp. 311-315

Tantam, D. (2003). The challenge of adolescents and adults with Asperger syndrome. *Child and Adolescent Psychiatric Clinics of North America,* Vol. 12, No. 1, pp. 143–163

Taylor, J.L., & Seltzer, M.M. (In press.) Changes in the mother-child relationship during the transition to adulthood for youth with autism spectrum disorders. *Journal of Autism and Developmental Disorders.*

Taylor, J.L., & Seltzer, M.M. (2011). Employment and post-secondary educational activities for young adults with autism spectrum disorders during the transition to adulthood. *Journal of Autism and Developmental Disorders,* Vol. 41, No. 5, pp. 566-574

Taylor, J.L., & Seltzer, M.M. (2010). Changes in the autism behavioral phenotype during the transition to adulthood. *Journal of Autism and Developmental Disorders,* Vol. 40, No. 12, (December 2010), pp. 1431-1446

Tobias, A. (2009). Supporting students with autistic spectrum disorder (ASD) at secondary school: A parent and student perspective. *Educational Psychology in Practice,* Vol. 25, No. 2, (June 2009), pp. 151-165

Townson, L. Macauley, S., Harkness, E., Docherty, A., Dias, J., Eardley, M., & Chapman, R. (2007). Research project on advocacy and autism. *Disability & Society,* Vol. 22, No. 5, pp. 523 - 536

Van Bergeijk, E., Klin, A., & Volkmar, F. (2008). Supporting more able students on the autism spectrum: College and beyond. *Journal of Autism and Developmental Disorders,* Vol. 38, No. 7, pp. 1359-1370

Wasserman, S., Weisman, A.D.M., & Mundy, P. (2010). Parents' criticisms and attributions about their adult children with high functioning autism or schizophrenia. *Autism,* Vol. 14, (March 2010), pp. 127-138

Whitby, P.J.S., & Mancil, G.R. (2009). Academic achievement profiles of children with high functioning autism and Asperger syndrome: A review of the literature. *Educational and Training in Developmental Disabilities,* Vol. 44, No. 4, pp. 551-560

White, S.W., Ollendick, T.H., & Bray, B.C. (In press). College students on the autism spectrum: Prevalence and associated problems. *Autism.*

White, S. W., & Robertson-Nay, R. (2009). Anxiety, social deficits, and loneliness in youth with autism spectrum disorders. *Journal of Autism and Developmental Disorders,* Vol. 39, No. 7, pp. 1006-1013

Whitehouse, A. J., Durkin, K., Jaquet, E., & Ziatas, K. (2009). Friendship, loneliness and depression in adolescents with Asperger's syndrome. *Journal of Adolescence,* Vol. 32, No. 2, (April 2009), pp. 309-322

Wolf-Wendel, L., Ward, K., & Kinzie, J. (2009). A tangled web of terms: The overlap and unique contribution of involvement, engagement, and integration to understanding college student success. *Journal of College Student Development,* Vol. 50, No. 4, (July/August 2009), pp. 407-428

Yang, Y., Raine, A., Lencz,T., Bihrle, S., & Lacasse, L. (2005) Prefrontal white matter in pathological liars. *British Journal of Psychiatry,* Vol. 187, No. 4, pp. 320-325

Yechiam, E., Arshavsky, O., Shamay-Tsoory, S.G., Yaniv, Shoshana, & Aharon, J. (2010). Adapted to explore: Reinforcement learning in autistic spectrum conditions. *Brain and Cognition,* Vol. 72, No. 2, (March 2010), pp. 317-324

Zager, D., & Alpern, C.S. (2010). College-based inclusion programming for transition-age students with autism. *Focus on Autism and Other Developmental Disabilities,* Vol. 25, No. 3, (September 2010), pp. 151-157

Zwickel, J., White, S.J., Coniston, D., Senju, A., & Frith, U. (In press.) Exploring the building blocks of social cognition: Spontaneous agency perception and visual perspective taking in autism. *Social Cognitive and Affective Neuroscience.*